IMPLANT DENTISTRY

A Practical Approach

SECOND EDITION

IMPLANT DENTISTRY

A PRACTICAL APPROACH

ARUN K. GARG, DMD

Visiting Professor
College of Dentistry
University of Florida
Gainesville, Florida

Former Professor of Surgery
Division of Oral/Maxillofacial Surgery
University of Miami School of Medicine
Miami, Florida

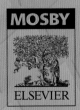

MOSBY

ELSEVIER

3251 Riverport Lane
Maryland Heights, Missouri 63043

IMPLANT DENTISTRY: A PRACTICAL APPROACH   ISBN: 978-0-323-05566-6
Copyright © 2010 by Mosby, Inc., an affiliate of Elsevier Inc.
Copyright © 1995 by Arun K. Garg

Vice President and Publishing Director: Linda Duncan
Executive Editor: John Dolan
Developmental Editor: Brian S. Loehr
Publishing Services Manager: Julie Eddy
Project Manager: Rich Barber
Design Direction: Karen Pauls
Cover Designer: Tony Reiss
Text Designer: Kim Scott

Printed in China

Last digit is the print number: 9 8 7 6 5 4 3 2 1

Preface

While teaching dental implant courses throughout the years, I became aware of how general dentists and dental specialists needed a practical book or manual that would guide them, step by step, through the processes that I taught them. The realization that clinicians had no such tool available motivated me to write the first edition of *Implant Dentistry: A Practical Approach*, a book that quickly became a must for dentists nationwide, especially to those who found in dental implantology a remarkable and professionally gratifying field.

To me, it has been exceedingly satisfying to know that thousands of dentists have benefited from my first edition of this practical, exceptionally detailed, and graphic approach.

Just as this second edition's predecessor, *Practical Implant Dentistry* came about as a result of my seminars and teachings, this one has evolved in a similar manner. Throughout the years, the technique and science of implant dentistry have evolved. My courses have evolved. Dental implant science has become more comprehensive, concepts have changed, and some have even disappeared. In order to keep up with the science and the times, I suddenly found myself giving my dentists several updated guides, instead of one, so they could firmly grasp all the important concepts and lessons. Very soon, it became clear to me that we now needed a single guide that effectively compiled all the information and detailed images from my seminars.

This was the genesis of this edition. It is intended to be one single source of invaluable information, resources, techniques, and strategies aimed not only for those dentists who time and again take my courses, but to all those that have found in dental implantology the most gratifying, fulfilling, and lucrative area of dentistry today.

The book starts by looking at the historical development of dental implants, followed by a step-by-step guide to bone grafting, implantology, and restorative dentistry.

One of the highlights of the book includes immediate loading of dental implants, bone biology, and a detailed, one-of-a-kind list of guidelines for handling complications. This guide is a must-have for all dentists, regardless of their specialty.

I hope this book inspires dentists to place and restore more implants and gives them the information needed to effectively enhance the health and well-being of their patients. This is, after all, the most gratifying and rewarding part of our profession!

Arun K. Garg, DMD

Acknowledgments

The creation of this book was made possible thanks to the dedication and commitment to excellence by the people at Elsevier who constantly pushed me to be my best. I especially want to thank publisher, John Dolan, and editor, Brian Loehr.

I also what to thank the team at Implant Seminars and the team at the Center for Dental Implants for their fantastic support in helping me complete this second edition of *Implant Dentistry*. They constantly took the weight off my shoulders, giving me the time to complete this important project.

My deepest appreciation and love goes to my wife, Heather, whose loyalty and selflessness were vital in giving me the time to spend at the computer. Her energy and support have been instrumental to developing the teachings and clinical care enjoyed by doctors and patients.

And finally, thanks to my three adored children, who are my biggest inspirations.

New to this Edition

Outstanding photos and illustrations!

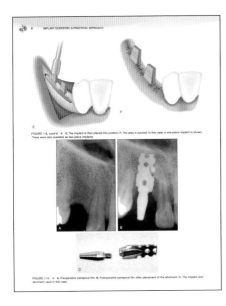

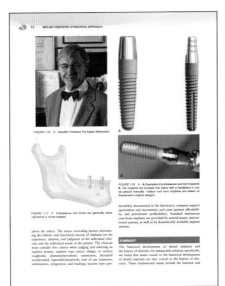

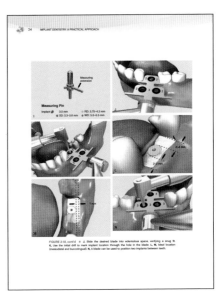

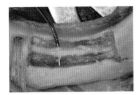

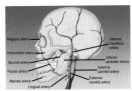

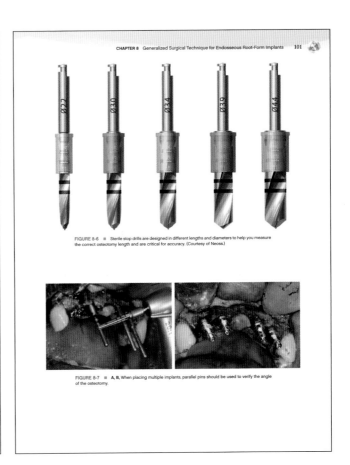

Keep up with the innovations, techniques, and procedures of oral implantology with these new chapters!

Chapter 15: Immediate Loading of Implants in the Edentulous Patient

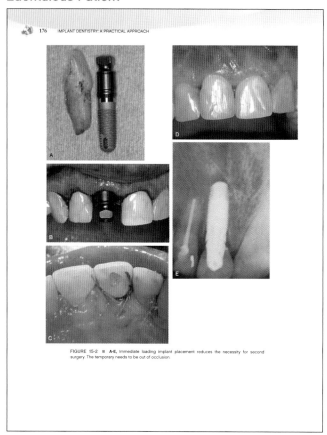

FIGURE 15-2 ■ A-E, Immediate loading implant placement reduces the necessity for second surgery. The temporary needs to be out of occlusion.

Chapter 16: Bone Biology, Osseointegration, and Bone Grafting

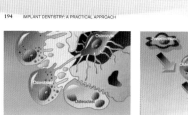

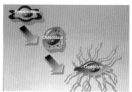

FIGURE 16-1 ■ Osteoclasts resorb bone as it ages, while osteoblasts deposit new bone simultaneously and adjacently. Once the osteoblasts deposit bone and become encapsulated, they are known as osteocytes.

FIGURE 16-2 ■ Pre-osteoblasts mature into osteoblasts, which then mature into osteocytes.

Bone Biology

A study of bone biology includes elements related to bone cells, metabolism, structure, and repair.

Bone Cells

Three different types of cells—osteoblasts, osteocytes, and osteoclasts—are related to bone metabolism and physiology. The three are closely related to each other and are derived from similar precursors (Figure 16-1).

Osteoblasts, which are associated with the process of osteogenesis, are located in two general areas next to the bone surfaces where they deposit bone matrix. Therefore, they frequently are referred to as endosteal osteoblasts or periosteal osteoblasts. The cytoplasm of osteoblasts is intensely basophilic, which suggests the presence of ribonucleoproteins related to bone matrix protein component synthesis. Fine granules, which can be observed in the cytoplasm, are closely related to the site of active matrix deposit (Figure 16-2).

When osteoblasts become embedded in the bone matrix, they transform into osteocytes, which have a slightly basophilic cytoplasm. Prolongations of this cytoplasm extend from the osteocyte, through a network of fine canaliculi that emerge from the lacunae, to a specific distance. During bone formation, these prolongations extend beyond their normal limit, and a direct contiguity, or continuity, with adjacent osteocytes is evident. In mature bone, almost no extension of these prolongations is seen, but the canaliculi continue to function as a means of metabolic and biochemical messenger exchange between the blood system and the osteocytes.

The system of canaliculi connects the osteocyte lacunae with each other and the tissue spaces. Tissue fluid in these spaces mixes with fluid from the canaliculi, allowing a metabolic and biochemical messenger exchange between the bloodstream and the osteocytes. This mechanism allows the osteocytes to remain alive, regardless of the calcified intercellular substance that surrounds them. However, this duct system is not functional if it is located more than 0.5 mm from a capillary, which is why such an abundant blood supply is found in bone through capillaries that run through Haversian systems and Volkmann's canals.

Osteoclasts are fused monocytes that appear histologically as multinucleated giant cells located in shallow excavations (Howship's lacunae) along the mineralized surface.[3] The cytoplasm of osteoclasts is slightly basophilic and granular, with characteristic vacuoles. Osteoclasts are responsible for bone resorption and form in response to parathyroid hormone. After the process of local bone resorption is complete, osteoclasts disappear, probably by degeneration.

Bone Metabolism

Bone, the primary reservoir of calcium, has a tremendous turnover capability for responding to the metabolic needs of the body and is critical for maintaining a stable serum calcium level.[1,2] Because calcium participates in many reactions, it has an essential life support function. It works in conjunction with the lungs and kidneys to help maintain the pH balance of the body through the production of additional phosphates and carbonates, as well as by electrical charge conduction in nerve and muscle, including cardiac muscle. In addition, the metabolic environment is an extremely important component of the biomechanical structure of bone. Bone undergoes continuous turnover in response to metabolic reactions, with the skull and jaws unquestionably affected by this turnover.

The structural integrity of bone may be compromised in times of normal metabolic calcium need and in disease

Chapter 19: Guidelines for Handling Complications Associated with Implant Surgical Procedures

so cylindrical implants are recommended.[47,50,51] The use of a resorbable membrane as a cushion between the implant and the nerve may help to protect the nerve.[52]

Other complications that occur much less commonly with nerve repositioning include infection (typically associated with graft material placed in the region), mandibular fracture, and implant loss (particularly when fracture occurs).[48]

Sinus Membrane Perforations

Sinus membrane perforation is the most common complication of sinus augmentation (Figure 19-5). This membrane, also known as the Schneiderian membrane, lines the sinus cavity and is firmly attached to the bordering bone of the maxillary sinus. When intact, the membrane and its periosteum supply blood to the graft. Although perforations do not necessarily require aborting the surgery, they are a concern because the maxillary sinus communicates with all other sinuses in the respiratory system, and infection can spread quickly. Sinus pneumatization can occur in this area.

The most common cause of sinus membrane perforation is overly vigorous reflection in one area of the osteotomy site without adequate freeing up and elevating of the adjacent membrane area.[41] Perforations can occur during infracture of the lateral wall. Perforations usually occur at the level of the greenstick fracture (when the infracture technique is used), at the level of the superior osteotomy line, and in the inferomedial part of the membrane.

To cover small perforations (1 to 2 mm diameter), a small piece of collagen, a resorbable cellulous membrane, Collatape, Gelfoam, or Surgicel may be used. This should extend over the unaffected membrane by at least 3 mm in all directions. A resorbable collagen wound dressing can be placed below antral lacerations to provide a temporary interface between the antrum and the graft material to be placed.

For larger perforations (greater than 2 mm diameter), the torn membrane can be elevated off the medial wall, folded onto itself to approximate the lacerated membrane of the lateral wall, and then covered with a resorbable collagen wound dressing. This requires the membrane to be of adequate consistency.

If the defect is too large and the margins of the membrane surrounding the perforation have been well elevated, resorbable suture material (5.0 or 6.0) can be used to close the defect. This suturing technique can be unpredictable and very difficult, however, if the membrane cannot be elevated around the margins of the perforation. This may require perforating the bone surrounding the osteotomy to provide a site through which to suture.

Another alternative is to stop the procedure and then suture the outer soft tissues. After 2 to 3 months of healing, the sinus elevation procedure can be performed again. This approach is difficult and is not always practical.

If all else fails, a final—although not always stable—approach to repairing large perforations is to shape and place a large lamellar bone sheet within the osteotomy site, thereby creating a pouch over the perforate region. Graft material is placed along the borders of the bone sheet to stabilize it and then in the middle of the sheet over the perforation.

To prevent sinus membrane perforation, a split-thickness flap design is suggested and a brushstroke type of contact should be used to penetrate the bone when the lateral wall of the sinus membrane is osteotomized. This allows good access while minimizing perforation risk. A No. 8 surgical diamond round bur is recommended for this procedure.

The osteotomy design should consist more of a rounded edge rectangle involving a complete osteotomy on the lateral and inferior walls, as opposed to a hinged-door type of osteotomy window.[42] The osteotomy design should be changed if extensive bony septa are discovered because reflection over these membrane-adhering septa increases the risk for perforation.

Fractured Mandible

Mandibular fracture after implant placement is rare but has been reported in conjunction with severely resorbed edentulous mandibles.[54] The risk is particularly high when numerous implants are placed, and when the bone has been mechanically weakened.[47] The risk for mandibular fracture also increases following nerve repositioning with implant placement.[48]

Patients with fracture tend to present with pain and swelling in the mandible and chin area. Occasionally, they report sensory disturbances of the lower lip and chin.

If a pathologic fracture occurs after implant placement, certain things must be considered in determining how to proceed. The basic goals for all fracture treatment approaches are reduction and immobilization to restore form and function.[45]

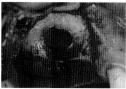

FIGURE 19-5 ■ Sinus membrane perforation can occur from vigorous reflection of the membrane area. A collagen membrane is used to repair 1- to 2-mm sinus membrane perforations.

Practical information for you and your patients!

Delicious postoperative recipes to offer your patients!

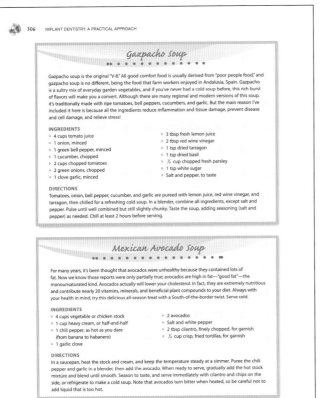

306   IMPLANT DENTISTRY: A PRACTICAL APPROACH

Gazpacho Soup

Gazpacho soup is the original "V-8." All good comfort food is usually derived from "poor people food," and gazpacho soup is no different, being the food that farm workers enjoyed in Andalusia, Spain. Gazpacho is a sultry mix of everyday garden vegetables, and if you've never had a cold soup before, this rich burst of flavors will make you a convert. Although there are many regional and modern versions of this soup, it's traditionally made with ripe tomatoes, bell peppers, cucumbers, and garlic. But the main reason I've included it here is because all the ingredients reduce inflammation and tissue damage, prevent disease and cell damage, and relieve stress!

INGREDIENTS

- 4 cups tomato juice
- 1 onion, minced
- 1 green bell pepper, minced
- 1 cucumber, chopped
- 2 cups chopped tomatoes
- 2 green onions, chopped
- 1 clove garlic, minced

- 3 tbsp fresh lemon juice
- 2 tbsp red wine vinegar
- 1 tsp dried tarragon
- 1 tsp dried basil
- ¼ cup chopped fresh parsley
- 1 tsp white sugar
- Salt and pepper, to taste

DIRECTIONS

Tomatoes, onion, bell pepper, cucumber, and garlic are pureed with lemon juice, red wine vinegar, and tarragon, then chilled for a refreshing cold soup. In a blender, combine all ingredients, except salt and pepper. Pulse until well combined but still slightly chunky. Taste the soup, adding seasoning (salt and pepper) as needed. Chill at least 2 hours before serving.

Mexican Avocado Soup

For many years, it's been thought that avocados were unhealthy because they contained lots of fat. Now we know those reports were only partially true; avocados are high in fat—"good fat"—the monounsaturated kind. Avocados actually will lower your cholesterol. In fact, they are extremely nutritious and contribute nearly 20 vitamins, minerals, and beneficial plant compounds to your diet. Always with your health in mind, try this delicious all-season treat with a South-of-the-border twist. Serve cold.

INGREDIENTS

- 4 cups vegetable or chicken stock
- 1 cup heavy cream, or half-and-half
- 1 chili pepper, as hot as you dare (from banana to habanero)
- 1 garlic clove

- 2 avocados
- Salt and white pepper
- 2 tbsp cilantro, finely chopped, for garnish
- ¼ cup crisp, fried tortillas, for garnish

DIRECTIONS

In a saucepan, heat the stock and cream, and keep the temperature steady at a simmer. Puree the chili pepper and garlic in a blender, then add the avocado. When ready to serve, gradually add the hot stock mixture and blend until smooth. Season to taste, and serve immediately with cilantro and chips on the side, or refrigerate to make a cold soup. Note that avocados turn bitter when heated, so be careful not to add liquid that is too hot.

A detailed glossary devoted to implantology terminology.

Glossary

A

Aberrant deviating from the norm or the usual.

Abrade to grind, rub, scrape, or wear away the surface of a part by friction.

Abrasion a surface or a part worn away by natural or artificial means.

Abscess an abscess is an enclosed collection of pus on the body as a result of the body's defensive reaction to an infection. Most abscesses can occur anywhere in the body.

Absorbable See: BIOABSORBABLE.

Absorption the reception of substances through, by, or into biological tissue.

Abutment the portion of an implant or implant component(s) above the neck of the implant that serves to support and/or retain a fixed, fixed-detachable, or removable dental prosthesis.

Abutment attachment a mechanical device for the fixation, retention, or stabilization of an implant-borne dental prosthesis.

Abutment clamp 1. any device used for positioning a dental implant abutment upon a dental implant body. 2. forceps used to assist in the positioning of an abutment on the implant platform.

Abutment connection a procedure for securing an abutment to an implant.

Abutment level impression the impression of an abutment either directly (using conventional impression techniques) or indirectly (using an abutment impression coping). See: IMPLANT LEVEL IMPRESSION.

Abutment screw a screw used to secure the abutment to the implant, usually torqued to a final seating position.

Abutment selection the decision during prosthodontic treatment concerning the type of abutment used for the restoration, based on implant angulation, interarch space, soft tissue (mucosal) height, planned prosthesis, occlusal factors (e.g., opposing dentition, parafunction), and esthetic and phonetic considerations.

Abutment swapping See: PLATFORM SWITCHING.

Abutment transfer device See: ORIENTATION JIG.

Access hole the channel in a screw-retained implant prosthesis that receives the abutment or prosthetic screw, usually through the occlusal or lingual surface of the prosthesis.

Accessory ostium occasional opening of the maxillary sinus either into the infundibulum or directly in the wall of the middle meatus. See: OSTIUM (MAXILLARY SINUS).

Acellular having no cells.

Acellular dermal allograft a substitute for autogenous soft tissue grafts in root coverage procedure that replaces lost dermis and is used as a synthetic or biosynthetic material. Also referred to as skin grafts.

Acid-etched implant external surface of an implant body modified by the chemical action of an acidic medium intended to enhance osseointegration.

Acid-etched surface an implant surface treated with acid to increase the surface area by subtraction. See: SUBTRACTED SURFACE.

Acrylic resin a self-cured or heat-cured plastic consisting of monomers (usually liquid) and polymers (usually powders).

Actinobacillus actinomycetem comitans a species of gram-negative, facultatively anaerobic spherical or rod-shaped bacteria; frequently associated with some forms of human periodontal disease as well as subacute and chronic endocarditis; occurs with actinomycetes in actinomycotic lesions.

Actonel an oral bisphosphonate; brand name for active ingredient risedronate sodium; used to treat Paget's disease of the bone, and to prevent and treat postmenopausal osteoporosis and ucocorticoid-induced osteoporosis in men and women. Several cases of bisphosphonate-related osteonyelitis (BON, also referred to as osteonecrosis of the jaw) have been associated with the use of the oral bisphosphonates (Fosamax [alendronate], Actonel [risedronate] and Boniva [ibandronate]) for the treatment of osteoporosis; these patients may have had other conditions that could put them at risk for developing BON.

Added surface syn: Additive surface treatment; alteration of an implant surface by addition of material. See: SUBTRACTED SURFACE, TEXTURED SURFACE.

Additive surface treatment See: ADDED SURFACE.

Adduct to pull or draw medially.

Adhesion the sticking together of dissimilar materials.

Adjustment a modification of a restoration of a tooth or of a prosthetic after insertion in the mouth.

245

Consent forms for your practice.

appendix B

Consent Form: Dental Implant(s)

Part 1—Patient and Doctor Information

Patient Name: _____

Doctor Name: _____

In order for me to make an informed decision about undergoing a procedure, I should have certain information about the proposed procedure, the associated risks, the alternatives, and the consequences of not having it. The doctor has provided me with this information to my satisfaction. The following is a summary of this information. This form is meant to provide me with the information I need to make a good decision; it is not meant to alarm me.

Part 2—Details of Consent

Condition

My doctor has explained the nature of my condition to me: Missing tooth or teeth.

Procedure—Dental Implant

My physician has proposed the following procedure to treat or diagnose my condition: Dental implant This means: Surgically place an implant into the supporting jawbone.

We believe that patients have a right to be informed about any treatment, but the law requires extensive disclosure of the risks of surgery and anesthesia, many of which are extremely unlikely to occur. These can be alarming for the patient. Please feel free to ask the doctor about the frequency of any risks or complications disclosed herein that might apply to you (based on our clinical experience and that of other oral surgeons and implantologists).

1. After a careful oral examination and study of my dental condition, the doctor has advised me that my missing tooth or teeth may be replaced with artificial teeth supported by an implant. I hereby authorize and direct the doctor and his authorized associates and assistants to treat my condition.

2. The procedure I choose to treat this condition is understood by me to be the placement of root form implant(s). Additional treatment procedures may include a bone graft including materials of human, animal, or plant origin. I understand that the purpose of this procedure is to allow me to have more functional artificial teeth by the implants providing support, anchorage, and retention for these teeth.

3. I understand that this is nonetheless an elective procedure, that such procedures are performed to improve function, and that an alternative option, although less desirable, is to not undergo surgery and do nothing. I have also

293

Contents

chapter 1

The Historical Development of Dental Implants

THE HISTORICAL DEVELOPMENT OF DENTAL IMPLANTS can be understood properly only in the context of the history of dentistry. We may define a dental implant as a device surgically placed underneath the gingiva within the alveolar bone, to which is attached a permanent or removable single artificial tooth or teeth. Issues important to the historical development of dental implants are issues important to the history of dentistry. These issues include, fundamentally, only two: the function and esthetics of a patient's teeth. Related issues include preventive dentistry, anesthesiology, pathobiology, and orthopedics, specifically, the anatomy of the mandible and maxilla, and subcategories such as bone grafting and radiology.

The historical development of implants before the modern era in dentistry began (since approximately 1700) can be discussed only tangentially, and we must be careful not to apply modern methods of thinking—especially regarding technological skill—to ancient practices, because only in the twentieth century have nonautologous materials existed that could be fashioned for medical use to avoid their rejection by the human body.[1] Only since the end of the first quarter of the twentieth century have modern dental implants been developed and widely used. These implants fall roughly into two major categories: subperiosteal implants (which rest on alveolar bone beneath the gingiva

1

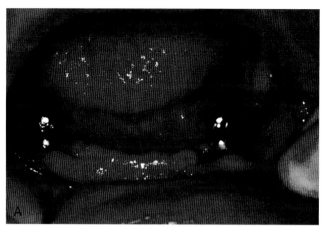

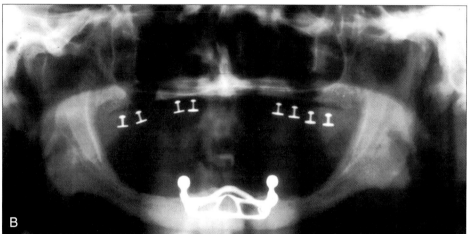

FIGURE 1-1 ■ **A,** Clinical view of a subperiosteal implant in the mandible. **B,** Radiograph of a subperiosteal implant in the anterior mandible.

and usually are not attached to the severely resorbed jawbone for which these implants were designed) and endosseous implants (which are placed within the alveolar bone) (Figure 1-1). Variations of the endosseous implant include the blade implant (which, as its name implies, is a thin, elongated, flat device designed to be secured in narrow, even knife-edged alveolar bone) (Figure 1-2), the ramus frame implant (which is designed for the completely edentulous mandible and is secured anteriorly in a single point, as well as posteriorly on each side of the jaw), the transosseous implant (which penetrates the entire jaw and emerges below the jaw, where it is secured), and the root-form implant or cylindrical implant (which resembles an actual tooth root and can be threaded or simply cylindrical with no threads). Therefore, only within the context of the twentieth and twenty-first centuries can a discussion of the historical development of dental implants be practically undertaken, and always within the confines of the two crucial issues of tooth function and esthetics for individual patients.

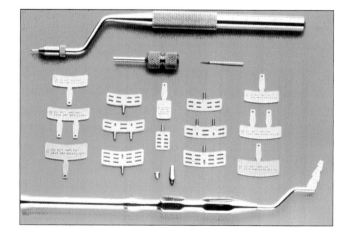

FIGURE 1-2 ■ Examples of blade implants.

Dentistry and Dental Implants in the Pre-Modern Era

Pain Relief, Better Function, and Pretty Smiles

With important exceptions, the modern definition of a dental implant can be used to describe the kinds of devices used for centuries as replacements for missing teeth. For example, the American Dental Association defines dental implants as "manufactured devices that are placed surgically in the upper or lower jaw, where they function as anchors for replacement teeth. Implants are made of titanium and other materials that are compatible with the human body."[2] Except for the word "titanium" and the phrase "compatible with the human body," this definition describes tooth replacement options available since the dawn of time.

The ancient Egyptians referred to toothaches in their medical texts 5,500 years ago. Clay tablets dating to approximately 2,500 BC and attributed to ancient Sumerians in the Mesopotamian city of Ur refer not only to toothaches but to their origin: worms that cause tooth decay. Of course, these ancient dentists had a variety of cures to apply to the disease, including medicines, "surgical" procedures, and prayers—all of which should remind the modern dentist of how, in many ways, little has changed over the past 5,000 years regarding doctors' need to eliminate their patients' pain and discomfort.

A variety of other ancient cultures have provided us with evidence of the practice of dentistry, fundamentally to maintain or restore patient function or esthetics. These ancient dental practitioners included Hindus (who treated gum disease and used a variety of dental instruments, including those for extraction and for drilling to place gold in teeth); Chinese and Japanese (who used acupuncture to treat toothache); Hebrews (who used gold and silver to replace missing teeth), Phoenicians (who used the teeth extracted from slaves to replace those of the more worthy!); Etruscans (who used gold to fashion bands used for dental bridges); Greeks and Romans (who used a variety of dental instruments, developed theories of mouth disease, used bridges to replace missing teeth, and practiced rudimentary forms of orthodontics); and Mayans (who used stones and metal inlays to decorate teeth) (Figure 1-3).

The first "true dental replacements," according to Malvin E. Ring, can be attributed to the early Etruscans, who, as already noted, experimented not only with dental bridges but with tooth replacements fashioned from oxen bones.[3] The first endosseous implant is probably of Mayan origin (7th century AD) and was constructed of sea shells and placed in the mandible. A mandibular implant fashioned of stone has been verified as attributable to a Honduran civilization, circa 800 AD (Figure 1-4).[3]

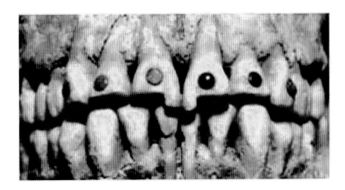

FIGURE 1-3 ■ Mayan jaw with stones and metal inlay decorations still intact on the teeth.

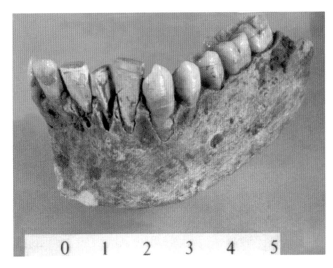

FIGURE 1-4 ■ This mandible, dated 800 AD, was found in Honduras. This jaw shows three carved, implanted incisors made from carved sea shells. Calculus formation on these three implants indicates this was not a burial ceremony, but a fixed, functional, and esthetic tooth replacement. (Courtesy of the Peabody Museum of Archaeology and Ethnology, 33-19-20/254.0).

From the fall of Rome until the European Renaissance, dentistry underwent few advances, although some Arab medical practitioners advocated particular elements of tooth care and cleansing, as well as tooth transplantation. Studies of anatomy during the Renaissance (including a mid-16th century text on tooth anatomy) helped advance the study of dentistry; this same century saw some French practitioners performing rudimentary dental surgery and advocating the use of tooth replacements manufactured from bone and from wood.

Scientific and Technical Advancements

The first quarter of the eighteenth century saw the publication of *The Surgeon Dentist* by Pierre Fauchard, considered by most historians to be the father of modern dentistry.

The development of artificial teeth made of porcelain and of mineral paste was a direct result of the interest in dental practice generated by Fauchard and others. Other European advances in dentistry included knowledge of tooth growth and anatomy based on actual scientific experimentation and practice, made available through the publication of a number of volumes devoted exclusively to dental practice. Instrumentation, which became more specialized, included the English key (turnkey), developed specifically for tooth extraction.

Nineteenth century advances in dentistry paved the way for the development of true implants in the early twentieth century. For example, in 1806, Giuseppe Angelo Fonzi used metal pins to attach artificial teeth (colored to look like natural teeth) to a denture base. Other major advances included the use of porcelain crowns and the development, in the last quarter of the century, of the electrical dental drill. Of course, the single most important dental—and medical—advancement in the nineteenth century was probably the use of anesthesia. In the 1840s, American dentists Horace Wells and William Morton developed means for anesthetizing dental patients using nitrous oxide (Wells) or ether (Morton).

As the practice of dentistry became more respectable and accepted by the masses, dental schools began to form, particularly after mid-century, following, in 1839, the establishment of the first dental school in the world, the Baltimore College of Dental Surgery. Establishment of not only dental schools but also dental societies and dental journals spread in the nineteenth century from America to Europe. Scientific advancements in the nineteenth century that clearly and significantly affected the practice of dentistry included American dentist Greene Vardiman Black's invention of the foot-powered dental drill (1858), Louis Pasteur's theories concerning germs (1860), Robert Koch's experiments with bacterial growth specifically related to the study of tooth decay, and biochemist Willoughby Dayton Miller's experiments showing the connection between sugar and tooth decay (1890). The late nineteenth century discovery of X-rays by Wilhelm Conrad Roentgen led to the use of radiography to treat impacted teeth and other jaw disorders (Figure 1-5).

Early twentieth-century discoveries important to the development of dentistry and of implantology include the development of materials more malleable than plaster for the taking of dental impressions. Albert Einhorn's development of Novocaine as a local anesthetic led to the replacement of the use of general anesthetics for drilling and extractions (Figure 1-6).

Increasing knowledge of the importance of oral hygiene to general health, the discovery and widespread use of fluoride in water supplies, and surveys of the general dental community conducted by the Carnegie Foundation in 1921 all led to significant advances in preventative dentistry, including the development of dental school curricula, to arm the modern dentist and, increasingly, the general public, with means for treatment to avoid the otherwise painful and esthetic complications that may result from improper tooth care. Modern drilling instruments, with diamond bits and carbide burs, which were developed in the second

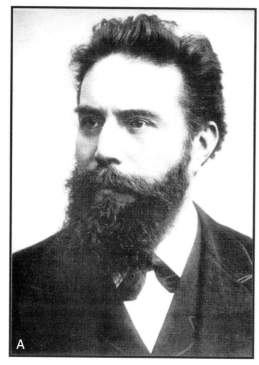
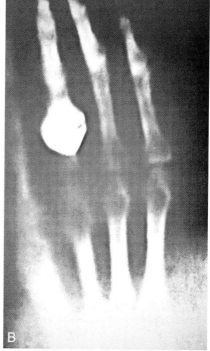

FIGURE 1-5 ■ **A,** Wilhelm Conrad Roentgen. **B,** The first x-ray image.

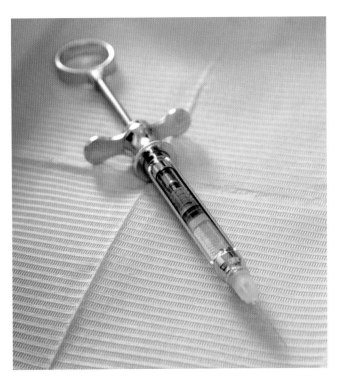

FIGURE 1-6 ■ Novocaine was developed as a local anesthetic solution to substitute the use of general anesthesia for dental procedures.

quarter of the century, led to much more precise, reliable, and convenient dental surgery. More recently, computer aided design–computer assisted manufacturing technologies enable three-dimensional models for the fashioning of man-made and hybrid materials, not only for implant placement and prosthetics, but also for bone repair and augmentation.

Modern History of Implants: 1700-1900

A major obstacle to the development of implants by innovators such as J. Maggiolo in the first decade of the nineteenth century, and Dieu Blanc and Hillicher in the past two decades, was inadequate biomaterials.[4] For example, Maggiolo inserted a gold implant tube in a fresh extraction site, allowing it to heal passively; a crown was later added. Inflammation of the gingiva, however, was the natural result. Maggiolo describes the attempt in his book, *Le Manuel de l'Art du Dentiste*. A similar result was inevitable given the use of other nonautologous materials, including gold, platinum, porcelain, rubber, and silver, by other early experimenters.

M.E. Ring catalogues a remarkable number of practitioners in the late nineteenth century who used a variety of materials and techniques to effect successful substitutions for missing teeth. These innovators included Dr. J.M. Younger, who placed a dried tooth into an extraction socket; Dr. Herbst, who implanted an extracted tooth and supported it with a rubber dam; Dr. S.M. Harris, who used a porcelain post with a roughened lead surface to support

a porcelain crown inserted into an artificial socket; Dr. W.G.A. Bonwill, who inserted gold or iridium tubes into an artificial socket; and Dr. C.T. Gramm, who experimented with dogs as recipients of pure lead implants.[3]

Modern History of Implants: 1900-1980

On January 28, 1913, E.J. Greenfield, D.D.S., of Wichita, Kansas, presented a paper entitled "Implantation of Artificial Crown and Bridge Abutments" at the monthly meeting of the Academy of Stomatology of Philadelphia, in which he described how a "hollow, latticed cylinder of iridio-platinum, No. 24 gage, soldered with 24-karat gold" could be used as an "artificial root" to "fit exactly the circular incision or socket made for it in the jaw-bone of the patient."[5] By means of a slot on the top of this root, an artificial tooth was fitted.

After Greenfield, brothers Alvin and Moses Strock experimented in the 1930s with Vitallium orthopedic screw fixtures, implanting them in both dogs and human subjects to restore individual teeth; their work is notable for the concentration on overcoming the problems of choosing a metal most compatible with human tissue.

Some attribute the Strock brothers with being the first to place an endosteal implant successfully, and later with the first successful use of an endodontic stabilizer and a single submerged root-form implant placed in the anterior maxilla[4] (Figure 1-7). Also noteworthy at this time is the 1938 patent by Dr. P.B. Adams of an "Anchoring Means for False Teeth," essentially an internally and externally threaded cylinder endosseous implant that bears remarkable similarities to root-form implants marketed today.[6]

A variety of implant designs were attempted in the mid-twentieth century, including those by Seger-Dorez (a four-part implant with a bone-buried shaft and internal threads for reception of a screw, neck, and prosthesis post), Lehman (a tantalum arch implant designed specifically for fresh extraction sites), Pretto (a "trombone" implant designed to allow bone growth within its buried shaft), and Ted Lee (a narrow post design with extension to encourage blood flow and bone growth around the implant).[7]

The Italian Manlio S. Formiggini, the so-called "Father of Modern Implantology," and a colleague, Zepponi, designed a post-type endosseous implant in the 1940s, whose spiral stainless steel or tantalum wires provided for the ingrowth of bone. Spaniard Perron Andres modified the basic Formiggini spiral design to include a solid shaft.[4] The Frenchman Raphael Cherchere developed the spiral design and complemented the implant by designing burs and taps to facilitate its insertion for the best possible fit. Italian Giordano Muratori continued to develop the spiral design in the 1960s by using a shaft with internal threading.

Leonard Linkow's vent-plant implant design (1963) was an adaptation of the basic spiral design into a flat plate implant, manufactured in various configurations to accommodate the type of bone and the area requiring restored dentition (Figure 1-8).

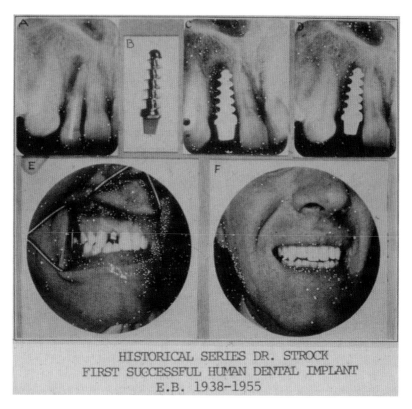

HISTORICAL SERIES DR. STROCK
FIRST SUCCESSFUL HUMAN DENTAL IMPLANT
E.B. 1938-1955

FIGURE 1-7 ■ The first endosteal implant of the modern era is attributed to the Strock brothers. Endosseous implants from 1938 bear remarkable similarities to the roof-form implants marketed today.

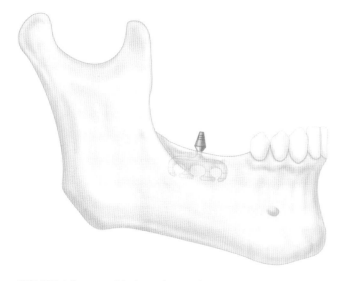

FIGURE 1-8 ■ A blade implant is depicted here. The steps of the procedure are shown in Figure 1-9.

A unique variation in implant design about this time was Jacques Scialom's tripod implant, whose three-pin design enabled the clinician to use a very stable implant with acrylic-fused separate sections that would form an area for the fitting of a prosthesis. Linkow's blade implant was another implant innovation: an implant designed originally to accommodate into knife-edge ridges, where bone

width was at a minimum (Figure 1-9). The blade design took advantage of the relative abundance of bone lengthwise in the alveolar bone, and it was available in different designs to accommodate different areas of the mandible and maxilla[7] (Figure 1-10).

A number of innovators can be attributed with the development of the subperiosteal implant in the 1940s: Dahl first used the implant in 1940 in Sweden, followed by mucosal inserts in 1942, and his work was carried on in the United States with variations in surgical procedure and design by Gershkoff and Goldberg (1948) and Weinberg (1947).[4]

Development of the subperiosteal design, including the use of direct bone impressions (Lew, Bausch, and Berman in 1950) and the use of a single superstructure (Sol and Salogaray in 1957), continued in the 1950s (Figures 1-11, 1-12). Ramus implants were developed in the 1970s by Roberts, and in 1972, the ramus frame increased options for patients who could not use a blade implant or a subperiosteal implant for anatomical reasons[4]. Small, in 1975, continued to increase the options for restoring severely compromised dentition through his introduction of the transosteal mandibular staple bone plate, which was later modified by Hans Booker (Figures 1-13, 1-14).

Modern History of Implants: 1980-Present

The rapid increase in the acceptability of dental implants as regular treatment in the late twentieth and early twenty-

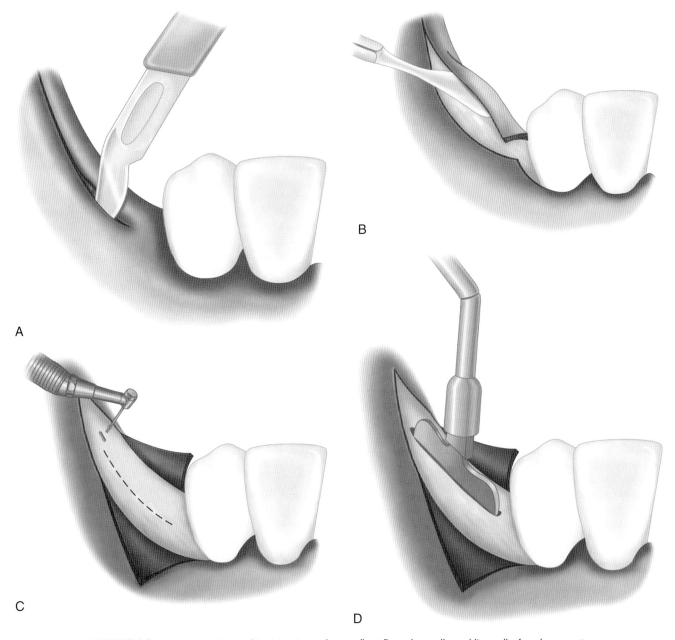

FIGURE 1-9 ■ **A,** A midcrestal incision is made to reflect flaps, buccally and lingually, for placement of a blade implant. **B,** Flap reflection. **C,** Cutting a trough for the placement of a blade implant. **D,** The blade implant is being tried in. The trough is modified and/or the implant is modified by cutting it, as needed, to fit. *Continued*

first centuries is largely attributable to Swedish Professor Per-Ingvar Brånemark (Figure 1-15), an orthopedic surgeon who turned an accidental discovery into a dental revolution.[8] In the late 1950s, the young Brånemark worked at Lund University studying blood flow in vivo by placing a titanium chamber in the femur of a rabbit; over time, the chamber became firmly attached to the bone and could not be extracted.

Brånemark's genius and pioneering spirit were revealed years later, when he decided that tooth anchoring would be the clinical area in which to apply the attachment principle he coined "osseointegration."[9] In 1982 in Toronto, the dental medical community formally accepted the evidence he presented after years of controlled clinical studies. All endosteal root-form and cylindrical implants used today are based on Brånemark's original designs (Figure 1-16). Some have even referred to the mid-1980s as the "Dawn of New Era" in the practice of not only implantology but dental practice in general, mainly because of the contributions of Brånemark to establish the legitimacy of implants for treatment, especially for high-risk or previously only marginally treatable patients.[10]

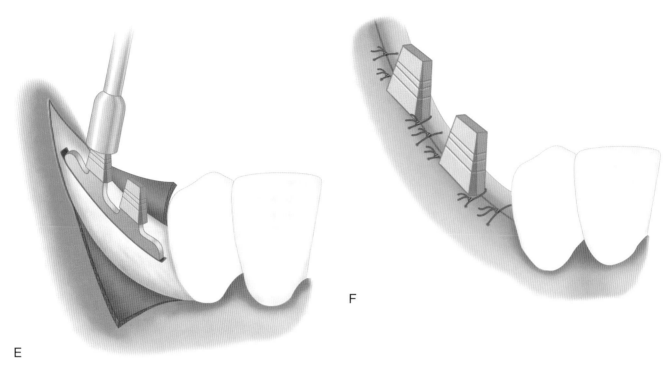

E

F

FIGURE 1-9, cont'd ■ **E,** The implant is then placed into position. **F,** The area is sutured. In this case, a one-piece implant is shown. These were also available as two-piece implants.

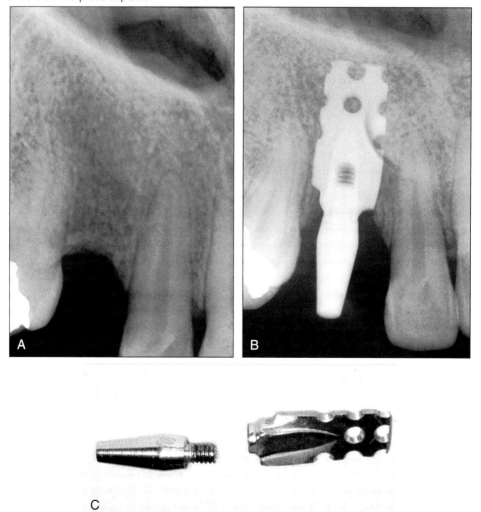

A

B

C

FIGURE 1-10 ■ **A,** Preoperative periapical film. **B,** Postoperative periapical film after placement of the abutment. **C,** The implant and abutment used in this case.

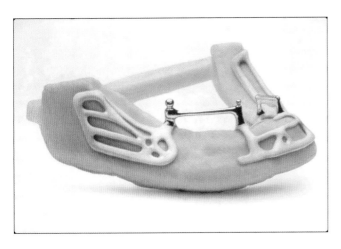

FIGURE 1-11 ■ To avoid the need to take an impression, CT scans were used from which a three-dimensional model was fabricated. The subperiosteal implant framework was then fabricated.

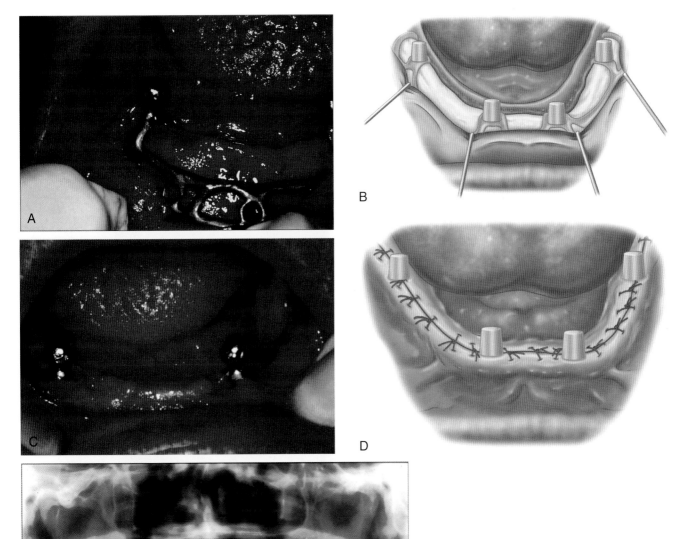

FIGURE 1-12 ■ A, B, Placement of a subperiosteal implant framework onto the bone after flap reflection. C, D, Flap closure after the subperiosteal implant is placed. E, Panoramic radiograph after placement of an anterior subperiosteal implant.

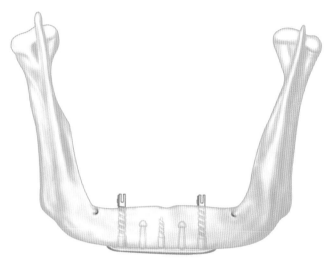

FIGURE 1-13 ■ Facial view of mandible with Small's transosteal mandibular staple bone plate.

Another pioneer of modern implantology was Dr. André Schroeder, who along with Dr. Straumann of the Institute Straumann in Waldenburg, Switzerland, was engaged in development of a dental implant system in the 1970s and 1980s, mainly through experiments with metal products for use in orthopedic surgery. One account, in fact, suggests that Schroeder's experiments at Straumann may have been the first to provide histological evidence of osseointegration.[11] Although Brånemark and Schroeder have received much of the acclaim, dental implantology in the twentieth century began long before; in fact, beginning at the turn of the twentieth century, a number of implant pioneers preceded these late twentieth century innovators, as has been chronicled by a number of authors and was discussed previously.[3,4,7,12,13]

Since the mid-1980s, endosseous root-form implants have become the standard implants used by clinicians. Although blade implants, subperiosteal implants, and transosseous implants still have occasional utility, they essentially have been replaced by the more predictable and easier to use root-form implants. Several decades of research have

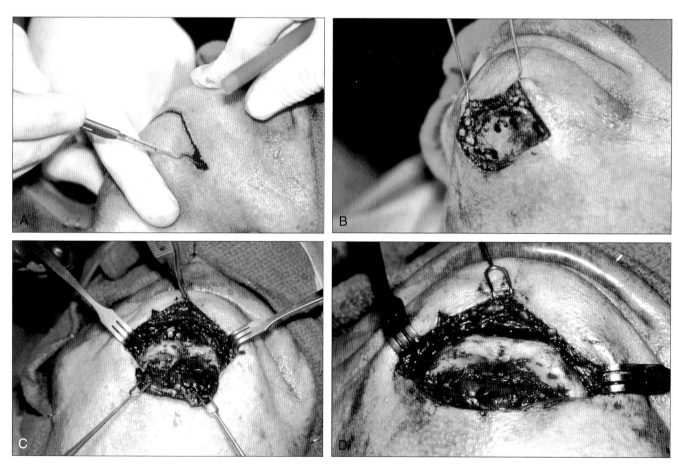

FIGURE 1-14 ■ **A,** A transcutaneous incision for placement of a transmandibular implant. The surgery is performed under general anesthesia. **B,** Exposure of the underlying fat pad. This can be excised if necessary, for esthetic reasons. **C,** Dissection is further carried out to the inferior border of the mandible. **D,** The area for implant placement is exposed and evaluated in preparation for drilling the osteotomies.

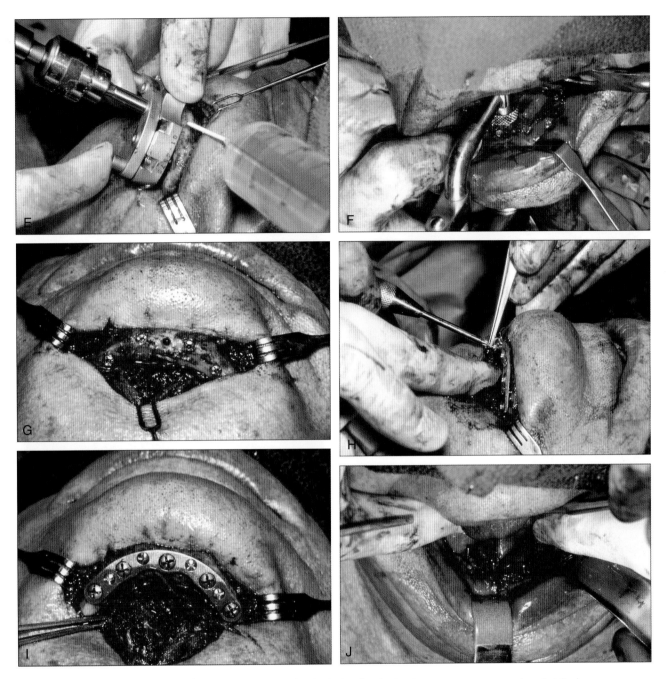

FIGURE 1-14, cont'd ■ **E,** Using a guide, the holes for the implant posts are screwed and drilled. Sterile saline is used as an irrigant to prevent overheating of the bone. **F,** The intraoral area is checked to ensure that the drilling will be done midcrestally. **G,** The fixation screws are tried in. **H,** The inferior plate is fixated with the fixation screws. **I,** The posts are then placed through the plate and through the superior crest of the mandible. **J,** The appearance of the intraoral implant posts.

confirmed their superiority over other forms of implants (Figures 1-17, 1-18).

Because so many different implant systems are available (nearly 100 different root-form implants are now on the market), selecting one or more of them requires the clinician to consider many different factors. Many systems are considered major, international systems, readily available and expected to remain so for the long term. Additionally,

some individual countries have a few domestically available implant systems, many of which copy or modify the major systems.

No particular endosseous root-form implant brand is clearly superior to all others, nor is there any definitive documentation that a particular surface or prosthetic attachment or surgical placement is vastly superior, although several commercially available brands stand out

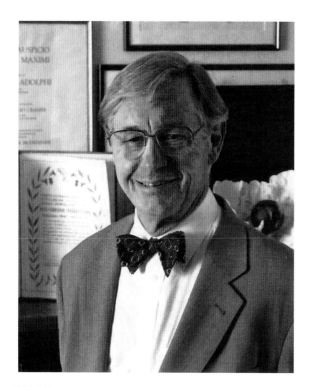

FIGURE 1-15 ■ Swedish Professor Per-Ingvar Brånemark.

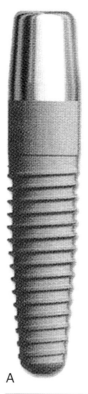
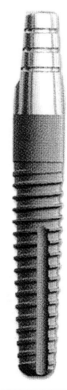

A

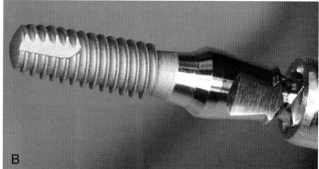

B

FIGURE 1-16 ■ **A,** Examples of endosseous root form implants. **B,** The implants are screwed into place with a handpiece or can be placed manually. Today's root form implants are based on Branemark's original designs.

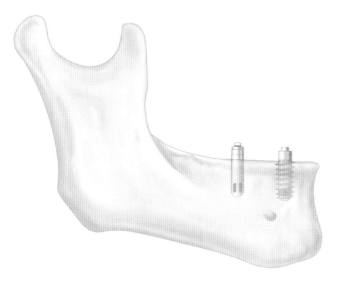

FIGURE 1-17 ■ Endosseous root forms are generally either cylindrical or screw shaped.

above the others. The major overriding factors determining the esthetic and functional success of implants are the experience, abilities, and judgment of the individual clinician and the individual needs of the patient. The clinician must consider five criteria when judging and selecting an implant system: implant type (micro design, or surface roughness; abutment/prosthetic connection; threaded/nonthreaded; tapered/nontapered); ease of use (insertion, stabilization, integration, and loading); success rates (pre-dictability documented in the literature); company support (guarantees and warranties); and costs (patient affordability and practitioner profitability). Standard endosseous root-form implants are provided by several major, international systems, as well as by domestically available implant systems.

SUMMARY

The historical development of dental implants and the history of dentistry are inseparable subjects; specifically, we noted that issues crucial to the historical development of dental implants are also crucial to the history of dentistry. These fundamental issues include the function and

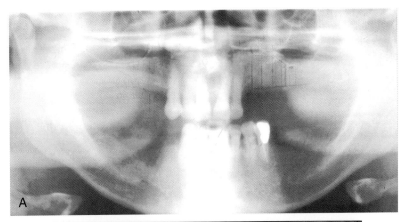

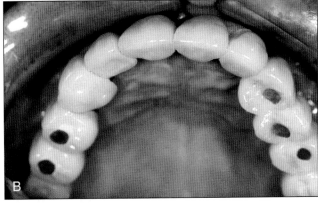

FIGURE 1-18 ▪ **A,** A preoperative Panorex of a patient treatment planned for dental implants in the early 1980s. **B,** Final prosthetic reconstruction.

esthetics of patients' teeth. It has been noted that one of the most significant developments in implant dentistry, and in the study of osseointegration, over the past 20 years has been the expansion of treatment indications, spanning patients' conditions ranging from the fully edentulous lower jaw to the single missing tooth.[14] This observation is noteworthy in that—from "ancient" implants to the most modern, covering the entire history of dentistry—the emphasis has always been and should always remain the dentist's obligation to satisfy the needs of patients for fully functional and attractive dentition, no matter the individual patient's circumstance.

REFERENCES

1. Becker MJ: Ancient "dental implants": a recently proposed example from France evaluated with other spurious examples, *Int J Oral Maxillofac Implants* 14(1):19-29, 1999.
2. Missing a tooth? A single-tooth implant may be for you, *JADA* 135:1499, 2004.
3. Ring ME: A thousand years of dental implants: a definitive history—part 1, *Compend Contin Educ Dent* 16(10):1060, 1062, 1064, 1995, passim.
4. Linkow LI, Dorfman JD: Implantology in dentistry: a brief historical perspective, *N Y State Dent J* 57(6):31-35, 1991.
5. Greenfield EJ: Implantation of artificial crown and bridge abutments, *Int J Oral Implantol* 7(2):63-68, 1991.
6. Burch RH: Dr. Pinkney Adams—a dentist before his time, *Ark Dent* 68(3):14-15, 1997.
7. Smollon JF: A review and history of endosseous implant dentistry, *Georgetown Dent J* 63(1):33-45, 1979.
8. American Dental Association: ADA survey reveals increase in dental implants over five-year period (News release on the Internet). 2002 Apr (cited 2004 Oct 27). Available at: http://www.ada.org/public/media/releases/0204_release01.asp
9. Darle C: Honoring a pioneer, *Int J Periodontics Restorative Dent* 23(4):311, 2003.
10. Reiss RM: Osseointegration—the transition during 40 years of practice, *Compend Contin Educ Dent* 20(4):346-348, 350, 352, 1999, passim.
11. Laney WR: In recognition of an implant pioneer: Professor Dr. Andre Schroeder, *Int J Oral Maxillofac Implants* 8(2):135-136, 1993.
12. Ring ME: A thousand years of dental implants: a definitive history—part 2, *Compend Contin Educ Dent* 16(11):1132, 1134, 1136, 1995, passim.
13. Waite DE: Overview and historical perspective of oral reconstructive surgery, *Oral Surg Oral Med Oral Pathol* 68(4 Pt 2):495-498, 1989.
14. Sullivan RM: Implant dentistry and the concept of osseointegration: a historical perspective, *J Calif Dent Assoc* 29(11):737-745, 2001.

chapter 2

Basic Armamentarium for Implant Surgery

THE PURPOSE OF THIS CHAPTER IS TO INTRODUCE the manual instruments that are required to perform routine implant surgical procedures. The discussion will not include motorized/electrical instruments (e.g., drills) or any specialized instruments associated with any specific implant system (e.g., osteotomes). The instruments described in this chapter are used for a wide variety of soft tissue and hard tissue surgical procedures that are involved in implant placement; this includes the extraction of teeth. This chapter deals primarily with the description of these instruments; in subsequent chapters, their uses will be discussed. A typical setup of dental implant surgical instruments consists of retractors, bite block, scalpel, elevators, forceps, curette, hemostat, needle holder, and scissors. For convenience, the instruments are discussed alphabetically.

Instruments generally are designed for a specific use, but experienced clinicians sometimes can give instruments the use that is more convenient in their hands. Also, different types of instruments may be designed for the same purpose. This variation can be appreciated when one compares instruments designed and named by different clinicians and manufactured by different companies. With time and experience, a surgeon will learn to distinguish and choose the best one for a specific purpose and will start to develop preferences. Some instruments should never be absent during a specific procedure.

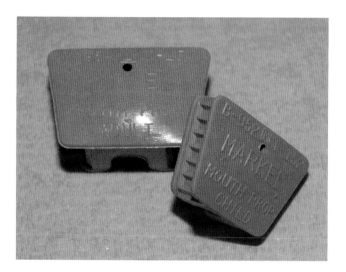

FIGURE 2-1 ■ Bite blocks are used to maintain a patient's mouth open, particularly during long procedures.

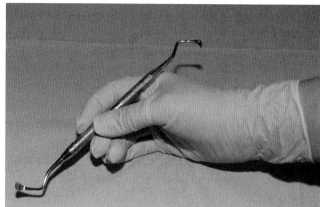

FIGURE 2-2 ■ A curette is used to remove soft tissue from a bony surface.

Therefore, all surgeons should have at least a basic kit for each procedure. These basic kits can be enhanced later by the addition of more sophisticated instrumentation that can make the surgical procedure easier and/or faster with a better final result. In this chapter, we will focus on the basic instrumentation.

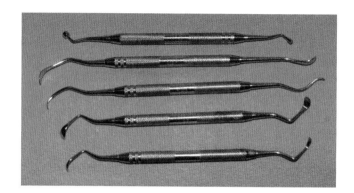

FIGURE 2-3 ■ Set of sinus lift curettes.

Bite Block

Blocks made from rubber, with serrated areas designed for teeth to rest on without slipping, are very helpful for keeping the patient's mouth open, especially during long procedures or for patients who have problems maintaining an appropriate opening (Figure 2-1). The bite block also helps to stabilize the bite when the patient experiences tremors as the result of muscle fatigue. The rubber bite block has a trapezoidal shape and is placed with the narrower end toward the back of the mouth and the flat, closed side toward the cheek. This allows one to control the amount of opening by sliding it back or forth. This rubber bite block comes in adult (S-M-L) and child sizes. An adult with a very small mouth could require a child-size bite block.

When the patient is required to hold the mouth open for prolonged periods of time, the bite block can be used. The bite block is generally a rubber block upon which the patient can rest the teeth. The patient opens his or her mouth to a comfortably wide position, and the rubber bite block is inserted, which holds the mouth in the desired position. Should the surgeon need the mouth to open wider, the patient must open wider, and the bite block can be positioned more to the posterior of the mouth. Bite blocks are also available as plastic rods that can be cut and shaped to fit the oral cavity as needed. Wadded gauze can also be used as a bite block.

Curette

The curette, also called a periapical, surgical, or bone curette, is an angled, double-ended instrument that is used to remove soft tissue from bony defects (Figure 2-2). The active part of this instrument is a spoon-like tip with sharp edges that varies in diameter. The most common sizes for bone grafting range from 3 mm to 5 mm, but some wider diameters can be useful. In its function as an instrument for dental implant surgery, a curette fits the general definition of such an instrument, that is, its working end is scoop- or spoon-shaped, and it is used to remove soft tissue from a bony surface or cavity. The working end of the curette typically is forged from stainless steel, and the handle (solid or hollow) is composed of stainless steel or aluminum. Curettes can be straight (Molt) or angled (Lucas, Miller), and generally are 7 to 9 inches long (Figure 2-3). Periapical curettage generally is defined as the removal with a curette of diseased pathological soft tissues in the bony crypt surrounding a tooth root apex and smoothing of the apical surface of a tooth without excision of the tooth tip.

The periapical curette is significantly different from the periodontal curette in both design and function. The purpose of the periodontal curette is to remove calculus deposits from teeth. As such, it is a debridement instrument, typically a universal curette, which can be used on all tooth surfaces, anteriorly and posteriorly. Periodontal curettes come in sets as well, for use when working in specific areas of dentition. Series names include Gracey, Kramer-Nevins, and Turgeon.

Elevator

An elevator is an instrument for tooth extraction that consists of a straight, thick handle with variations in the active tip according to the area where it will be applied. The most common design in elevators is the straight-channeled one, which can be thin, medium, or thick. You also will find the same channeled design but with an angle. With this, you encounter infinite variations consisting of longer or shorter versions with more or less pronounced curves, different angulations, and sharper or more blunt tips (Figure 2-4). Another type of handle found in elevators is the "T" handle. With this, a myriad of combinations can be found in the market, from which the clinician should start with the simplest common versions and let experience dictate the preference in more exotic designs.

An elevator consists of a single, stainless steel blade with an aluminum, stainless steel, or phenolic handle; it is used as a lever or as a wedge. Routinely, the clinician places the elevator between a tooth and a bone and turns the elevator on its long axis to dislodge or luxate the tooth or the tooth root. Straight elevators include Coupland's elevators and Warwick James elevators; angled elevators include Cryer's elevators. Periotomes are very thin elevators that can be used to sever the periodontal ligament attachment of teeth; other uses include atraumatic extractions, especially in the esthetic zone.

Coupland's elevator comes in three sizes. The elevator blade resembles a forceps blade. The socket of a tooth to be extracted can be dilated when the clinician uses the elevator blade as a wedge, driving vertically along the long axis between the socket and the root. Cutting the periodontal fibers dilates the bony socket both buccally and lingually. Forceps can be used to finish the procedure.

The Cryer's elevator consists of pairs that have a triangular blade, which projects from the handle at right angles. The device can be inserted into the empty socket next to a molar in the mandible when an adjacent molar has been removed and the clinician wishes to retain one of the roots; when used in this way, the elevator's point can remove the inter-radicular bone to the root. The Warwick James elevator comes in one straight and two angled, fine versions and is used in ways similar to Coupland's and Cryer's.

Dental elevators are used to luxate teeth; this may require extraction before or in conjunction with dental implant placement. By luxating the teeth before applying the forceps, the surgeon can minimize the incidence of broken roots and teeth. Finally, the luxation of teeth before forceps application facilitates the removal of a broken root (should it occur) because the root will be loose in the dental socket. Elevators can also be used to elevate roots. Scoop elevators can be used to separate the tuberosity from the distal area of the tooth.

Forceps

Generally speaking, forceps are surgical instruments designed to grasp, hold, or occlude hard or soft tissues. Categories of surgical forceps include bone-holding forceps, dressing forceps, hemostats, and tissue forceps and extraction forceps (Figure 2-5). Forceps designed for tooth extraction are constructed of two continued handle-blade parts

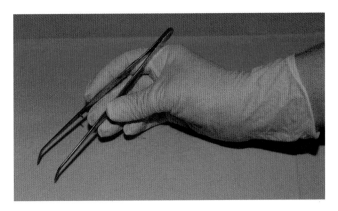

FIGURE 2-4 ■ Elevators come in different sizes.

FIGURE 2-5 ■ Cotton pliers, which are generally not useful for surgical procedures.

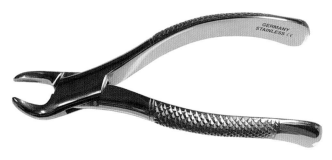

FIGURE 2-6 ■ Extraction forceps.

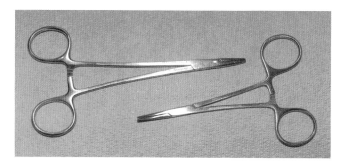

FIGURE 2-8 ■ Hemostats.

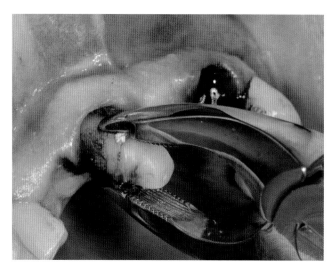

FIGURE 2-7 ■ Extraction forceps are used to grasp the tooth as apically as possible on the root.

that cross at a third of the instrument's length, so that the active blades face and oppose each other, creating an active grasping area (Figure 2-6).

 ## Extraction Forceps

Extraction forceps are used to grasp the tooth as apically as possible on the root; universal forceps usually are used for this purpose, but a variety of types of extraction forceps are available. Sharp-edge blades can be used to sever periodontal fibers; they also can be used as a wedge to dilate the tooth socket. The inner sections of the blades, or beaks, are concave for proper grasping of the root; the blades also have sharp edges for cutting periodontal ligament fibers (Figure 2-7). Their wedge shape can be used to dilate the tooth socket. Different forceps are used for removing different types of teeth. For example, upper anterior teeth usually are extracted when the clinician uses straight-handle, contoured forceps of approximately 14 cm to 17 cm.

 ## Hemostat

A hemostat (also referred to as hemostatic forceps) is a surgical instrument used to clamp, compress, or otherwise constrict a blood vessel to reduce or to stop blood flow (Figure 2-8). Commonly known as Mosquitoes, these instruments resemble a small pair of scissors. The hemostat usually has fully serrated jaws for constricting a blood vessel. These jaws are located directly above the box lock of the instrument, which is above the instrument's shanks. Directly above the finger rings of the hemostat, and at the base of the shanks, is a ratchet to control the degree of restriction on the engaged blood vessel. Hemostats exist in a wide variety of designs that go from straight to curved and are available in different sizes.

Needle Holder

Suture needles come in a large variety of shapes and sizes. Needles can be straight or curved, can come with eyes (for attaching suture material) or eyeless (suture material connected via swaged attachment).

The needle holder is an instrument with a locking handle and a short, stout beak that is used to hold and to guide suture needles during suturing of tissues (Figure 2-9). For intraoral placement of sutures, a 6-inch needle holder usually is recommended. The beak of the needle holder is shorter and stronger than the beak of the hemostat, and the jaws are typically milled so the needle does not slip. The face of the beak of the needle holder is crosshatched to allow for a positive grasp of the suture needle. The hemostat, by contrast, has parallel grooves on the face of the beaks, thereby decreasing control over the needle. Therefore, the hemostat should not be used for suturing. The needle should be held approximately two-thirds of the distance between the tip and the end of the needle. This technique allows enough of the needle to be exposed to the tissue, while allowing the needle holder to grasp the needle at its strongest portion to prevent bending of the needle. Generally, the size of the

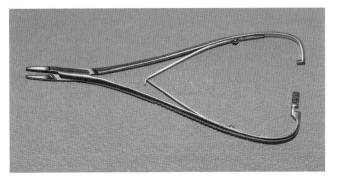

FIGURE 2-9 ■ A needle holder can be found in a variety of shapes and sizes.

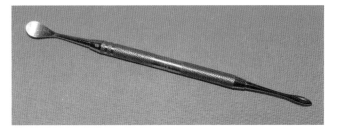

FIGURE 2-10 ■ The #9 Molt periosteal elevator used for flap reflection.

needle dictates the size of the needle holder. So the smaller the needle, the smaller are the jaws of the needle holder; this would avoid slippage or stress of the needle.

Periosteal Elevator

A #9 Molt periosteal elevator is the classic instrument for flap reflection that is used most commonly to reflect the mucosa and periosteum from the underlying bone after an incision (Figure 2-10). When such a mucoperiosteal incision is made, the scalpel blade should be pressed down firmly, so the incision penetrates both the mucosa and the periosteum in the same stroke. The #9 Molt periosteal elevator has a sharp, pointed end and a broader flat end. Usually, the pointed end is used to start lifting the soft tissue flap and directing it toward the bone, and the broader end is used to continue dissecting the soft tissue from the underlying bone. The clinician should alternate between both tips according to the area. The pointed end is used to reflect the tissue from between the teeth, and the broad end is used to elevate the tissue from the bone.

The periosteal elevator can be used to reflect soft tissue by three methods:

1. The pointed end can be used in a prying motion to elevate soft tissue.
2. The broad end of the instrument can be slid underneath the flap, thus separating the periosteum of the underlying bone. This is the most efficient stroke ("push stroke"), and the one which that be used most frequently.
3. The pull stroke, or scrape stroke, can be used occasionally for some areas but tends to shred or tear the periosteum unless it is done very carefully.

The periosteal elevator can also be used as a retractor. Once the periosteum has been elevated, the broad blade of the periosteal elevator is pressed against the bone, with the mucoperiosteal flap elevated into its reflective position.

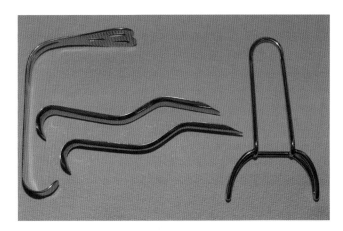

FIGURE 2-11 ■ Several different styles of retractors. A retractor for implant surgery is typically hand-held.

Retractor

Retractors are surgical instruments used to hold back the cheeks, the tongue, or a flap, permitting visibility of the surgical site (Figure 2-11). Typically, they are self-retaining (equipped with a ratchet with lock handles) or hand-held. Size and location of the incision determine the size and type of retractor needed. Several different retractors are useful for implant surgery.

The Minnesota retractor can be used to retract the cheek and the mucoperiosteal flap simultaneously (Figure 2-12, A). Before the flap is created, the retractors are held loosely in the cheek, and once the flap is reflected, the retractor is placed on the bone and then is used to retract the flap.

The Selding retractor is longer and straighter than the Minnesota retractor and is more useful for small flaps. The instrument most commonly used to retract the tongue is the Weider tongue retractor (Figure 2-12, B). This instrument has a broad, heart-shaped area with grooves and perforations that help pull the tongue apart when needed. It comes in various sizes, the smaller one being the most convenient for oral surgeries. When this retractor is used, one must take care not to position it so far posteriorly that it causes gagging.

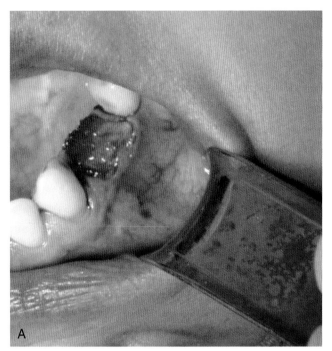

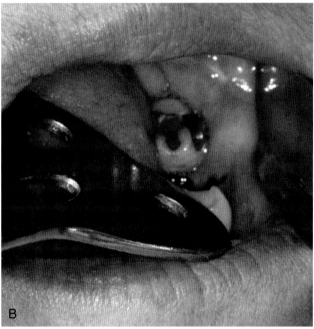

FIGURE 2-12 ■ **A,** Minnesota retractor, which is generally used for the lips. **B,** Weider retractor, which is generally used for the tongue.

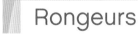

Rongeurs

Rongeur forceps are used most commonly for snipping bone (Figure 2-13). These instruments have sharp blades that are squeezed together by the handles. The forceps have a spring between the handles so that when hand pressure is released, the instrument will open. This feature allows the surgeon to make repeated cuts of bone without making special efforts

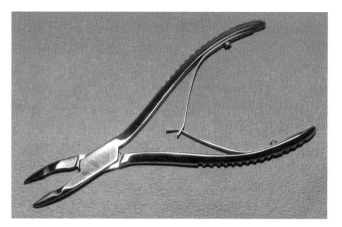

FIGURE 2-13 ■ A Rongeur forceps is used for cutting bone and is not to be used for extracting teeth.

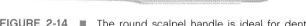

FIGURE 2-14 ■ The round scalpel handle is ideal for dental implant surgery.

to reopen the instrument. The major design used is one that provides for both side cutting and end cutting. The blades are concave toward the inside, permitting bits of bone to be contained as it is removed. Rongeurs can be used to remove large amounts of bone efficiently and quickly, but because rongeurs are relatively delicate instruments, the surgeon should not use these forceps to remove large amounts of bone in single bites. Rather, small amounts of bone should be removed, and each in multiple bites. Similarly, rongeurs should not be used to remove teeth, since the edges are designed to cut more than to grasp, and this practice will quickly dull and destroy the instrument. Rongeurs generally are expensive, so care should be taken to keep them in good working order. Another type of rongeur is the Kerrison forceps, which has a very specialized application, generally for sinus window surgery.

Scalpel

The instrument used for making an incision is the scalpel, which is composed of a handle (Figure 2-14) and a sharp blade. The classic handle is the #3 flat scalpel handle, which sometimes can come with a metric ruler carved on the handle; this is very useful for measuring specimens obtained for grafting. The preferred handle in implant surgery is the round handle #5, but occasionally, the flat #3 will be used. The tip of the scalpel handle is prepared to receive a variety of differently shaped scalpel blades that can be inserted by sliding them so the slot in the blade fits the receiver portion of the handle. The most commonly used scalpel blade for implant surgery is the #15 blade or the #15C blade, and occasionally a #12 blade. The scalpel blade is loaded carefully onto the handle with a needle holder to avoid cutting the operator's fingers. The blade is held with the needle holder obliquely over the cutting portion and never covering the slot. Then it is placed over the receiving portion of the handle, making sure that the diagonal inferior portion of the blade will meet correctly with the diagonal resting portion of the handle. The knife blade then is slid onto the handle until it clicks into position.

The knife is unloaded by reversing this process: the needle holder grabs the cutting portion of the blade, sliding it away from you while the lower noncutting portion of the blade is lifted with a finger. This has to be done while making sure that no one is standing in front of you, as the force with which the blade will disengage sometimes is difficult to control. The used blade should always be discarded immediately into a ridged-sided "sharps" container. The scalpel blades are designed for single patient usage and are not to be re-sterilized. They are easily dulled when they come into contact with hard tissues such as bones and teeth, so it may be necessary to have several blades handy during a single surgical procedure to ensure that the cuts will be precise.

Scissors

Several different types of scissors are used for dental implant surgery: straight, curved, angled, serrated, nonserrated, and

so on. In addition to their use as cutting instruments, scissors can be used for dissecting. Suture scissors usually have relatively long handles, as well as thumb and finger rings. The thumb and ring fingers are inserted through the rings. The index finger is held along the length of the scissors to steady and direct them. The index finger should not be put through the finger ring because such action usually results in a dramatic decrease in control. Suture scissors (also known as Dean scissors) usually have short cutting edges since their sole purpose is to cut sutures. Dean scissors are very useful for cutting sutures during the surgical procedure and at suture removal as well.

An additional type of scissors, known as the Metzenbaum scissors, are similar but have a blunt nose as opposed to a sharp tip. These can be used for dissecting soft tissue, as well as for cutting. A third type of scissors that is very useful during implant surgery is the Iris scissors. The Iris scissors are small, delicate tools used for fine work (Figure 2-15).

Tissue Forceps

When the clinician performs soft tissue surgery, it frequently is necessary to stabilize soft tissue flaps to pass the suture needle through soft tissue, or to hold a flap while cutting it or attempting to retrieve a soft tissue graft. The instrument most commonly used for this purpose is the Adson forceps (Figure 2-16). These are delicate forceps with small teeth that can be used to hold tissue gently, thereby stabilizing it or picking it up. This is the reason why these instruments are commonly known as "pick ups." When Adson forceps are used, care should be taken not to grasp the tissue too tightly and thereby crush it. Adson forceps are available with and without teeth. The DeBakey forceps are similar to the Adson but are longer and allow better access for deep areas. Russian tissue forceps are large, round-ended tissue forceps that are very gentle on soft tissues but are very useful for picking up fragments and covering screws or other devices. The round end allows a positive grip so that tissue is not likely to slip out of the instrument's grip, as commonly occurs with the hemostat. The Russian forceps are also used for placing gauze in the mouth when the surgeon is isolating a particular area for surgery.

Suction Tips

Suction tips are an important part of the surgical armamentarium in any oral surgery because good appropriate suction of fluids (e.g., blood, saliva, irrigation solutions) can guarantee perfect visualization of the surgical site (Figure 2-17). The ideal suction tip is one that permits control of suction force with the existence of a relief hole, like the Frazier suction tip. This type of tip comes with an opening that can

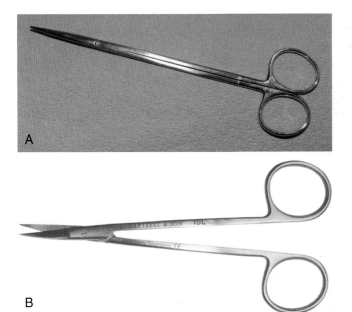

FIGURE 2-15 ■ **A,** Metzenbaum scissors. **B,** Iris scissors.

be covered with the index finger to control the amount of suction. Leaving it uncovered lets it function as an exhaust hole for air to escape through; this permits less suction; therefore, soft tissues will not be picked up by the tip if this is not desired at a given moment and only fluids are to be aspirated. On the other hand, occluding the exhaust hole will permit picking up of soft tissues with the aspirating action and pulling them as desired at any moment of a procedure. This suction tip is long, permitting good access inside the oral cavity.

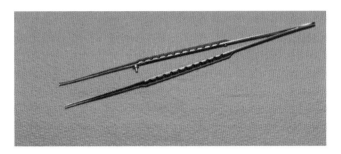

FIGURE 2-16 ■ DeBakey tissue forceps. The tissue forceps are instruments commonly known as "pick ups."

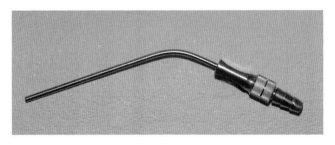

FIGURE 2-17 ■ Frazier suction tip. A suction tip guarantees perfect visualization of the surgical suite.

Implant Guiding System

The Implant Guiding System will ensure correct implant location (buccolingual and mesiodistal) while also helping determine the optimal implant diameter during placement (Figure 2-18). The IIT Guidance System is universal and can be used with any dental implant system on the market.

The Guidance System is comprised of:

Titanium blades – will accurately determine appropriate implant diameter and position for one or two implants.

Titanium measuring pins with extensions – will guide position and diameter of implants in edentulous arches.

Titanium parallel pins – used for ensuring parallel placement of implants and to check positioning.

Blade handle – Provides the ability to securely maneuver and position the blades throughout the mouth.

Tray – Sturdy, autoclavable housing for all Guiding System parts.

Surgical Technique

1. The blades are used to place one or two implants, in an edentulous space or two implants between teeth. Choose the size of blade by approximating to the diameter of implant and slide it into the handle following the safety latch.

2. Slide the desired blade into edentulous space to verify a snug fit. Proper insertion will be achieved when lateral extensions touch vestibular faces of adjacent teeth. Always present the blade through the buccal aspect. Note: if the selected blade does not achieve a snug fit, then repeat the steps with different blades until an accurate measurement is obtained.

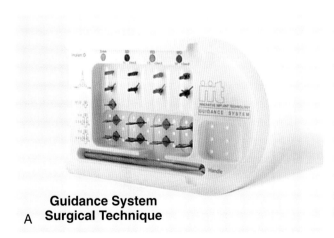

Guidance System
A **Surgical Technique**

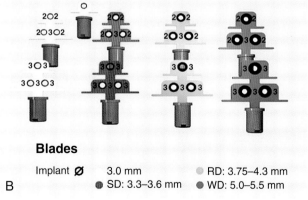

Blades

Implant ∅   3.0 mm   ● RD: 3.75–4.3 mm
             ● SD: 3.3–3.6 mm   ● WD: 5.0–5.5 mm
B

FIGURE 2-18 ■ **A,** The ITT Guiding System is designed to be used in place or in conjunction with a surgical stent when placing implants. **B,** Chart of titanium blades.

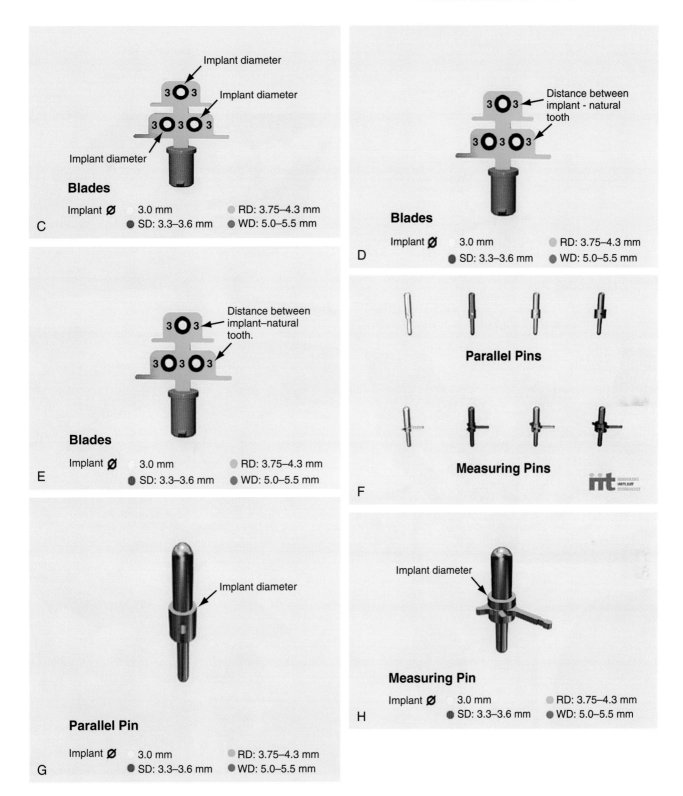

FIGURE 2-18, cont'd ■ **C,** Each blade will determine the appropriate implant diameter and position for one or two implants. **D, E,** The blades will measure the distance between implant and natural tooth. **F,** Parallel and measuring pins. **G,** Titanium parallel pins are used for ensuring parallel placement of implants and to check positioning. **H, I,** Measuring pins with extensions will guide position and diameter of implants in edentulous arches.

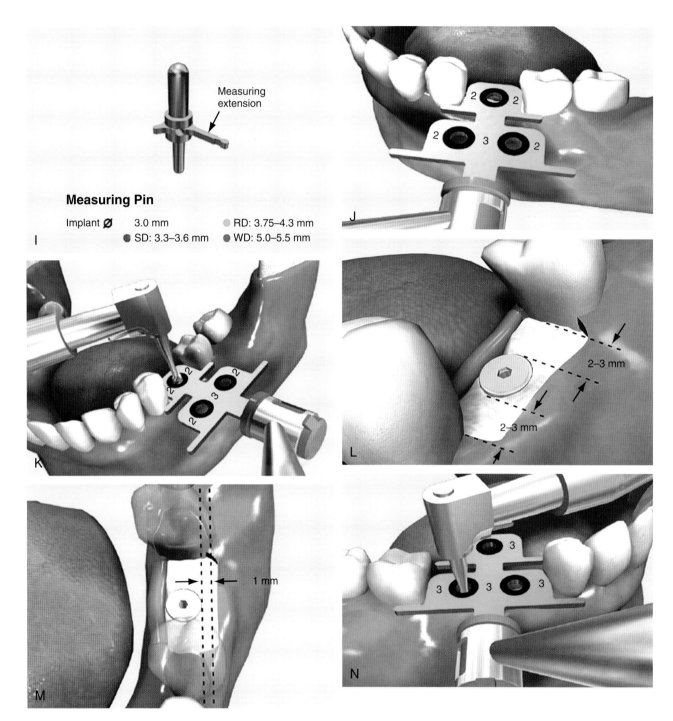

Measuring Pin

Implant Ø   3.0 mm   ● RD: 3.75–4.3 mm
              ● SD: 3.3–3.6 mm   ● WD: 5.0–5.5 mm

Measuring extension

2–3 mm

2–3 mm

1 mm

FIGURE 2-18, cont'd ■ **J,** Slide the desired blade into edentulous space, verifying a snug fit. **K,** Use the initial drill to mark implant location through the hole in the blade. **L, M,** Ideal location (mesiodistal and buccolingual). **N,** A blade can be used to position two implants between teeth.

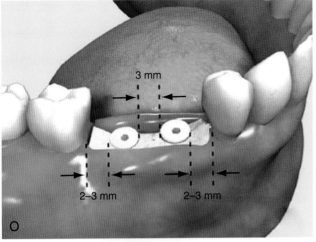

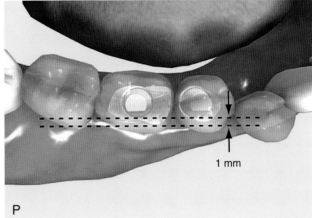

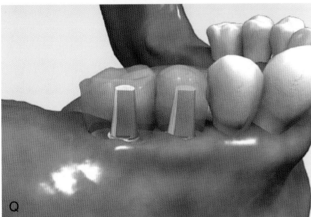

FIGURE 2-18, cont'd ■ **O, P,** Ideal positioning of two implants (mesiodistal and buccolingual). **Q,** Healing abutments in place. (Courtesy of Innovative Implant Technology, Aventura, Fla.)

3. Implant diameter is decided and perfect positioning is achieved.
4. Utilize your initial drill to mark the implant location through the hole in the blade. Note: the blade is only used to guide the positioning of the implant and should be removed once the bone is marked.
5. An ideal location (mesiodistal and buccolingual) and implant diameter will provide desired esthetic and functional outcomes.

SUMMARY

Implant dentistry involves not only the surgical placement of implants, but also adjunctive hard and soft tissue augmentation procedures. Such an array of procedures requires the clinician to utilize proper surgical armamentarium. Instruments are intended for specific usage; however, an experienced surgeon may choose to use instruments for purposes outside their original design.

For each surgical procedure, the clinician should have at least a basic kit, which includes the following: retractors, bite block, scalpel, elevator, forceps, curette, hemostat, needle holder, and scissors. When it comes to actual implant placement, surgery can often be facilitated with the use of an implant guided system. Using a system of measuring blades and pins, such a surgeon will be able to properly place implants in their desired location.

REFERENCES

1. Block MS: *Color atlas of dental implant surgery*, St. Louis, 2007, WB Saunders.
2. Kapczynski H: *Surgical instruments 101: an introduction to KMedic certified instruments*, Northvale, NJ, 1997, KMedic Inc.
3. Nield-Gehrig JS: *Fundamentals of periodontal instrumentation*, ed 6, Philadelphia, 2007, Lippincott Williams & Wilkins.
4. Pedlar J, Frame JW: *Oral and maxillofacial surgery: an objective-based textbook*, ed 2, Edinburgh, 2008, Churchill Livingstone.

chapter 3

Patient Medical History for Dental Implant Surgery

TREATMENT PLANNING FOR IMPLANTS can begin only when the clinician has determined that the patient is in good general health and is psychologically, functionally, anatomically, and medically a good candidate for implants. The ascendancy of implant therapy as the prosthetic standard of care for many dental conditions can be maintained only if clinicians develop comprehensive case selection criteria.[1] Patient selection criteria should include a determination as to whether conventional dentures or fixed partial prostheses may be preferable to dental implants for patients with certain medical conditions (e.g., epilepsy, oral carcinoma, myocardial infarction, scleroderma, Parkinson's disease, tardive dyskinesias).[2] In addition to classifying patients as totally or partially edentulous, the clinician must evaluate patients' current dental condition through intraoral examinations, charting, diagnostic casts, photographs, periapical and panoramic radiographs, and other diagnostic aids. These are needed to determine not only the quality and quantity of alveolar bone but also the existence of malocclusion, caries, periapical lesions, and periodontal disease.[3-5] Information gathered during the clinical examination is of great importance, and this examination should be done meticulously and routinely with every patient. It should always start with assessment of the patient's extraoral conditions and palpation of the face and neck, with attempts to detect any abnormalities in glands or lymph nodes. Intraoral examinations should include visualization of every single area of the oral cavity lined with mucosa—the tongue, the throat—and, finally, an evaluation of the condition of the teeth. All this important information should be written in the patient's chart immediately after the examination.

Additionally, the implantologist must obtain a complete patient medical history in order to determine proper treatment planning.[2,6-9] Many dentists use the classification of physical status established by the American Society of Anesthesiology (ASA) to determine the planning and treatment of patients affected by systemic disease and sequelae.[9] Very few medical conditions preclude implant placement, provided that the patient's general health is adequate to withstand the required surgical and reconstructive procedures. However, specific medical conditions can minimize implant success, so the clinician must be diligent in obtaining factual information about patient history through an inclusive dental (Figure 3-1) and medical history form (Figure 3-2), patient interview, and consultation with the patient's physicians and therapists. A review of how and why this patient information is gathered can help the dental practitioner more clearly understand the importance of the patient's medical history to the success of dental implant procedures.

Dental and Medical History Form

The purpose of the dental and medical history form is to obtain information from the patient that will enable the clinician to provide dental care compatible with the patient's general health. The patient must be convinced and confident that providing accurate information is essential, because incorrect information could endanger not only the successful outcomes of dental procedures but also the patient's health. Of course, practitioner confidence, based on sound diagnostic practice and guidelines, can directly mirror patient confidence. For example, a 2005 study in Australia investigated the confidence in diagnosis and management of periodontal disease by dental practitioners, to determine if national guidelines on periodontal record keeping were being followed and to improve the periodontal knowledge of dentists.[10] Although the study concluded that most dentists surveyed were confident when diagnosing periodontal disease, as well as treating the more common types of the disease, some dentists were not following minimum standards for periodontal record keeping. Therefore, thoroughness in dental record keeping can be an important factor in instilling patient and practitioner confidence. Additionally, along with clinician knowledge and experience, communication skills can play a key role in building patient trust in clinical procedures and practice.[11]

The patient's physical status will determine whether routine dental therapies can be undertaken with or without

modifications, limitations, or other special considerations regarding, for example, the duration of therapy,[12] asepsis and sterilization preventative measures,[13] and use of sedation.[14-16] Patient medical history is just one of many factors often included during patient treatment to determine the increased risk for complications, along with other categories such as demographics, implant specifics, anatomical considerations, prosthetics, and reconstruction.[12]

It is also important for the practitioner to realize that patients of advanced age may present the dental team with several concerns not necessarily related to general health.[9] The clinician must be aware of the physical, metabolic, and endocrine changes associated with aging and how these changes may affect implant treatment.[17-19] Persons over 65 (and the fastest growing segment of the population, those between 85 and 100) often are affected by medical conditions that prevent them from exercising proper oral hygiene. Such diseases include Parkinson's disease, cerebrovascular accident, Alzheimer's disease, and major depressive disorder.[9]

The patient medical form generally contains three categories of information: general, medical history, and dental history.

General Information

General demographic information includes the patient's contact information (name, address, phone number, e-mail, and so on) and personal information (sex, age, marital status, employment, insurance information, financial information, contact information for nearest relative, and so on). Accurate general information is essential for notifying the patient, of course, but also for notifying relatives or employers regarding emergencies.

Medical History

General medical conditions that minimize implant success include metabolic disorders (diabetes 1 and 2), osteoporosis, osseous metabolic disturbances (e.g., osteomalacia, osteitis deformans, Paget's disease, osteogenesis imperfecta, osteopetrosis), hematologic disorders (e.g., anemia), disorders involving leukocytes (e.g., leukemia), disorders involving the blood clotting system (e.g., hemophilia), cardiac and circulatory diseases, collagen disorders (e.g., scleroderma), current medications (e.g., corticosteroids, immunosuppressives, antibiotics), and age-related elements (e.g., still-growing patients, advanced age)[4] (Figure 3-3). Specific medical conditions that minimize implant success include uncontrolled diabetes, alcohol addiction, drug addiction, blood dyscrasias, and regular intake of corticosteroid or immunosuppressive drugs. Consequently, the following question areas should be included on the form: changes in health within the last year, last physical examination, current physician care and medication (including regularly taken herbal medications or drugs—legal or illegal—ingested

---

DENTAL HISTORY

Name _____   Date _____

Part I. Dental Experiences and Symptoms

1. **What is the main reason for your visit?**
    _____

2. **When you look inside your mouth, do you know what to look for?**

	Yes	No
Tooth Decay	☐	☐
Oral Cancer	☐	☐
Gum Disease	☐	☐
Cold Sores	☐	☐

3. **Have you had dental x rays in the past 2 years?**
    ☐ Yes   Type _____   ☐ No

4. **Have you had any complications or negative experiences associated with previous dental treatment?**

    ☐ Yes   Explain _____
    ☐ No

5. **Generally, how have you felt about your previous dental appointments?**
    ☐ Very anxious and afraid   ☐ Don't care one way or the other
    ☐ Somewhat anxious and afraid   ☐ Look forward to it

6. **How much do you agree or disagree with this statement: oral health affects general health.**

    ☐ Strongly agree   ☐ Agree   ☐ Disagree   ☐ Strongly disagree

7. **Are you experiencing any of the following symptoms?**
    (please check all that apply)

☐ Sensitive teeth	☐ Sore jaw	☐ Toothache	☐ Sore gums
☐ Bleeding gums	☐ Difficulty chewing	☐ Filling fell out	☐ Dry mouth
☐ Bad breath	☐ Burning sensation	☐ Abscess	☐ Recession
☐ Swelling inside mouth	☐ Tartar buildup	☐ Yellowing teeth	
☐ Sinus problems	☐ Difficulty swallowing		

8. **Do you clench or grind your teeth in the daytime or at night?**
    ☐ Yes   ☐ No
    If yes, do you wear a bite guard? _____   For how long? _____

9. **In the past two years, have you been concerned about your breath or the appearance of your teeth or face?**

    (If yes, please check all that apply)

☐ Yellowing/graying teeth	☐ Spacing between teeth	☐ Bad breath
☐ Stains	☐ Gums	
☐ Crowded, crooked teeth	☐ Facial profile	

10. **Have you experienced any injuries to your teeth, face and jaw?**
    ☐ Yes   Explain _____
    ☐ No

11. **Have you experienced any of the following?**

☐ Root planing	☐ Gum surgery	☐ Severe pains of face/head
☐ Tooth extractions	☐ Orthodontics/braces	☐ Bad reaction to a local anesthetic
☐ Dental implants	☐ Head and neck radiation therapy	☐ Prolonged bleeding after dental treatment
☐ Root canals	☐ Jaw surgery	☐ Other

FIGURE 3-1 ■ Dental history form. (From Darby ML, Walsh MM: *Dental hygiene: theory and practice* ed 3, Saunders, St Louis, 2010.)

Part II.   Oral Self-Care

1.   **Check the following you regularly use at home:**

☐ Soft toothbrush   ☐ Dental floss   ☐ Floss threader   ☐ Fluoride rinse or gel
☐ Hard toothbrush   ☐ Special brush   ☐ Toothpick   ☐ Flourideted drops/tablets
☐ Medium toothbrush   ☐ Floride toothpaste   ☐ Mouth rinse   ☐ Fluoridated water
☐ Oral irrigator   ☐ Rubber tip   ☐ Whitening products   ☐ Fluoridated water at day care
☐ Denture adhesive   ☐ Powered interdental cleaner   ☐ Bottled water
☐ Denture cleaner   ☐ Power brush   ☐ Other _____

2.   **Check the type of toothpaste you use:**

☐ Fluoride   ☐ Tartar control   ☐ Gum benefit   ☐ Multiple benefit
☐ Sensitivity protection   ☐ Baking soda   ☐ Peroxide

3.   **Estimate how long it takes you to clean your teeth and gums each time:**
      Please indicate your best and most reliable estimate.

           Brushing _____   Flossing _____
                      (time)   (time)

4.   **About how many times each day/week do you brush and floss?**

           brush about _____ times per day OR _____ times per week
           floss about _____ times per day OR _____ times per week

5.   **Do you find it difficult to maintain an oral hygiene schedule due to your job or other**
      reasons ?
           ☐ Yes   ☐ No

6.   **Do any conditions make it difficult for you to adequately clean your teeth?**
      (If yes, please check all that apply)
           ☐ Hold a toothbrush   ☐ Use dental floss   ☐ Brush/floss for any length of time   ☐ Poor vision

7.   **Do you perform a monthly self-exam for oral cancer?**   ☐ Yes   ☐ No

Part III. Between-Meal Snacks

Please check which sweets and starches you eat between meals frequently

Food	Frequency	Food	Frequency
☐ Breath mints	_____	☐ Canned/bottled beverages	_____
☐ Cough drops	_____	☐ Sugared liquids	_____
☐ Chewing gum	_____	☐ Chips	_____
☐ Dried fruits	_____	☐ Crackers	_____
☐ Cookies	_____	☐ Others	_____

FIGURE 3-1, cont'd.

within the last 48 to 72 hours), treatment for cardiovascular ailments (rheumatic fever, heart murmur, pacemaker, angina) and hypertension, stomach or intestinal disease, blood-related ailments (abnormal blood pressure, anemia), pulmonary ailments (asthma, hay fever), cancer (radiation, chemotherapy), diabetes, hepatitis, kidney disease, sexually transmitted disease (STD) (venereal disease, AIDS), stroke, convulsions, arthritis, allergies to medications (local anesthetics, antibiotics, aspirin, iodine), major operations, head and neck injury, smoking and chewing tobacco, alcohol, or drug addiction, mental status (psychiatric care, counseling), and, for women, current pregnancy, nursing, menstrual conditions, birth control pills/chemicals, and menopause. Intravenous administration of bisphosphonates (to treat osteoporosis, Paget's disease, certain symptoms of multiple myeloma, and so on) has resulted in particularly alarming side effects, prompting the U.S. Food and Drug administration to warn health professionals in 2005 that patients taking bisphosphonates should not undergo invasive dental procedures: since 2003, 217 patients taking bisphospho-

nates have developed osteonecrosis of the jaw (gum infection, drainage, and poor healing; numbness, heaviness, pain, or swelling in the jaw; and exposed bone). Oral lesions associated with bisphosphonate use resemble osteonecrosis from radiation. Reports in the scientific literature have indicated a risk for development of osteonecrosis in patients taking intravenous and oral drugs for osteoporosis. The question remains as to the risk associated with oral forms of drugs for osteoporosis, including alendronate (Fosamax; Merck Co, West Point, VA), risedronate (Actonel), and ibandronate (Boniva; Roche Laboratories Inc, Nutley, NJ).

In addition to the above questions, the patient should be asked if anything not covered should be brought to the dentist's attention. Changes in health status should be reported to the dental office. A 2005 retrospective cohort study attempted to determine guidelines for treatment planning based on rates of dental implant failure.[20] To determine risk factors, the study examined data regarding patient gender and age, implant location, bone quality and volume,

Text continued on p. 35

Center for Dental Implants
of South Florida
ARUN K. GARG, D.M.D.

IMPLANT CONSULTATION

This questionnaire was designed to provide important facts regarding the history of your pain or condition. The information you provide will assist in reaching a diagnosis and determining the best treatment. Please take your time and answer each question as completely and honestly as possible.

PATIENT INFORMATION   TODAY'S DATE:_____

☐MR. ☐MS ☐MISS ☐MRS. ☐DR. Name:_____
                          FIRST   MIDDLE INITIAL   LAST
AGE: _____ DATE OF BIRTH: _____☐MALE ☐FEMALE

ADDRESS:_____ CITY/STATE/ZIP:_____

E-MAIL ADDRESS:_____

MOBILE TELEPHONE NUMBER:_____

HOW LONG AT CURRENT ADDRESS? _____ (IF LESS THAN 3 YEARS, PLEASE GIVE PREVIOUS ADDRESS.)

PREVIOUS ADDRESS:_____

EMPLOYED BY:_____ OCCUPATION:_____

ADDRESS:_____

REFERRED BY:_____

SS#: _____ HOME PHONE: _____ WORK PHONE: _____

ADDRESS IF DIFFERENT FROM PATIENT:_____

FAMILY PHYSICIAN:_____

ADDRESS:_____

FAMILY DENTIST/Previous Dentist:_____

ADDRESS:_____

2999 NE 191ST STREET SUITE 210   AVENTURA, FLORIDA 33180

FIGURE 3-2 ■ Medical history form from the author's practice.

Center for Dental Implants
of South Florida

ARUN K. GARG, D.M.D.

DO ANY OF THE FOLLOWING CHIEF COMPLAINTS APPLY TO YOU

Yes ☐ No ☐ Diet limited to semisolid food or soft foods   Yes ☐ No ☐ Jaw locks
                                                                                ☐ upper ☐ lower
Yes ☐ No ☐ Mouth sores   Yes ☐ No ☐ Limited opening of jaw
Yes ☐ No ☐ Diet limited to liquid foods   Yes ☐ No ☐ Teeth do not meet properly
Yes ☐ No ☐ Numbness in lower lip   Yes ☐ No ☐ Loss of teeth
Yes ☐ No ☐ Difficulty chewing   Yes ☐ No ☐ Poorly fitting dental appliance
Yes ☐ No ☐ Numbness in jawbone   Yes ☐ No ☐ Pain in jaw joint
Yes ☐ No ☐ Difficulty speaking   Yes ☐ No ☐ Gagging easily
Yes ☐ No ☐ Tingling in jawbone   Yes ☐ No ☐ Pain when swallowing
Yes ☐ No ☐ Difficulty swallowing   Yes ☐ No ☐ Head pain
Yes ☐ No ☐ Nutritional disorders   Yes ☐ No ☐ Pain when chewing
Yes ☐ No ☐ Digestive problems   Yes ☐ No ☐ Jaw clicks
Yes ☐ No ☐ Pain in jaw bone   Yes ☐ No ☐ Other
Yes ☐ No ☐ Facial pain

Yes ☐ No ☐ Are you currently in pain _____

Yes ☐ No ☐ Do you feel your oral condition is affecting your general health in any way _____

LIST ANY MEDICATIONS/SUBSTANCES THAT HAVE CAUSED AN ALLERGIC REACTION:

Y ☐ N ☐ Antibiotics   Y ☐ N ☐ Metals
Y ☐ N ☐ Aspirin   Y ☐ N ☐ Plastic
Y ☐ N ☐ Barbiturates   Y ☐ N ☐ Sedative
Y ☐ N ☐ Codeine   Y ☐ N ☐ Sleeping pill
Y ☐ N ☐ Lidocaine
Y ☐ N ☐ Latex
Y ☐ N ☐ Local anesthetics
Y ☐ N ☐ Sulfa drugs
Y ☐ N ☐ Other

LIST ANY MEDICATIONS/SUPPLEMENTS CURRENTLY BEING TAKEN:

Y ☐ N ☐ Antibiotics   Y ☐ N ☐ Cortisone
Y ☐ N ☐ Insulin   Y ☐ N ☐ Sulfa drugs
Y ☐ N ☐ Anticoagulants   Y ☐ N ☐ Ginko Biloba
Y ☐ N ☐ Muscle relaxants   Y ☐ N ☐ Diet pills
Y ☐ N ☐ Barbiturates   Y ☐ N ☐ Heart medication
Y ☐ N ☐ Nerve pills   Y ☐ N ☐ Tranquilizers
Y ☐ N ☐ Blood thinners   Y ☐ N ☐ Medications for osteoporosis
Y ☐ N ☐ Pain medication   Y ☐ N ☐ Bisphosphonates
Y ☐ N ☐ Codeine   Y ☐ N ☐ Herbal supplements
Y ☐ N ☐ Sleeping pills
Y ☐ N ☐ Other _____ _____ _____

FIGURE 3-2, cont'd.

Center for Dental Implants
of South Florida

ARUN K. GARG, D.M.D.

PLEASE LIST OTHER HEALTHCARE PRACTITIONERS SEEN IN THE LAST 9 MONTHS:

Practitioner   Specialty   Treatment & Approximate date

_____

_____

MEDICAL HISTORY(Please indicate dates on questions checked YES)

Y ☐ N ☐ Abnormal bleeding after surgery or injury   Y ☐ N ☐ Heart disorder
Y ☐ N ☐ Anemia   Y ☐ N ☐ Heart pacemaker
Y ☐ N ☐ Allergic rhinitis   Y ☐ N ☐ Heart valve replacement
Y ☐ N ☐ Arteriosclerosis   Y ☐ N ☐ Hemophilia
Y ☐ N ☐ Asthma   Y ☐ N ☐ Hepatitis
Y ☐ N ☐ Autoimmune disorders   Y ☐ N ☐ Hypoglycemia
Y ☐ N ☐ Bleeding easily   Y ☐ N ☐ Immune system disorder
Y ☐ N ☐ Bloating   Y ☐ N ☐ Insomnia
Y ☐ N ☐ Blood pressure ☐ High ☐ Low   Y ☐ N ☐ Intestinal disorders
Y ☐ N ☐ Bruising easily   Y ☐ N ☐ Jaw joint surgery
Y ☐ N ☐ Cancer   Y ☐ N ☐ Kidney problems
Y ☐ N ☐ Chemotherapy   Y ☐ N ☐ Liver disease
Y ☐ N ☐ Chronic bronchitis   Y ☐ N ☐ Menstrual cramps
Y ☐ N ☐ Chronic fatigue   Y ☐ N ☐ Multiple sclerosis
Y ☐ N ☐ Chronic mouth dryness   Y ☐ N ☐ Muscle aches
Y ☐ N ☐ Cold hands & feet   Y ☐ N ☐ Muscle shaking (tremors)
Y ☐ N ☐ Colitis   Y ☐ N ☐ Muscle spasms or cramps
Y ☐ N ☐ Current pregnancy   Y ☐ N ☐ Muscula dystrophy
Y ☐ N ☐ Depression   Y ☐ N ☐ Nasal stuffiness in the morning
Y ☐ N ☐ Diabetes   Y ☐ N ☐ Nervousness
Y ☐ N ☐ Dizziness   Y ☐ N ☐ Neuralgia
Y ☐ N ☐ Emphysema   Y ☐ N ☐ Osteoporosis
Y ☐ N ☐ Epilepsy   Y ☐ N ☐ Ovarian cysts
Y ☐ N ☐ Excessive thirst   Y ☐ N ☐ Parkinson's disease
Y ☐ N ☐ Fainting spells   Y ☐ N ☐ Poor circulation
Y ☐ N ☐ Fluid retention   Y ☐ N ☐ Prior orthodontic treatment
Y ☐ N ☐ Frequent cough   Y ☐ N ☐ Psychiatric treatment
Y ☐ N ☐ Frequent illnesses   Y ☐ N ☐ Rheumatoid arthritis
Y ☐ N ☐ Frequent stressful situations   Y ☐ N ☐ Rheumatic fever
Y ☐ N ☐ Glaucoma   Y ☐ N ☐ Scarlet fever
Y ☐ N ☐ Gout   Y ☐ N ☐ Seizures
Y ☐ N ☐ Hay fever   Y ☐ N ☐ Shortness of breath
Y ☐ N ☐ Headaches   Y ☐ N ☐ Slow healing sores
Y ☐ N ☐ Hearing impairment   Y ☐ N ☐ Sickle cell anemia
Y ☐ N ☐ Heart murmur   Y ☐ N ☐ Sinus problems
Y ☐ N ☐ Injury to   Y ☐ N ☐ Speech difficulties
  ☐ Face ☐ Neck ☐ Mouth ☐ Teeth   Y ☐ N ☐ Stomach ulcers
Y ☐ N ☐ Needing extra pillows to help breathing at   Y ☐ N ☐ Stroke
  night   Y ☐ N ☐ Swelling of ankles
Y ☐ N ☐ Tumors   Y ☐ N ☐ Tendency for frequent colds
Y ☐ N ☐ Urinary disorders   Y ☐ N ☐ Tuberculosis
Y ☐ N ☐ Other medical/dental history_____

FIGURE 3-2, cont'd.

Center for Dental Implants
of South Florida

ARUN K. GARG, D.M.D.

Do you take aspirin regularly? ☐ Yes ☐ No   Smoke tobacco? ☐ Yes ☐ No

Has any close relative had a serious illness or condition _____

Emotional or nervous disturbances? ☐ Yes ☐ No

If yes, please explain _____

Patient Signature _____ **Date**_____

FIGURE 3-2, cont'd.

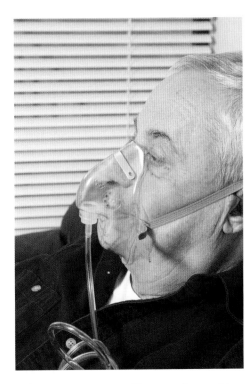

FIGURE 3-3   ■   Patients over 60 years of age with respiratory problems need special attention during dental implant treatment.

and medical history. Although the study concluded that the overall failure of dental implants is low and that no contraindications to implant placement can be considered absolute, certain conditions nonetheless were associated with significantly increased risk for failure; the conditions that dentists should consider during treatment planning and should include in the process of patient informed consent include being over 60 years of age, smoking, having a history of diabetes or radiation to the head and neck, and being menopausal and receiving hormone replacement therapy.[20]

Another later 2005 study provides conclusions based on a literature review centered on the success or failure of dental implants.[21] The purpose of the study was to aid the dentist in recommending patients for implant placement. Implant success predictors included bone quantity and quality, age of the patient, experience of the dentist, implant location, implant length, axial loading of the implant, and maintenance of oral hygiene. The main predictors for implant failure included poor bone quality, chronic periodontitis, systemic disease, smoking, caries or infection that was unresolved, advanced age, location of the implant, short implants, acentric loading, inadequate implant number, parafunctional habits, and the absence or loss of integration related to hard and soft tissue conditions.

Diabetes Mellitus

Diabetes mellitus (Type 1, insulin dependent; Type 2, non-insulin dependent; and gestational) is a systemic

disorder whose sequelae include alterations in wound healing; therefore, the effects of diabetes mellitus on osseointegration of implants have received considerable attention in the literature (Figure 3-4). As life expectancy continues to rise in populations worldwide, particularly in the developed world, dentists are more and more likely to treat patients who have developed diabetes mellitus. Studies have been inconclusive, showing rival failure rates between controlled diabetics and non-diabetic controls.[22] One prospective study's assessment of dental implants in type 2 diabetic patients showed no statistically significant difference in rates of failure of three different implants systems;[23] another study conducted the same year (2000), however, revealed that Type 2 diabetic patients appear to have more implant failures than non-diabetic ones.[24] A 2002 study concluded that diabetes mellitus should no longer be considered a contraindication for the placement of implants as long as the patient maintains control of blood sugar levels and is willing to follow a proper oral hygiene regimen[25] (Table 3-1).

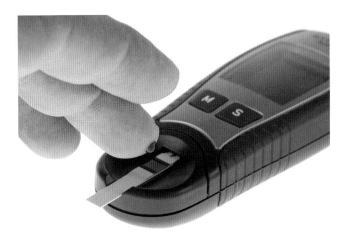

FIGURE 3-4   ■   The idea that patients with controlled diabetes are not good candidates for dental implants is a myth. (© 2009 Jupiter Images Corporation.)

TABLE 3-1	HbA1c Values vs. Blood Glucose Levels
HBA1C(%)	*AVERAGE BLOOD SUGAR (MG/DL)*
6	*120*
7	*150*
8	*180*
9	*210*
10	*240*
11	*270*
12	*300*

A histomorphometric evaluation of new bone formation in diabetic rats into which were placed temporary implants revealed that new bone formation in cortical and periosteal regions did not differ significantly between the control group and the diabetic group; however, significant differences did result in medullar canal and in the bone-to-implant contact in the medullar portion.[26] Another 2005 study using diabetic rats confirmed the inhibiting effects of diabetes on osseointegration, and further showed that the adverse effects could be marginalized to a significant extent by the use of aminoguanidine systemically, and by the use of doxycycline to a much lesser extent.[27] A 2005 study to evaluate histologically the bone-to-implant contact in diabetes-induced rats after osseointegration had begun (uncontrolled diabetes vs. insulin-controlled) showed that bone-to-implant contact was maintained in the insulin-controlled cohort over four months; there was a decrease in contact, however, in the rats whose diabetes remained uncontrolled.[28]

Dental patients with diabetes mellitus should be treated according to guidelines that include a morning appointment, non-interruption of lifestyle, a good breakfast, patient-administered insulin, stress (anxiety, pain) reduction in the dental office, breaks during treatment, patient observation for hypoglycemic event, antibiotics for active infections, postoperative diet restrictions, insulin adjustment, and the absence of aspirin for postoperative pain.[9]

To explain what the A1c test is, think in simple terms. Sugar sticks, and when it's around for a long time, it's harder to get it off. In the body, sugar also sticks, particularly to proteins. The red blood cells that circulate in the body live for about 3 months before they die. When sugar sticks to these cells, it gives us an idea of how much sugar has been around for the preceding 3 months. In most labs, the normal range is 4% to 5.9 %. In poorly controlled diabetes, its 8.0% or above, and in well-controlled patients it's less than 7.0%. The benefits of measuring A1c is that is gives a more reasonable view of what's happening over the course of time (3 months), and the value does not bounce as much as finger-stick blood sugar measurements.

There is a correlation between A1c levels and average blood sugar levels as follows:

Although there are no guidelines to use A1c as a screening tool, it gives a physician a good idea that someone is diabetic if the value is elevated. Right now, it is used as a standard tool to determine blood sugar control in patients known to have diabetes.

The American Diabetes Association currently recommends an A1c goal of less than 7.0%.

Of interest, studies have shown that there is a 10% decrease in relative risk for every 1% reduction in A1c. So, if a patients starts off with an A1c of 10.7 and drops to 8.2, even though they are not yet at their goal, they have managed to decrease their risk of microvascular complications by about 20%. The closer to normal the A1c, the lower the absolute risk for microvascular complications.

Blood Dyscrasias

An assortment of blood dyscrasias can affect healing in the dental patient (Figure 3-5). Definitions of blood dyscrasias include neutropenia, severe neutropenia, thrombocytopenia, hemolytic anemia, aplastic anemia, pancytopenia, and bicytopenia.[29] The risk for severe blood dyscrasia (fivefold increases) has been associated with antibiotic use, including cephalosporins (highest risk), macrolides, penicillins, and quinolones.[29] Various blood dyscrasias have been associated with other systemic disorders (diabetes mellitus, hormonal changes, HIV infection) affecting the course and severity of periodontal disease due to subsequent alteration of inflammatory responses in the oral cavity.[30] Of particular concern for the dentist is the association of blood dyscrasias with mouth ulcerations.[31] Despite the potential complications from bleeding related to surgical and restorative procedures associated with dental implants, patients with classic hemophilia can experience unimpaired function through the use of serial extractions and chairside temporization, allowing the dental surgeon to place implants with precision.[32]

Regular Intake of Corticosteroid or Immunosuppressive Drugs

Corticotherapy can be used to treat a variety of autoimmune connective tissue diseases, cancer, blood dyscrasias, and patients who have undergone transplantation. Acute adrenal cortical failure could result from the stress of dental treatment for some patients; prevention and alternative corticoid therapies are possible remedies for the dental patient.[33] The history of liver transplantation since the mid-1980s has seen the increased use of immunosuppressive drugs to boost the success rate of such operations; however,

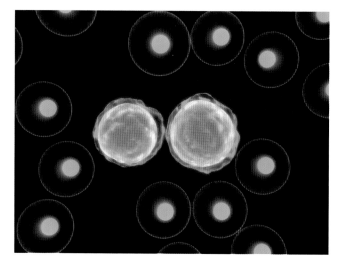

FIGURE 3-5 ■ Blood dyscrasias like leukemia can affect a patient's healing.

studies have documented that the use of immunosuppressors such as cyclosporine and tacrolimus can adversely affect the buccodental health of liver transplant patients, including gingival overgrowth, gingival recession, and dental mobility.[34,35] Immunosuppressive therapy can also affect bone metabolism.

A 2001 rabbit study investigated the results on bone surrounding titanium implants after the administration and withdrawal of cyclosporin A (CsA)/nifedipine, to determine changes and their reversibility, suggesting a significant decrease in treated animals within the bone area within the limits of the threads of the implant.[36] A 2003 rabbit study attempted to evaluate the influence of the administration of CsA on the bone tissue around titanium implants; the study's intergroup analysis showed that the removal torque and the percentage of bone contact with the implant surface for the CsA group were significantly lower than for the cytotoxic T lymphocyte (CTL) group after 12 weeks, suggesting that long-term administration of CsA may negatively influence bone healing around implants.[37] However, the aim of another 2003 study was to evaluate the influence of the administration and withdrawal of CsA/nifedipine on bone density in a lateral area adjacent to implants placed in rabbits; it was determined that short-term immunosuppressive therapy may not negatively influence the density of the preexisting bone around titanium implants.[38]

Cardiovascular Ailments and Hypertension

Because cardiac disease remains the leading cause of death in the United States, a patient's indication of a history of cardiac disease should lead the dentist to conduct a thorough inquiry into the patient's present cardiac status; further questioning and the dentist's knowledge of types of cardiac disease will help determine the peri-operative treatment planning for implant placement[39] (Figure 3-6). Four general categories of cardiac disease include ischemic, valvular, arrhythmic, and myopathic; cardiac status can be measured in a number of ways, including pulse rate and rhythm, blood pressure, respiratory rate, cyanosis, clubbing of fingernails, and pedal edema.[39] Contraindications for implant surgery may include recent myocardial infarction and congestive heart failure, unstable coronary syndrome, unstable angina pectoris, significant arrhythmia, and severe valvular disease.[9] A 1998 study focusing on the detection of medically compromised dental patients in The Netherlands classified patients according to the ASA risk score system, modified for dental treatment; an inventory of the number and nature of medical problems and the modified ASA risk score revealed that conditions that increased with age included hypertension and cardiovascular disease.[6] A retrospective study of medically compromised patients (1,000 outpatients who visited a Tokyo University Clinic for oral

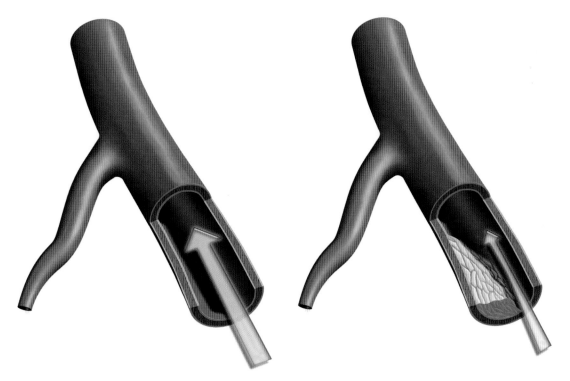

FIGURE 3-6 ■ The clinician must complete the patient's medical history. Be sure to ask if the patient has any cardiac or cardiocirculatory diseases such as atherosclerosis. Atherosclerosis can decrease perfusion to the heart.

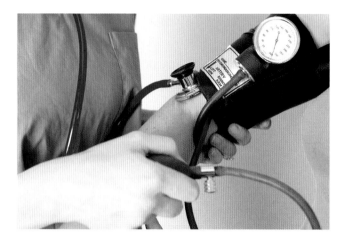

FIGURE 3-7 ■ Hypertension could be an obstacle for proper coagulation.

implants between April 1995 and June 1998) revealed that 35.3% of the outpatients were medically compromised, and that the greatest number of medically compromised patients was in the 50 to 59 age group; furthermore, the highest ratio of medically compromised patients was in the 60 to 69 age group (48.2%). Among the 35% of medically compromised patients, 68 cases involved the insertion of implants, and among those, patients with cardiovascular disease were the most numerous (33.9%), followed by metabolic and digestive tract diseases.[7]

Hypertension in the United States is increasing, and although 2005 National Health and Nutrition Examination Survey data show an improvement in awareness, treatment, and control of hypertension, less than a third of adults with hypertension control the condition (Figure 3-7). To complicate matters for the dental implant surgeon, hypertension is common in patients with diabetes.[40] Patients with stage 3 hypertension (due to the higher risk for an ischemic event) can present a contraindication for oral implant surgery.[9,41] A number of studies have revealed the importance of the dental professional's knowledge of the role that hypertension can play in diagnosis and treatment planning.[42-46] Therapies for treating hypertension have been modified over the years, and some therapies have been accepted historically but only through unsupported anecdotal information on dental management; therefore, guidelines for managing the dental patient are necessary.[42] In fact, dentists can help detect patients with hypertension and can refer them accordingly for medical diagnosis and treatment, so that dental procedures can commence. Typically, a large number of patients who are aware of their high blood pressure control it medically, and patients in this category who are seeking dental procedures are at risk for complications, including stroke, heart disease, kidney disease, and retinal disease; additionally, stressful dental procedures require patients with acute hypertension to be monitored during certain procedures (e.g., oral surgery, periodontal surgery, dental implant surgery).[43]

With some exceptions due to genetics and the environment, blood pressure consistently increases with age.[44] The National Heart, Lung, and Blood Institute publishes recommendations on the prevention, detection, evaluation, and treatment of high blood pressure, and dental professionals should use these recommendations as part of their diagnostic and treatment procedures. Because hypertension affects a significant number of Americans and is closely associated with cardiovascular disease, dentists, along with their fellow health care providers, should be aware of the diagnosis, treatment, and control of hypertension, in order to decrease instances of undetected and untreated hypertension.[44,45]

Cancer Therapies: Radiation, Chemotherapy

Because cancer therapy survival rates are often high, and because success rates for osseointegration therapies are generally favorable, patients who have received radiation therapy should not be excluded immediately from implant therapy. In fact, loss and damage to tissue as a result of therapy for head and neck malignancies often leave the patient with no viable alternative for oral rehabilitation other than dental implants, with failure rates occurring less often in the mandible than in the maxillary region.[47] Similar dental implant therapies of choice are selected by patients with Parkinson's disease, because of their effects on the oropharyngeal musculature, which result in problems with oral function (speaking, chewing, swallowing) when traditional dentures are impractical or impossible to use.[48]

A retrospective study performed in 2005 evaluated implant survival for hundreds of osseointegrated implants placed in irradiated cancer patients over 25 years, beginning in 1979; implant failure rates were higher after previous radiotherapy when compared with a control group.[49] The study documented high implant failures from high-dose radiotherapy, long after irradiation. Although all craniofacial regions were affected, the highest failure rates occurred in frontal bone, zygoma, mandible, and nasal maxilla; the lowest in the oral maxilla. The following therapies helped to lower the rate of failure: the use of long fixtures, fixed retention, and hyperbaric oxygen. The study also concluded that noncontributing factors for implant survival included gender, age, smoking habits, tumor type and size, surgical oncologic treatment, and the osseointegration surgery itself.[49] Although some researchers have suggested that adjunctive therapies are not required for successful osseointegration of implants in irradiated patients,[50] hyperbaric oxygen therapy is often suggested for dental patients who have received head and neck cancer treatments, and who experience delayed complications from radiation therapy; soft tissue injury from radiation often occurs in the area of subsequent dental implantation, and hyperbaric oxygen therapy has been shown to reduce implant failure rates.[51]

A study conducted in 1999 documented a significantly improved implant survival rate in irradiated patients who had previously lost most implants placed before they subsequently received hyperbaric oxygen therapy and new implants (34 of 43 implants lost vs. 5 of 42 lost).[52]

Alcohol, Drug, and Tobacco Addiction

In addition to lack of bone support, some of the factors most closely associated with implant failure include heavy smoking habits, bruxism, depression, and addiction to cigarettes, alcohol, and/or narcotics[53] (Figure 3-8). As early as 1970, the adverse clinical effects of smoking on oral wound healing had been noted.[54] Subsequent studies revealed the connection between smoking and impaired wound healing, seen in clinical results from plastic and reconstructive surgery, periodontal therapy, and tobacco cessation programs.[55-63] The connection between implant failure and smoking[64-78] and, more specifically, between smoking and implant failure in sinus lift procedures has been noted in the literature.[79-81] Smoking may be only one of many factors that contribute to impaired wound healing in patients who undergo intraoral bone grafting and the simultaneous placement of implants.[64]

Although some researchers have found that a significantly higher percentage of dental implant failures occurred in smokers, the exception for the differences occurred in the posterior mandible, suggesting that sufficient bone quantity and quality may negate the higher instances of implant failure among smokers.[65] One study revealed a similar finding of no detrimental effects attributable to smoking for implants in the mandible, while noting that failures attributable to smoking in the maxilla were significant (31% for smokers vs. 4% for nonsmokers).[67] Significantly, failures for nonsmokers generally were associated with poor bone quality. Some researchers list smoking as one of at least 15 factors associated with failure of osseointegrated oral implants, although it is not the most common.[68] Generally, studies reveal the detrimental effect that smoking can have on implant success, especially in the maxilla, and that such losses may also be attributed to less than good bone quality.[70] Although some have noted an implant failure rate of 16.5% for smokers versus 6.9% for nonsmokers, also noted is the importance of longer implant length for reduction of failure in smokers.[71] Some researchers conclude that long-term failure of implants occurs more significantly in smokers than in nonsmokers, but that these failures are not the result of impaired healing or osseointegration but rather are caused by exposure of peri-implant tissue to tobacco smoke.[72] It has been concluded that smoking seems to adversely affect cancellous bone more seriously than cortical bone.[75] Similarly, meta-analyses that evaluated the effects of smoking and implant failure concluded that there was no difference between smoking and nonsmoking groups in terms of implant success rates; rather, differences in success rates were attributable to implant types.[76] Use of surface-modified dental implants can result in no significant differences in success rates for smokers and nonsmokers (97% in smokers vs. 98.4% in nonsmokers).[77]

Regarding the effects of smoking on implant failure for procedures involving the grafted maxillary sinus, researchers note that smoking seems unfavorable for the success of such implants, listing a 82.7% success rate in nonsmokers versus a 65.3% success rate in smokers.[79] However, although some researchers note that higher implant failures in the augmented maxillary sinus seem to correlate with smoking, an assortment of augmentation materials were used, including autogenous, allogenic, and alloplastic bone, as well as combinations thereof.[80] Other researchers emphasize the significant differences in success rates of implants placed in augmented ridges for nonsmokers (100%) versus smokers (43%).[81] Another study concluded that higher failure rates in grafted maxillary sinuses were attributable to a combination of smoking, the use of nonthreaded implants, and poor oral hygiene.[79]

Pregnancy, Nursing, Menstrual Conditions, Birth Control Pills/Chemicals, and Menopause

Pregnancy and menopause could present challenges to implant placement. For example, inflammatory response may be heightened during pregnancy as the result of increased hormonal production (estrogen, progesterone); additionally, the dentist may decide that dental surgery should be performed during the second trimester, thus

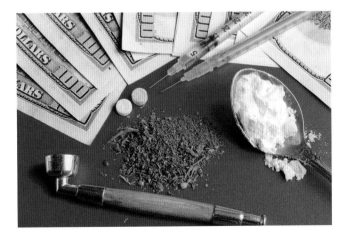

FIGURE 3-8 ■ It is important to review the patient medical history and to question the patient regarding use of recreational drugs, tobacco, or alcohol.

avoiding possible adverse conditions associated with the other stages of pregnancy (first trimester: heartburn, regurgitation, reflex hypersalivation; third trimester: physical discomfort, patient trauma, and preterm delivery concerns).[9] The major concern for dentists regarding patients experiencing menopause relates to the development of osteoporosis, which occurs most often in postmenopausal women.[9]

Osteoporosis

Osteoporosis, a systemic disease associated with decreased bone mass and density, leaves patients, especially the elderly, susceptible to bone fracture because of the resulting porous and brittle condition of bones. As the patient ages, calcium is drawn from internal sources of the bone to adjust for losses due to reduced calcium consumption, absorption failures, and transport deficiencies. The literature is inconclusive concerning whether osteoporosis and osteoporosis-like conditions contraindicate the placement of implants, although alveolar bone is as much affected by the condition's processes as are other bones of the body.[82-85] For example, the purpose of a 2001 retrospective study was to follow patients with osteoporosis of the axial or appendicular skeleton, including the jaw bone, who received oral implant therapy.[84] An adapted bone site preparation technique and extended healing periods were used, and the study showed that successful implant placement may result over a period of several years in patients whose average bone density showed osteoporosis in both the lumbar spine and hip, as well as poor local bone texture. A 2004 rabbit study that attempted to gauge how osteoporosis-like bone conditions affect osseointegration of implants concluded that although the osseointegration characteristics of implants were affected, long-term biomechanical stability under masticatory forces remained uncertain.[85] An important clinical element in this study was that osteoporosis-like conditions were created by intramuscular injections of glucocorticoids.

Patients on medications for osteoporosis should consult with their physician before any surgical procedures, including tooth extraction and dental implants, as the healing can be severely compromised and bone necrosis is possible. Specifically, patients on pamidronate (Aredia; Novartis Pharmaceuticals, East Haverford, NJ), zoledronate (Zometa; Novartis Pharmaceuticals), and alendronate or other bisphosphonates for osteoporosis (as well as some types of cancer involving bone metabolism) should be referred for evaluation before undergoing any surgical procedure because of the significant potential for avascular necrosis of bone.[86-95]

Bisphosphonates are nonhormonal medications (e.g., pamidronate, alendronate, risedronate, zoledronate, clodronate)[89] used to prevent and treat osteoporosis because they inhibit bone resorption by both reducing bone removal and improving bone formation. Bisphosphonates mimic the structure of pyrophosphate, which is a naturally occurring element of bone; they inhibit osteoclast activity, allowing bone growth to occur.

Intravenous administration of bisphosphonates (to treat, for example, Paget's disease and certain symptoms of multiple myeloma) has resulted in particularly alarming side effects, prompting the U.S. Food and Drug Administration to warn health professionals in 2005 that patients taking bisphosphonates should not undergo invasive dental procedures: since 2003, 217 patients taking bisphosphonates have developed osteonecrosis of the jaw (gum infection, drainage, and poor healing; numbness, heaviness, pain, or swelling in the jaw; and exposed bone).[91] Oral lesions associated with bisphosphonate use resemble osteonecrosis from radiation.[93] Some believe that the masticatory stress created in the maxilla and mandible make them susceptible to necrosis, because an effect of the bisphosphonates prevents microdamage and microfracture in the alveolar bone from healing through uninhibited bone remodeling.[93] Slightly higher incidences of necrosis have been reported for the mandible.[94]

Prevention of refractory bone exposure in the jaw—a complication of the use of bisphosphonates—is not possible.[93] However, a study has shown that pre-therapy dental care can reduce the incidence of this complication, and nonsurgical dental procedures (antibiotics/chlorhexidine) can prevent new cases.[92] Prevention of osteonecrosis involves identifying patients at risk: those who have received therapy with bisphosphonates (particularly intravenously) before receiving dental surgery.[95] Additionally, comorbid factors (e.g., systemic ailments such as diabetes mellitus) may exacerbate the effects of bisphosphonates in the oral cavity, so it is essential that the dentist obtain a thorough oral and medical history of prospective surgical patients.[93]

Dental History

Questions pertaining to dental history should include whether the patient ever experienced fainting, abnormal bleeding, allergic reaction, or any other complications as the result of any previous dental treatment. The patient should also be asked if gums bleed during brushing and if food ever is caught between the teeth. Other questions can include the following areas: brushing and flossing frequency, use of fluoride supplement, current satisfaction with appearance of teeth, jaw/teeth trauma, current dental appliances, apprehension about dental treatment, gag reflex, difficulty chewing food, pain during brushing or flossing, swollen or sensitive gums, tooth movement (shifting, moving), tooth sensitivity (heat, cold, pressure, aching), teeth grinding or clenching, pain or clicking in the jaw or in the area around the ear, sore jaw muscles, and sores or growths in the oral cavity. The patient's dental history will also include information about any previous dental treatments that may be evident in the actual oral condition.

Patient Interview

Although a great deal of data can be gathered through the medical and dental history form (as well as through clinical examination) regarding dental caries, periodontal and mucosal disease, oral infection and cancer, temporomandibular disorders, and craniofacial disorders, the clinician should never discount the importance of the patient interview for gathering essential patient data as part of the diagnostic and treatment planning stage (Figure 3-9). The patient's general appearance and behavior can speak volumes concerning proper treatment options. It is advised that a written record should be made during or immediately after the interview.

The clinician should assure the patient that disclosure of his or her medical and dental conditions is standard procedure in the dental practice. The patient should also be assured that the information shared with the clinician is confidential. This information will be placed in the patient's dental records in the office and is protected by law.

The interview, in fact, can cover much of the same information requested on the dental and medical history form, such as medical conditions, recent medical treatment, allergies, and medications. The clinician can explain that gathering this information through an interview is not "repetition" but "confirmation" of information obtained through the forms. Gathering this information through conversation with the patient gives the clinician an opportunity to observe and evaluate the patient's features while he or she speaks, as well as to obtain valuable information pertaining to facial dimensions, muscle tone, symmetry, smile line, and so on. The interview also provides the clinician with an opportunity to determine the level of expectations and desires that the patient may have regarding treatment. The clinician can assure the patient that even though some medical or dental information may not seem important enough to mention, the patient nevertheless should feel free to discuss such information with the clinician. Safety and avoiding risks are necessary outcomes of full information disclosure by the patient.

In addition to currently prescribed medications that the patient is taking, the clinician should also be made aware of any recent course of medication, as well as any regular medication taken for day-to-day complaints. Over-the-counter medications and herbal remedies taken regularly should also be discussed. Of course, recreational drug use should be discussed, although the patient may be reluctant to divulge such information. Patients taking antidepressants should make the clinician aware because some local anesthesias could interfere with the proper functioning of certain types of antidepressants, and alternative anesthesia may be necessary. Patients may be concerned about anesthetics and often need to be reassured that local anesthesia is the most common and safest option in regular practice. Patients also should be urged to discuss any allergies to medications (e.g., penicillin), foods, or materials (e.g., latex gloves, suture material).

Women should inform the clinician about any oral contraceptives that are being taken, because their effectiveness could be impaired by antibiotics prescribed by the clinician. Pregnant patients may have to be told that dental treatment should begin only after delivery of the baby.

Asthma patients should be identified and told to make sure an inhaler is brought to each session. The clinician should be notified concerning the onset of any asthmatic symptoms during the session. Asthma patients are often poor candidates for general anesthesia or sedation.

Patients with heart ailments (e.g., heart murmur, rheumatic fever) can be told that they may receive antibiotics approximately 1 hour before any dental treatment involving bleeding (e.g., tooth extraction, implant placement) is provided, to help lessen the opportunity for infection of the heart valves; furthermore, the local anesthetic may be different to lessen the chances of aggravating the heart condition.

Chemotherapy patients should be urged to complete dental work before undergoing chemotherapy treatments, if at all possible. Chemotherapy can lead to problems with swallowing and taste, as well as with the gums, including ulcers and bleeding. Radiation therapy can affect the salivary glands and cause dry mouth, increasing the chances for tooth decay and osteoradionecrosis. Patients with epilepsy must inform the dentist of this condition so that staff members can be prepared to handle illness during treatment sessions, which can be triggered by anxiety about dental treatment.

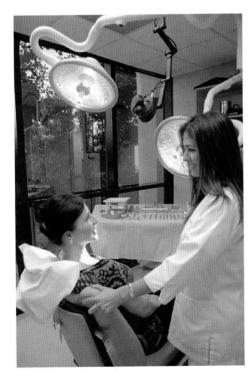

FIGURE 3-9 ■ The patient interview is your best opportunity to ask the tough questions for which patients are most likely to offer false information.

Patients with HIV or hepatitis B or C may have to be told that they will be treated, but only when special treatment conditions are available, particularly if the disease is not under control. Such blood-borne infection risks require dentists and their staffs to follow rigid policies and procedures to prevent cross-infection. Obviously, the dentist must work in close collaboration with the HIV patient's physician. To reduce the numbers of pathogens and postoperative complications, the clinician should employ aseptic and atraumatic techniques. Patients with a history of bleeding tendencies or poor healing must be accommodated, and improvements in oral hygiene before and after treatment are essential.

Depending on the patient's medical and dental history, he or she may have to be informed that hospitalization may be necessary to optimize medical and dental care, particularly patients with blood or heart disorders (e.g., hemophilia), and those with acute asthma or uncontrolled diabetes. Diabetic patients can suffer from severe periodontal disease, requiring regular oral care. Slow healing may be a result of diabetes, as may lower resistance to infection and increased risk for heart disease, requiring antibiotics for some dental treatments. The clinician should emphasize that hospital personnel are trained to handle such medical conditions, and that the dental professional may deem such hospitalization necessary for patient safety.

Medical Consultation

Proper assessment of oral health involves not only an evaluation of the patient's general health, but also coordination with any number of previous and current health care providers. Diagnostic studies should be obtained from previous medical and dental care procedures, including, for example, biopsies of lesions sent to pathology. A system for tracking and charting such studies will help ensure clinician consideration for consulting the physician or dentist who had previously treated the patient. For example, patients who have received radiation therapy to the jaws may be subject to osteoradionecrosis and should be treated with caution only after the dentist consults with the patient's radiotherapist. Once the patient has granted permission, the clinician may wish to consult with the patient's medical doctor concerning any particularly difficult or risky dental procedures.

SUMMARY

Implant success can be directly affected by the overall medical condition of the patient; therefore, the dental clinician must diligently obtain accurate data concerning the patient's medical and dental history. An inclusive dental and medical history form, patient interview, and consultation with the patient's physicians and therapists enable the clinician to confidently begin treatment planning for implants; these tools help the clinician to determine not only that the patient is in good general health, but that he or she is psychologically, functionally, anatomically, and medically suitable for implants. Classifying patients correctly (totally or partially edentulous), performing intraoral examinations, and using other diagnostic elements (e.g., casts, photographs, periapical and panoramic radiographs) enable the clinician to diagnose a patient's condition accurately; however, obtaining a complete patient medical history through forms, interviews, and consultations completes the necessary stages for proper treatment planning.

REFERENCES

1. McNutt MD, Chou CH: Current trends in immediate osseous dental implant case selection criteria, *J Dent Educ* 67(8):850-859, 2003.
2. Sugerman PB, Barber MT: Patient selection for endosseous dental implants: oral and systemic considerations, *Int J Oral Maxillofac Implants* 17(2):191-201, 2002.
3. Barbosa F: Patient selection for dental implants. Part 1: data gathering and diagnosis, *J Indiana Dent Assoc* 79(1):8-11, 2000.
4. Barbosa F: Patient selection for dental implants. Part 2: contraindications, *J Indiana Dent Assoc* 80(1):10-12, 2001.
5. Julian JM: Diagnosis and treatment planning for implant placement, *Dent Today* 23(4):104-109, 2004.
6. Smeets EC, de Jong KJ, Abraham-Inpijn L: Detecting the medically compromised patient in dentistry by means of the medical risk-related history: a survey of 29,424 dental patients in The Netherlands, *Prev Med* 27(4):530-535, 1998.
7. Nagao H, Tachikawa N, Uchida W, Taira K, Shiota M, Enomoto S: Clinical study on risk management for dental implant treatment—Part 1: clinical retrospective study on the medically compromised patients at clinic for oral implant, *Kokubyo Gakkai Zasshi* 67(1):18-22, 2000.
8. Beikler T, Flemmig TF: Implants in the medically compromised patient, *Crit Rev Oral Biol Med* 14(4):305-316, 2003.
9. Marder MZ: Medical conditions affecting the success of dental implants, *Compend Contin Educ Dent* 25(10):739-742, 744, 746, 2004, passim; quiz 772, 795.
10. Darby IB, Angkasa F, Duong C, Ho D, Legudi S, Pham K, Welsh A: Factors influencing the diagnosis and treatment of periodontal disease by dental practitioners in Victoria, *Aust Dent J* 50(1): 37-41, 2005.
11. Hannah A, Millichamp CJ, Ayers KM: A communication skills course for undergraduate dental students, *J Dent Educ* 68(9): 970-977, 2004.
12. McDermott NE, Chuang SK, Woo VV, Dodson TB: Complications of dental implants: identification, frequency, and associated risk factors, *Int J Oral Maxillofac Implants* 18(6):848-855, 2003.
13. Klinge B, Hultin M, Berglundh T: Peri-implantitis, *Dent Clin North Am* 49(3):661-676, vii-viii, 2005.
14. Roelofse J: Overview of pharmacological aspects of sedation—Part I, *SADJ* 55(7):387-389, 2000.
15. Zuniga JR: Guidelines for anxiety control and pain management in oral and maxillofacial surgery, *J Oral Maxillofac Surg* 58 (10 suppl 2):4-7, 2000.
16. Silverman MD: Benefits and protocols of oral sedation for implant surgery, *Dent Implantol Update* 14(6):41-45, 2003.
17. Garg AK, Winkler S, Bakaeen LG, Mekayarajjananonth T: Dental implants and the geriatric patient, *Implant Dent* 6(3):168-173, 1997.

18. Vidjak FM, Zeichner-David M: Immediate-loading dental endosteal implants and the elderly patient, *J Calif Dent Assoc* 31(12):917-924, 2003.

19. Engfors I, Ortorp A, Jemt T: Fixed implant-supported prostheses in elderly patients: a 5-year retrospective study of 133 edentulous patients older than 79 years, *Clin Implant Dent Relat Res* 6(4):190-198, 2004.

20. Moy PK, Medina D, Shetty V, Aghaloo TL: Dental implant failure rates and associated risk factors, *Int J Oral Maxillofac Implants* 20(4):569-577, 2005.

21. Porter JA, von Fraunhofer JA: Success or failure of dental implants? A literature review with treatment considerations, *Gen Dent* 53(6):423-432, 2005; quiz 433, 446.

22. Ashley ET, Covington LL, Bishop BG, Breault LG: Ailing and failing endosseous dental implants: a literature review, *J Contemp Dent Pract* 4(2):35-50, 2003.

23. Olson JW, Shernoff AF, Tarlow JL, Colwell JA, Scheetz JP, Bingham SF: Dental endosseous implant assessments in a type 2 diabetic population: a prospective study, *Int J Oral Maxillofac Implants* 15(6):811-818, 2000.

24. Morris HF, Ochi S, Winkler S: Implant survival in patients with type 2 diabetes: placement to 36 months, *Ann Periodontol* 5(1):157-165, 2000.

25. Abdulwassie H, Dhanrajani PJ: Diabetes mellitus and dental implants: a clinical study, *Implant Dent* 11(1):83-86, 2002.

26. Ottoni CE, Chopard RP: Histomorphometric evaluation of new bone formation in diabetic rats submitted to insertion of temporary implants, *Braz Dent J* 15(2):87-92, 2004. Epub 2005 Mar 11.

27. Kopman JA, Kim DM, Rahman SS, Arandia JA, Karimbux NY, Fiorellini JP: Modulating the effects of diabetes on osseointegration with aminoguanidine and doxycycline, *J Periodontol* 76(4):614-620, 2005.

28. Kwon PT, Rahman SS, Kim DM, Kopman JA, Karimbux NY, Fiorellini JP: Maintenance of osseointegration utilizing insulin therapy in a diabetic rat model, *J Periodontol* 76(4):621-626, 2005.

29. Huerta C, Garcia Rodriguez LA: Risk of clinical blood dyscrasia in a cohort of antibiotic users, *Pharmacotherapy* 22(5):630-636, 2002.

30. Michelberger D, Matthews D: Periodontal manifestations of systemic diseases and their management, *J Can Dent Assoc* 62(4):313-314, 317-321, 1996.

31. Scully C, Porter S: Orofacial disease: update for the dental clinical team: 2. ulcers, erosions and other causes of sore mouth, Part II, *Dent Update* 26(1):31-39, 1999.

32. Gornitsky M, Hammouda W, Rosen H: Rehabilitation of a hemophiliac with implants: a medical perspective and case report, *J Oral Maxillofac Surg* 63(5):592-597, 2005.

33. Lorenzo-Calabria J, Grau D, Silvestre FJ, Hernandez-Mijares A: Management of patients with adrenocortical insufficiency in the dental clinic, *Med Oral* 8(3):207-214, 2003.

34. Heckmann SM, Heckmann JG, Linke JJ, Hohenberger W, Mombelli A: Implant therapy following liver transplantation: clinical and microbiological results after 10 years, *J Periodontol* 75(6):909-913, 2004.

35. Diaz-Ortiz ML, Mico-Llorens JM, Gargallo-Albiol J, Baliellas-Comellas C, Berini-Aytes L, Gay-Escoda C: Dental health in liver transplant patients, *Med Oral Patol Oral Cir Bucal* 10(1):72-76, 66-72, 2005.

36. Duarte PM, Nogueira Filho GR, Sallum EA, de Toledo S, Sallum AW, Nociti Junior FH: The effect of an immunosuppressive therapy and its withdrawal on bone healing around titanium implants: a histometric study in rabbits, *J Periodontol* 72(10):1391-1397, 2001.

37. Sakakura CE, Margonar R, Holzhausen M, Nociti FH Jr, Alba RC Jr, Marcantonio E Jr: Influence of cyclosporin A therapy on bone healing around titanium implants: a histometric and biomechanic study in rabbits, *J Periodontol* 74(7):976-981, 2003.

38. Duarte PM, Nogueira Filho GR, Sallum EA, Sallum AW, Nociti Junior FH: Short-term immunosuppressive therapy does not affect the density of the pre-existing bone around titanium implants placed in rabbits, *Pesqui Odontol Bras* 17(4):362-366, 2003. Epub 2004 Apr 19.

39. Lifshey FM: Evaluation of and treatment considerations for the dental patient with cardiac disease, *N Y State Dent J* 70(8):16-19, 2004.

40. Andros V: Uncontrolled blood pressure in a treated, high-risk managed care population, *Am J Manag Care* 11(7 suppl): S215-S219, 2005.

41. Maulaz AB, Bezerra DC, Michel P, Bogousslavsky J: Effect of discontinuing aspirin therapy on the risk of brain ischemic stroke, *Arch Neurol* 62(8):1217-1220, 2005.

42. Muzyka BC, Glick M: The hypertensive dental patient, *J Am Dent Assoc* 128(8):1109-1120, 1997.

43. Little JW: The impact on dentistry of recent advances in the management of hypertension, *Oral Surg Oral Med Oral Pathol Oral Radiol Endod* 90(5):591-599, 2000.

44. Riley CK, Terezhalmy GT: The patient with hypertension, *Quintessence Int* 32(9):671-690, 2001.

45. Herman WW, Konzelman JL Jr, Prisant LM: Joint National Committee on Prevention, Detection, Evaluation, and Treatment of High Blood Pressure: New national guidelines on hypertension: a summary for dentistry, *J Am Dent Assoc* 135(5):576-584, 2004; quiz 653-654.

46. Aubertin MA: The hypertensive patient in dental practice: updated recommendations for classification, prevention, monitoring, and dental management, *Gen Dent* 52(6):544-552, 2004; quiz 553, 527-528.

47. Shaw RJ, Sutton AF, Cawood JI, Howell RA, Lowe D, Brown JS, Rogers SN, Vaughan ED: Oral rehabilitation after treatment for head and neck malignancy, *Head Neck* 27(6):459-470, 2005.

48. Heckmann SM, Heckmann JG, Weber HP: Clinical outcomes of three Parkinson's disease patients treated with mandibular implant overdentures, *Clin Oral Implants Res* 11(6):566-571, 2000.

49. Granstrom G: Osseointegration in irradiated cancer patients: an analysis with respect to implant failures, *J Oral Maxillofac Surg* 63(5):579-585, 2005.

50. Andersson G, Andreasson L, Bjelkengren G: Oral implant rehabilitation in irradiated patients without adjunctive hyperbaric oxygen, *Int J Oral Maxillofac Implants* 13(5):647-654, 1998.

51. Adkinson C, Anderson T, Chavez J, Collier R, MacLeod S, Nicholson C, Odland R, Vellis P: Hyperbaric oxygen therapy: a meeting place for medicine and dentistry, *Minn Med* 88(8):42-45, 2005.

52. Granstrom G, Tjellstrom A, Branemark PI: Osseointegrated implants in irradiated bone: a case-controlled study using adjunctive hyperbaric oxygen therapy, *J Oral Maxillofac Surg* 57(5):493-499, 1999.

53. Ekfeldt A, Christiansson U, Eriksson T, Linden U, Lundqvist S, Rundcrantz T, Johansson LA, Nilner K, Billstrom C: A retrospective

analysis of factors associated with multiple implant failures in maxillae, *Clin Oral Implants Res* 12(5):462-467, 2001.

54. Christen AG: The clinical effects of tobacco on oral tissue, *J Am Dent Assoc* 81(6):1378-1382, 1970.

55. Mosely LH, Finseth F, Goody M: Nicotine and its effect on wound healing, *Plast Reconstr Surg* 61(4):570-575, 1978.

56. McCann D: Tobacco use and oral health, *J Am Dent Assoc* 118(1):18-25, 1989.

57. Cuff MJ, McQuade MJ, Scheidt MJ, Sutherland DE, Van Dyke TE: The presence of nicotine on root surfaces of periodontally diseased teeth in smokers, *J Periodontol* 60(10):564-569, 1989.

58. Reus WF 3rd, Colen LB, Straker DJ: Tobacco smoking and complications in elective microsurgery, *Plast Reconstr Surg* 89(3):490-494, 1992.

59. Silverstein P: Smoking and wound healing, *Am J Med* 93(1A): 22S-24S, 1992.

60. Stafne EE: The role of the dental office in tobacco cessation: a practical approach, *Northwest Dent* 72(1):17-21, 1993.

61. Luomanen M, Tiitta O, Heikinheimo K, Leimola-Virtanen R, Heinaro I, Happonen RP: Effect of snuff and smoking on tenascin expression in oral mucosa, *J Oral Pathol Med* 26(7): 334-338, 1997.

62. Campanile G, Hautmann G, Lotti T: Cigarette smoking, wound healing, and face-lift, *Clin Dermatol* 16(5):575-578, 1998.

63. Jones RB: Tobacco or oral health: past progress, impending challenge, *J Am Dent Assoc* 131(8):1130-1136, 2000.

64. Jones JK, Triplett RG: The relationship of cigarette smoking to impaired intraoral wound healing: a review of evidence and implications for patient care, *J Oral Maxillofac Surg* 50(3):237-279, 1992; discussion 239-240.

65. Bain CA, Moy PK: The association between the failure of dental implants and cigarette smoking, *Int J Oral Maxillofac Implants* 8(6):609-615, 1993.

66. Gorman LM, Lambert PM, Morris HF, Ochi S, Winkler S: The effect of smoking on implant survival at second-stage surgery: DICRG Interim Report No. 5, Dental Implant Clinical Research Group, *Implant Dent* 3(3):165-168, 1994.

67. De Bruyn H, Collaert B: The effect of smoking on early implant failure, *Clin Oral Implants Res* 5(4):260-264, 1994.

68. Esposito M, Hirsch JM, Lekholm U, Thomsen P: Biological factors contributing to failures of osseointegrated oral implants: (I) success criteria and epidemiology, *Eur J Oral Sci* 106(1):527-551, 1998.

69. Zitzmann NU, Scharer P, Marinello CP: Factors influencing the success of GBR: smoking, timing of implant placement, implant location, bone quality and provisional restoration, *J Clin Periodontol* 26(10):673-682, 1999.

70. Hultin M: Factors affecting peri-implant tissue reactions (thesis), Department of Periodontology, Institute of Odontology, Karolinska Institute, Stockholm, Sweden, 2001. Available at: http://diss.kib.ki.se/2001/91-628-4761-9/thesis.pdf.

71. Wallace RH: The relationship between cigarette smoking and dental implant failure, *Eur J Prosthodont Restor Dent* 8(3):103-106, 2000.

72. Lambert PM, Morris HF, Ochi S: The influence of smoking on 3-year clinical success of osseointegrated dental implants, *Ann Periodontol* 5(1):79-89, 2000.

73. Schwartz-Arad D, Samet N, Samet N, Mamlider A: Smoking and complications of endosseous dental implants, *J Periodontol* 73(2):153-157, 2002.

74. Elsubeihi ES, Zarb GA: Implant prosthodontics in medically challenged patients: the University of Toronto experience, *J Can Dent Assoc* 68(2):103-108, 2002.

75. Nociti FH Jr, Cesar NJ, Carvalho MD, Sallum EA: Bone density around titanium implants may be influenced by intermittent cigarette smoke inhalation: a histometric study in rats, *Int J Oral Maxillofac Implants* 17(3):347-352, 2002.

76. Bain CA, Weng D, Meltzer A, Kohles SS, Stach RM: A meta-analysis evaluating the risk for implant failure in patients who smoke, *Compend Contin Educ Dent* 23(8):695-699, 702, 704, 2002, passim; quiz 708.

77. Nociti Junior FH, Cesar Neto JB, Carvalho MD, Sallum EA, Sallum AW: Intermittent cigarette smoke inhalation may affect bone volume around titanium implants in rats, *J Periodontol* 73(9): 982-987, 2002.

78. Kumar A, Jaffin RA, Berman C: The effect of smoking on achieving osseointegration of surface-modified implants: a clinical report, *Int J Oral Maxillofac Implants* 17(6):816-819, 2002.

79. Kan JY, Rungcharassaeng K, Kim J, Lozada JL, Goodacre CJ: Factors affecting the survival of implants placed in grafted maxillary sinuses: a clinical report, *J Prosthet Dent* 87(5):485-489, 2002.

80. Olson JW, Dent CD, Morris HF, Ochi S: Long-term assessment (5 to 71 months) of endosseous dental implants placed in the augmented maxillary sinus, *Ann Periodontol* 5(1):152-156, 2000.

81. Mayfield LJ, Skoglund A, Hising P, Lang NP, Attstrom R: Evaluation following functional loading of titanium fixtures placed in ridges augmented by deproteinized bone mineral: a human case study, *Clin Oral Implants Res* 2(5):508-514, 2001.

82. Friberg B: Treatment with dental implants in patients with severe osteoporosis: a case report, *Int J Periodontics Restorative Dent* 14(4):348-353, 1994.

83. Winkler S, Mekayarajjananonth T, Garg AK, Tewari DS: Nutrition and the geriatric implant patient, *Implant Dent* 6(4):291-294, 1997.

84. Friberg B, Ekestubbe A, Mellstrom D, Sennerby L: Branemark implants and osteoporosis: a clinical exploratory study, *Clin Implant Dent Relat Res* 3(1):50-56, 2001.

85. Keller JC, Stewart M, Roehm M, Schneider GB: Osteoporosis-like bone conditions affect osseointegration of implants, *Int J Oral Maxillofac Implants* 19(5):687-694, 2004.

86. Degidi M, Piattelli A: Immediately loaded bar-connected implants with an anodized surface inserted in the anterior mandible in a patient treated with diphosphonates for osteoporosis: a case report with a 12-month follow-up, *Clin Implant Dent Relat Res* 5(4):269-272, 2003.

87. Marx RE: Pamidronate (Aredia) and zoledronate (Zometa) induced avascular necrosis of the jaws: a growing epidemic, *J Oral Maxillofac Surg* 61(9):1115-1117, 2003.

88. Carter GD, Goss AN: Bisphosphonates and avascular necrosis of the jaws, *Aust Dent J* 48(4):268, 2003.

89. Robinson NA, Yeo JF: Bisphosphonates—a word of caution, *Ann Acad Med Singapore* 33(4 suppl):48-49, 2004.

90. Melo MD, Obeid G: Osteonecrosis of the maxilla in a patient with a history of bisphosphonate therapy, *J Can Dent Assoc* 71(2): 111-113, 2005.

91. Wooltorton E: Patients receiving intravenous bisphosphonates should avoid invasive dental procedures, *CMAJ* 172(13):1684, 2005. Epub 2005 Jun 1.

92. Marx RE, Sawatari Y, Fortin M, Broumand V: Bisphosphonate-induced exposed bone (osteonecrosis/osteopetrosis) of the jaws: risk factors, recognition, prevention, and treatment, *J Oral Maxillofac Surg* 63(11):1567-1575, 2005.

93. Migliorati CA, Casiglia J, Epstein J, Jacobsen PL, Siegel MA, Woo SB: Managing the care of patients with bisphosphonate-associated osteonecrosis: an American Academy of Oral Medicine position paper, *J Am Dent Assoc* 136(12):1658-1668, 2005.

94. Markiewicz MR, Margarone JE 3rd, Campbell JH, Aguirre A: Bisphosphonate-associated osteonecrosis of the jaws: a review of current knowledge, *J Am Dent Assoc* 136(12):1669-1674, 2005.

95. Melo MD, Obeid G: Osteonecrosis of the jaws in patients with a history of receiving bisphosphonate therapy: strategies for prevention and early recognition, *J Am Dent Assoc* 136(12): 1675-1681, 2005.

chapter 4

Anatomic Considerations in Oral Implantology

I N ALL DISCIPLINES OF DENTISTRY, and particularly in the field of oral implantology, the anatomical characteristics of the patient's oral cavity play a key role in successful achievement of treatment goals.[1-4] Even when treatment is considered clinically successful, damage to anatomical structures related to implant placement may lead to legal action against the clinician.[5] After natural tooth loss or tooth extraction, resorption of the alveolar ridges is a continuing process that precipitates anatomical and functional changes in the patient, both vertically and horizontally.[6,7] Thus, the space relationships of the different anatomical structures change.[8] Each dental implant case must be individually planned according to the wide variations among patients in bone height and density,[9,10] nerve positions,[11-15] and blood supply[16-24] (Figure 4-1). Although dental implant clinicians have relied on various forms of imaging techniques (e.g., radiography) to identify anatomical structures for treatment planning,[25-28] in the past decade, a number of dental implant systems have come to rely more and more on such forms of imaging to develop effective dental implant guides and templates to help ensure correct anatomical placement of implants.[29,30] In addition, the clinician must take into consideration the patient's general dental and health condition. Potential implant patients can be categorized as fully dentate (periodontally involved dentition), partially edentulous (one tooth missing, or two or more teeth missing), or fully

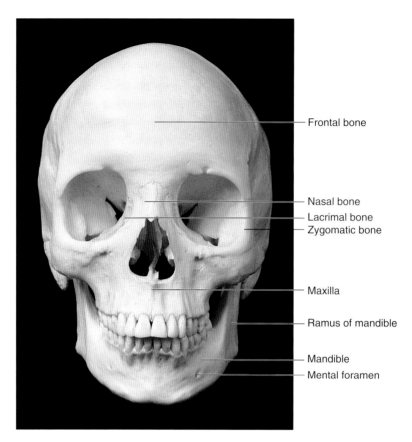

- Frontal bone

- Nasal bone
- Lacrimal bone
- Zygomatic bone

- Maxilla

- Ramus of mandible

- Mandible
- Mental foramen

FIGURE 4-1 ■ Skull, from the front. (Modified from Abrahams PH, Hutchings RT, Marks SC Jr: *McMinn's color atlas of human anatomy*, ed 4, Mosby, St Louis, 1998.)

edentulous (all teeth missing).[31] The bone structures (e.g., maxilla, mandible), the sensory and motor innervations (e.g., the trigeminal and facial nerves), and the vasculature (e.g., the facial and maxillary arteries and veins and their branches) of the oral cavity have a direct impact on oral implantology.

Bone Structures of the Oral Cavity

Maxilla

The maxillary bone comprises the maxillae, which are the second largest bones of the face.[32] Their union forms the whole of the upper jaw. The maxillary bone, or maxilla, has a quadrilateral shape that is slightly flattened from the outside in, and is made up of an external face, an internal face, four borders, and four angles.[33] The body of the maxilla can be described as a four-sided pyramid with its base facing the medial aspect of the skull. It lies in an almost horizontal axis, the apex being elongated laterally in relation to its base.[1] The body of the maxilla is hollowed by

a large pyramidal cavity known as the maxillary sinus, or the antrum of Highmore. The sinus is oriented in the same direction as the body of the maxilla. The floor of the sinus, formed by the alveolar process, has several conical processes that correspond to the roots of the teeth. All of the interior walls of the sinus are covered by a mucous membrane (Figure 4-2).

The anterior maxilla has usually represented a supreme challenge to the placement of dental implants for clinicians: no other area receives so much esthetic focus for the patient; additionally, the preexisting anatomy of the anterior maxilla often presents difficult obstacles.[34] The clinician must review the potential for implant failure in the region, including bone height and width, implant positioning, proper implant selection, multiple/single tooth replacement, bone grafting, wound closure, and adequate osseointegration intervals before loading.[2]

The maxillary sinus is of particular concern when the clinician is deciding on the type of implant treatment (of which there are several)[35-37] (Figure 4-3) to be used in a posteriorly edentulous patient. When teeth are lost in the posterior maxilla, pneumatization of the sinuses occurs. This process frequently minimizes or completely eliminates the amount of vertical bone available for implant placement. However, this problem can be overcome by grafting bone on the maxillary

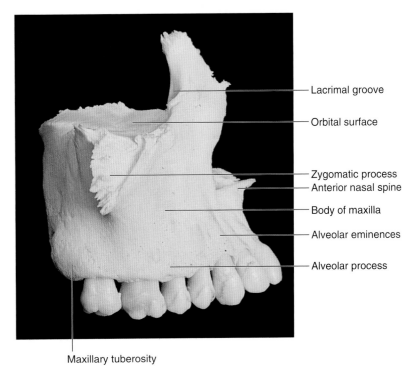

Lacrimal groove

Orbital surface

Zygomatic process
Anterior nasal spine
Body of maxilla
Alveolar eminences
Alveolar process

Maxillary tuberosity

FIGURE 4-2 ■ Right maxilla, from the lateral side. (Modified from Abrahams PH, Hutchings RT, Marks SC Jr: *McMinn's color atlas of human anatomy*, ed 4, Mosby, St Louis, 1998.)

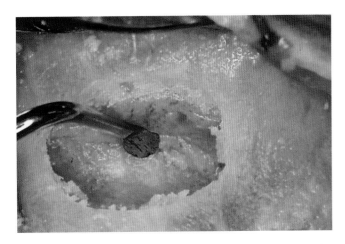

FIGURE 4-3 ■ Sinus lift procedure whereby the lining of the maxillary sinus is lifted in an atrophic posterior maxillary region and augmented.

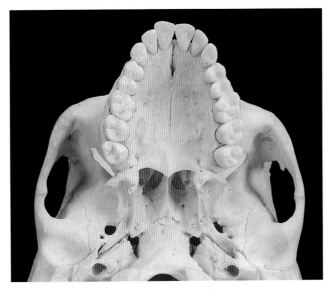

FIGURE 4-4 ■ Occlusal view of the maxilla. Note the relationship between this structure and the zygomas, which form the anterior aspect of the cheek. The lateral portion is supported by the zygomatic arch. (Modified from Abrahams PH, Hutchings RT, Marks SC Jr: *McMinn's color atlas of human anatomy*, ed 4, Mosby, St Louis, 1998.)

anterior floor to increase the alveolar height.[2,38,39] The four surfaces of the maxilla make up the anterior (facial), posterior (intratemporal), superior (orbital), and medial (nasal) sections. The four borders or processes of the maxilla are the zygomatic, frontal, alveolar, and palatine.[32] The anterior and posterior surfaces of the maxilla, which are separated by the zygomatic process, form the skeleton of the anterior part of the cheek[40] (Figure 4-4).

On the inferior aspect of the anterior surface, a series of eminences correspond to the positions of the roots of the

teeth (Figure 4-5, *A*). Superomedial to these eminences is a depression of the incisive fossa, and lateral to the incisive fossa is the larger and deeper canine fossa.[32] Near the upper inner corner of the canine fossa is the infraorbital foramen, the opening to the infraorbital canal[1] (Figure 4-5, *B*).

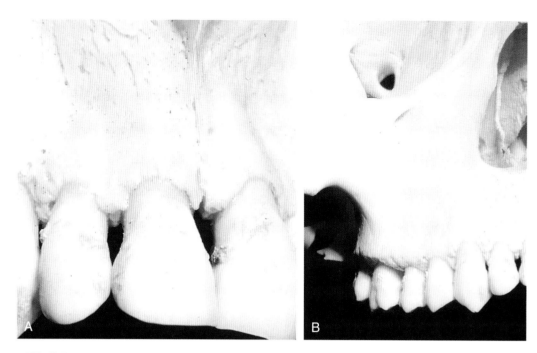

FIGURE 4-5 ■ **A,** Inferior portion of the anterior face of the maxilla. The eminences corresponding to the roots of the anterior teeth can be appreciated, as can the incisive and canine fossae. **B,** Anterior surface of the maxilla. Note the close relationship between the alveolar process, the infraorbital foramen, the piriform rim, and the floor of the orbit.

The convex posterior surface of the maxillary body (the maxillary tuberosity, or tuber) forms part of the anterior walls of the intratemporal fossa.[1] The alveolar process, which originates at the midline and terminates posterior to the tuberosity, is the thickest and the most spongy part of the maxilla. Its arched form is broader posteriorly than anteriorly, and it has eight deep cavities, or sockets, for reception of the teeth.[32]

The maxillary teeth lie oblique to the vertical axis of the cranium. As a result, the roots in the upper arch are more closely spaced than the crowns of the teeth, which usually have the appearance of tilting slightly outward. The axes of the incisor teeth deviate by approximately 3.0 degrees, and those of the molar teeth by 1.5 to 2.0 degrees. It is important to maintain this anatomical relationship whenever dental implants are inserted.

Mandible

The mandible, the largest and strongest of the facial bones, consists of a horseshoe-shaped body (which contains the lower teeth) and the rami (processes on either side that project upward from the posterior part of the body).[1] In the context of oral implantology, the mandibular body is the main concern, although some aspects of the rami are also discussed.

The body of the mandible has an anterior and a posterior surface and a superior and an inferior border.[33] The external surface is marked at the midline by the symphysis menti, which is the union line of both halves of the man-

dible as seen in the fetus.[32] Adjacent to the midline, the anterior surface of the body projects to form a triangular prominence (the mental protuberance, or bony chin). A depression, the mental fossa, lies laterally on either side of the chin.[1] The mental foramen, an opening through which the mental nerve and vessels pass, lies on the lateral surface of the mandibular body, inferior to the second premolar, midway between the lower border of the mandible and the alveolar ridge[33] (Figure 4-6).

On the internal surface of the mandibular body, the main concern is the sublingual fossa, which supports a salivary gland of the same name. The sublingual fossa is located along the mylohyoid line, which extends posteriorly from the mental spines on each side of the symphysis. Superior to the anterior part of this line is the smooth, triangular sublingual fossa, and inferior to the posterior part of the line are the oval, submandibular fossae.[32] During implant surgery, the clinician must keep these structures in mind to avoid accidentally perforating them as a result of angulation of the burs (Figure 4-7).

The alveolar process, better known as the alveolar ridge, is another important mandibular structure when implant placement is considered. From a superior view, it can be seen clearly that the alveolar process, stemming from the upper border of the body of the mandible, has a sharper curvature than the bulk of the body itself (see Figure 4-6, *B*). Thus, although the mandibular body continues posterolaterally, the alveolar process turns inward toward the sagittal plane. Because of this feature, the posterior end of the alveolar process juts strongly in from the arch of the mandibular body.[1] As in the

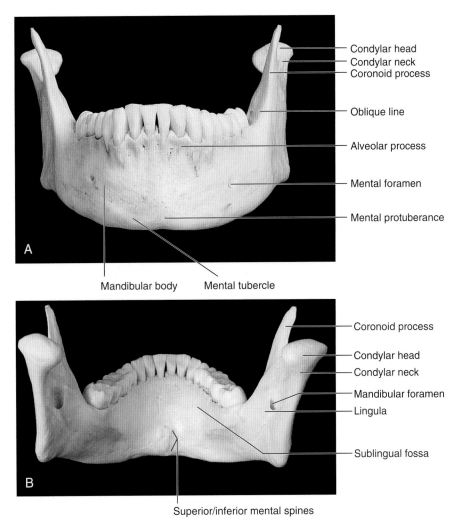

Condylar head
Condylar neck
Coronoid process

Oblique line

Alveolar process

Mental foramen

Mental protuberance

Mandibular body   Mental tubercle

Coronoid process

Condylar head

Condylar neck

Mandibular foramen

Lingula

Sublingual fossa

Superior/inferior mental spines

FIGURE 4-6 ■ Anterior **(A)** and posterior **(B)** aspects of the mandible. (Modified from Abrahams PH, Hutchings RT, Marks SC Jr: *McMinn's color atlas of human anatomy*, ed 4, Mosby, St Louis, 1998.)

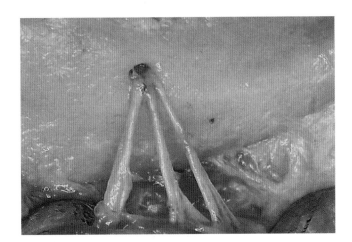

FIGURE 4-7 ■ The mental foramen, an opening through which the mental nerve passes on the lateral surface of the body of the mandible.

maxilla, the mandibular alveolar process is hollowed into sockets for the reception of 16 teeth. These sockets, or alveoli, are the ones that form the so-called alveolar arch.

The retromolar triangle is located distal to the posteriormost limit of the mandibular alveolar process. It is formed at the point where the body of the mandible meets the ramus and corresponds to the retromolar tuberculum of the maxilla (Figure 4-8). In adolescent patients, under certain circumstances, it can be considered as a site for insertion of an implant, because the mandibular canal runs approximately 8 mm mediocaudally to its floor with a normal mandibular angle, or 120 degrees.

The mandibular teeth are inclined inward relative to the vertical axis of the cranium such that their crowns, on opposite sides of the jaw, lie closer than the roots. This feature means that the cortical bone is thicker lingually than buccally. However, the alveolar walls of the adult mandible are more completely differentiated both lingually and buccally than are the corresponding structures of the maxilla.[1]

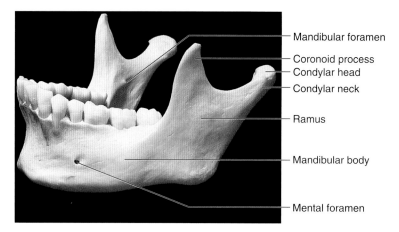

FIGURE 4-8 ■ Lateral view of the mandible. (Modified from Abrahams PH, Hutchings RT, Marks SC Jr: *McMinn's color atlas of human anatomy*, ed 4, Mosby, St Louis, 1998.)

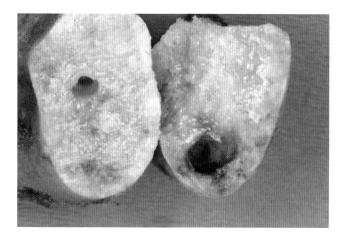

FIGURE 4-9 ■ Transverse sections of the endentulous mandible. The *left portion* shows the position of the canal in the area of the second bicuspid, and *the right* shows the area corresponding to the second molar.

The mandibular foramina are located on the medial surface of the mandibular rami, near the midline (see Figure 4-6, *B*). The mandibular foramen has a prominent ridge and an anterior sharp spine known as the lingual mandibula. The foramen marks the beginning of the mandibular canal, which courses obliquely downward and forward carrying the inferior alveolar vessels and nerve. After reaching the mandibular body, the canal continues forward horizontally under the alveoli, communicating with them through small openings.[32] When the canal reaches the area of the second bicuspid, it divides into the mental canal, which passes laterally and upward and terminates at the mental foramen, and the incisive canal, which provides innervation and blood supply to the anterior teeth[33] (Figure 4-9).

The distance between the roof of the mandibular canal and the floor of the dental alveoli is 3 mm to 4 mm in the region of the third molar, and approximately 8 mm under the first molar. These relationships, however, will be modified by the atrophy of the mandibular alveolar process, as determined by the loss of teeth and patient age.[7] After the loss of teeth, the alveolar ridge atrophies. In addition, during aging, severe degenerative changes can occur in the basal part, involving the lingual aspect to a greater extent than the buccal.[40] This process leads to thin knife-edge ridges and a short vertical distance between the top of the alveolar process and the mandibular canal.

Sensory and Motor Innervations of the Oral Cavity

The Trigeminal Nerve (V)

The trigeminal nerve (cranial nerve V), the largest of the cranial nerves, consists of a greater somatic sensory portion and a smaller motor section[1] (Figure 4-10). It is the major cutaneous sensory nerve of the face, with the sensory portion carrying afferent impulses from the skin, mucous membranes, and other internal structures of the head. The motor nerve innervates the masticatory muscles.[32] The trigeminal nerve divides into three branches: the ophthalmic nerve (V_1), the maxillary nerve (V_2), and the mandibular nerve (V_3) (Figure 4-11).

The ophthalmic nerve is entirely sensory and supplies the upper eyelid, the entire dorsum, and upper parts of the sides of the nose, forehead, and scalp as far back as the interauricular line. This branch of the trigeminal nerve, however, does not play a role in the concerns of oral implantology.

The maxillary nerve, which arises from the middle of the trigeminal ganglion, is intermediate in size and is positioned between the ophthalmic and mandibular branches. Similar to the ophthalmic nerve, the maxillary nerve is entirely sensory.[32] It has three cutaneous branches that supply the area of the skin derived from the embryonic maxillary

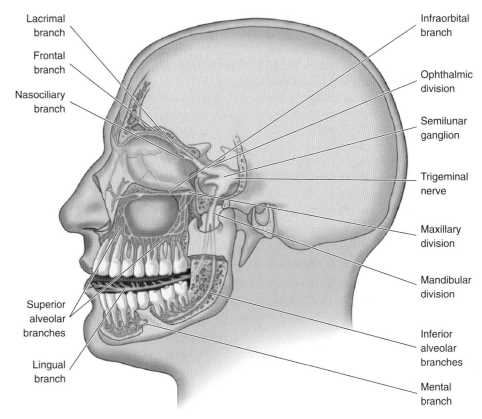

FIGURE 4-10 ■ Distribution of the trigeminal nerve. (Modified from Nelson SJ, Ash MM: *Wheeler's dental anatomy, physiology, and occlusion*, ed 9, Saunders, St Louis, 2010.)

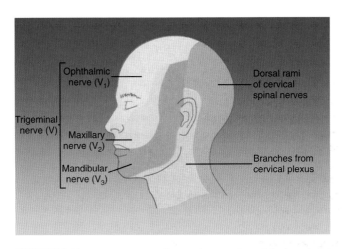

FIGURE 4-11 ■ Sensory and motor innervation of the head and neck.

prominence (process), the middle portion of the face, lower eyelid, side of the nose, and upper lip; the mucous membrane of the nasopharynx, maxillary sinus, soft palate, tonsils, and roof of the mouth; and the upper gingiva and teeth.[32,41]

The three cutaneous branches of the maxillary nerve are (1) the infraorbital nerve, which passes through the infraorbital foramen and supplies the skin of the ala (left wing) of the nose, the upper lip, and the lower eyelid; (2) the zygomaticofacial nerve, which emerges from the zygomatic bone through a small foramen with the same name as the nerve and supplies the skin of the face over the zygomatic bone; and (3) the zygomaticotemporal nerve, which emerges from the zygomatic bone through a small foramen of the same name as the nerve and supplies the skin over the temporal region. The mandibular nerve, the third and largest division of the trigeminal nerve, is a mixed nerve that contains sensory branches and the entire motor portion of the trigeminal nerve[1]. The four sensory branches of the mandibular nerve usually separate from each other approximately 5 mm to 10 mm below the base of the skull. The internal branches comprise the buccal and lingual nerves, which supply large areas of the oral mucosa. The intermediate branch (the inferior alveolar nerve) supplies the mandibular teeth, the skin and mucous membrane of the lower lip, and the skin of the chin (Figure 4-12). The external branch (the auriculotemporal nerve) supplies the external surface of the face, specifically, the posterior part of the cheek and the posterior area of the temporal region, including parts of the outer ear.[1] The motor fibers of the mandibular nerve, which stimulate contraction of the masticatory muscles responsible for chewing, make up the masseteric nerve, the posterior and anterior deep temporal nerves, the medial pterygoid nerve, and the lateral pterygoid nerve.[1]

The lingual and mental nerves have the most clinical importance in this division, as their fibers are the most vulnerable if the area where they lay is invaded during surgery. The lingual nerve will pass very close to the retromolar pad and will continue near the roots of the third molar in the soft tissue. It later continues anteriorly in a sublingual direction, where it comes down and hooks under the duct of the submandibular salivary gland. Some variation may occur in the level of position of this nerve, so it is very important to keep all incisions buccal to a midline of the retromolar pad. The mental nerve is also very important during implant surgery. In a panoramic radiograph, it can be visualized between the first and second mandibular premolars, but care has to be taken when the mental nerve forms a loop anterior to the foramen. This area of the loop can be invaded easily during drilling if it is not previously identified for its avoidance.

The Facial Nerve (VII)

The facial nerve (cranial nerve VII) emerges from the skull through the stylomastoid foramen between the mastoid process and the styloid process of the temporal bone, and it almost immediately enters the parotid gland. It runs superficially within the parotid gland before giving rise to five terminal branches (temporal nerve, zygomatic nerve, buccal nerve, marginal mandibular nerve, and cervical nerve). All of these divisions of the facial nerve emerge from the superior, anterior, or inferior margins of the parotid gland.[41]

The facial nerve comprises the motor, sensory, and parasympathetic portions. The motor nerves innervate the muscles of facial expression, the muscles of the scalp and external ear, and the buccinator, platysma, stapedius, stylohyoid, and posterior belly of the digastric muscles. The sensory portion supplies taste sensation to the anterior two-thirds of the tongue and general sensation to parts of the external acoustic meatus, soft palate, and adjacent pharynx. The parasympathetic part supplies secretomotor fibers for the submandibular, sublingual, lacrimal, nasal, and palatine glands.[32]

The trajectory of the facial nerve does not put it at risk during basic implant placement. Any damage to this nerve during implant placement or intraoral block grafting could occur only in a very aberrant procedure that would involve proximity to the area of the parotid gland, where it lies. A transient facial paralysis could occur during a mandibular block if the needle goes too far down to the angle of the mandible.

Vasculature of the Oral Cavity

Two main branches of the external carotid artery, the facial and maxillary arteries, provide the blood supply to the maxillae and the mandible. The facial and maxillary veins provide venous drainage.

The Facial Artery

The facial artery arises at the lower border of the mandible.[32] Before appearing on the external surface of the mandible, the facial artery passes through the lower mandibular border and gives off the submental artery, which runs forward beneath the chin to the mental tubercle[1] (Figure 4-13). Before reaching the corner of the lip, the facial artery gives off the inferior labial artery, which passes medially into the lower lip and anastomoses with the same artery from the contralateral side.[42] Another branch of the facial artery, the superior labial artery, goes to the upper lip and anastomoses with its corresponding artery from the contralateral side. Thereafter, the facial artery runs along the side of the

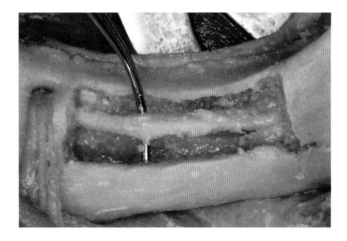

FIGURE 4-12 ■ The inferior alveolar nerve courses through the mandible before exiting the mental foramen, and often there is inadequate height of bone to allow for implant placement in the posterior mandible without a nerve lateralization or bone grafting procedure in conjunction with implant placement.

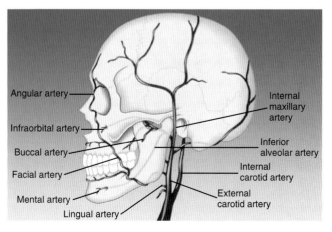

FIGURE 4-13 ■ The major arterial blood supply to the maxillofacial region and neighboring structures.

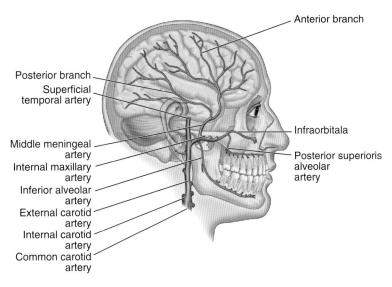

FIGURE 4-14 ■ Projection of the maxillary artery and its branches in relation to the brain, skull, and mandible, including the teeth. (Modified from Nelson SJ, Ash MM: *Wheeler's dental anatomy, physiology, and occlusion*, ed 9, Saunders, St Louis, 2010.)

nose toward the medial angle of the eye, where it becomes the angular artery.[41] The angular artery may terminate by anastomosing with a terminal branch of the ophthalmic artery; however, in some patients, the angular artery is very poorly developed or even absent.[33]

The Maxillary Artery

The maxillary artery arises as one of the terminal branches of the external carotid artery at the posterior border of the mandibular ramus, passing forward almost horizontally medial to the ramus and below the level of the neck mandible (Figure 4-14). The maxillary artery has numerous branches. Close to its origin is the small, deep auricular artery, which supplies the temporomandibular joint (TMJ) and the external acoustic meatus.[32] More anteriorly, the maxillary artery gives rise to two large branches: the middle meningeal and inferior alveolar arteries. The middle meningeal artery runs upward to enter the skull through the foramen spinosum. The inferior alveolar artery runs downward across the medial pterygoid and passes between the mandible and the sphenomandibular ligament to reach the mandibular foramen. Just before entering the foramen, it gives off the mylohyoid branch, which runs downward in the mylohyoid groove to the mylohyoid muscle.[1] Within the mandibular canal, the inferior alveolar artery branches to the teeth until it reaches the mental foramen, where it emerges as the mental branch.

As the maxillary artery reaches the lower border of the lateral pterygoid muscle, it joins the masseteric artery. As it runs through the lateral pterygoid muscle, it gives off the temporal and buccal arteries. The maxillary artery then passes deeply through the pterygomaxillary fissure into the pterygopalatine foramina, where it gives off the posterior

alveolar artery. The posterior superior alveolar artery runs downward on the posterior surface of the maxilla, enters the foramina forward of the alveolar process, and supplies the dental branches to the posterior teeth.[32]

Other terminal branches of the maxillary artery are the tiny artery of the pterygoid canal and the pharyngeal branch to the pharynx. A large descending palatine artery appears on the palate as greater and lesser palatine arteries and as a sphenopalatine artery, passing straight medially from the pterygopalatine fossa into the nasal cavity.[42]

The Facial Vein

The upper end of the facial vein, the angular vein, lies immediately adjacent to the angular artery. It often has no obvious origin; however, when traced upward, it frequently is a continuation of the veins of the forehead. Because it lies beside the nose, the angular vein receives drainage from the small veins of the nose and both eyelids.[1] As the facial vein descends past the mouth, it receives drainage from the superior and inferior labial veins. Because it lies on the buccinator muscle, it also receives venous flow from the deep facial vein, which emerges deep from the ramus of the mandible adjacent to the buccal artery and the buccal branch of the mandibular nerve. Superior to this location, the facial vein also receives drainage from the front end of the intraorbital vein. At its terminal end, the facial vein receives venous flow from the submental vein and then drains into the internal jugular vein (Figure 4-15).

The Maxillary Vein

Numerous venous branches, including the inferior ophthalmic vein, middle meningeal vein, pterygoid plexus, superior

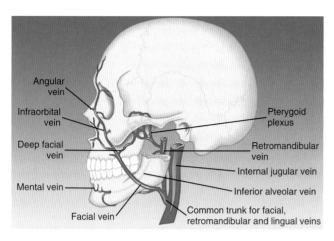

FIGURE 4-15 ■ Major venous drainage from the maxilla and mandible.

alveolar veins, and inferior alveolar vein, drain into the maxillary vein. All of these venous branches course along the same anatomical pathways as their corresponding arteries, as was previously described. The maxillary vein forms the retromandibular vein, which descends posteriorly to the ramus and usually divides into posterior and anterior parts before reaching the angle of the mandible. The posterior branch joins the posterior auricular vein to form the external jugular vein, and the anterior branch joins the facial vein in emptying into the internal jugular vein.

SUMMARY

Resorption of the alveolar ridges after tooth extraction is a continuing process that manifests itself through anatomical and functional changes in the patient. The anatomical changes occur in a vertical as well as a horizontal plane. The final result is an alteration of the space relationships of the different anatomical structures. As the mandibular ridge resorbs, the residual ridge migrates toward many of the muscles that originate or insert into the mandible, and, at the same time, the neurovascular structures become more superficial. In the maxillary arch, the loss of teeth also encourages resorption of the remaining alveolar bone, which is thinner and of a poorer quality than the mandibular bone. With advancing age, the maxillary sinus pneumatizes, increasing in breadth at the expense of the remaining alveolar bone. In addition, the amount of bone between the crest of the ridge and the floor of the nose decreases. Because of these and many other factors, a clear understanding and awareness by the implant dentist of the human oral anatomy and the changes it undergoes with age are critical to ensure successful treatment and functional rehabilitation of dental implant patients.

REFERENCES

1. Dubrul E: *Oral anatomy*, St. Louis, 1992, IshiyaKu EuroAmerica, Inc.
2. Block MS: *Color atlas of dental implant surgery*, Philadelphia, 2001, WB Saunders.
3. Machado CL, Babbush CA, Rathburn A: Surgical anatomic considerations for dental implant reconstruction. In: Babbush CA, editor: *Dental implants: the art and science*, Philadelphia, 2001, WB Saunders, pp 19-33.
4. Pedlar J, Frame JW: *Oral and maxillofacial surgery: an objective-based textbook*, Edinburgh, 2001, Churchill Livingstone.
5. Neiva RF, Gapski R, Wang HL: Morphometric analysis of implant-related anatomy in Caucasian skulls, *J Periodontol* 75(8):1061-1067, 2004.
6. Denissen HW, Kalk W, Veldhuis HA, van Waas MA: Anatomic consideration for preventive implantation, *Int J Oral Maxillofac Implants* 8(2):191-196, 1993.
7. Stellingsma C, Vissink A, Meijer HJ, Kuiper C, Raghoebar GM: Implantology and the severely resorbed edentulous mandible, *Crit Rev Oral Biol Med* 15(4):240-248, 2004. Review.
8. Misch CE: *Contemporary implant dentistry*, St. Louis, 1999, Mosby Year Book, Inc.
9. Marx RE, Garg AK: Bone structure, metabolism, and physiology: its impact on dental implantology, *Implant Dent* 7(4):267-276, 1998. Review.
10. Fanuscu MI, Chang TL: Three-dimensional morphometric analysis of human cadaver bone: microstructural data from maxilla and mandible, *Clin Oral Implants Res* 15(2):213-218, 2004.
11. Morrison A, Chiarot M, Kirby S: Mental nerve function after inferior alveolar nerve transposition for placement of dental implants, *J Can Dent Assoc* 68(1):46-50, 2002.
12. Yamamoto R, Nakamura A, Ohno K, Michi KI: Relationship of the mandibular canal to the lateral cortex of the mandibular ramus as a factor in the development of neurosensory disturbance after bilateral sagittal split osteotomy, *J Oral Maxillofac Surg* 60(5):490-495, 2002.
13. Jacobs R, Mraiwa N, van Steenberghe D, Gijbels F, Quirynen M: Appearance, location, course, and morphology of the mandibular incisive canal: an assessment on spiral CT scan, *Dentomaxillofac Radiol* 31(5):322-327, 2002.
14. Kraut RA, Chahal O: Management of patients with trigeminal nerve injuries after mandibular implant placement, *J Am Dent Assoc* 133(10):1351-1354, 2002.
15. Mraiwa N, Jacobs R, van Steenberghe D, Quirynen M: Clinical assessment and surgical implications of anatomic challenges in the anterior mandible, *Clin Implant Dent Relat Res* 5(4):219-225, 2003. Review.
16. Noreau G, Landry PP, Morais D: Arteriovenous malformation of the mandible: review of literature and case history, *J Can Dent Assoc* 67(11):646-651, 2001. Review.
17. Weibrich G, Foitzik CH, Kuffner H: Life threatening oral hemorrhage after implantation into the distal right mandible, *Mund Kiefer Gesichtschir* 6(6):442-445, 2002. Epub 2002 Jul 30. German.
18. Gultekin S, Arac M, Celik H, Karaosmaoglu AD, Isik S: Assessment of mandibular vascular canals by dental CT, *Tani Girisim Radyol* 9(2):188-191, 2003. Turkish.
19. Harn SD, Durham TM: Anatomical variations and clinical implications of the artery to the lingual nerve, *Clin Anat* 16(4):294-299, 2003.
20. Flanagan D: Important arterial supply of the mandible, control of an arterial hemorrhage, and report of a hemorrhagic incident, *J Oral Implantol* 29(4):165-173, 2003.

21. Persky MS, Yoo HJ, Berenstein A: Management of vascular malformations of the mandible and maxilla, *Laryngoscope* 113(11):1885-1892, 2003.

22. Isaacson TJ: Sublingual hematoma formation during immediate placement of mandibular endosseous implants, *J Am Dent Assoc* 135(2):168-172, 2004. Review.

23. Kalpidis CD, Setayesh RM: Hemorrhaging associated with endosseous implant placement in the anterior mandible: a review of the literature, *J Periodontol* 75(5):631-645, 2004. Review.

24. Flanagan D: Implants and arteries, *J Am Dent Assoc* 135(5):566, 2004.

25. Gogarnoiu D, Cavanaugh RR: Three-dimensional CT scan analysis for implant-supported fixed prostheses, *Compend Contin Educ Dent* 20(9):855-860, 862, 864, 1999, passim; quiz 868.

26. Bou Serhal C, Jacobs R, Persoons M, Hermans R, van Steenberghe D: The accuracy of spiral tomography to assess bone quantity for the preoperative planning of implants in the posterior maxilla, *Clin Oral Implants Res* 11(3):242-247, 2000.

27. Gahleitner A, Hofschneider U, Tepper G, Pretterklieber M, Schick S, Zauza K, Watzek G: Lingual vascular canals of the mandible: evaluation with dental CT, *Radiology* 220(1):186-189, 2001.

28. Salvolini E, De Florio L, Regnicolo L, Salvolini U: Magnetic resonance applications in dental implantology: technical notes and preliminary results, *Radiol Med (Torino)* 103(5-6): 526-529, 2002. English, Italian.

29. Sammartino G, Della Valle A, Marenzi G, Gerbino S, Martorelli M, di Lauro AE, di Lauro F: Stereolithography in oral implantology: a comparison of surgical guides, *Implant Dent* 13(2):133-139, 2004.

30. Casap N, Wexler A, Persky N, Schneider A, Lustmann J: Navigation surgery for dental implants: assessment of accuracy of the image guided implantology system, *J Oral Maxillofac Surg* 62(9 suppl 2):116-119, 2004.

31. Garg AK, Reiche OJ: Principles for the placement of endosteal implants in the patient, *Implant Soc* 3(1):6-8, 1992.

32. Clemente C: *Anatomy of the human body by Henry Gray*, Philadelphia, 1984, Lea & Febiger.

33. Testut L, Latarjet A: Compendio de anatomia descriptiva, Barcelona, Spain, 1984, *Salvat Editores.*

34. Buser D, Martin W, Belser UC: Optimizing esthetics for implant restorations in the anterior maxilla: anatomic and surgical considerations, *Int J Oral Maxillofac Implants* 19(suppl):43-61, 2004. Review.

35. Lee SP, Paik KS, Kim MK: Anatomical study of the pyramidal process of the palatine bone in relation to implant placement in the posterior maxilla, *J Oral Rehabil* 28(2):125-132, 2001.

36. Woo I, Le BT: Maxillary sinus floor elevation: review of anatomy and two techniques, *Implant Dent* 13(1):28-32, 2004.

37. Rodoni LR, Glauser R, Feloutzis A, Hammerle CH: Implants in the posterior maxilla: a comparative clinical and radiologic study, *Int J Oral Maxillofac Implants* 20(2):231-237, 2005.

38. Reiche O, Garg AK: Grafting of the maxillary sinus for the placement of endosteal implants, *Implant Soc* 2(3):1, 14-16, 1991.

39. Small SA, Zinner ID, Panno FV, Shapiro HJ, Stein JI: Augmenting the maxillary sinus for implants: report of 27 patients, *Int J Oral Maxillofac Implants* 8(5):523-528, 1993.

40. Schroeder A, Sutter F, Krekele G: *Oral implantology—Basics of the ITI hollow cylinder system*, New York, 1991, Thieme Medical Publishers, Inc.

41. Moore K: Clinically oriented anatomy, Baltimore, 1999, Williams and Wilkins.

42. Clemente C: Anatomy: A regional atlas of the human body, Baltimore, 1997, Williams & Wilkins.

chapter 5

Sterilization, Disinfection, and Asepsis in Implantology

THE IMPORTANCE OF ASEPSIS in the long-term success of dental implant procedures cannot be overemphasized. Although dental infection control programs should have the dual goals of reducing risks for health care–associated infection for patients and for dental health care personnel,[1] the focus of this chapter will be on protecting the dental patient. Maintaining an aseptic field—one that is free from infection, septic material, or contact with microorganisms—during placement of implants in the oral cavity is critical for preventing postoperative infection and rejection of the fixtures by the body. To achieve this goal, dental surgeons are obligated to provide a clean and safe operating environment for their patients. Today, most dental implant surgeries are performed on an elective, outpatient basis. The procedure can be planned carefully because it is not an emergency, and it is done with local, regional, or general anesthesia without the need to hospitalize the patient overnight (Figure 5-1). Concerns related to asepsis include the operating room, surgical instruments, the dental team, and the patient.

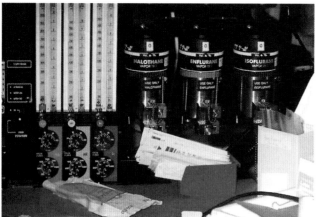

FIGURE 5-1 ■ Appropriate anesthesia may include, in some cases, general anesthesia.

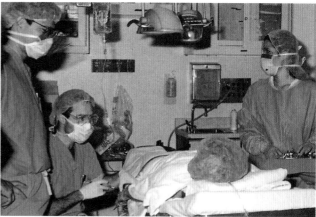

FIGURE 5-2 ■ After the patient has been seated comfortably and the patient's hair has been covered with a surgical cap, appropriate anesthesia is provided.

Operating Room

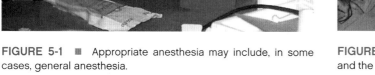

Most postoperative wound infections are caused by seeding of endogenous bacteria; however, exogenous bacteria also have been frequently implicated. Sources of exogenous bacteria include operating personnel, anesthesia equipment, the operating table, operating room lights, wall and floor surfaces, furniture, instruments, supplies, and the air in the surgical suite. Certain areas in the operating room can become heavily contaminated with pathogens because they are difficult to clean, often because of poor access. Operating room surfaces should be cleaned and disinfected on the basis of certain common sense considerations, including how likely it is for the patient to come into direct contact with such surfaces, how frequently the surfaces are contacted by hand, and how likely it is that body substances or other microorganisms will come into contact with the surfaces.[1]

The operating room should be not only clean but also free of dust (Figure 5-2). Airborne counts should not exceed one bacterium per square foot. Dust usually can be controlled by improving air filtration. In addition, phenolic detergents are recommended for wet vacuuming the floors. Ideally, the floor should have a homogenous surface free of grooves and fissures.

Effective and efficient air conditioning systems should be used to eliminate airborne microbial contamination. Studies have shown that airborne bacteria account for 98% of the bacteria found in wounds postoperatively when the surgery was performed in a conventionally ventilated room.[2] The use of unidirectional airflow within the operating room and occlusive surgical clothing reduces airborne bacteria by about 100 times and wound contamination by 30 times.[2] Air conditioning systems must be properly and regularly maintained. Otherwise, inefficient ventilation systems and poor filtration can result in rebreathing of contaminated air, leading to upper respiratory tract infections. Although the use of ultraclean air has been proposed as a method for limiting airborne infection of wounds,[3] other researchers suggest that directing air away from the wound rather than toward it is perhaps an even more important consideration.[4,5]

Surgical Instrument Care

To prevent postoperative infection or patient cross-contamination, implant surgical instruments should be handled and stored in accordance with strict sterilization procedures and controls. Although the threat of such infections is real, public fears of postoperative infection are fueled by the rise in cases among those infected by human immunodeficiency virus (HIV) and living with and dying from acquired immunodeficiency syndrome (AIDS). According to The Joint United Nations Programme on HIV/AIDS (UNAIDS), the total number of people living with HIV/AIDS in 2007 was 30 to 36 million. AIDS deaths in 2007 numbered between 1.8 and 2.3 million.[6] These numbers continue to fuel patient anxiety regarding infections received from other patients or health care personnel, and these fears persist despite the facts that the transmission of HIV is most likely to occur from patient to dental health care personnel, and no HIV transmission from dental health care personnel to patients has occurred since 1992.[1]

The Centers for Disease Control and Prevention (CDC) has proposed three categories of infection control related to surgical instruments.[1] These categories are Critical, Semicritical, and Noncritical. Critical items are defined as those that penetrate soft tissue, contact bone, or enter into or contact the bloodstream or other normally sterile tissue; such items include periodontal scalers, scalpel blades, and surgical burs. These items should be sterilized by heat. Semicritical items are defined as those items that contact mucous membranes or nonintact skin; such items include the mouth

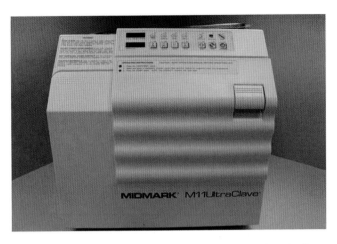

FIGURE 5-3 ■ A typical autoclave found in the dental office.

mirror, amalgam condenser, and reusable impression trays. These items should be sterilized by heat unless heat sensitive; if so, high-level disinfection can be used. Noncritical items are defined as those that contact intact skin; such items include a radiograph head/cone, blood pressure cuff, and facebow. For these items, cleaning is adequate unless the item is visibly soiled, and cleaning should be followed by disinfection with an Environmental Protection Agency (EPA)-registered hospital disinfectant.[1]

Sterilization is the complete destruction or elimination of all living microorganisms, accomplished by physical methods (dry or moist heat), chemical agents (ethylene oxide, formaldehyde, alcohol), irradiation (ultraviolet, cathode), or mechanical methods (filtration). Disinfection, which reduces or eliminates infectious organisms, does not necessarily kill all of the microbes. After instruments have been used on one patient, they must be thoroughly cleaned before they can be sterilized.[7-9] If an item cannot be cleaned properly, it cannot be sterilized. Special care must be given to surgical burs because of their intricate shapes. Bone drills can serve as reservoirs for microorganisms that subsequently could be inoculated directly into a patient during bone drilling.[10,11]

Sterilization methods rather than disinfection alone must be used to process these instruments.[12] Among the suppliers of quality dental equipment, dental handpieces are relatively similar when a number of parameters are evaluated, including ability to withstand multiple cleanings and sterilizations; so, maintaining performance and longevity is critical for instruments properly heat sterilized between patient uses.[13]

Autoclaves produce moist heat in the form of saturated steam under pressure and provide the crucial elements of asepsis (sterilization and disinfection) (Figure 5-3). Often, during surgery, rapid sterilization of an instrument is required when an instrument has been inadvertently omitted from the surgical pack, or when it has been dropped on the floor accidentally. A small steam sterilizer provides a highly effective means of emergency sterilization that is far superior to the relatively ineffective and potentially compromising method of cold sterilization.

Before sterilization, the instrument should be washed with a brush and soapy water, placed unpacked in the perforated metal tray on the shelf of the sterilizer, and locked in the machine. Steam enters the machine for 40 seconds until the temperature rises. During operation, steam pressure of 27 psi is maintained. After 3 minutes, the steam is released and the instrument is ready for use. Sterilizers must be monitored constantly with temperature sensors or biological indicators to ensure their efficacy.

Although universal precautions dictate sterilization of all invasive surgical equipment, many of the current methods of sterilization are not compatible with the delicate, intricate instruments used during implantation that require a quick turnaround. The time-honored method of steam sterilization cannot be used for items that do not tolerate heat. Ethylene oxide (ETO) gas can be used for these delicate items. However, complete sterilization and aeration of items to remove residual ETO gas requires 10 to 24 hours, and this modality is rarely available outside of a hospital setting.[14] Thus, the dental surgeon could consider other methods of sterilization that are available besides steam, heat, and ETO. Those that could be applied to oral implant instruments include electron beam sterilization, sterilization filtration, ultraviolet irradiation, ionizing irradiation, and peracetic acid (one of the newest methods of sterilization available).[14-16]

Dental Team

Asepsis protocol for the dental team includes proper surgical scrub and attire (Figure 5-4).

Surgical Scrub

According to the CDC, "Hand hygiene ... substantially reduces potential pathogens on the hands and is considered the single most critical measure for reducing the risk of transmitting organisms to patients and HCP (health care personnel)."[1] The CDC lists the methods of hand washing (routine and antiseptic) and antiseptic hand rub as indicated before and after a clinician treats a patient, after touching objects that could be contaminated by blood or saliva, before leaving the dental operating room or laboratory, when soiled, and before regloving once damaged gloves are removed. Surgical antisepsis is indicated before the surgeon dons sterile gloves for surgery.

Transient or resident skin flora include β-hemolytic streptococci, *Staphylococcus aureus*, *Pseudomonas*, *Escherichia coli*, and *Klebsiella*, among others. *S aureus* is the most common resident flora. Hand scrubbing with a disinfectant agent most readily removes transient flora, but resident flora are more difficult to remove. For optimal effect, 5 to 10 minutes of hand scrubbing is recommended.

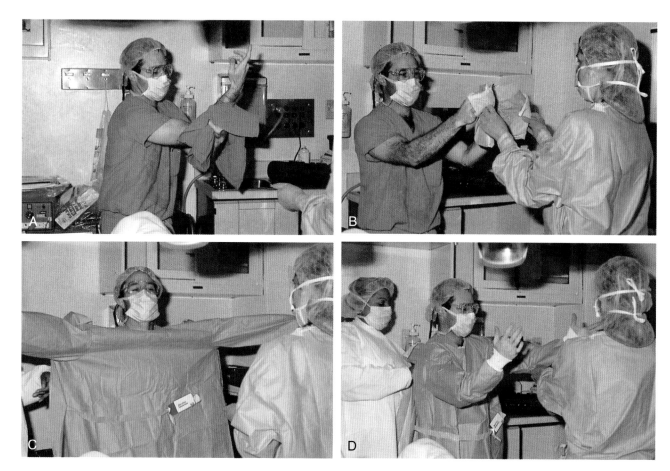

FIGURE 5-4 ■ **A,** Washing, scrubbing, rinsing, and drying procedures can be used with a standard protocol. **B,** The sterile assistant can assist the doctor with his or her gown and gloves. **C,** A second assistant is necessary to tie the gown in the back. **D,** The sterile assistant and the circulating assistant can assist the doctor during the preoperative stage as well as during surgery.

Antiseptics widely used for hand scrubbing include iodophors (Betadine; Purdue Products LP, Stamford, CT), chlorhexidine (Hibiclens; Mölnlycke Health Care US, LLC, Norcross, GA), and hexachlorophene.

The following protocol should be used by the surgical team to disinfect the fingernails, fingers, arms, and elbows. This should be done before a sterile gown and gloves are donned:

1. Hands, arms, and elbows should be washed with soap and water using a sterile brush to remove surface fats, debris, and cells.
2. A nail file should be used to clean fingernails meticulously under running water.
3. A sterile brush should be impregnated with a disinfectant solution, and the entire surface of the fingers, fingernails, hands, arms, and elbows should be scrubbed, in that order.
4. All excess solutions should be washed away by thorough rinsing under running water. Excess water should be allowed to drip by holding the hands above flexed elbows.
5. The scrubbing and rinsing procedures should be repeated.

Surgical Attire

One of the most important advances in surgery in the last century was the realization that a significant number of postoperative infections could be prevented by combining the intraoperative use of sterile techniques and garments. The most common source of infection during surgery is the operating room personnel. Thus, emphasis is placed on keeping the skin microorganisms of the surgical team away from the surgical site.[17-19]

A study performed in 1999 concluded that reusable cloth gowns had a high strikethrough rate; as a result, most surgeons found them unacceptable.[20] Better protection came from reinforced disposable gowns. These gowns had the highest strikethrough rates at cuffs, forearms, and thighs, and these points of vulnerability require new designs for surgical gowns. Regarding the use of surgical masks, a 2003 study recommended that the reason health care personnel wear masks has shifted from protection of the patient to protection of the personnel.[21] The study goes on to say that there is little evidence to support the contention that wearing a surgical mask adequately protects health care personnel from all the hazards likely encountered in an acute health care setting; consequently, the study recommends that a respirator and face shield should replace a mask, depending on the circumstances.

An aseptic barrier can be defined as any material placed between the surgical incision and a possible source of bacteria, with the intention of preventing passage into the sterile zone. All surgical personnel must wear sterile, disposable caps and masks to minimize the possibility of introducing bacteria-laden droplets from the nasal and oral cavities and desquamated epithelium and dandruff from the hair and scalp into the operating room environment. Because clothing gives off lint and dust, sterile, disposable gowns (traditionally made of 140-thread cotton muslin) are used to minimize contamination of the surgical field. Gloves made of latex are used during surgery. Any time a glove suffers a slight prick or catch, it should be treated as a tear in the glove, and the glove should be changed.

Other measures that can be taken to minimize the risk for infection include having the surgical team keep their movements and speech to a minimum and restricting visitors in the operating room.

Patient Preparation

Patient preparation includes preoperative and perioperative care.

Preoperative Preparation

Preoperative preparation of patients undergoing surgical placement of dental implants is aimed at reducing the number of pathogens at the surgical site. Doing so eliminates or minimizes the sources of contamination, prevents infection, and improves the patient's general resistance. The patient should be free of remote infections (e.g., periodontal disease, acute or chronic respiratory tract infection, chronic sinusitis in the head or neck region) that could significantly increase the risk for infection of operated wounds if left untreated.[22] It is also prudent to ensure that patients have received adequate medical treatment for associated noninfectious conditions, such as diabetes mellitus and cirrhosis of the liver, which could delay or impede wound healing and repair.

Preparation of the Surgical Field

After the patient is seated comfortably in the operating room, specific steps are taken to help keep the surgical field clean and free of contamination. The surgical field comprises the patient's entire face, extending from the infraorbital region, across the periauricular region, over the angle of the mandible, and down to the clavicles (Figure 5-5). The patient's hair should be covered with a surgical cap. The head then is draped with a sterile towel to ensure that the hair, ears, and eyes are covered, and towels are placed at the sides of the patient's head to collect excess disinfectant.

The concept of preparing a patient's skin for surgery was first introduced more than a century ago. However, despite advances in our knowledge of skin flora and the effects of antiseptics on infection, the procedures for skin preparation remain basically the same today as when they were first originated. In the "Recommended Practices for Skin Preparation of Patients" put forth by the Association of Operating Room Nurses (AORN), the stated goals of preoperative skin preparation are to decrease the risk for postoperative wound infection by removing soil and transient microorganisms from the skin, reduce the residual microbial count to subpathogenic quantities in a short time with the least amount of tissue irritation, and inhibit the rapid rebound growth of microorganisms.[23,24]

Although approximately 20% of the resident skin cannot be removed by surgical scrubs and antiseptics, it is not possible to sterilize the skin without damaging it.[25] Therefore, the most that can be done to minimize contamination of wounds is for health care personnel to disinfect the skin while wearing sterile gloves. Transient flora are usually superficial and can be removed by washing the skin with soap and water or with a mild disinfectant. Resident flora, however, are deep-seated and adherent, requiring stringent disinfection. Commonly used disinfecting agents include iodine, povidone-iodine, chlorhexidine gluconate, and 70% isopropyl alcohol (Figure 5-6).

A 1993 study reported that when povidone-iodine alcohol solutions were used to disinfect the skin, a higher reduction factor was noted in the total resident flora, and the solution was a reasonable and effective antibacterial agent for preoperative skin preparations.[26] Much more recent studies continue to examine the best systems, processes, and combinations of antiseptic agents for effective asepsis in surgery.[27,28]

The "prep-table" should be covered with a sterile drape and supplied with gloves, towels, sponges, and a bowl of disinfectant. A scrubbed and ungowned surgeon or assistant should remove the surface dirt, loose skin, and debris from the surgical site (excluding the oral cavity) by scrubbing the patient's skin with soap and water. The surgical field should be scrubbed in a circular fashion—from the center to the periphery—and dried with sterile, disposable paper towels. Next, the patient's skin should be disinfected with sterile sponges and the previously mentioned disinfectant agents. The skin should be "painted" from the center of the surgical field to the periphery and allowed to air dry. After donning a sterile gown and gloves, the surgeon drapes the patient to demarcate the surgical field and to keep the patient warm. The surgery can then proceed.

SUMMARY

All surgical procedures, including dental implantation, involve certain risk factors. One of the most common is

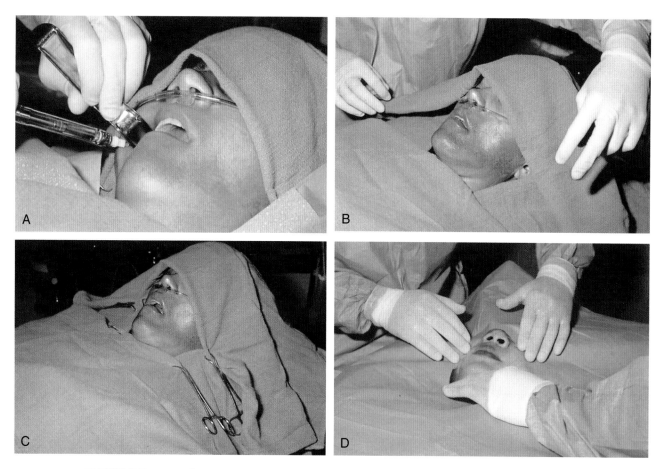

FIGURE 5-5 ■ **A,** The patient can now be anesthetized. **B,** The appropriate surgical field is draped. **C,** The drapes can be clamped. **D,** The entire field is draped with an appropriately designed surgical drape.

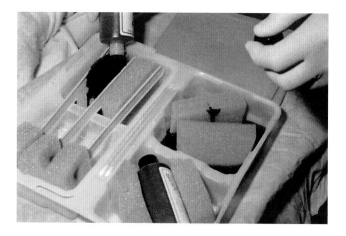

FIGURE 5-6 ■ Disinfecting agents such as povidone-iodine can be used.

postoperative infection. The harsh realities of today's medical environment—such as the threat of blood-borne pathogens and transmissible infections, increased costs of hospitalization, and the increase in malpractice lawsuits against surgeons—make it imperative that all surgeons follow safe and sterile surgical protocols that reduce the

chance for infection and ensure satisfactory results. As recommended by the CDC, all dental practices should have a written program for infection control to reduce and prevent (when possible) the risk for disease transmission.[1]

REFERENCES

1. Kohn WG, Collins AS, Cleveland JL, Harte JA, Eklund KJ, Malvitz DM; Centers for Disease Control and Prevention (CDC): Guidelines for infection control in dental health-care settings—2003, *MMWR Recomm Rep* 52(RR-17):1-61, 2003.
2. Whyte W, Hambraeus A, Laurell G, Hoborn J: The relative importance of the routes and sources of wound contamination during general surgery, II. airborne, *J Hosp Infect* 22(1):41-54, 1992.
3. Dharan S, Pittet D: Environmental controls in operating theatres, *J Hosp Infect* 51(2):79-84, 2002.
4. Chow TT, Yang XY: Ventilation performance in operating theatres against airborne infection: review of research activities and practical guidance, *J Hosp Infect* 56(2):85-92, 2004.
5. Persson M, van der Linden J: Wound ventilation with ultraclean air for prevention of direct airborne contamination during surgery, *Infect Control Hosp Epidemiol* 25(4):297-301, 2004.
6. 2008 Report on the global AIDS epidemic, UNAIDS/WHO, July 2008. Cited July 2008. Available at: http://www.unaids.org/en/KnowledgeCentre/HIVData/GlobalReport/2008/

7. Crow S, Rayfield S: *Asepsis: the right touch: something old is now new*, Bossier City, LA, 1990, Everett Publishing.

8. Clappison RA: Cross contamination control and the dental handpiece, *J Prosthet Dent* 73(5):492-494, 1995.

9. Young JM: Keys to successful handpiece maintenance, *Tex Dent J* 114(12):15-19, 1997.

10. Rutala WA, Weber DJ, Thomann CA: Outbreak of wound infections following outpatient podiatric surgery due to contaminated bone drills, *Foot Ankle* 7(6):350-354, 1987.

11. Muscarella LF: Are all sterilization processes alike? *AORN J.* 67(5):966-970, 973-976, 1998.

12. Rutala WA: Disinfection and sterilization of patient-care items, *Infect Control Hosp Epidemiol* 17(6):377-384, 1996.

13. Leonard DL, Charlton DG: Performance of high-speed dental handpieces subjected to simulated clinical use and sterilization, *J Am Dent Assoc* 130(9):1301-1311, 1999.

14. Crow S: Sterilization processes: meeting the demands of today's health care technology, *Nurs Clin North Am* 28(3):687-695, 1993.

15. Rutala WA, Weber DJ: New disinfection and sterilization methods, *Emerg Infect Dis* 7(2):348-353, 2001.

16. Harte JA, Miller CH: Sterilization update 2003, *Compend Contin Educ Dent* 25(1 suppl):24-29, 2004.

17. Laufman H, Eudy WW, Vandernoot AM, Harris CA, Liu D: Strike-through of moist contamination by woven and nonwoven surgical materials, *Ann Surg* 181(6):857-862, 1975.

18. Rutala WA, Weber DJ: A review of single-use and reusable gowns and drapes in health care, *Infect Control Hosp Epidemiol* 22(4):248-257, 2001.

19. Association of Perioperative Registered Nurses: Recommended practices for selection and use of surgical gowns and drapes, *AORN J* 77(1):206-210, 213, 2003.

20. Pissiotis CA, Komborozos V, Papoutsi C, Skrekas G: Factors that influence the effectiveness of surgical gowns in the operating theatre, *Eur J Surg* 163(8):597-604, 1997.

21. Lipp A: The effectiveness of surgical face masks: what the literature shows, *Nurs Times* 99(39):22-24, 2003.

22. Pedlar J, Frame JW: *Oral and maxillofacial surgery: an objective-based textbook*, Edinburgh, 2001, Churchill Livingstone.

23. Jepsen OB, Bruttomesso KA: The effectiveness of preoperative skin preparations: an integrative review of the literature, *AORN J* 58(3):477-479, 482-484, 1993.

24. Association of Operating Room Nurses: Recommended practices for skin preparation of patients, *AORN J* 75(1):184-187, 2002.

25. Mackenzie I: Preoperative skin preparation and surgical outcome, *J Hosp Infect* 11(suppl B):27-32, 1988.

26. Arata T, Murakami T, Hirai Y: Evaluation of povidone-iodine alcoholic solution for operative site disinfection, *Postgrad Med J* 69(suppl 3):S93-S96, 1993.

27. Seal LA, Paul-Cheadle D: A systems approach to preoperative surgical patient skin preparation, *Am J Infect Control* 32(2):57-62, 2004.

28. Hibbard JS: Analyses comparing the antimicrobial activity and safety of current antiseptic agents: a review, *J Infus Nurs* 28(3):194-207, 2005.

chapter 6

Radiographic Modalities for Dental Implants

SUCCESSFUL ORAL IMPLANTATION is highly dependent on proper preoperative treatment planning, in which appropriate radiographic evaluation of the edentulous ridge and potential implant site(s) plays a key role.[1,2] The American Academy of Oral and Maxillofacial Radiology recommended in 2000 that clinicians employ cross-sectional imaging when planning implant cases; additionally, the Academy noted that conventional cross-sectional tomography should be the preferred method for obtaining this information for most implant patients.[3] Modern imaging techniques are facilitating the trend toward nonspecialist placement of implants in the dental office; the dentist can choose the appropriate radiographic modality—digital or film—that enables him or her to plan treatment, place the implants, perform restoration and proper postoperative treatment, and use intraoral and panoramic images—both linear and complex motion tomography, as well as computed tomography.[4,5] A thorough radiograph examination should enable the surgeon to assess the quantity and quality of the bone present and to visualize the locations and relationships between critical internal anatomical structures.[6-9]

Before implant placement and during treatment planning, the surgeon must be able to measure the height and width of the alveolar process to ensure adequate bone and to select appropriately sized implants. In addition, the surgeon

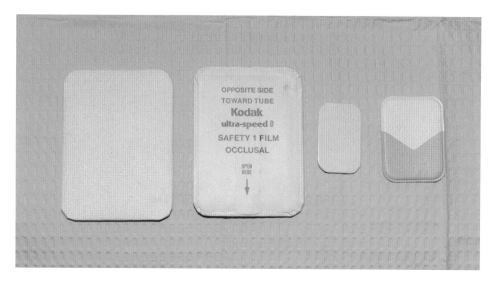

FIGURE 6-1 ■ Different sizes of intraoral films.

must know the precise location of the mandibular canal (injury to the neurovascular bundle within the canal can result in facial paresthesia) and the maxillary sinuses (perforation of the sinuses creates the possibility of antral infection and increases the likelihood of implant failure).

Multiple views of the proposed implant site should be taken; this often requires the use of different imaging procedures. Various radiographic modalities, including intraoral films (i.e., periapical and occlusal radiographs), panoramic radiographs, cephalometric radiographs, plain (conventional) tomography, computed tomography (CT), digital subtraction radiography (DSR), and magnetic resonance imaging (MRI), are available to the clinician.

Intraoral Films

Periapical radiographs provide excellent images of whole teeth, bone trabeculae, and surrounding dental structures and gums; such radiographs also supply detailed information on small sections of the buccolingual width and the occlusoapical height, so that the available bone can be observed and measured with minimal distortion (Figure 6-1).

Radiographic film in a protective casing is placed in the patient's mouth and normally is held in position behind the teeth to be x-rayed. This procedure can present certain difficulties if the patient has a very sensitive gagging reflex. Correct positioning of the film is more difficult in edentulous regions of the mandible, where the floor of the patient's mouth can be very shallow and not deep enough to give room for placement of the film other than above the edentulous mandibular ridge. In addition, the presence of ana-

tomical variations (such as mandibular tori) makes this procedure difficult. If the implant position has not been determined, the film should be placed parallel to the lingual cortical plate bone, because angulation of the implant osteotomy is sometimes dependent on this structure.[10] The specific needs and treatment objectives of the patient, as the literature notes, determine the radiographic imaging choices made by the clinician for the planning of implant placement in this and similar cases,[11] including general dental practice (diagnostic and preventative services)[12] and dental habilitation surgery.[13] Biological risks to the dental patient (i.e., dose measurements) should also be a concern for the clinician in radiographic decision planning.[14]

Periapical radiographs, however, have a number of limitations because of the small size of the film, which restricts the view to specific sections of the dental arch. It is difficult to interpret the anatomical details that are out of the scope of this small film, and it is impossible to ensure adequate width of the bone. The restricted field of view also makes orientation difficult in completely edentulous spans.[6] In addition, the location of the mandibular canal is often difficult to determine, and the mental foramen is visible in only 50% of periapical films of that region (Figure 6-2).

An occlusal radiograph can be used to visualize the mandible and maxilla in an axial view. After the film is placed intraorally parallel to the plane of occlusion, the beam is directed perpendicular to the film, above it for the maxilla or below it for the mandible. The patient's head is oriented so that the film is taken at a right angle (90 degrees) to the mandibular dental arch.[7] This view provides substantive information on the buccolingual width of the mandible, which is depicted on the film as the distance between the points located on the extreme boundaries of the buccal and lingual cortical plates. However, the three-dimensional

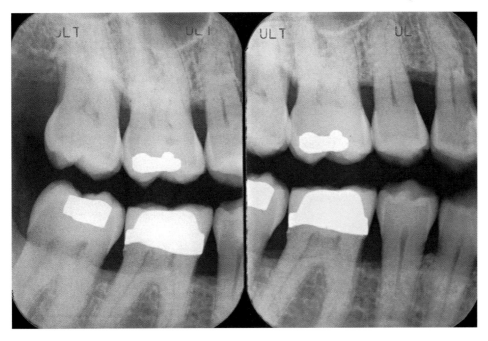

FIGURE 6-2 ■ Periapical radiographs have limitations when used for an implant diagnosis. The film doesn't show important anatomic structures to be considered during the implant placement.

structure of the bone, particularly in the exterior and interior areas of the mandible, is not always easy to evaluate with this type of film. The inclinations and curvatures that the mandible presents, especially in its inner aspect, will not be apparent on an occlusal film. In addition, the maxilla is often distorted on occlusal films; superimposition of structures between the nasal bones and the maxilla will be apparent on the film, and the view may be less helpful for determining the width of the arch.

Because of the stated disadvantages of periapical and occlusal radiographs, they are of limited use in implant treatment planning and are recommended as an additional evaluation tool, primarily in cases of single implant placement.[15] Even for a single implant site, the periapical and occlusal films should be complements to a panoramic film. For a single site, several periapical views and at least one properly positioned occlusal radiograph should be taken to provide optimal image detail of the implant site with minimal geometric distortion. Intraoral radiographs can help the clinician estimate the approximate height of the bone, as well as the location of the proposed site relative to critical anatomic structures.[16]

Panoramic Radiographs

The panoramic radiograph, currently the most used radiographic modality in implant dentistry, produces a single two-dimensional image of the maxilla and mandible and their supporting anatomical structures in a frontal plane[7,17]

(Figure 6-3). A panoramic image is very helpful when one is planning multiple implant sites, and, when properly positioned, can provide useful information for single implant site selection; the literature suggests that limited site radiography may best be performed with intraoral radiography.[18] The panoramic radiograph provides a wide-field view, whereby the gross anatomy of the maxilla and mandible, the opposing structures within the jaw, and related pathologic findings are easily identified and evaluated. Comparisons can be made to contralateral landmarks, and existing conditions (e.g., odontogenic lesions, condylar changes) that might interfere with implant placement or jeopardize the success of the procedure can be visualized.[7] In addition, the vertical height of the bone can be readily assessed, and the procedure can be performed conveniently and rapidly, with minimal exposure of the patient to radiation. When a patient presents with a highly atrophic mandible, particularly with unfavorable imaging conditions, rotational panoramic radiographs can yield results more useful to the clinician than those of limited intraoral radiographs for peri-implant bone loss evaluation.[19] The clinician should note that manufacturers' instructions for positioning dentate patients during panoramic radiography may yield errors in positioning on the panoramic radiographs of edentulous patients, unless modifications are made. As with all radiographic treatment, appropriate training of dental staff is essential, as is the use of proper technique when panoramic films are exposed and developed for proper diagnosis and planning of implants for edentulous patients.[20,21]

Several disadvantages are associated with the use of panoramic radiographs with regard to implantology. The

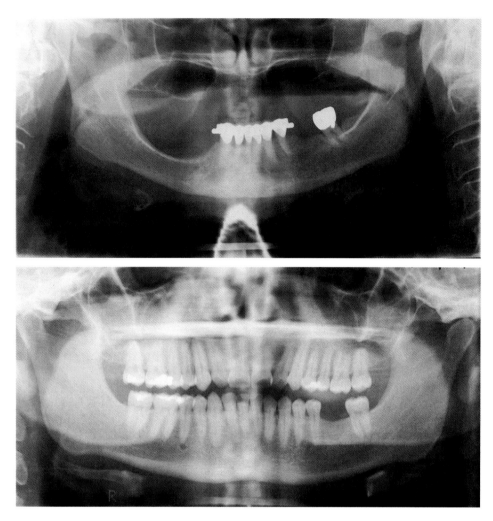

FIGURE 6-3 ■ **A, B,** Panoramic x-rays are essential for a thorough dental examination. They allow a broad overview of the entire mouth, including the upper and lower jawbones, sinuses, and other hard and soft tissues around the head and neck. It is the standard for evaluation for dental implant surgery.

image does not produce the fine anatomical resolution seen with other types of radiographs. In addition, no information is provided in terms of bone thickness, and the use of a panoramic image alone can lead to errors in estimating or determining bone width.[7] Superimposition or overlapping of structures can result in poor image quality. The presence of metallic restorations, metal frameworks, or base metal implants can cause metallic artifacts and streaking to appear on the image. Nonuniform magnification is an inherent problem with panoramic films (Figure 6-4).[6,22,23]

The major disadvantage associated with the use of panoramic radiographs is their extreme sensitivity to errors in patient position,[24-26] which can result in significant geometric distortion of the image. This distortion can be divided into vertical and horizontal components. The dimensions of the vertical image are dependent on the x-ray source as the focus, with the degree of distortion determined by the distance from the patient's arch to the film. The horizontal dimensions are affected by the rotation center of the beam

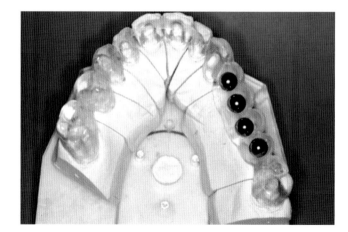

FIGURE 6-4 ■ Metallic balls can potentially help calculate magnification distortion percentages in panoramic x-rays.

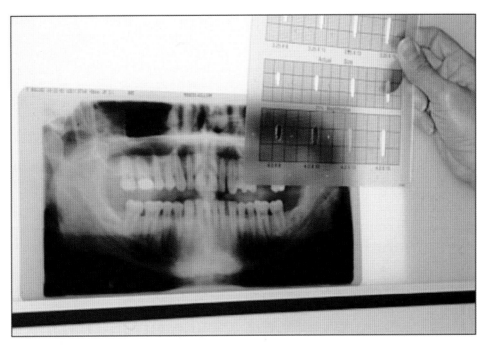

FIGURE 6-5 ■ Implant companies generally provide templates to help clinicians choose the correct implant length.

as the focus, and they change dramatically in relation to object-film distance.[27] It has been reported that panoramic images can produce a 50% to 70% horizontal distortion and a 10% to 32% vertical distortion.[17,28-30] This distortion factor and the inconsistency in enlargement make accurate assessment and determination of implant length based on longitudinal measurements from the panoramic radiograph extremely difficult.[6]

Before the advent of newer, more sophisticated imaging modalities (e.g., plain tomography, CT), surgeons had to rely solely on clinical assessment of bone width, and it was not unusual to discover during surgery that bone for implant placement was inadequate. Because of the limitations of panoramic films and the availability of adjunctive radiographic procedures, panoramic radiography should no longer be the only imaging modality used during the preoperative treatment planning phase for oral implants. Although not always commercially available when developed during the early 1990s, new technologies were being developed to create digital images from conventional panoramic radiography.[31-35] Over time, these innovations helped to decrease the procedure's sensitivity and reduce the problems associated with patient positioning. Recent literature has shown the equivalency, in most cases, of digital panoramic radiographs and film-based images.[36]

Various commercially available implant systems provided templates that could be placed over the panoramic x-ray to help calculate the area that the implant would occupy in a particular site (Figure 6-5). These templates came with the implants depicted with an estimate of the magnification expected in a panoramic film. To help determine proper placement of the implants, the clinician obtained the pan-

oramic radiograph with a surgical stent in place. A stent is a clear resin duplicate of the diagnostic wax-up of the patient's denture, which provides information regarding optimum implant sites and desired angulation of the prosthesis.[17,37] Guiding grooves or holes are placed in conjunction with cutouts or flat plane surfaces in potential implant sites, with radiopaque metallic ball bearings of known diameter luted over placement sites on the stent. On the panoramic image, the metallic spheres will appear "suspended" over potential implant sites. The distortion factor at each site can be determined by dividing the actual diameter of the sphere by its diameter on the radiographic image. The true height of the residual ridge at the site can be calculated on the radiograph by measuring the distance from the ridge crest to the superior aspect of the mandibular canal (or to the inferior border of the mandible in the symphysis region, or the inferior aspect of the maxillary sinus in the maxilla) and multiplying this result by the distortion factor.[17] This information can be of considerable help in selecting the correct implant length. When the radiographic treatment planning has been completed, the ball bearings are removed and the stent is cut out and grooved for implant surgery.

Lateral Cephalometric Radiographs

Generally, lateral cephalometric radiographs are not very useful when one is planning for implant placement because of the number of superimposed images that will make visualization of the anatomical area of interest very difficult. Nevertheless, a lateral cephalometric radiograph can be used in treatment planning of implants for or near the midsagittal region of the maxilla and mandible, where the trajectory and angulation of the residual bone are well visualized.[6,38] Magnification ranges from 6% to 15%, providing a more accurate representation than the panoramic radiographs of vertical height, width, and angulation at the bone at the midline. In addition, a lateral projection of the skull can help in evaluating factors such as loss of bone in the vertical dimension, skeletal arch interrelationships, anterior crown-to-implant ratio, and anterior tooth position in the prosthesis.

One technique for evaluating bony changes in the anterior edentulous maxilla involves a modification of the traditional cephalometric analysis. A comparison is made of the measurements of the patient's initial (baseline) analysis versus the patient's follow-up radiographic analysis; results can be used to identify bone loss amounts occurring between examinations.[39] Oblique lateral cephalometric radiographs have been found to be effective for measuring mandibular height in longitudinal studies of patients with and without implants.[40]

This technique can be enhanced by soft tissue projection correction, which can significantly reduce the variation between radiographs caused by soft tissue positions.[41] Other studies have concluded that superimposition of oblique cephalometric radiographs can be used effectively to determine tooth movement in implant cases.[42]

Plain (Conventional) Tomography

In plain tomography, the x-ray head and x-ray film move simultaneously in opposite directions, with the resulting film showing only the body part or section under study as a cross-sectional image or "slice" of the section. Because the x-ray head and film are positioned so the tissue is in focus at one depth only, all background and foreground structures appear blurred.

For implant site selection, plain tomograms provide an image focused on a selected parasagittal plane. The procedure was used initially to obtain cross-sectional views of the maxilla and mandible. Valuable information on the quality and quantity of bone at the implant site can be obtained, and the layers of cortical bone and trabecular bone and anatomical structures at the location can be accurately evaluated.[43-45] The presence of adequate bone at the precise implant site can be directly measured from the tomogram.[30] Some have advocated plain tomograms as the most cost-effective radiographic modality for assessing implant site.[46] However, this technique has certain limitations in the treatment planning of oral implants because the distance between

cross-cuts is large, the images are blurry, and the contrast is poor. Unfamiliarity of the dentist with reading conventional tomograms made of dental implant sites has been noted in the literature, and the dentist often needs aid in identifying normal anatomical landmarks on cross-sectional slices for correlation with sagittal slices.[47,48] Tomograms can have as much as a 40% enlargement factor, and superimposition of structures out of the plane of focus (although not as much of a problem as with other radiographic procedures) can result in a "smearing" of the image under study.[6] Plain tomography is very labor intensive when used to evaluate multiple implant sites.[7]

These limitations have been addressed effectively with the introduction and availability of computed tomography (CT), which produces extremely accurate, highly detailed images.

Computed Tomography

The CT scanner, first introduced to the medical field in 1972, exemplifies the significance of the computer's contribution to medical imaging. In CT scanning, multiple beams of x-rays are passed through the body part being examined, and their degree of absorption is recorded by sensors. The scanner moves around the patient, emitting and recording x-ray beams from every point of the circle; in this way, data on the density characteristics of the object under study are obtained. Using information produced by the scanner, a computer constructs cross-sectional images of the object. These images are the visual equivalent of bloodless slices of anatomy, with each scan being a single slice. Images can be manipulated electronically to obtain the best view of the area of interest. Adjacent two-dimensional slices can be reconstructed to produce three-dimensional representations, as well as images in different planes. In this way, a CT scan can provide coronal or frontal views, lateral or sagittal views, and axial or horizontal views (Figure 6-6).

Numerous advantages have been attributed to the use of CT scans in oral implantology.[49-51] Computed tomography images are rapidly processed and highly detailed, and reconstruction of the image is possible. No superimposition or overlapping of images occurs, and no distortion is seen, as with other radiographic procedures (e.g., panoramic radiographs). Automatic calculation of bone height and width and precise estimation of available bone are possible. Information pertaining to the quality of the cancellous bone and the thickness of the cortical plates is available (Figure 6-7).

Commercially available, specialized software, in conjunction with CT scans in the early 1990s, became one of the newest tools in radiographic planning in oral implantology.[52-54] Programs generate three-dimensional volume imaging that can be viewed from any angle and surface, or sliced panoramic views and vertical cross-sectional images of the jaw, encompassing the entire arch of the alveolar

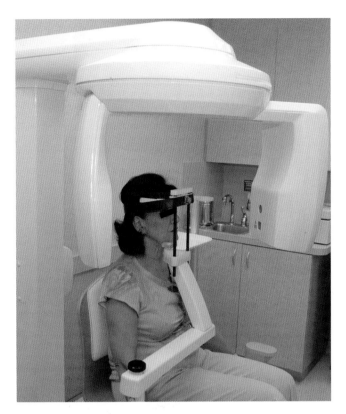

FIGURE 6-6 ■ The CT scanner fits easily in a dental office with similar space requirements as a panorex unit.

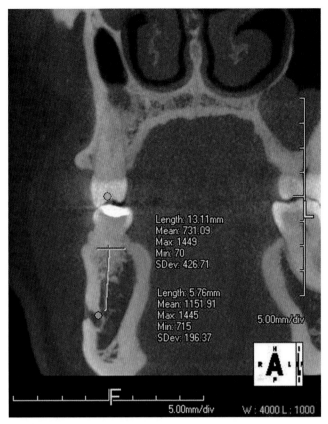

FIGURE 6-7 ■ The use of cone beam imaging aids the clinician in planning implant surgery and ensures the success of the surgery.

ridge. The software produces axial images of the maxilla and the mandible from a variety of CT scans and makes life-size (i.e., 1:1 ratio) three-dimensional images that show bone width, height, and depth at the proposed implant site (Figures 6-8 to 6-12).

The dimensions of the residual ridges and bone height relative to critical anatomical structures can be measured directly from the scan. The mandibular canal, maxillary sinuses, nasal cavities, mental foramen, and incisive canal can be located precisely. Residual ridge trajectory and angulation are readily visualized, as are the submandibular fossa and unsuspected irregularities in ridge structure, thus eliminating any guesswork about the size or configuration of the patient's anatomical structures.

It is most important to note that the ability to reconstruct three-dimensional images allows for interactive placement of simulated root-form implants in the reformatted images. With this capability, it is possible to know exactly, simultaneously in all three dimensions, how each implant affects the patient's oral anatomy. The clinician is able to prepare and evaluate several treatment plans before surgery and to select the one best suited for the patient. In this way, no unwelcome surprises are noted at the time of surgery and prosthetic restoration. Computed tomography scanning, with its two- and three-dimensional reconstruction capabilities, is currently the most useful and precise radiographic modality for treatment planning in oral implantology, espe-

cially when multiple implant sites in the maxilla and/or mandible are being evaluated[7] (see Figure 6-12).

A very promising area of dental implantation and CT scanning involves transferring planning to the surgical field through the use of computer-aided design (CAD)/computer-aided manufacturing (CAM) techniques such as stereolithographic rapid prototyping, to build surgical guides to aid in the precision of implant placement.[55]

Although the literature suggests that improved placement is often the result of using such surgical guides, the technique needs further exploration, particularly involving guide stability during implantation, and in cases of unilateral bone-supported and non–tooth-supported conditions.[56]

Cone Beam CT

The literature supporting the efficacy of CT scans in implant dentistry reaches back decades.[49,57,58] Time and practice have demonstrated the benefits of preoperative imaging that reaches beyond the two-dimensional images provided by panoramic and periapical radiography, particularly for the functional and esthetic demands of implant dentistry.[59-61] One of the newest developments in CT imaging technology

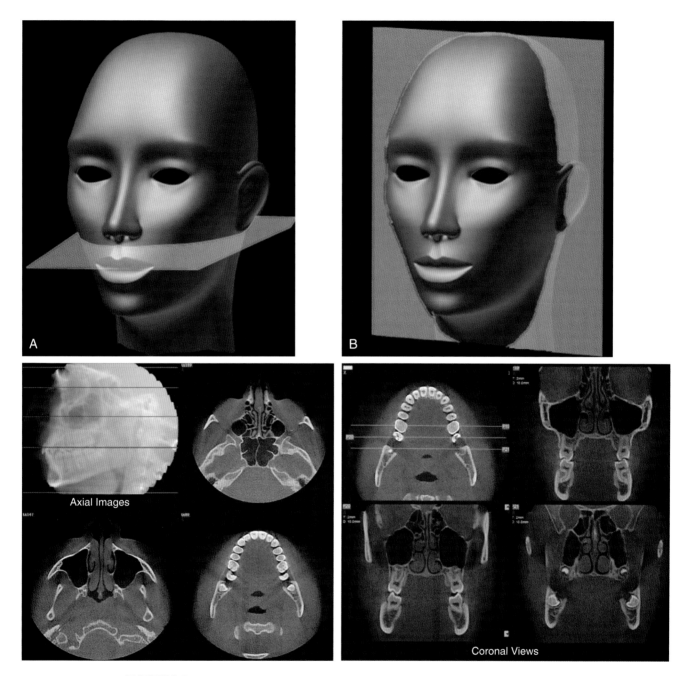

FIGURE 6-8 ■ **A, B,** A CT scan can be used to view images in different planes as slices.

is cone beam imaging, which can potentially reduce the size and cost of CT scanners[62] (see Figure 6-8). This technology yields images with isotropic submillimeter spatial resolution; as a result, its use is suited perfectly for dental and maxillofacial cases. A wide range of dental and maxillofacial diagnoses and surgeries can be accomplished with the aid of this high-resolution imaging, as opposed to conventional CT fan-beam scanning.

In addition, numerous studies attest to the geometric accuracy of the cone beam CT.[63-66] For example, the aim of one study was to evaluate the accuracy of linear measurements obtained from cone beam CT (CBCT) images.[65] A caliper was used to obtain 13 measurements in dry skulls (internal and external anatomical sites). These real measurements then were compared with measurements gained from CBCT imaging examinations. Real measurements were always larger than CBCT images, but the examiners considered these differences significant only for measurements of the internal structures of the skull base. Differences are considered significant only for the skull base, so measure-

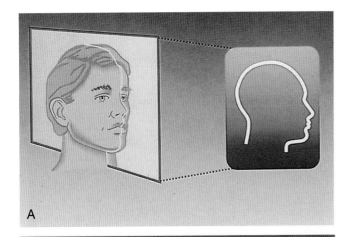

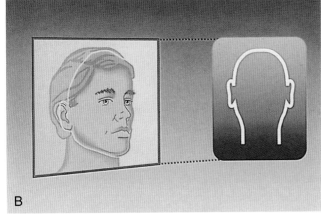

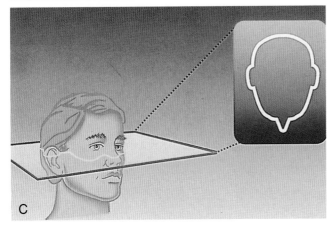

FIGURE 6-9 ■ **A-C,** A slice in the sagittal, coronal, and axial planes.

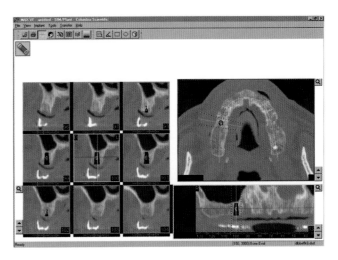

FIGURE 6-10 ■ Using specialized software, the clinician can visualize the implant in all the affected anatomy.

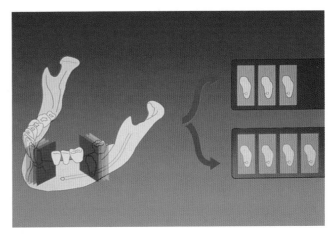

FIGURE 6-11 ■ A series of cross-sectional views in the mandible, which show the width and angulation of bone (in addition to height).

ments were reliable for linear evaluation of other structures essential for dentomaxillofacial imaging.

In another study, researchers attempted to determine the geometric accuracy of digital volume tomograms to assess their usability for implant planning.[66] This study employed a measuring object with 216 exactly known geometric measuring points. The cone beam scanner was used to develop images of the object for comparison with known measure-

ments. Results showed that when all three coordinate axes were considered, the digital volume tomographic images were geometrically correct, with only slight geometric deviations, and so were suitable for three-dimensional implant planning.

Other studies attest to the advantages of cone beam CT scanning in terms of lower dosages of radiation absorbed by the patient.[67-69] In one study, the purpose was to measure the tissue-absorbed dose and calculate the effective dose. Comparisons were made with existing reports on dose measurement and effective dose estimates for similar, conventional CT examinations for dental implants.[67] Thermoluminescent dosimeters were used in the study, and dose measurements were obtained after single and double exposures. Results showed that the effective dose with the cone beam CT scanner (CBCT) was significantly lower than with

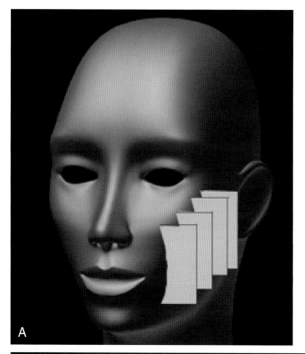

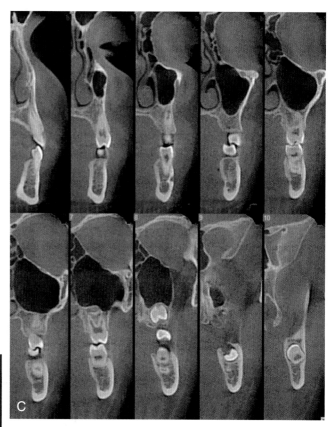

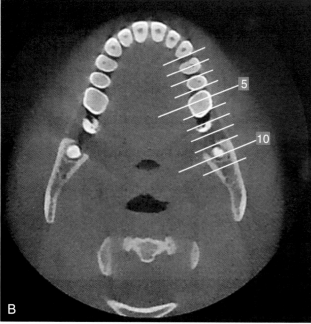

FIGURE 6-12 ■ **A-C,** A series of radiographic cross-sectional views of the mandible and maxilla.

traditional CT imaging. In another study, radiation doses were determined to balance risks against usefulness of the different modalities available for imaging of the facial skeleton, and these values revealed that exposure levels of CBCT systems fell between those of CT and conventional radiography, suggesting that clinicians should select the imaging system that is most appropriate when considering delivered doses of radiation and the image quality required for the clinical case.[68]

It is perhaps when employed as a means for developing surgical guides for implant dentistry that CBCT scanning finds one of its best uses.[56,70-72] For example, one study describes a technique to facilitate precise dental implant placement using a barium-coated template with external guide wires in conjunction with a CT scan and interactive software.[70] Computed tomography scan image measurements are transferred to the template via a precision-milled cylinder placed into the template. The template thus provides the surgeon with optimal position for implants. In a similar study, the purpose was to illustrate how a CT-derived template could successfully treat a completely edentulous patient through the use of flapless surgery and a transitional prosthesis.[71] Other researchers showed how an interactive imaging program allows CT images to place dental implants virtually and construct a precise guide splint and final prosthesis for delivery during implant placement.[72] The guide splint and final prosthesis were returned to the clinical site for implant placement, and an implant map was provided for each patient, indicating diameter and length of implants and abutments. The prosthesis was delivered after flapless surgery. The study concluded that this interactive computer imaging system can allow precise planning for implant position, and that images can be used successfully for guide splint and final prosthetic fabrication.

Finally, the aim of another study was to evaluate the match between positions and axes of planned and placed implants when a stereolithographic surgical guide is used.[56] This study employed six surgical guides in four patients, and investigators concluded that computer-aided rapid prototyping of surgical guides could be useful, but that additional clinical studies with a greater patient complement are needed to clarify certain issues.

The PreXion is the latest development in cone beam imaging for the maxillofacial region. State-of-the-art characteristics include very low radiation exposure for patients. In fact, it offers 10 to 20 times less radiation than is provided by other cone beam systems because of its scanner, which uses a unique "pulse" system that activates the x-ray only at essential times, thus giving fewer than 6 seconds of total full-scan exposure. Other systems employ x-rays during the entire scan. Because the system can provide a single low dose to create an accurate reconstruction of a 3D model of the patient's skull or any portion of the maxillofacial region, better evaluation is possible for a number of cases, including temporomandibular joint (TMJ), bone relationships, impacted teeth, retained root tips, paranasal sinus passages, and so on (Figure 6-13).

The PreXion employs "Smart Beam" technology to increase safety for adults and children. The imaging system virtually eliminates incorrect exposures through automatic and continuous monitoring. Radiation levels are set automatically during scout interviews through evaluation of the patient's anatomical density. Although an adult patient receives a very low level of radiation exposure with the system, a child will receive up to 40% less.

3G: Variable and Multiple Fields of View

The PreXion imaging system, with its variable field of view, is ideal for a variety of maxillofacial needs, from orthodon-

tics to endodontics. The PreXion can provide a full cephalometric image at the 12″ field of view, as well as increased resolution at 9″ and 6″ fields. Even though the system offers volumetric cephalometrics, the fixed 9″ field of view system can be used effectively for implantology and oral surgery.

The PreXion also offers multiple fields of view. The PreXion scanner is considered "full size," meaning that it delivers a volume size of 8.5″, in addition to displaying increased resolution in fields of view of volume sizes 6.5″ and 4.1″. Voxel sizes from the 3G range from .2 mm to .4 mm and are enabled by the 3G's 12-bit 1024 × 1024 acquisition matrix.

The PreXion scan provides unlimited imaging, so a single low-dose scan can yield several high-quality images, from cephalometrics, to panoramics, to cross-sectionals, to a series of cross-sectionals and 3Ds. Additionally, the system provides for multiple reconstructions. Thus, any plane can be chosen for primary reconstruction. Reconstructions for the occlusal plane or the mandibular plane can be compiled from the same scan. The PreXion software can deliver high-quality images for user-defined templates that are available on paper or film, or in digital form. Third-party software can be accommodated as well, because the PreXion software can provide date to Digital Imaging and Communications in Medicine (DICOM) format.

Cone beam CT will continue to be used to plan dental implant surgery, so the clinician can accurately assess the locations of anatomical structures and bone suitability. The relatively small doses of radiation and the effective imaging CT scans that are offered by systems such as the 3G system will enable implantologists to provide patients with the comfort, function, and esthetics that they increasingly demand (Figure 6-14).

Digital Subtraction Radiography

Although CT is the best radiographic modality for the treatment planning phase of implant therapy, the procedure is limited after implant placement because of implant artifacts from the metallic objects and radiopaque streaking, both of which can obscure details.[73] After implant placement is complete, the clinician is faced with new diagnostic concerns to determine the success or failure of the procedure. Detecting initial saucerization or the formation of an angular defect around the implants is very difficult on radiographs. In addition, because of the sharp contrast between the bone and the implant surface, spreading bone loss along the threads of a root-form implant is often difficult to visualize.[74] Digital subtraction radiography (DSR), however, has been applied to postoperative evaluation of implants to address the problems associated with detecting these changes with radiographs.[75,76]

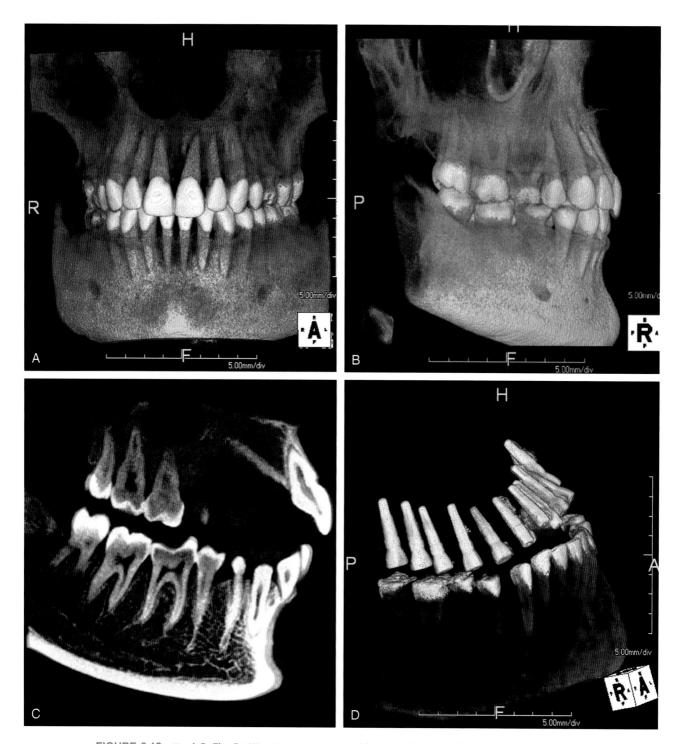

FIGURE 6-13 ■ **A-D,** The PreXion imaging system, with its variable field of view, is ideal for a variety of maxillofacial needs, from orthodontics to endodontics, in addition to dental implant surgery.

With the use of DSR, a computer digitizes and manipulates radiographic images to "subtract" (i.e., remove) unwanted distracting background detail between two images to produce a clear image. The digitization process converts the traditional radiographic film to a digital image consisting of a series of discrete numbers that correspond to the gray scale of the original radiograph. A computer-imaging device known as a digitizer then forms a grid over the original radiograph, creating small squares or picture elements (pixels). Each pixel is converted to a number that corresponds to its gray level.[74] By the clinician's subtracting all of the anatomical structures that have not changed between

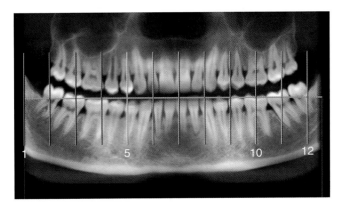

FIGURE 6-14 ■ Computed tomography scan, reformatted into a panoramic image.

radiographic examinations, any variations are plainly demonstrated against a neutral gray background or are superimposed on the original radiograph itself, and the clinician is able to easily visualize changes that have taken place.

DSR has been found to be an effective method for detecting and quantifying experimentally produced external root resorptive defects in teeth, especially when compared with conventional radiographic methods.[77,78] Other techniques for employing DSR include the accurate assessment of alveolar bone grafts,[79] as well as enhancement of the accuracy of alveolar crestal bone loss detection, especially because DSR requires fewer resources than conventional radiography, and the skills needed to operate the equipment are readily acquired with relatively minimal training.[80] DSR has also been found to be more accurate than panoramic radiographs in the detection of simulated osteophytic lesions of the mandibular condyle.[81]

Detecting periodontal bone changes as part of the long-term maintenance of Class II furcation defects has proven to be an effective use of DSR, especially when compared with conventional radiography; specifically, when evaluating the criteria of bone gain, bone loss, unchanged appearance, and areas impossible to visualize, visual interpreters of digital subtraction images were less subjective and more accurate when detecting periodontal bone changes in Class II furcation defects in mandibular molars than were interpreters of conventional radiographs.[82]

Methods for making digital subtraction radiology more accessible to researchers and practicing dentists include batch mode implementation (to enable the processing of large volumes of data) and restricting a region of interest and improving feature extraction.[83] Most digital subtraction methods for registration use manual landmarks; however, researchers have developed an automatic registration method that restricts geometric matching of images to a specific area, allowing comparison of the cross-correlation coefficient only between those areas, thus increasing accuracy up to 17% over manual methods.[84]

Magnetic Resonance Imaging

Magnetic resonance imaging (MRI) is similar to CT in that it produces images that are the visual equivalent of a slice of anatomy. Instead of using ionizing radiation, MRI generates images by detecting and processing radio signals emitted by protons, which are subjected to a very strong magnetic field and pulsed radio waves. Although MRI scans may look similar to CT scans, MRI scans generally provide much greater contrast between normal and abnormal soft tissue caused by differences in water content within these tissues.

When used in conjunction with CT scanning and new optoelectronic and ultrasonically based systems, MRI can produce unprecedented three-dimensional human jaw modeling and animation.[85]

Magnetic resonance imaging has limited use in implant dentistry, although radiation is totally absent with this modality, and no special reformatting programs are needed.[86,87] Early studies suggested that MRI could provide adequate information concerning amount of bone and anatomical limitations for placement of endosseous implants in both the mandible and the maxilla.[88,89] When used for presurgical implant assessment of available bone, MRI along with an acrylic surgical template with reference markers allows accurate identification of implant sites at surgery.[90] Extensive retrospective and prospective studies of internal derangements of the temporomandibular joint have been performed with MRI technology, as have imaging assessments of the salivary glands, paranasal sinuses, and cerebrovascular disease.[91]

The use of MRI is hindered by several drawbacks.[88] First, interpreting the quality of cortical and trabecular bone is very difficult. Second, as with CT scans, the presence of metal restorations causes artifacts.[92,93] However, some studies suggest that selection of specific dental casting alloys based on elemental compositions could minimize the detection of metal artifacts in MRI now caused by titanium alloys.[94]

SUMMARY

Early in the development of implant technology, it became apparent that conventional dental imaging techniques were limited in evaluating the patient for implant surgery. During the treatment planning phase, the recipient bed is routinely assessed by visual examination and palpation, as well as by periapical and panoramic radiology. These two imaging modalities provide a two-dimensional image of the mesiodistal and occlusoapical dimensions of the edentulous regions where implants might be placed.

When adequate occlusoapical bone height is available for endosteal implants, the buccolingual width and angulation of the available bone are the most important criteria for implant selection and success. However, neither buccolingual width nor angulation can be visualized on most traditional radiographs. Although clinical examination and traditional radiographs may be adequate for patients with wide residual ridges that exhibit sufficient bone crestal to the mandibular nerve and maxillary sinus, these methods do not allow for precise measurement of the buccolingual dimension of the bone or assessment of the location of unanticipated undercuts.

Because of these concerns, it is necessary to view the recipient site in a plane through the arch of the maxilla or mandible in the region of the proposed implants. Implant surgeons soon recognized that, for the optimum placement of implants, cross-sectional views of the maxilla and mandible served as the ideal means of providing necessary preoperative information.

Today, the two most often used and most applicable radiographic studies for implant treatment planning are the panoramic radiograph and tomography. Although distortion can be a major problem with panoramic radiographs, when performed properly, they can provide valuable information and are readily accessible and cost efficient. To help localize potential implant sites and assist in obtaining accurate measurement, it is recommended that surgical stents be used with panoramic radiographs. In simple cases where a limited number of implants are to be placed, panoramic radiography and/or plain tomography can be used to obtain a view of the arch of the jaw in the area of interest.

For complex cases in which multiple implants are required, the CT scan imaging procedure is recommended. Because of its ability to reconstruct a fully three-dimensional model of the maxilla and mandible, CT provides a highly sophisticated format for precisely defining jaw structure and locating critical anatomical structures. The use of CT scans in conjunction with software that renders immediate "treatment plans" using the most real and accurate information provides the most precise radiographic modality currently available for the evaluation of patients for oral implants.

DSR can be very helpful for following patients after implant surgery because it addresses the limitations of other radiographic modalities in detecting postoperative changes. By eliminating unchanged information, DSR allows the clinician's eye to focus on the actual changes that have occurred between the recordings of two images.

REFERENCES

1. Caswell CW, Clark AE: Tissue-integrated prosthesis for the edentulous patient: Brånemark (NoblePharma) system. In: *Dental implant prosthodontics*, Philadelphia, 1991, JB Lippincott.

2. McKinney RV: Evaluation and selection of the endosteal implant patient. In: *Endosteal dental implants*, St. Louis, 1991, Year Book Medical.

3. Tyndall AA, Brooks SL: Selection criteria for dental implant site imaging: a position paper of the American Academy of Oral and Maxillofacial Radiology, *Oral Surg Oral Med Oral Pathol Oral Radiol Endod* 89(5):630-637, 2000.

4. Parks ET, Williamson GF: Digital radiography: an overview, *J Contemp Dent Pract* 3(4):23-39, 2002.

5. Mupparapu M, Singer SR: Implant imaging for the dentist, *J Can Dent Assoc* 70(1):32, 2004.

6. SanGiacomo TR: Topics in implantology, 3. radiographic treatment planning, *RI Dent J* 23(4):5, 7-11, 1990.

7. Miles DA, Van Dis ML: Implant radiology, *Dent Clin North Am* 37(4):645-668, 1993.

8. Tugnait A, Clerehugh V, Hirschmann PN: Use of the basic periodontal examination and radiographs in the assessment of periodontal diseases in general dental practice, *J Dent* 32(1):17-25, 2004.

9. Pretty IA, Maupome G: A closer look at diagnosis in clinical dental practice: part 3, effectiveness of radiographic diagnostic procedures, *J Can Dent Assoc* 70(6):388-394, 2004.

10. Petrikowski CG, Pharoah MJ, Schmitt A: Presurgical radiographic assessment for implants, *J Prosthet Dent* 61(1):59-64, 1989.

11. Reiskin AB: Implant imaging: status, controversies, and new developments, *Dent Clin North Am* 42(1):47-56, 1998.

12. Brennan DS, Spencer AJ: Provision of diagnostic and preventive services in general dental practice, *Community Dent Health* 20(1):5-10, 2003.

13. Shashua D, Omnell ML: Radiographic determination of the position of the maxillary lateral incisor in the cleft alveolus and parameters for assessing its habilitation prospects, *Cleft Palate Craniofac J* 37(1):21-25, 2000.

14. Dula K, Mini R, van der Stelt PF, Buser D: The radiographic assessment of implant patients: decision-making criteria, *Int J Oral Maxillofac Implants* 16(1):80-89, 2001.

15. Garg AK, Vicari A: Radiographic modalities for diagnosis and treatment planning in implant dentistry, *Implant Soc* 5(5):7-11, 1995.

16. BouSerhal C, Jacobs R, Quirynen M, van Steenberghe D: Imaging technique selection for the preoperative planning of oral implants: a review of the literature, *Clin Implant Dent Relat Res* 4(3):156-172, 2002.

17. Hobo S, Ichida E, Garcia LT: *Osseointegration and occlusal rehabilitation*, Chicago, 1989, Quintessence.

18. Molander B: Panoramic radiography in dental diagnostics, *Swed Dent J Suppl* 119:1-26, 1996.

19. Zechner W, Watzak G, Gahleitner A, Busenlechner D, Tepper G, Watzek G: Rotational panoramic versus intraoral rectangular radiographs for evaluation of peri-implant bone loss in the anterior atrophic mandible, *Int J Oral Maxillofac Implants* 18(6):873-878, 2003.

20. Glass BJ, Seals RR Jr, Williams EO: Common errors in panoramic radiography of edentulous patients, *J Prosthodont* 3(2):68-73, 1994.

21. Goren AD, Lundeen RC, Deahl ST 2nd, Hashimoto K, Kapa SF, Katz JO, Ludlow JB, Platin E, Van Der Stelt PF, Wolfgang L: Updated quality assurance self-assessment exercise in intraoral and panoramic radiography, American Academy of Oral and Maxillofacial Radiology, Radiology Practice Committee, *Oral Surg Oral Med Oral Pathol Oral Radiol Endod* 89(3):369-374, 2000.

22. Samfors KA, Welander U: Angle distortion in narrow beam rotation radiography, *Acta Radiol Diagn (Stockh)* 15(5):570-576, 1974.

23. White S, Pharoah M: *Oral radiology: principles and interpretation*, St. Louis, 2003, Mosby.

24. Schiff T, D'Ambrosio J, Glass BJ, Langlais RP, McDavid WD: Common positioning and technical errors in panoramic radiography, *J Am Dent Assoc* 113(3):422-426, 1986.

25. Lanlang OE, Langlais RP, McDavid WD, et al: Troubleshooting errors in panoramic techniques. In: *Panoramic radiology*, Philadelphia, 1989, Lea & Febiger.

26. Glass BJ: *Successful panoramic radiography*, Rochester, NY, 1999, Eastman Kodak.

27. Yosue T, Brooks SL: The appearance of mental foramina on panoramic and periapical radiographs, II. experimental evaluation, *Oral Surg Oral Med Oral Pathol* 68(4):488-492, 1989.

28. Lund TM, Manson-Hing LR: A study of the focal troughs of three panoramic dental x-ray machines, Part I, the area of sharpness, *Oral Surg Oral Med Oral Pathol* 39(2):318-328, 1975.

29. Manson-Hing LR, Lund TM: A study of the focal troughs of three panoramic dental x-ray machines, Part II, image dimensions, *Oral Surg Oral Med Oral Pathol* 39(4):647-653, 1975.

30. Engelman MJ, Sorensen JA, Moy P: Optimum placement of osseointegrated implants, *J Prosthet Dent* 59(4):467-473, 1988.

31. Arai Y, Araki M, Ohgame Y, et al: A fundamental study on digital panoramic tomography, 8th International Congress of Dento-Maxillo-Facial Radiology, San Antonio, TX, IADR, 1988.

32. McDavid WD, Dove SB, Welander U, Tronje G: Electronic system for digital acquisition of rotational panoramic radiographs, *Oral Surg Oral Med Oral Pathol* 71(4):499-502, 1991. Erratum in *Oral Surg Oral Med Oral Pathol* 71(6):762, 1991.

33. Sinoda K, Arai Y, Hashimoto K, et al: Clinical trial of the new digital panoramic tomography, 9th International Congress of Dento-Maxillo-Facial Radiology, Budapest, Hungary, OMIKK, 1991.

34. Arai Y, Shinoda K, Hashimoto K, et al: Development of digital panoramic radiography: trial of multi-layer digital tomographic image, 2nd Symposium on Digital Imaging in Dental Radiology, Amsterdam, Holland, ACTA, 1992.

35. Dove SB, McDavid WD: Digital panoramic and extraoral imaging, *Dent Clin North Am* 37(4):541-551, 1993.

36. Molander B, Grondahl HG, Ekestubbe A: Quality of film-based and digital panoramic radiography, *Dentomaxillofac Radiol* 33(1):32-36, 2004.

37. Zinner ID, Small SA, Panno FV: Presurgical prosthetics and surgical templates, *Dent Clin North Am* 33(4):619-633, 1989.

38. Fernandes RJ, Azarbal M, Ismail YH, Curtin HD: A cephalometric tomographic technique to visualize the buccolingual and vertical dimensions of the mandible, *J Prosthet Dent* 58(4):466-470, 1987.

39. Scott RF, Barber HD, Maxson BB: A technique for evaluating bony changes in the anterior edentulous maxilla: a modification of a cephalometric analysis, *Oral Surg Oral Med Oral Pathol* 71(2):250-251, 1991.

40. Verhoeven JW, Cune MS: Oblique lateral cephalometric radiographs of the mandible in implantology: usefulness and accuracy of the technique in height measurements of mandibular bone in vivo, *Clin Oral Implants Res* 11(1):39-43, 2000.

41. Ruijter JM, Verhoeven JW, van der Linden JA, Cune MS, Terlou M: Image processing and analysis program for measurement of bone density changes in reference and follow-up standardized extraoral oblique lateral cephalometric radiographs of the mandible, *Dentomaxillofac Radiol* 32(6):379-384, 2003.

42. Sakima MT, Sakima CG, Melsen B: The validity of superimposing oblique cephalometric radiographs to assess tooth movement: an implant study, *Am J Orthod Dentofacial Orthop* 126(3):344-353, 2004.

43. Fredholm U, Bolin A, Andersson L: Preimplant radiographic assessment of available maxillary bone support: comparison of tomographic and panoramic technique, *Swed Dent J* 17(3):103-109, 1993.

44. Monahan R, Furkart AJ: Technical note: sagittal tomography as an adjunct to cross-sectional evaluation of select implant sites, *Dentomaxillofac Radiol* 25(5):298-301, 1996.

45. Thunthy KH, Yeadon WR, Nasr HF: An illustrative study of the role of tomograms for the placement of dental implants, *J Oral Implantol* 29(2):91-95, 2003.

46. Kassebaum DK, Stoller NH, Goshorn BI: Radiographic techniques for presurgical assessment of dental implant sites, *Gen Dent* 40(6):502-505, 509-510, 1992.

47. Thunthy KH, Yeadon WR: Normal anatomy on tomograms for dental implants, *Gen Dent* 51(2):134-140, 2003.

48. Peltola JS, Mattila M: Cross-sectional tomograms obtained with four panoramic radiographic units in the assessment of implant site measurements, *Dentomaxillofac Radiol* 33(5):295-300, 2004.

49. Schwarz MS, Rothman SL, Chafetz N, Rhodes M: Computed tomography in dental implantation surgery, *Dent Clin North Am* 33(4):555-597, 1989.

50. Abrahams JJ: Dental CT imaging: a look at the jaw, *Radiology* 219(2):334-345, 2001.

51. Siessegger M, Schneider BT, Mischkowski RA, Lazar F, Krug B, Klesper B, Zoller JE: Use of an image-guided navigation system in dental implant surgery in anatomically complex operation sites, *J Craniomaxillofac Surg* 29(5):276-281, 2001.

52. Rothman SL, Chaftez N, Rhodes ML, Schwarz MS: CT in the preoperative assessment of the mandible and maxilla for endosseous implant surgery: work in progress, *Radiology* 168(1):171-175, 1988. Erratum in *Radiology* 169(2):581, 1988. Schwartz MS [corrected to Schwarz MS].

53. Abrahams J: CT assessment of dental implant planning, *Oral Maxillofac Surg Clin North Am* 4:1-7, 1992.

54. Yune HY: Two-dimensional-three-dimensional reconstruction computed tomography techniques, *Dent Clin North Am* 37(4):613-626, 1993.

55. Sarment DP, Sukovic P, Clinthorne N: Accuracy of implant placement with a stereolithographic surgical guide, *Int J Oral Maxillofac Implants* 18(4):571-577, 2003.

56. Di Giacomo GA, Cury PR, de Araujo NS, Sendyk WR, Sendyk CL: Clinical application of stereolithographic surgical guides for implant placement: preliminary results, *J Periodontol* 76(4):503-507, 2005.

57. Fjellstrom CA, Strom C: CT of the edentulous maxilla intended for osseo-integrated implants, *J Craniomaxillofac Surg* 15(1):45-46, 1987.

58. Andersson L, Kurol M: CT scan prior to installation of osseointegrated implants in the maxilla, *Int J Oral Maxillofac Surg* 16(1):50-55, 1987.

59. Gher ME, Richardson AC: The accuracy of dental radiographic techniques used for evaluation of implant fixture placement, *Int J Periodontics Restorative Dent* 15(3):268-283, 1995.

60. Iplikcioglu H, Akca K, Cehreli MC: The use of computerized tomography for diagnosis and treatment planning in implant dentistry, *J Oral Implantol* 28(1):29-36, 2002.

61. Tischler M: Interactive computerized tomography for dental implants: treatment planning from the prosthetic end result, *Dent Today* 23(3):90, 92-93, 2004.

62. Sukovic P: Cone beam computed tomography in craniofacial imaging, *Orthod Craniofac Res* 6(suppl 1):31-36, 2003; discussion 179-182.

63. Enciso R, Memon A, Mah J: Three-dimensional visualization of the craniofacial patient: volume segmentation, data integration and animation, *Orthod Craniofac Res* 6(suppl 1):66-71, 2003; discussion 179-182.

64. Carano A, Velo S, Incorvati C, Poggio P: Clinical applications of the Mini-Screw-Anchorage-System (M.A.S.) in the maxillary alveolar bone, *Prog Orthod* 5(2):212-235, 2004.

65. Lascala CA, Panella J, Marques MM: Analysis of the accuracy of linear measurements obtained by cone beam computed tomography (CBCT-NewTom), *Dentomaxillofac Radiol* 33(5):291-294, 2004.

66. Marmulla R, Wortche R, Muhling J, Hassfeld S: Geometric accuracy of the NewTom 9000 Cone Beam CT, *Dentomaxillofac Radiol* 34(1):28-31, 2005.

67. Mah JK, Danforth RA, Bumann A, Hatcher D: Radiation absorbed in maxillofacial imaging with a new dental computed tomography device, *Oral Surg Oral Med Oral Pathol Oral Radiol Endod* 96(4):508-513, 2003.

68. Schulze D, Heiland M, Thurmann H, Adam G: Radiation exposure during midfacial imaging using 4- and 16-slice computed tomography, cone beam computed tomography systems and conventional radiography, *Dentomaxillofac Radiol* 33(2):83-86, 2004.

69. Rustemeyer P, Streubuhr U, Suttmoeller J: Low-dose dental computed tomography: significant dose reduction without loss of image quality, *Acta Radiol* 45(8):847-853, 2004.

70. Kopp KC, Koslow AH, Abdo OS: Predictable implant placement with a diagnostic/surgical template and advanced radiographic imaging, *J Prosthet Dent* 89(6):611-615, 2003.

71. Fortin T, Isidori M, Blanchet E, Perriat M, Bouchet H, Coudert JL: An image-guided system-drilled surgical template and trephine guide pin to make treatment of completely edentulous patients easier: a clinical report on immediate loading, *Clin Implant Dent Relat Res* 6(2):111-119, 2004.

72. Parel SM, Triplett RG: Interactive imaging for implant planning, placement, and prosthesis construction, *J Oral Maxillofac Surg* 62(9 suppl 2):41-47, 2004.

73. Brooks SL: Computed tomography, *Dent Clin North Am* 37(4):575-590, 1993.

74. Reddy MS, Jeffcoat MK: Digital subtraction radiography, *Dent Clin North Am* 37(4):553-565, 1993.

75. Engelke W, de Valk S, Ruttimann U: The diagnostic value of subtraction radiography in the assessment of granular hydroxylapatite implants, *Oral Surg Oral Med Oral Pathol* 69(5):636-641, 1990.

76. Jeffcoat MK, Reddy MS, van den Berg HR, Bertens E: Quantitative digital subtraction radiography for the assessment of peri-implant bone change, *Clin Oral Implants Res* 3(1):22-27, 1992.

77. Kravitz LH, Tyndall DA, Bagnell CP, Dove SB: Assessment of external root resorption using digital subtraction radiography, *J Endod* 18(6):275-284, 1992.

78. Heo MS, Lee SS, Lee KH, Choi HM, Choi SC, Park TW: Quantitative analysis of apical root resorption by means of digital subtraction radiography, *Oral Surg Oral Med Oral Pathol Oral Radiol Endod* 91(3):369-373, 2001.

79. Maruko EY, Forbes DP: Digital subtraction radiography for assessing alveolar bone grafts: diagnostic accuracy and sensitivity, *Northwest Dent Res* 4(1):21-23, 1993.

80. Nummikoski PV, Steffensen B, Hamilton K, Dove SB: Clinical validation of a new subtraction radiography technique for periodontal bone loss detection, *J Periodontol* 71(4):598-605, 2000.

81. Masood F, Katz JO, Hardman PK, Glaros AG, Spencer P: Comparison of panoramic radiography and panoramic digital subtraction radiography in the detection of simulated osteophytic lesions of the mandibular condyle, *Oral Surg Oral Med Oral Pathol Oral Radiol Endod* 93(5):626-631, 2002.

82. Cury PR, Araujo NS, Bowie J, Sallum EA, Jeffcoat MK: Comparison between subtraction radiography and conventional radiographic interpretation during long-term evaluation of periodontal therapy in Class II furcation defects, *J Periodontol* 75(8):1145-1149, 2004.

83. Yoon DC: A new method for the automated alignment of dental radiographs for digital subtraction radiography, *Dentomaxillofac Radiol* 29(1):11-19, 2000.

84. Yi WJ, Heo MS, Lee SS, Choi SC, Lee SB, Huh KH: Automatic noise robust registration of radiographs for subtraction using strategic local correlation: an application to radiographs of dental implants, *Comput Biol Med* 35(3):247-258, 2005.

85. Enciso R, Memon A, Fidaleo DA, Neumann U, Mah J: The virtual craniofacial patient: 3D jaw modeling and animation, *Stud Health Technol Inform* 94:65-71, 2003.

86. Gray CF, Redpath TW, Bainton R, Smith FW: Magnetic resonance imaging assessment of a sinus lift operation using reoxidised cellulose (Surgicel) as graft material, *Clin Oral Implants Res* 12(5):526-530, 2001.

87. Imamura H, Sato H, Matsuura T, Ishikawa M, Zeze R: A comparative study of computed tomography and magnetic resonance imaging for the detection of mandibular canals and cross-sectional areas in diagnosis prior to dental implant treatment, *Clin Implant Dent Relat Res* 6(2):75-81, 2004.

88. Zabalegui J, Gil JA, Zabalegui B: Magnetic resonance imaging as an adjunctive diagnostic aid in patient selection for endosseous implants: preliminary study, *Int J Oral Maxillofac Implants* 5(3):283-287, 1990.

89. Gray CF, Redpath TW, Smith FW: Magnetic resonance imaging: a useful tool for evaluation of bone prior to implant surgery, *Br Dent J* 184(12):603-607, 1998.

90. Gray CF, Redpath TW, Smith FW: Pre-surgical dental implant assessment by magnetic resonance imaging, *J Oral Implantol* 22(2):147-153, 1996.

91. Matteson SR, Deahl ST, Alder ME, Nummikoski PV: Advanced imaging methods, *Crit Rev Oral Biol Med* 7(4):346-395, 1996.

92. Devge C, Tjellstrom A, Nellstrom H: Magnetic resonance imaging in patients with dental implants: a clinical report, *Int J Oral Maxillofac Implants* 12(3):354-359, 1997.

93. Abbaszadeh K, Heffez LB, Mafee MF: Effect of interference of metallic objects on interpretation of T1-weighted magnetic resonance images in the maxillofacial region, *Oral Surg Oral Med Oral Pathol Oral Radiol Endod* 89(6):759-765, 2000.

94. Shafiei F, Honda E, Takahashi H, Sasaki T: Artifacts from dental casting alloys in magnetic resonance imaging, *J Dent Res* 82(8):602-606, 2003.

chapter 7

Implant Surgical Templates in Implant Dentistry

A NUMBER OF DIFFERENT FACTORS—including restrictive factors—influence the accuracy of implant surgery when computer-aided surgical templates are considered. Today's image-guided templates can be manufactured to allow the implantologist to place implants precisely and reliably. However, although computer-aided implant dentistry (which involves image scanning, template manufacture, and template guidance during surgery) is necessarily more expensive than conventional dentistry, its significant error reduction (particularly in areas of sensitive anatomy) and reliability in the placement of functional and esthetically pleasing implants usually warrant the extra cost. The use of surgical templates in esthetically critical areas, such as the edentulous maxilla, often allows immediate placement of implants when sufficient bone is available for primary stability. In such cases, surgical guides can aid the dental team in treatment planning, placement of implants for immediate provisionalization, and prosthodontic therapy. In particular, surgical guides facilitate the positioning of implants optimally with existing teeth. The management of implants surgically and prosthodontically becomes a reliable process when relationships between alveolar bone, existing dentition, and implants are clearly established by the tomographic/surgical template.

Surgical Templates: The Literature

The literature on surgical templates for implants is best explored by examining the general development of surgical templates, the stability factor of surgical templates, and the specific use of surgical templates for cases involving the edentulous maxilla/mandible and immediate loading.

The Development of Surgical Templates

As early as 1989, surgical templates were used to aid the surgeon in optimal placement of implants in the mandible in a two-stage surgery, preceded by prosthodontic planning and followed by temporary and final prosthetic appliances; in addition, the importance of teamwork between the surgeon and the restorative dentist for such procedures became clear.[1] Computed tomography (CT) scans for prosthetic planning have been used since the early 1990s to provide a surgical template for the predictable, reliable placement of osseointegrated implants in the mandible. Such scans provide a three-dimensional view of alveolar bone, so the dental team can establish the position, angle, and depth of the implant. One study refers to the "positioner" template developed by the team to reduce errors associated with perforating the mandible.[2] Positioning errors can be determined by a second CT. CT scanning also aids the restorative dentist's prosthodontic reconstruction (Figure 7-1).

In 1995, software programs were being used regularly to obtain reformatted CT images of the mandible and maxilla for planning of fixed and removable prosthetic suprastructures, including radiopaque prosthetic templates for optimal positioning of implants in edentulous patients.[3] In addition, magnetic resonance imaging (MRI) was used to assess bone for presurgical implant, because its tomographic modality provided accurate three-dimensional information on the anatomy of structures in the mandible and maxilla.[4] MRI markers placed on an acrylic surgical template permitted identification of potential implant sites. MRI technology proved superior in many respects to CT and similar techniques because of the ease of adjusting angulation and offsetting of the scan plane; MRI tolerance of metal pins and amalgam fillings was an additional advantage.[4] MRI technology reveals cancellous bone and cortical bone detail through thin slice, high-resolution images that show not only bone quality and thickness, but also the position of relative structures (e.g., inferior dental nerve, nasal sinuses). MRI images can be used successfully when complemented by rotational panoramic X-rays for the planning and placement of implants.[4] Thus, a diagnostic template could be

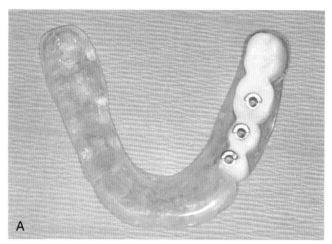

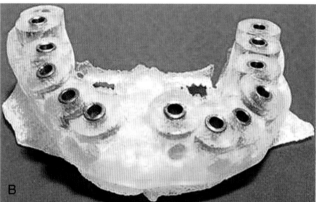

FIGURE 7-1 ■ A, B, Surgical templates can be fabricated and have been used to accurately place the implant during surgery.

manufactured from radiographic markers by using MRI and CT scans, and data from the study of the template images could be transferred to the laboratory for construction of a surgical template, enabling the surgeon to map implant sites three dimensionally.[5]

By 1998, the literature contained numerous studies on a variety of implant surgical template designs and imaging techniques for presurgical assessment of dental implant sites, but precision was not always reliable unless three-dimensional imaging techniques were used to develop the template. Some efforts to increase accuracy included the use of telescoping metal tubes as radiographic markers and as implant drill guides.[6]

By the end of the century, other attempts to increase the accuracy of templates included complementing the imaging techniques with a simple mechanical system to transfer a preoperatively defined implant position to the surgical site.[7] In such cases, bone availability was a concern in terms of placement and the final restorative prosthesis. Such use of the surgical template enabled precise placement in otherwise contraindicated anatomical sites, as well as elimination of manual errors. Evaluation of transfer error for the position of implants from imaging scans to a surgical template has been an ongoing concern, but patient outcomes regularly demonstrated that such errors were clinically irrelevant.[8]

The dental team approach is often at the heart of the use of the dental surgical template, especially in difficult cases involving grafted bone, in which precise implant placement is even more crucial than usual. For example, one method for ensuring accuracy involves the complementary use of Kirschner wires, inserted into the alveolar ridge through the mucosa before mucoperiosteal flap elevation to fixate the implant position and angulation.[9] Bone is exposed after the wires are inserted, and implant sites are prepared with a trephine drill guided by wires alone or by a special guidance cylinder.

Some practitioners have extended template technology to include reconstruction of the osseous support for a missing interdental papilla between adjacent implants by means of an interimplant papillary template—a first-stage titanium housing or stent that carried a bone grafting mixture to protect osteogenesis during healing, and to eliminate harvesting of oral bone.[10] Other innovations for ideal plate construction and sequence with larger, partially edentulous cases include a technique with a template constructed of hard acrylic with holes slightly larger than the 3.0-mm drill, commonly used for this surgery; with this technique, dentist and surgeon consultation precedes wax-up creation and implant location decisions before appliance construction.[11]

By the beginning of the new millennium, the literature contained general praise for how computer-guided surgery and computer-milled surgical templates could enable precise implant placement, planned and executed by an entire implant team.[12] Radiographic templates could be converted more easily into surgical templates using the information from tomogram analysis. Implant position and angulation were transferred to an indexed and sectioned cast, and realignment with the correct position allowed modification into a surgical template.[13] Such fabrication of a dual-purpose radiographic surgical template is accomplished by the transfer of radiographic information to the surgical template.[14] Typical steps include a prosthesis that is fabricated and duplicated in acrylic resin to serve as a scanning template. Axial images from a CT scan are transferred to software that provides real three-dimensional information to determine implant position. The planning software helps to determine implant size and any anatomical complications. The scanning template is drilled to reflect the planning and is used as a drilling and placement guide during surgery[15] (Figure 7-2).

Refinements of surgical template techniques include the increasing use of cone beam tomography instead of the relatively expensive and high radiation producing CT, enabling transfer of the preoperative implant axis planned on three-dimensional imagery to a surgical template.[16] Other benefits include those associated with the use of a precision template: flapless surgery, prosthesis preparation before surgery

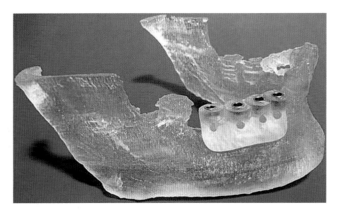

FIGURE 7-2 ■ Surgical template fabricated on a three-dimensional model of the mandible.

used for immediate loading, avoidance of critical anatomical structures, and elimination of errors associated with manual placement of implants.

Furthermore, because successful implant placement requires preoperative radiographic assessment of the topography of the mandible and maxilla, innovative radiopaque materials have been developed as radiographic markers instead of using traditional materials (such as barium sulfate and lead foil). For example, lipiodol ethiodized oil mixed with the monomer of autopolymerizing acrylic resin can yield an acrylic template that shows the contour of the future prosthesis, angulation of the future implant, and soft tissue thickness.[17] Because the template is transparent, it can be modified to become the surgical guide for implant placement and implant position registration during surgery. The simplicity of construction and low expense recommend it for routine dental implantation. Another technique uses a barium-coated template with external guide wires in conjunction with a CT scan and interactive software for diagnosis, treatment planning, and fabrication of a surgical template.[18] Additionally, surgical templates in dental implantology have been used effectively in conjunction with orthodontic procedures. Simple methods have been proposed to fabricate a surgical template that can provide good visual access, as well as flexibility for the clinician and template stability, especially for multidisciplinary cases that involve fixed orthodontic devices.[19] Finally, the reliability of surgical guides may be enhanced by the use of computer-aided rapid prototyping, although it has been acknowledged that better stability is needed during surgery in cases of unilateral bone–supported and non–tooth-supported guides[20] (Figure 7-3).

The current literature attests to the predictability of computer-aided implant surgery—a predictability that appears to justify the additional radiation dose, effort, and costs (e.g., CT imaging, fabrication of a registration template, intraoperative referencing for bur tracking, image-guided manufacturing of a surgical template) associated with the technique.[21]

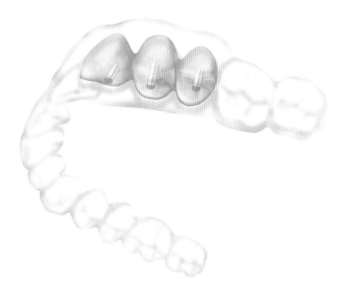

FIGURE 7-3 ▪ Radiograph markers can be incorporated into the surgical template. (Courtesy of Zimmer Dental. All rights reserved.)

Stability of the Surgical Template

One problematic area for the use of surgical templates involves the stability of the template during surgery, particularly in critical areas of function and esthetics. For example, a fixed surgical template using microimplants has been developed to facilitate the creation of a complete implant-supported prosthesis in the maxilla for a patient with slight resorption of the alveolar ridge and a high lip line.[22] Such cases require highly precise implant placement to ensure proper esthetics, phonetics, and function. The study compared a fixed surgical template versus a conventional movable surgical template, concluding that the fixed template offered considerably higher precision.[22]

Dental surgical templates can also be stabilized through the use of palatal implants to establish stationary anchorage. As with the placement of implants that eventually will receive restorations, use of a three-dimensional surgical template stabilized by palatal implants can help to eliminate faulty implant placement, reduce chair time, and minimize trauma to the tissues while enhancing osseointegration.[23] With yet another stabilization technique, surgical guides for edentulous patients can be stabilized to ensure accurate implant placement and predictable esthetic results through the use of transitional implants, which can guide placement of permanent implants.[24] Use of transitional implants for stabilization has been described as a simple, noninvasive, cost-effective technique for surgical template stabilization, because transitional implants can be placed the same day as the definitive implants.[25] During such procedures, transitional implants act, essentially, as surgical fixation screws to orient a surgical template predictably during the

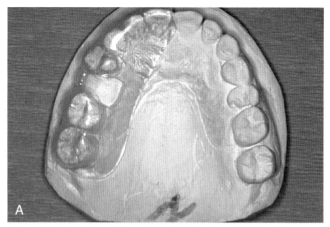

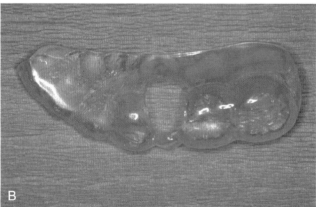

FIGURE 7-4 ▪ **A, B,** A vacuum–form template can be fabricated on the partially edentulous model that can be used at the time of surgery to determine the ideal mesiodistal, buccolingual, and long-axis orientation of the implant. However, when the opening is cut too large (as shown), the template provides minimal benefit.

placement of implants, for example, in the anterior mandible for an implant-supported bar-retained overdenture[26] (Figure 7-4).

Additional template accuracy techniques are often necessary for the positioning of implants in important areas such as the inferior alveolar nerve and the maxillary sinus. In such cases, a predictive equation can provide an extra margin of security.[27] The literature contains a report of a partial denture surgical template with a tube technique using a Coen's drill guide in combination with a mathematical equation to find the clinical-radiographic discrepancy to help ensure accuracy of placement.[27]

Although computer-assisted fabricated surgical templates are considered the static method for accurate placement of implants—as opposed to intraoperative image-guided navigation as the dynamic method (e.g., VectorVision2; BrainLAB, Heimstetten, Germany)—for transfer of three-dimensional preoperative planning, the former is still preferable because of the uncomplicated handling and low resource demands.[28]

The Edentulous Maxilla/ Mandible and Immediate Loading

Although surgical templates can be used effectively for the placement of single or multiple implants, they find their most popular use in the edentulous mandible and maxilla. For example, the technique of using a template to determine the angle and position of implants can be applied to the case of an anterior single-tooth implant, including the steps of using a pilot osteotomy and abutment guide.[29] Esthetics is a major concern in this area of dentition, and the template allows the dentist to assess and modify the angulation of the implant in the available space for restoration. Once angulation and sufficient room for the prosthesis are established with the use of the template, the surgeon can place the implant as planned.[29] Additionally, radiographic templates, diagnostic templates, and surgical templates are of particular importance in single-tooth and partially edentulous cases because of the crucial need to place the correct number of implants in the correct position and angulation to support the surrounding bone and proper esthetics.[30] So, placement of dental implants in the esthetic zone, particularly for a single tooth, can be one of the most challenging tests for clinicians because of the patient's esthetic needs, as well as the preexisting anatomy. Options for highly demanding surgical cases have been documented with the use of computer-guided implant placement and immediate provisionalization. Of particular concern with such techniques is making sure that implant placement and fixed restoration complement soft tissue esthetics.[31]

Nevertheless, it is in the edentulous patient that the surgical template finds its widest use. Precise placement of implants is particularly important for an implant-supported prosthesis, to provide functional and esthetic reconstruction in the challenging area of the edentulous anterior maxilla, where bone support can be problematic. Computed tomography and surgical guides can help to meet this challenge. The template can serve not only as a surgical guide but in preliminary work as a guide for radiographic evaluation, after which it is modified for surgery.[32]

The edentulous patient's need for immediate provisionalization and loading of implants is another reason why the surgical template has become popular in this area of implantology; in addition, immediate placement can be ideal for a patient with a nonrestorable dentition. In such cases, fabrication and use of a stable surgical template by means of staged tooth extraction can facilitate predictable immediate implant placement.[33] A variation of the surgical template can involve the use of three-dimensional planning software to fabricate a drilling template that contains high-precision drilling sleeves fitted on the jawbone; such a method can allow advance preparation of a fixed definitive prosthesis to be placed when surgery is complete.[34] Advantages of imme-

diate loading protocols with surgical templates include flapless surgery, predetermined placement of implants, and prefabricated provisional restorations, particularly in the maxilla, where bone availability is often challenging and failure rates for implants are higher.[35] Studies have indicated the clinical predictability of dental implant placement using an image-guided system to provide a patient implant in the maxilla. Steps include an acrylic template fabricated on a patient model, a software-produced treatment plan based on CT scans, and fabrication of the surgical template with the use of a dedicated drilling machine. During surgery, the template is used to drill the first osteotomy, then the template is removed for completion of osteotomy and standard implant placement.[36] In many cases, the edentulous maxilla can be restored via flapless surgery and immediate function by means of such systems as the Teeth-in-an-Hour concept (Nobel Biocare AB, Goteborg, Sweden); this process can be successful not only for fully edentulous patients, but also for those with staged surgery and partial edentulism.[37] In some cases of immediate loading of the edentulous maxilla, the immediate provisional prosthesis can be used as a surgical and restorative guide[38] (Figure 7-5).

For immediate restoration, the steps taken when a surgical template and a fabricated provisional restoration are used include determining the mesiodistal inclination of the implant, the buccolingual dimension of the alveolar ridge, and the proper position of the implant; fabricating the surgical guide, and the provisional restoration; and placing the implant implants and provisional restoration.[39] Immediate loading in the mandible can require a five-step procedure: (1) building a scannographic template, (2) performing a CT scan, (3) planning an implant with the use of SurgiCase software (Materialise NV, Leuven, Belgium), (4) placing an

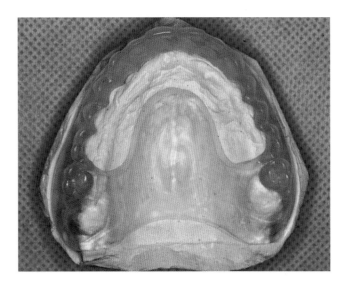

FIGURE 7-5 ■ The acrylic material in the palate gives the surgical template the proper stability, especially in an edentulous anterior ridge. Again, when the opening is too large, the benefit is minimized.

implant with the use of a drill guide created by stereolithography, and (5) placing the prosthesis, with definitive restoration after 3 months.[40] Immediate loading of the edentulous mandible using a surgical template has become a popular option.[41]

Teeth-in-an-Hour (Nobel Biocare, Yorba Linda, CA) dental implants for edentulous patients represents an increasingly popular choice. Immediately loaded implants are placed with a computer-aided design (CAD)/computer-aided manufacturing (CAM)-derived surgical template using a flapless surgical technique, then are loaded with a prefabricated restorative prosthesis.[42] Such techniques utilize the implant-retained overdenture in a technique for the fabrication of a surgical template for an implant-retained overdenture in the mandible.[43] So, for completely edentulous patients, the advantages of a surgical template include flapless surgery and use of a transitional prosthesis that is fabricated before surgery; an image-guided system fabricates a surgical guide based on a preoperative three-dimensional plan for accurately placing implants in bone.[44]

Surgical Templates: An Overview

The dental implant surgeon can use a surgical template as a positional guide for implant placement to determine ideal mesiodistal, buccolingual, and long-axis orientations of the implant. To be effective, surgical templates must be designed to provide stability and proper orientation after the tissue flaps have been raised. If lack of available bone or nonoptimal anatomical structures prevent ideal placement, long-axis orientation can be altered. In that case, the surgeon can choose a secondary site and can implement a backup treatment plan to place the implants in predetermined alternative sites. On the other hand, the surgeon may elect to place no implants if the required number, location, or axial orientation of the implants cannot be achieved, and such a situation will preclude the successful completion of the prosthetic reconstruction dictated by the treatment plan. Surgical templates can be traditionally fabricated for fully edentulous or for partially edentulous patients. Several computerized fabrication methods are available.

Surgical Templates for Fully Edentulous Patients

The traditional fabrication of surgical templates for fully edentulous patients should follow these steps:

1. The diagnostic denture wax-up: the patient's existing denture should be duplicated in crystal clear acrylic (Figure 7-6).
2. The palate and/or flange areas in the areas where the tissue flaps will be located should be removed to avoid impinging or compressing of the flaps to ensure proper orientation and stability of the stent (Figure 7-7).
3. The occlusal halves of the acrylic teeth should be removed to determine the mesiodistal and buccolingual orientation and to allow the drill access to the bone (Figure 7-8).

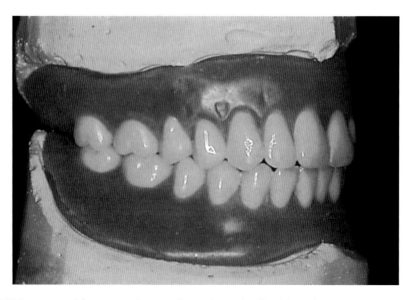

FIGURE 7-6 ■ For fabrication of surgical templates for the fully edentulous patient, a denture waxup should be used. The waxup denture should be duplicated in clear acrylic as a guide for implant placement.

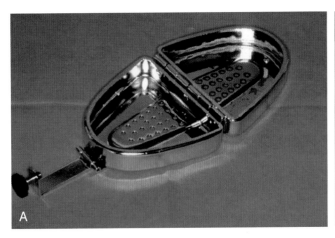
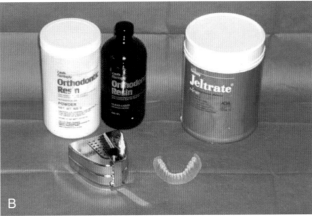

FIGURE 7-7 ■ **A,** Either the laboratory can duplicate a patient's denture waxup or it can be done in the office using a commercially available denture duplicator. **B,** Clear orthodontic resin can be used to duplicate the diagnostic denture waxup or the patient's existing denture. Ensure that the denture will fit within the borders.

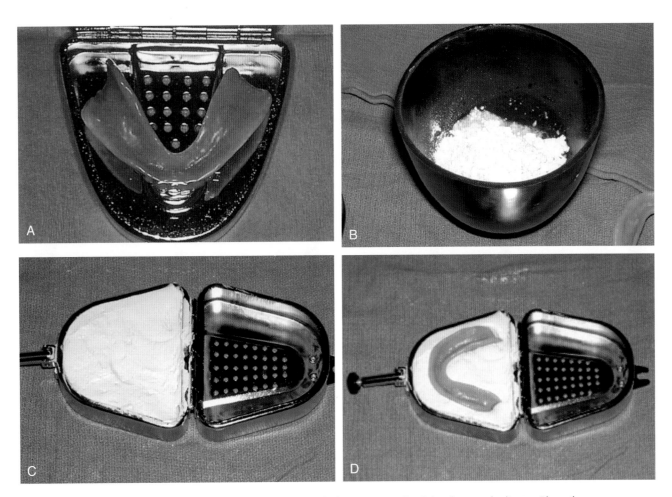

FIGURE 7-8 ■ **A-N,** Mix alginate material and place in one side of the denture duplicator. Place the denture to be duplicated into the alginate. With a wet finger, smooth out the impression material from the borders of the denture to the rim of the flask. Spray the denture and the impression material with silicone. Place impression material in the upper half of the flask. Use the rest of the impression material and carefully place alginate into the base of the denture in the lower half of the flask. With steady pressure, close the flask, secure the thumbscrew, and allow the material to set. Open the flask slowly. Fill in with clear orthodontic resin and close the flask tightly until the resin sets. Then open the flask and remove the clear acrylic.

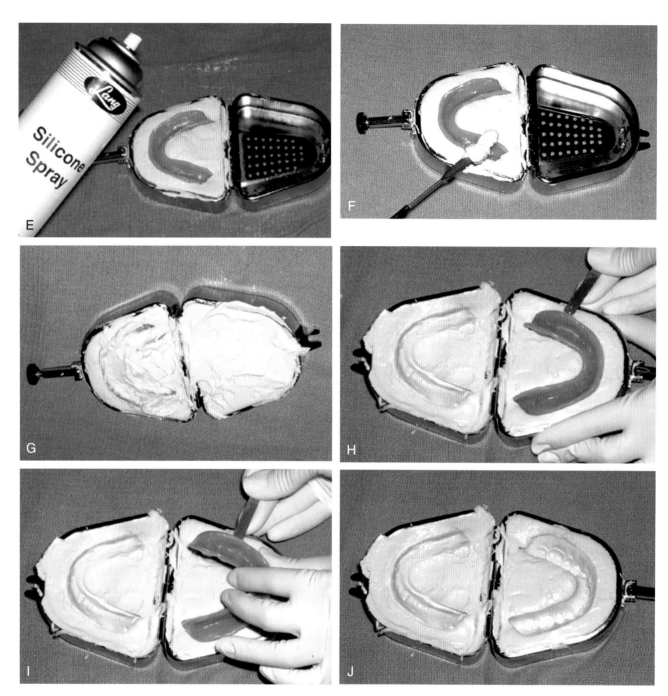

FIGURE 7-8, cont'd.

4. Holes should be drilled through the acrylic in the areas where implant placement is desired, with the use of a drill with the same diameter as the final surgical spade drill. As an alternative, a slot, rather than individual holes, can be placed in the template. The slots allow greater latitude in placement as compared with the holes.

Surgical Templates for Partially Edentulous Patients

Traditional fabrication of surgical templates for partially edentulous patients can follow one of two methods.

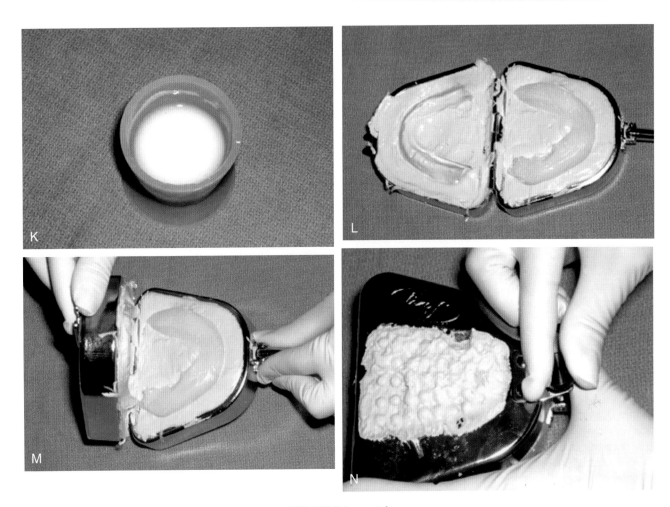

FIGURE 7-8, cont'd.

Method I

In this method, the patient's existing partial denture should be duplicated in crystal clear acrylic using a denture-duplicating flask as mentioned above. Then the areas of the surgical template that will impinge or compress tissue flaps should be removed to ensure proper orientation and stability of the stent. Next, if necessary, a sufficient area of the occlusal halves of the acrylic teeth should be removed to provide adequate access to the bone for the drill. Then, holes should be drilled through the acrylic in the areas where implant placement is desired, by using a drill with the same diameter as the final surgical spade drill.

Method II

In this second method, based on study models made from impressions of the patient's existing dentition, the teeth (or denture teeth) should be hand-waxed in the edentulous areas where implants are to be placed in occlusion with the opposing dentition. An impression of the study model should be made to produce a stone model, and then a 0.2-mm-thick temporary splint material should be vacuum-formed over the study model by means of a vacuum-forming machine and trimmed to the vestibules in the edentulous areas and to the height of contour on the existing teeth. The temporary splint material should be removed from the model. Areas where the tissue flaps will be raised should be removed to prevent impingement and compression of the tissue, which would prevent the proper orientation and stability of the stent. Next, holes should be drilled through the plastic form in the areas where implant placement is desired.

Computerized Surgical Template Systems

Computerized surgical template systems include the Compu-Guide Surgical Template System (Implant Logic Systems Ltd, Cedarhurst, NY), the SimPlant-SurgiGuide (Materialise NV), and the NobelGuide (Nobel Biocare USA LLC, Yorba Linda, CA).

The Compu-Guide Surgical Template System

According to the company literature, the Compu-Guide Surgical Template System takes the guesswork out of implant dentistry and offers many advantages over traditional implant surgery.

Specific advantages for the clinician include a more efficient, minimally invasive surgery. The precise implant placement helps to ensure that there are no surprises at the time of surgery; additionally, the system offers accurate immediate-load prosthetics. Advantages for the patient include less surgical trauma (because of the minimally invasive surgery and precise implant placement) and, as a direct consequence, less pain and faster healing times.

With this system, diagnostic casts are made by the doctor and are sent to Implant Logic Systems (Figure 7-9, A). A diagnostic waxup is performed there (Figure 7-9, B). Implant Logic Systems fabricates a CT scan appliance (Figure 7-9, C), and then a CT scan is taken with the patient wearing the CT scan appliance. The implant surgeon and the restorative doctor then create a SimPlant Plan (The SimPlant Academy, Leuven, Belgium; Figure 7-9, D). The CT scan appliance and the SimPlant Plan are sent to Implant Logic Systems for computer milling (Figure 7-9, E). The computer-milled appliance is converted into a Compu-Guide Surgical Template according to the SimPlant specifications (Figure 7-9, F).

The Compu-Guide Surgical Templates for this system include the basic, advanced, and temporary. The Compu-Guide Basic Template features a set of fixed-size drill guides used to create 2-mm pilot osteotomies with the exact location, angle, and depth as planned on the CT surgical simulation software. The Basic Template is shipped with a drilling report, which indicates the appropriate drilling depth for each of the implants.

The Compu-Guide Advanced Template uses a set of interchangeable, incrementally sized drill guide inserts to rigidly guide all the osteotomies necessary for complete implant placement, from the initial pilot osteotomy to the final placement of the implant through the template. The osteotomies will be made in the exact location, angle, and depth as planned on the CT surgical simulation software. A drilling report is supplied, which indicates the appropriate drilling depth for each implant.

The Compu-Temp Template can be fabricated optionally in a tooth-colored acrylic from basic or advanced surgical templates. After the surgical procedure has been completed, the surgeon can easily convert this surgical template into the provisional restoration.

SurgiGuides: The Bone-Supported Concept

The SimPlant-SurgiGuide concept converts the simulated implant's exact dimensions, including width, angulation, and depth, to a surgical guide. This SurgiGuide is made through a stereolithography process and is custom manufactured for each patient. During the operation, the SurgiGuide is placed on the jawbone (bone-supported SurgiGuide), on the mucosa (mucosa-supported SurgiGuide), or on the teeth (tooth-supported SurgiGuide). The SurgiGuide guides the surgeon's drill to the planned implant location. The surgeon places the implants into the drilled holes.

SurgiGuide types include the following: tooth-supported, bone-supported, mucosa-supported, and special implants. A tooth-supported SurgiGuide is a custom-manufactured drill guide made for a unique and stable fit on the remaining teeth; it guides the drill exactly to the planned position even if only a single tooth is missing. Tooth-supported SurgiGuides are indicated for surgery on partially edentulous patients. Tooth-supported SurgiGuides are perfect for minimally invasive surgery. Because all the planning has been done beforehand and the bone has been evaluated extensively, it is not necessary to make a bone flap to insert the drill and the implants. A small punched hole through the mucosa is sufficient to position the implants accurately. The user needs to send a plaster cast of the presurgical tooth situation to Materialise, together with the SimPlant plan. Materialise uses both pieces of information to produce an accurate SurgiGuide that fits onto the teeth in a unique and stable way and transfers the implant planning into the real surgery. This procedure allows some limited scatter in the CT images from teeth fillings or brackets.

A bone-supported SurgiGuide is a custom-manufactured drill guide made for a unique and stable fit on the jawbone of the patient. This type of SurgiGuide can be used for patients with edentulous and partially edentulous jaws. During surgery, a ridge incision is made, and mucoperiosteal flaps are raised to free the bone surface. The SurgiGuide is placed on the bone surface in the unique and stable position for which it was created, and it guides the drill into the planned position. Raising of the mucoperiosteal flaps also enables good visibility during the operation.

The mucosa-supported SurgiGuide is a custom-manufactured drill guide made for a unique and stable fit on the soft tissue of the patient's jaw. This type of SurgiGuide can be used for patients with edentulous jaws. A scan of the patient together with a scan prosthesis is obligatory. This also helps the clinician to visualize clearly the desired tooth setup on CT images for improved implant planning. During surgery, the SurgiGuide is placed on the soft tissue in the unique and stable position for which it was created; it guides the drill into the planned position. This technique leads to minimally invasive surgery.

The special implant SurgiGuide is a custom-manufactured drill guide used for placement of special implants, such as zygoma implants; bone-supported and mucosa-supported SurgiGuides for special implants can be manufactured. Good positioning and small angle deviation of these types of implants are extremely important. The preoperative planning is translated to the surgery by the

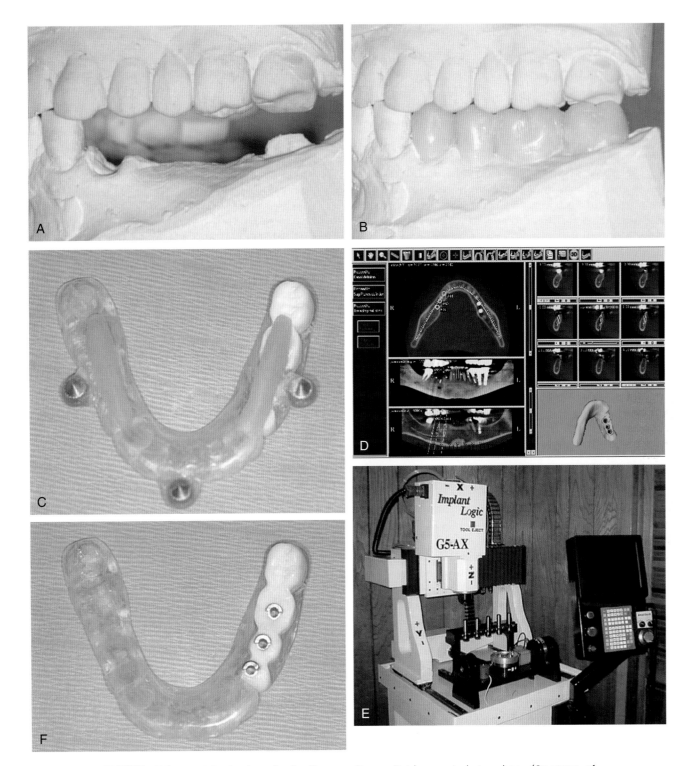

FIGURE 7-9 ■ A-F, Implant Logic System Compu-Guide surgical template. (Courtesy of BioHorizons.)

use of a SurgiGuide, to obtain the best possible results for implant placement. A model with color-planned implants is delivered together with the SurgiGuide. In this way, the surgeon can check and verify the planning and fit of the SurgiGuide.

NobelGuide

Nobel Biocare's NobelGuide is a planning and surgical concept that allows dentists to place implants in a single visit, so the patient leaves the office with a fully functioning tooth or teeth. NobelGuide uses Nobel Biocare's Procera surgical planning software and flapless surgery, alternatively described as "keyhole surgery." Using Procera software, dentists can plan complete implant treatment (number, length, and angulation).

CT or a plaster model taken of the patient's teeth and mouth provides the basis for determining the bone's shape and location. Planning data allow Nobel Biocare or a dental laboratory to create a surgical template, permitting less invasive, flapless surgery. The surgical template, secured over the patient's soft tissue, allows the dentist to drill directly into the bone through the soft tissue through guide holes. Teamwork between the dentist and the lab enables those using the NobelGuide to provide patients with a temporary or a final prosthetic solution once the implants are placed. These options can cut the conventional methods for implant placement and teeth restoration in half, from 10 patient visits to as few as 4.

How NobelGuide works:
1. The patient receives a CT scan, or a model of the mouth is created.
2. Aided by these complete views of the patient's bone structure, the dentist can use the Procera software system to derive a plan for implant placement, including the optimal length and angle of the implants.
3. A surgical template is fabricated, based on the Nobel Biocare CT data scans or on the dental laboratory's plaster model.
4. A temporary or permanent crown or bridge is prepared by the dental laboratory.
5. During surgery, the surgical template is used to place the implants and install the temporary or permanent restoration.

NobelGuide allows the simultaneous placement of implant, abutment, and restorative crown or bridge; furthermore, conventional or computer-aided three-dimensional design can be used to construct the surgical template to place implants in the exact position and depth needed for completion of the restorative plan.

SUMMARY

The implant dentist must consider a number of different factors when computer-aided surgical templates become a viable option in his or her practice. Implants can be placed precisely with surgical templates, but CT scanning, template manufacture, and template-guided surgery often lead to expenses well beyond those of conventional implant placement practice. The clinician must weigh the detriments of increased cost and time versus the benefits of significant error reduction and reliability in the placement of functional and esthetically pleasing implants. The weighing of detriments and benefits is particularly crucial when surgical templates are considered for use in esthetically critical areas, such as the edentulous maxilla, when immediate provisionalization and prosthodontic therapy are considered.

REFERENCES

1. Zinner ID, Small SA, Panno FV: Presurgical prosthetics and surgical templates, *Dent Clin North Am* 33(4):619-633, 1989. Review.
2. Modica F, Fava C, Benech A, Preti G: Radiologic-prosthetic planning of the surgical phase of the treatment of edentulism by osseointegrated implants: an in vitro study, *J Prosthet Dent* 65(4):541-546, 1991.
3. Besimo C, Lambrecht JT, Nidecker A: Dental implant treatment planning with reformatted computed tomography, *Dentomaxillofac Radiol* 24(4):264-267, 1995.
4. Gray CF, Redpath TW, Smith FW: Pre-surgical dental implant assessment by magnetic resonance imaging, *J Oral Implantol* 22(2):147-153, 1996.
5. Higginbottom FL, Wilson TG Jr: Three-dimensional templates for placement of root-form dental implants: a technical note, *Int J Oral Maxillofac Implants* 11(6):787-793, 1996.
6. Mizrahi B, Thunthy KH, Finger I: Radiographic/surgical template incorporating metal telescopic tubes for accurate implant placement, *Pract Periodontics Aesthet Dent* 10(6):757-765, 1998; quiz 766.
7. Fortin T, Champleboux G, Lormee J, Coudert JL: Precise dental implant placement in bone using surgical guides in conjunction with medical imaging techniques, *J Oral Implantol* 26(4):300-303, 2000.
8. Besimo CE, Lambrecht JT, Guindy JS: Accuracy of implant treatment planning utilizing template-guided reformatted computed tomography, *Dentomaxillofac Radiol* 29(1):46-51, 2000.
9. Minoretti R, Merz BR, Triaca A: Predetermined implant positioning by means of a novel guide template technique, *Clin Oral Implants Res* 11(3):266-272, 2000.
10. el-Salam el-Askary A: Inter-implant papilla reconstruction by means of a titanium guide, *Implant Dent* 9(1):85-89, 2000.
11. Small BW: Surgical templates for function and esthetics in dental implants, *Gen Dent* 49(1):30-32, 34, 2001.
12. Klein M, Abrams M: Computer-guided surgery utilizing a computer-milled surgical template, *Pract Proced Aesthet Dent* 13(2):165-169, 2001; quiz 170.
13. Sykaras N, Woody RD: Conversion of an implant radiographic template into a surgical template, *J Prosthodont* 10(2):108-112, 2001.
14. Wat PY, Chow TW, Luk HW, Comfort MB: Precision surgical template for implant placement: a new systematic approach, *Clin Implant Dent Relat Res* 4(2):88-92, 2002.
15. Fortin T, Bosson JL, Coudert JL, Isidori M: Reliability of preoperative planning of an image-guided system for oral implant placement based on 3-dimensional images: an in vivo study, *Int J Oral Maxillofac Implants* 18(6):886-893, 2003.
16. Fortin T, Champleboux G, Bianchi S, Buatois H, Coudert JL: Precision of transfer of preoperative planning for oral implants based on cone-beam CT-scan images through a robotic drilling machine, *Clin Oral Implants Res* 13(6):651-656, 2002.
17. Siu AS, Li TK, Chu FC, Comfort MB, Chow TW: The use of lipiodol in spiral tomography for dental implant imaging, *Implant Dent* 12(1):35-40, 2003.
18. Kopp KC, Koslow AH, Abdo OS: Predictable implant placement with a diagnostic/surgical template and advanced radiographic imaging, *J Prosthet Dent* 89(6):611-615, 2003.
19. Sukotjo C, Bocage V: Simplified fabrication of surgical template for orthodontic-implant treatment, *J Prosthodont* 15(1):59-61, 2006.

20. Di Giacomo GA, Cury PR, de Araujo NS, Sendyk WR, Sendyk CL: Clinical application of stereolithographic surgical guides for implant placement: preliminary results, *J Periodontol* 76(4):503-507, 2005.
21. Widmann G, Bale RJ: Accuracy in computer-aided implant surgery—a review, *Int J Oral Maxillofac Implants* 21(2):305-313, 2006.
22. Sicilia A, Enrile FJ, Buitrago P, Zubizarreta J: Evaluation of the precision obtained with a fixed surgical template in the placement of implants for rehabilitation of the completely edentulous maxilla: a clinical report, *Int J Oral Maxillofac Implants* 15(2):272-277, 2000.
23. Tosun T, Keles A, Erverdi N: Method for the placement of palatal implants, *Int J Oral Maxillofac Implants* 17(1):95-100, 2002.
24. Simon H: Use of transitional implants to support a surgical guide: enhancing the accuracy of implant placement, *J Prosthet Dent* 87(2):229-232, 2002.
25. Aalam AA, Reshad M, Chee WW, Nowzari H: Surgical template stabilization with transitional implants in the treatment of the edentulous mandible: a technical note, *Int J Oral Maxillofac Implants* 20(3):462-465, 2005.
26. Yeh S, Monaco EA, Buhite RJ: Using transitional implants as fixation screws to stabilize a surgical template for accurate implant placement: a clinical report, *J Prosthet Dent* 93(6):509-513, 2005.
27. Pramono C: Surgical technique for achieving implant parallelism and measurement of the discrepancy in panoramic radiograph, *J Oral Maxillofac Surg* 64(5):799-803, 2006.
28. Mischkowski RA, Zinser MJ, Neugebauer J, Kubler AC, Zoller JE: Comparison of static and dynamic computer-assisted guidance methods in implantology, *Int J Comput Dent* 9(1):23-35, 2006. English, German.
29. Shepherd NJ, Morgan VJ, Chapman RJ: Angulation assessment of anterior single tooth root form implants: technical note, *Implant Dent* 4(1):52-54, 1995.
30. Meijer HJ, Batenburg RH, Wietsma AK, Reintsema H, Raghoebar GM: Templates as an aid in implantology, *Ned Tijdschr Tandheelkd* 105(7):238-241, 1998. Dutch.
31. Sudbrink SD: Computer-guided implant placement with immediate provisionalization: a case report, *J Oral Maxillofac Surg* 63(6):771-774, 2005.
32. Cehreli MC, Sahin S: Fabrication of a dual-purpose surgical template for correct labiopalatal positioning of dental implants, *Int J Oral Maxillofac Implants* 15(2):278-282, 2000.

33. Al-Harbi SA, Verrett RG: Fabrication of a stable surgical template using staged tooth extraction for immediate implant placement, *J Prosthet Dent* 94(4):394-397, 2005.
34. van Steenberghe D, Naert I, Andersson M, Brajnovic I, Van Cleynenbreugel J, Suetens P: A custom template and definitive prosthesis allowing immediate implant loading in the maxilla: a clinical report, *Int J Oral Maxillofac Implants* 17(5):663-670, 2002.
35. Rocci A, Martignoni M, Gottlow J: Immediate loading in the maxilla using flapless surgery, implants placed in predetermined positions, and prefabricated provisional restorations: a retrospective 3-year clinical study, *Clin Implant Dent Relat Res* 5(suppl 1):29-36, 2003.
36. Blanchet E, Lucchini JP, Jenny R, Fortin T. An image-guided system based on custom templates: case reports, *Clin Implant Dent Relat Res* 6(1):40-47, 2004.
37. van Steenberghe D, Glauser R, Blomback U, Andersson M, Schutyser F, Pettersson A, Wendelhag I: A computed tomographic scan-derived customized surgical template and fixed prosthesis for flapless surgery and immediate loading of implants in fully edentulous maxillae: a prospective multicenter study, *Clin Implant Dent Relat Res* 7(suppl 1):S111-S120, 2005.
38. Cooper L, De Kok IJ, Reside GJ, Pungpapong P, Rojas-Vizcaya F: Immediate fixed restoration of the edentulous maxilla after implant placement, *J Oral Maxillofac Surg* 63(9 suppl 2):97-110, 2005. Review.
39. Di Sario F: A system for the diagnosis, placement, and prosthetic restoration of root form implants (U.S. Patent #5,769,636), *J Prosthodont* 12(1):2-7, 2003.
40. Tardieu PB, Vrielinck L, Escolano E: Computer-assisted implant placement. A case report: treatment of the mandible, *Int J Oral Maxillofac Implants* 18(4):599-604, 2003.
41. Pontual MA, Freire JN, Souza DC, Ferreira CF, Bianchini MA, Magini RS: A newly designed template device for use with the insertion of immediately loaded implants, *J Oral Implantol* 30(5):325-329, 2004.
42. Marchack CB: An immediately loaded CAD/CAM-guided definitive prosthesis: a clinical report, *J Prosthet Dent* 93(1):8-12, 2005.
43. Fakhry A: Fabrication of a surgical template for implant/bar-retained mandibular overdentures, *Int J Periodontics Restorative Dent* 25(4):401-407, 2005.
44. Fortin T, Isidori M, Blanchet E, Perriat M, Bouchet H, Coudert JL: An image-guided system-drilled surgical template and trephine guide pin to make treatment of completely edentulous patients easier: a clinical report on immediate loading, *Clin Implant Dent Relat Res* 6(2):111-119, 2004.

chapter 8

Generalized Surgical Technique for Endosseous Root-Form Implants

THE DESIGN, diameter, length, and quantity of implants will depend on the quality of available bone, the quantity of available bone, the location of available bone, and the type of prosthodontic application desired (Figure 8-1).

For stage 1 surgery, determine the anatomy of the available bone with the use of adequate radiographs, palpation, and direct visual inspection of the prospective implant site. Before you begin the dental implant procedure, establish the anatomical features that should be avoided. After proper aseptic technique, anesthetize the patient using routine procedures. Generally, when an implant is placed in the posterior mandible, infiltration into the buccal and lingual is used without the use of a block anesthesia.

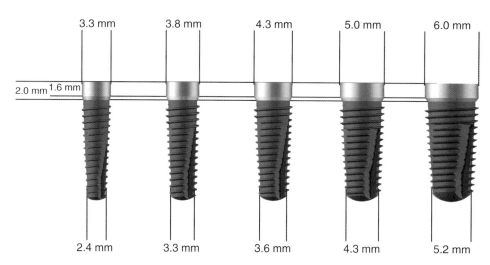

FIGURE 8-1 ■ Selecting the correct implant diameter is important before beginning the surgery. (Courtesy of Camlog.)

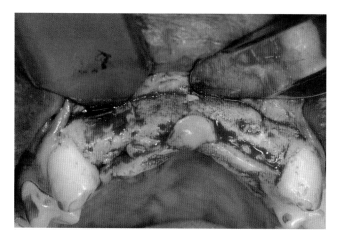

FIGURE 8-2 ■ The flap and incision design should be long enough to allow for an ample view of the surgical site.

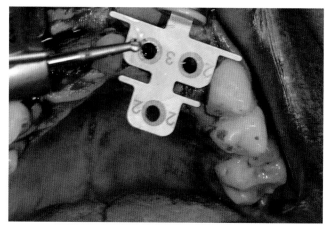

FIGURE 8-3 ■ Maintain a minimum of 3 mm from the implant to the natural tooth for optimum osseointegration.

Incision Design

Make an incision mesiodistally along the buccal side of the alveolar crest that extends through the mucoperiosteum and attached gingiva down to the bone. Flap and incision designs can vary because of the anatomical locations of the implant placement and remaining dentition. However, the incision should be long enough to permit adequate reflection of the flap without tearing the tissue and should provide an adequate view and access to the surgical site. Occasionally, a vertical releasing incision may be necessary. While using a sharp periosteal elevator, carefully reflect and lift the periosteum to expose the alveolar bone as necessary to provide an adequate surgical working area (Figure 8-2).

Use retractors or sutures to hold the tissues, and remove any sharp areas of the ridge or other bone irregularities with a large round or pear-shaped bur in a surgical drill. Alternatively, the rongeur forceps can be used to create as flat a bone plateau as possible (Figure 8-3).

Try to keep bone removal to a minimum in stage 1 surgery. The width of the ridge should allow at least 1 mm of bone to remain buccal to the implant and at least 1 mm lingual to the implant after placement. To optimize osseointegration, maintain a minimum of 3 mm to 6 mm (edge-to-edge) between implants, and a minimum of 3 mm from the edge of the adjacent natural dentition. Determine the appropriate length of the implant according to the occlusoapical height of the bone present. Palpate the ridge contour adequately to estimate an angle of insertion that will achieve parallelism not only with the other implants and natural tooth abutments, but with the angulation of the bone present and the opposing arch (Figure 8-4).

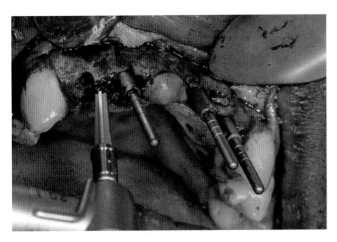

FIGURE 8-4 ▪ The osteotomy is enlarged by utilizing sequentially larger diameter burs.

Implant Handpiece Usage and Irrigation

Minimize the potential for overheating the bone by using a low-speed, high-torque, internally irrigated handpiece. Overheating the bone results in a layer of nonvital cells adjacent to the implant and possible fibrous encapsulation and loss of the implant. Appropriate speeds for commercially available implant systems vary but generally are in the range of 800 to 2,000 rpm. Use the appropriate speed to minimize excessive heat generation and to preserve the vitality of bone that is in contact with the implant.

Use profuse internal and/or external irrigation to keep the drill from clogging and to maintain minimal heating of the bone. To minimize the chance of overheating the bone, refrigerate the sterile saline bag before surgery; patients do not have a problem accepting this temperature of irrigation at the time of surgery. In addition, to accommodate external irrigation and to supplement internal irrigation, use several sterile saline-filled syringes.

Before drilling, confirm the accurate selections of proper implant body size and location. Do all drilling, particularly with the intermediate and final diameter drills, using a straight up-and-down motion to avoid creating an oval-shaped osteotomy site (Figure 8-5). To penetrate the dense cortical ridge crest, prepare a pilot hole using an extremely sharp, efficient, and relatively small-diameter pilot drill. This pilot hole establishes the ultimate location and angle of the implant, so prepare it with a surgical template, keeping in mind the complete prosthodontic treatment plan. Check and ensure the proper angulations. A drill extension is usually available to extend the cutting length if additional drill length is required and can be used with any standard latch-lock drill. It is important to clean the drill head often to remove debris and ensure a sharp cutting surface. Because of the dense bone in the symphysis, it is usually advisable to use a newer drill rather than a previously used and sterilized

one. Rotate the previously used and sterilized drill to the maxilla, where the bone is generally less dense.

Preparation of the Implant Bed

Prepare the implant bed in a clear field to allow the operator to view the actual site at all times to properly prepare and fit the implant. Keeping in mind the importance of the pilot hole, use an internally irrigated pilot drill to create a well-defined pilot hole of appropriate depth for the implant system. This depth corresponds to the length of the drill flutes. To establish parallelism and draw among implants, prepare the first pilot hole to the appropriate depth (Figure 8-6). Flush the pilot hole to remove bone debris. Insert into the prepared osteotomy site a paralleling instrument that corresponds in size to the pilot drill. Leave the paralleling instrument in the first pilot hole and move on to the next preparation, while referring to angularity and draw requirements established by the first implant site preparation (Figure 8-7, *A*). Continue to use the surgical template as a guide until all pilot holes have been drilled, leaving a paralleling instrument in each site as it is completed. Check each paralleling instrument for proper angulation before proceeding with the drill of next diameter (Figure 8-7, *B*). Use the internally irrigated intermediate drill to make a channel of the proper depth. Use an appropriate full-diameter final drill to complete the implant site preparation at each location. The diameter and length of each final drill must correspond to the specific implant body size. Be sure to use copious amounts of sterile saline and a low-speed drilling process in this step to prevent bone overheating and possible necrosis (Figure 8-8). Complete the final drilling using a straight up-and-down motion to avoid creating an oval-shaped site.

Refer to the surgical manual for the steps associated with a specific implant type.

Irrigate the completed implant receptor site with additional sterile saline. A depth gauge can be used to check the dimensions of the osteotomy. After placement of the implant, take a radiograph to check the implant placement. Carefully reposition the mucoperiosteal flap for maximum tissue adaptation, and then suture. Suturing materials and techniques are discussed in the following chapter.

Postoperative Course

Instruct the patient to follow a postsurgical regimen that includes biting firmly but gently on a gauze pad to stop the bleeding for about 15 to 30 minutes and using cold packs for the first 12 to 24 hours. Heat should be applied starting the following day and then for the next 12 to 24 hours. To minimize swelling and bleeding, the patient may want to keep the head elevated for the first 24 to 48 hours after surgery.

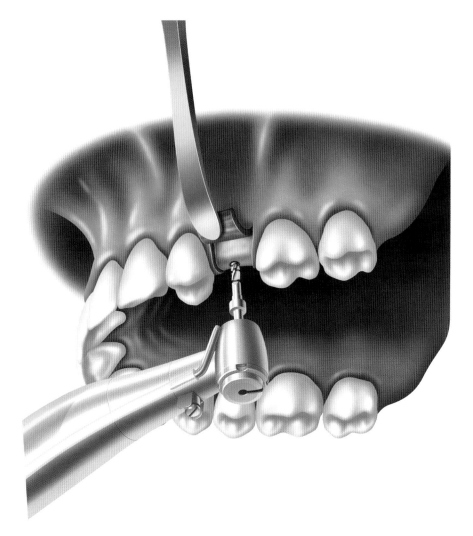

FIGURE 8-5 ■ Perform all drill procedures with a straight up-and-down motion to avoid creation of an oval osteotomy site. (Courtesy of Zimmer Dental. All rights reserved.)

Patients must make sure they relax as much as possible and avoid all strenuous activities for as long as 3 days following the dental implant surgery. They have to drink at least 8 glasses of water or fruit juice every day and should try to limit the diet to soft foods such as yogurt or soup during the first week of surgery. Patients should be asked to rinse their mouth with warm salt water solution—1 teaspoon of salt in 1 cup of water—about 3 to 4 times a day to further disinfect the area, starting on the day following the surgery. The patient has to make sure to spit carefully to avoid complications.

Prescribe the antibiotics of choice if necessary. Remove the sutures after 1 to 2 weeks. Relieve any removable prosthesis resting on the implant, and reline it using a soft tissue conditioner reline material (Lynal), encouraging the patient not to use the prosthesis for the first week. For the first 2 weeks postoperatively, a liquid or soft diet and saline mouth rinses should be prescribed. Depending on the patient's bone quality and quantity, allow a bonding period of bone to implant of approximately 3 to 4 months for the man-

dible and 5 to 6 months for the maxilla. It is important to leave the implants unloaded during the bonding period for optimum integration.

Exposure of the Implants

After the bonding period, uncover the implant healing screw (this is discussed in greater detail in a subsequent chapter). The location can be determined by palpating the soft tissue or using a periodontal probe. To surgically expose the cover screw, use a tissue punch (one-time use only) or a scalpel, taking care to preserve an adequate amount of keratinized gingiva. Remove the cover screw with the appropriate instrument. It is absolutely imperative that all bone and soft tissue be removed from the superior aspect of the implant body to guarantee complete seating of the abutment, because the presence of tissue or bone fragments between the implant and the abutment can lead to abutment loosening. Do not

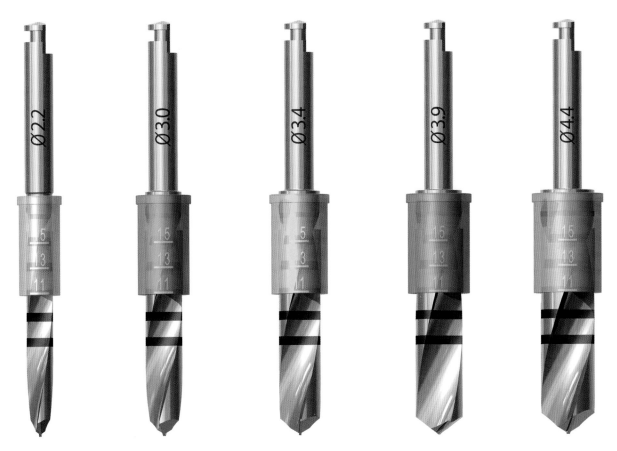

FIGURE 8-6 ■ Sterile stop drills are designed in different lengths and diameters to help you measure the correct osteotomy length and are critical for accuracy. (Courtesy of Neoss.)

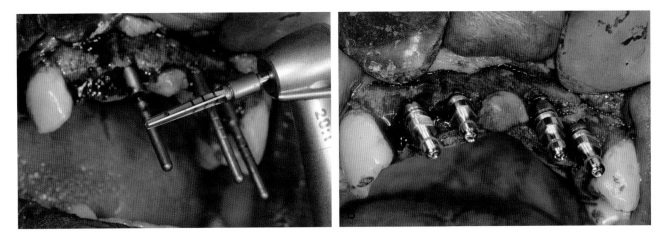

FIGURE 8-7 ■ **A, B,** When placing multiple implants, parallel pins should be used to verify the angle of the osteotomy.

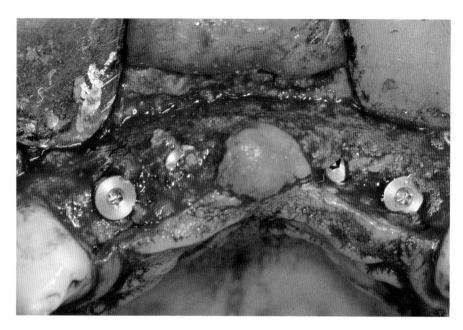

FIGURE 8-8 ■ After the osteotomy is done, make sure there is no tissue granulation on or in the site.

use a bur or other drilling instruments that can compromise the integrity of the implant or its coating. Screw the titanium healing collar cuff into the implant body and perform the final suturing. Restoration usually begins after the soft tissues have healed, generally 2 to 6 weeks later.

SUMMARY

The surgical techniques required to place dental implants are highly specialized and complex. Practitioners should attend courses on established techniques of oral implantology to avoid improper techniques that can cause implant failure and bone loss. Commercially available dental implants are intended to be used only with specially designed bone drills supplied in each particular kit and in accordance with strict manufacturers' guidelines for the particular system.

Excessive bone loss or infection may indicate implant failure. Remove as soon as possible any implant that shows signs of failure. In addition, if the implant becomes mobile at any point, it should be removed. If removal is necessary, curette the soft tissue from the implant site and allow the site to heal as if it were an atraumatic extraction.

By carefully following the instructions and using good surgical techniques, complications can be kept to a minimum. The following complications related to surgical procedure, although rare, can occur: dehiscence, delayed healing, paresthesia, hyperesthesia, edema, hematoma, infection, inflammation, and local and generalized allergic reaction. Therefore, it is important to be well versed in the placement and restoration of dental implants, as well as in the management of potential complications.

chapter 9

Wound Healing and Suturing Techniques in Dental Implant Surgery

SPECIFIC KNOWLEDGE OF THE WOUND HEALING PROCESS, as well as techniques in suturing and surgical knotting, must become part of the repertoire of many dental surgical clinicians, in particular, the implantologist. Over the past decade, plastic surgery techniques and materials have become more and more applicable to implant surgery.[1-4] The evolution in our understanding of wounds and wound treatment, as well as standard—and changing—availability of suturing materials, requires that surgeons have familiarity with surgical procedures essential for proper wound closure to decrease the potential for postoperative infection and to increase the successful esthetic and functional outcomes of implant surgery.[5]

Surgical Wounds and Wound Healing

A clear understanding of surgical wounds necessitates a discussion of types of wounds and wound healing, the wound healing process, and complications affecting the proper healing of wounds.

Types of Wounds and Wound Healing

Surgical wounds can be classified into four categories, based on the risk of infection during and after surgery: clean; clean-contaminated; contaminated; and dirty and infected.[6,7] Oral/dental surgery most often falls into the second or third category because of the flora associated with the oral cavity. Depending on the patient's condition before the time of surgery, oral surgery may also involve dirty and infected wounds if, for example, the surgical area includes abscesses.[7] Wound healing in oral mucoperiosteal tissues after surgical wounding has unique characteristics,[8-10] including how wound healing is affected by flap design (Figure 9-1).[11-13] Additionally, instead of the clinician approximating two vascular soft tissue surfaces for many bone grafting or implant surgery procedures, in some surgical procedures, one of the approximated surfaces is an avascular root surface previously exposed to the oral environment.[6] Generally, the clinician should aim for a trapezoidal shape for the flap design, with the wider portion at the base of the flap; such a shape facilitates blood supply to the tissue, as well as flexibility to help ensure nontension primary wound closure.[13] Properly placed vertical releasing incisions and appropriate flap reflection facilitate passive positioning of soft tissues, thereby reducing tears of flap edges during suturing and flap retraction.[1]

The types of wound healing (i.e., rate and pattern of wound healing) can be described in three categories, based on tissue type and closure issues: (1) healing by first intention (the four-stage process described below, involving the normal wound healing process: minimal edema, no local infection, no serious discharge, no separation of wound edges, minimal scarring); (2) healing by second intention (complicated and prolonged healing resulting from infection, trauma, lost tissue, or poor approximation of wound edges); and (3) healing by third intention, also known as delayed primary closure (the bringing together of two surfaces of granulation tissue, usually because of contaminated, traumatic wounds with high risk for infection).[7,14] Healing by first intention should be the goal in many implant surgical procedures, including first-stage dental implants, root coverage, bone grafting, and membranes used for tissue regeneration; healing by second intention occurs, for example, after a gingivectomy, and healing by third intention occurs

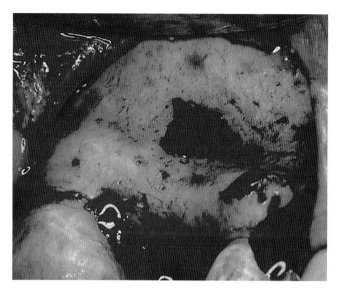

FIGURE 9-1 ■ The wound healing process is affected by the design of the flap.

in extraction sockets (unless a flap is advanced or a soft tissue graft is placed).[6]

The Wound Healing Process

Wound healing follows a step-by-step process, including hemostasis, inflammation, and repair; hemostasis includes fibrin formation, which leads to the formation of a protective wound scab, beneath which cell migration occurs along with movement of the wound edges[15] (Figure 9-2). Inflammation provides nutrients and facilitates removal of debris and bacteria, and repair includes epithelialization, fibroplasia, and capillary proliferation.[15]

When healthy tissues are punctured through injury or surgical incision, rapid blood clotting is triggered, along with movement of epidermal cells to the site. Many different types of cells and proteins work together to repair the wound, but the complementary nature of their roles is still the subject of much debate and research. For example, some researchers have suggested that separate genetic programs are responsible for each stage of the wound healing process.[16] Generally, however, four basic stages of cutaneous wound healing are known: hemostasis, inflammation, proliferation or granulation, and remodeling or maturation.[7,14,17,18]

Hemostasis

Once the skin is punctured, polymorphonucleocytes (PMNs), platelets, and plasma proteins enter the wound, which causes constriction of the blood vessels. Although platelets produce vasoconstrictors, they also help form a stable clot to seal punctured vessels. Adenosine diphosphate from surrounding tissues causes the platelets to gather and connect with nearby collagen; the platelets also release elements that help produce thrombin, leading to the produc-

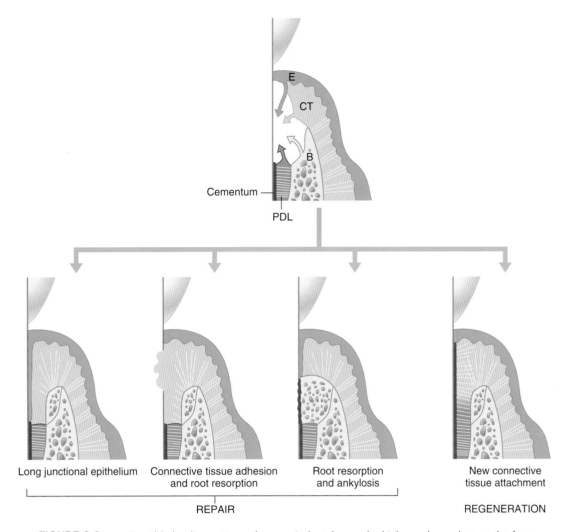

FIGURE 9-2 ■ Possible healing patterns for a periodontal wound, which are dependent on the four possible cell types that predominate that wound site. The downgrowth of epithelial cells (*E*) results in a long junctional epithelium. The proliferation of connective tissue (*CT*) may result in connective tissue adhesion ± root resorption. With the predominance of bone cells (*B*), there may be root resorption, ankylosis, or both. With the ingress of periodontal ligament (*PDL*) and perivascular cells from the bone, a regenerated periodontium with new cementum develops. (From Rose LF, Mealey BL: *Periodontics: Medicine, surgery, and implants*, St Louis, Mosby, 2004.)

tion of fibrin from fibrinogen. Platelets join with fibrin in the wound, and the platelets release platelet-derived growth factor (PDGF) and transforming growth factor (TGF)-beta, attracting PMNs and starting the inflammation stage (Figure 9-3).

Inflammation

Swelling and warmth (edema) are the clinical factors associated with this stage of healing. Macrophages replace PMNs after approximately 48 hours to continue the inflammation process, removing wound debris and releasing growth factors. This removal of wound debris is an essential element in the wound's ability to fight infection (Figure 9-4).

Proliferation (Granulation)

The proliferation stage begins about 72 hours after wound initiation. In this stage, fibroblasts, drawn to the wound by inflammatory cell growth factors, synthesize collagen. Clinical signs of this stage include granular red tissue in the base of the wound, dermal and subdermal tissue replacement, and wound contraction. In this stage, fibroblasts release collagen, which forms a framework for increased dermal growth. Angiogenesis also characterizes this stage of wound healing, involving the regeneration of capillaries. Additionally, keratinocytes control the process of epithelialization in the wound, leading to further wound contraction and the formation of a layered wound covering.

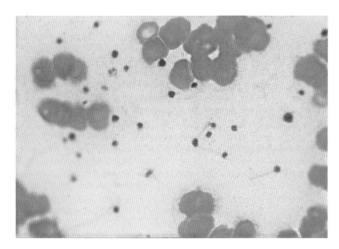

FIGURE 9-3 ■ The platelets are very important cells in the hemostasis process.

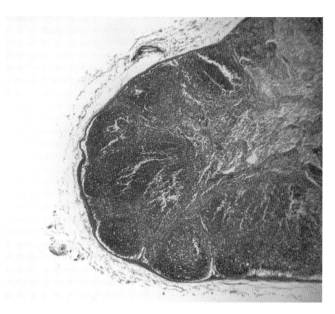

FIGURE 9-4 ■ The macrophages are responsible for the swelling and erythema in the wound healing process of the tissues.

Remodeling (Maturation)

The last stage of wound healing, remodeling, involves continued work of collagen as it restructures itself over the next several weeks to repair the skin. The tensile strength of the wound increases as dermal cells are remodeled, mainly by fibroblasts, over the next 18 to 24 months, and sometimes longer.

Factors Affecting Wound Healing

Numerous factors, including age (loss of tissue tone and elasticity, slower metabolism, poor circulation), weight (poor wound closure and blood supply due to excessive fatty tissue, increasing susceptibility to damage and infection), nutrition (e.g., vitamin and protein deficiencies impairing cell maintenance and the synthesis of collagen), dehydration (electrolyte imbalance leading to poor blood circulation), chronic disease (e.g., diabetes, which impairs blood supply to extremities), immune response (e.g., the impaired immune system of HIV patients, chemotherapy and radiation therapy patients, and patients allergic to medical materials such as sutures), and radiation therapy, affect wound healing and are directly related to the patient's health.[7]

Practicing sterilization and aseptic surgical technique is essential for helping to protect the surgical team or treatment area from infection, as is following surgical principles that include attention to length and direction of the incision, dissection techniques, tissue handling, hemostasis, tissue irrigation (during lengthy procedures), proper debridement, choice of closure materials, elimination of dead space in the wound (e.g., failure to approximate wound edges), tension of closure, and postsurgical wound stressors.[7]

Suture Materials

As repair and regeneration of bone and other supporting structures have become more and more the focus of implant surgery over the past decade, so has the study of suturing

techniques and materials that can facilitate such surgical procedures.[6] A primary goal of dental surgery is to establish nontension closure of primary wounds for all soft tissue flaps, so that wounds heal properly, whether the surgery is performed during traditional implant therapy, periodontal plastic cosmetic surgery, hard tissue grafting surgery, soft tissue regeneration, or excision of pathologic tissue.[1,13,19] Not only is nontension primary closure essential to implant success (for the implant itself and for any site requiring a bone graft), but several flap designs can facilitate surgical wound healing with no or few complications.[5,13] To reach this essential goal of positioning and securing surgical flaps to provide the best conditions for wound healing, practitioners must understand three areas of suturing in particular: types of sutures, suturing techniques, and surgical knotting techniques.[20]

Types of Sutures

A 2001 study of the effect of suture materials on most common complications in plastic surgery (tissue reactivity, infections, and wound dehiscence) revealed no substantial differences between the different suture materials and suturing techniques.[2] The study included 1,000 plastic surgery outpatients and consisted of an evaluation of the association of different suture materials, and of individual patient characteristics, surgeon skill, and wound site and length along with postoperative wound complications, revealing that patients' sex and age, as well as the length and site of wounds, were more responsible for wound complications than were suture materials.[2]

Each of the two basic categories of sutures—nonresorbable and resorbable—has advantages. For example, nonresorbable suture materials are naturally elastic, facilitating secure knotting; by contrast, resorbable sutures can lead to less postoperative inflammation.[20] Suture size refers to the diameter of surface material, measured from 1-0 to 10-0 and growing increasingly smaller in diameter and lower in tensile strength. Cost for suturing material generally increases as the size descreases.[6] Dental surgeons use 3-0 and 4-0 most commonly, reserving 5-0 and 6-0 for delicate mucogingival surgery.[20] The surgeon should use the smallest-diameter suture that will hold the wound tissue together during healing. Microsurgical suture materials (e.g., 7-0, 8-0) allow the clinician to increase the number of sutures without further restricting the blood supply; magnification devices usually are required for such suturing, to ensure proper manipulation of tissues.[5]

Nonresorbable Sutures. Nonresorbable sutures are made of silk (the filaments are twisted or braided together to form a strand) or polyester (monofilament type—most often nylon—and polytetrafluoroethylene, or PTFE, sutures). Silk sutures provide smooth tie-downs, and the natural elasticity of silk helps to promote knot security; however, nonresorbable sutures can lead to the "wicking effect," when the material draws bacteria and fluids into the wound site. Braided strands of polyester fibers can be coated with a lubricant (improving passage through tissues and knot tying but often leading to untying).[6]

Resorbable Sutures. Resorbable sutures (natural and synthetic) have become more popular in implant surgeries because they generally promote reduced postoperative inflammation; in addition, they are often preferred by patients because they don't require removal; clinicians note that resorbable sutures can reduce chairtime and patient anxiety.[1,20] Natural resorbable sutures include plain gut (mild tensile strength; 50% strength lost after 24 hours in oral cavity) and chromic gut materials (treated with chromium salt solution; resistant to body enzymes for 7 to 10 days). Resorbable sutures should not be used intraorally for patients who have suffered from epigastric reflux bulimia, esophagitis, or other conditions that facilitate suture breakdown.[20]

Synthetic resorbable sutures break down via hydrolysis. Polyglycolic acid (PGA) sutures consist of a polymer of lactide and glycolide that naturally exists in the body. PGA sutures resorb in 21 to 28 days intraorally. This is an inert suture material that causes little tissue reaction, and the suture has good tensile strength for use in situations involving muscle pull against the suture. Poliglecaprone 25 suture, another synthetic resorbable material, has a 90-day resorption rate with high tensile strength; however, its stiffness may feel abrasive against the tongue or cheek of the patient.[20]

Suturing Techniques

A variety of suturing techniques in dentistry allow the clinician to maximize healing via proper choices of suture positioning.[20] Sutures usually are placed distal to the last tooth, in interproximal spaces, and should be inserted first through the most mobile tissue flap with a circular needle. Suture needles should be grasped by needle holders only,

and the clinician should pull the suture only as tightly as needed to secure the flap without restricting blood supply. Furthermore, the clinician should avoid blanching the flaps during tying.[20] The clinician should grasp the needle in the center, a few millimeters from the tip of the needle holder, avoiding the needle and suture (swage) juncture. The needle entry should be made at right angles to the tissue. When multiple levels are sutured, the clinician should employ a periosteum-to-periosteum and tissue-to-tissue technique.[20] Because swelling generally occurs postoperatively for up to 48 hours, sutures should not be placed any closer than 2.0 mm to 3.0 mm from the edge of the flap, thus preventing flap tearing.

The most common suturing techniques use interrupted sutures, sling sutures, mattress sutures, continuous interlocking sutures, and anchor sutures.[6] These and other common suturing techniques are described below[20]:

- **Continuous sutures** (Figure 9-5): For securing flaps over several centimeters long, and for repositioning surgical flaps apically or coronally; for joining two or more interdental papillae of the same flap, generally when the clinician sutures the buccal flap separately from the lingual, with the needle penetrating the outer surface of the flap 3.0 mm from the edge, then the inner surface of the lingual flap coronal to the mucogingival junction, with the distance 5.0 mm between the needle penetration on the buccal and lingual sides. *Advantages:* minimize multiple knots, employ teeth to anchor flaps, enable precise flap placement, avoid periosteal sutures, and enable independent placement and tension (of buccal, lingual, and palatal flaps). *Disadvantages:* loose flaps or untied sutures. *Variations:* continuous locking suture (the needle, after being passed through the lingual flap, passes through the end loop of the suture and is pulled tightly for locking) and continuous horizontal mattress suture (needle passing through the outer surface of the buccal flap and then through the inner surface of the lingual flap, with the knot tied at the most distal end of the flap).

- **Figure 8 modification of interrupted suture** (Figure 9-6): Used in highly restricted areas, for coapting tissue and resembling the simple loop interrupted suture technique with second needle penetration through the outer surface of the lingual flap, with the knot tied at the buccal aspect of the flap after the needle passes back under the contact point.

- **Mattress suture:** Used for increased security and control of the flap, enabling more precise placement of the flap; often used with periosteal stabilization; used to resist muscle pull, to adapt flaps to bone, as regenerative barrier, implant, or tooth, and to avert the surgical flap edges. This technique also facilitates good papillary stabilization and placement.[20] *Variations:* vertical, coronally repositioned, horizontal, and vertical sling.

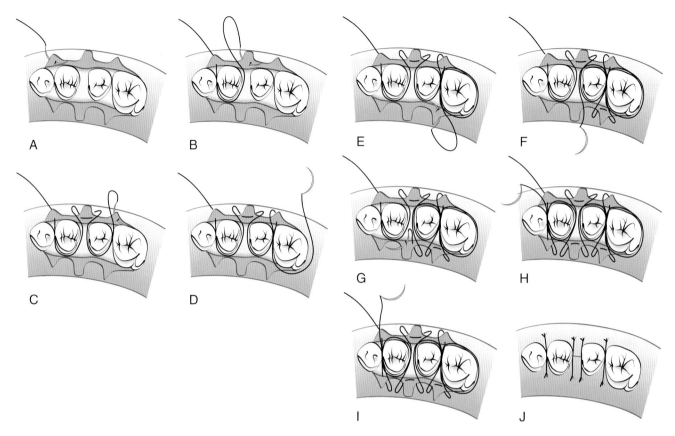

FIGURE 9-5 ■ **A**, Continuous, independent sling suture using a horizontal mattress suture around diastemata or wide interdental areas (**B and C**). This mattress suture is used on both the buccal (**D**) and the lingual (**E and F**) surfaces. Continuation of suture on lingual surfaces (**G, H, and I**) and completed suture (**J**). (From Newman MG et al: *Carranza's clinical periodontology*, ed 10, St. Louis, 2006, Saunders Elsevier.)

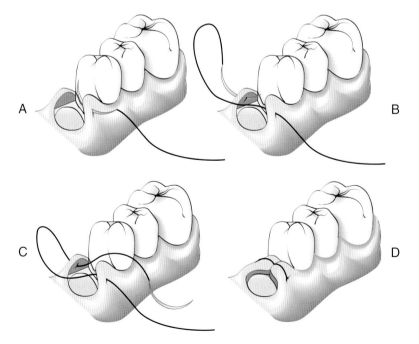

FIGURE 9-6 ■ Interrupted figure-eight suture is used to approximate the buccal and lingual flaps. The needle penetrates the outer surface of the first flap (**A**) and the outer surface of the opposite flap (**B**). The suture is brought back to the first flap (**C**), and the knot is tied (**D**). (From Newman MG et al: *Carranza's clinical periodontology*, ed 10, St. Louis, 2006, Saunders Elsevier.)

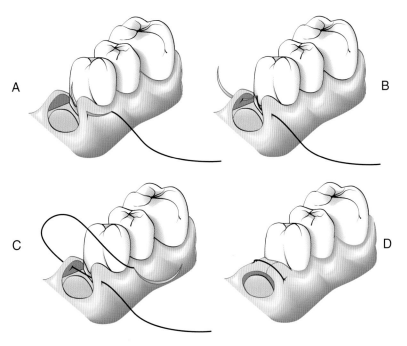

FIGURE 9-7 ■ Simple loop suture is used to approximate the buccal and lingual flaps. **A,** Needle penetrates the outer surface of the first flap. **B,** Undersurface of the opposite flap is engaged, and the suture is brought back to the initial side (**C**), where the knot is tied (**D**). (From Newman MG et al: *Carranza's clinical periodontology*, ed 10, St. Louis, 2006, Saunders Elsevier.)

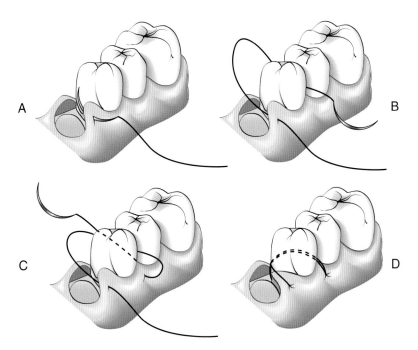

FIGURE 9-8 ■ Single, interrupted sling suture is used to adapt the flap around the tooth. **A,** Needle engages the outer surface of the flap and encircles the tooth (**B**). **C,** Outer surface of the same flap of the adjacent interdental area is engaged. **D,** Suture is returned to the initial site and the knot is tied. (From Newman MG et al: *Carranza's clinical periodontology*, ed 10, St. Louis, 2006, Saunders Elsevier.)

- **Periosteal suturing:** Penetrating the periodontal/peri-implant tissues and periosteum to the bone, and then rotating the needle back to the original direction, through the periosteum and keratinized tissue.
- **Simple loop modification of interrupted suture** (Figure 9-7): Used to approximate/coapt surgical flaps, not to create flap tension, with no placement of suture material between the tissue flaps.
- **Single interrupted sling suture** (Figure 9-8): Used for a flap elevated on one side of the arch or for positioning facial and lingual flaps at different levels; involves only two papillae to adapt the flap around tooth/implant, started on the mesial side of the site, with the needle encircling the tooth before being passed under the distal point.
- **Sling suture about single tooth:** Used primarily for a flap raised on one side of the tooth and involves only one or two adjacent papillae, most often in flaps positioned coronally and laterally, requiring one of the interrupted sutures, anchored about the adjacent tooth or slung around the tooth, for holding both papillae; the buccal or the lingual is reflected, and the clinician passes a 3/8 circle reverse cutting needle under the distal contact point of the most distal interdental papilla, then the inner side of the elevated surgical flap 3.0 mm from the papilla tip; the clinician then passes the needle under the next contact point in a mesial direction, before piercing the inner surface of the elevated surgical flap 3.0 mm from the tip of the interdental papilla.

Other suture techniques include the independent sling suture, the continuous independent sling suture (similar to vertical sling suture, used for a flap with three or more papillae on only one surface) and the cross (crisscross) suture (similar to a continuous mattress suture, with sutures placed horizontally).

Clinicians, of course, occasionally modify standard suturing techniques to accommodate special circumstances. For example, the ramp mattress suture was developed to obtain papillae between implants in the buccal area.[21] In this procedure, after a full-thickness flap is raised from the palatal to the vestibular side, it is stabilized with the ramp suture to apply pressure and tearing forces apicocoronally at the vestibular site and an opposite traction coronoapically at the palatal site; this technique helps to obtain a more coronal gingival margin. After 5 weeks of healing, the clinician performs a vestibular scalloped gingivectomy around the vestibular surface of the abutment, to create a scalloped gingival margin or interproximal papillae only, thus forming a gingival ramp palatovestibularly and reducing residual increased vestibular depth while creating better esthetics.[21] In another example of alternative suturing techniques, sulcus-deepening sutures have been used to create and maintain a lingual sulcus in patients requiring reconstruction by free tissue transfer (resections of the tongue, mouth floor, adjacent mandible).[22]

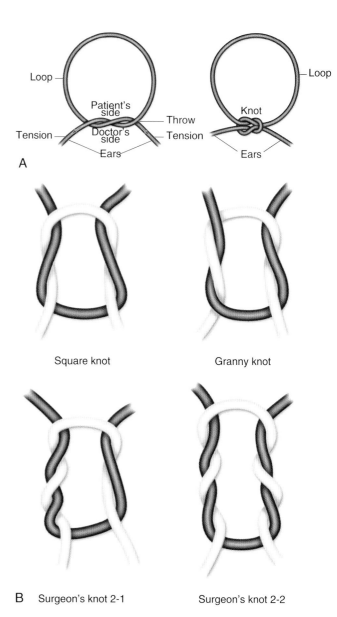

FIGURE 9-9 ■ **A,** Knot anatomy and its components. **B,** Different types of suturing knots.

Surgical Knotting Techniques

Only a limited number of more than 1,400 available knots are used in dentistry and implantology.[20] The clinician chooses the type of knot based on suture material, the nature of the incision (location and depth), and how much stress will be placed on the wound after surgery.[6] Specific knotting techniques are required for synthetic suture material.[20]

Certain knot tying criteria apply to all suture materials: firmness (to prevent slippage), simplicity, smallness, avoidance of instrument damage, correct tension, approximation (not strangulation) of tissues, proper traction at one end of the strand after the first loop to avoid loosening, a horizontal final throw, placement of a secure and flat knot, and avoidance of extra throws.[20] Synthetic multifilament or braided sutures are best for knot security, although variations are based on manufacturing. Key knots for the dental practitioner include the square knot, the slip knot, and the surgeon's knot (Figure 9-9).[20]

Square Knot. The square knot is a relatively simple knot: two overhand knots completed in opposite directions. First, the clinician makes a loop over the jaws of the needle holder, grabs the end of the suture, and pulls the knot to the flap. Next, the clinician makes a second overhand knot, placing a loop under the jaws of the needle holder again; the end of the suture is caught, and the two ends of the suture are pulled together.

Slip Knot. The slip knot is similar to the square knot: two single overhand knots made in the same direction. With the first, the clinician loops the suture over the needle holder, grabs the free end of the suture, and pulls it tight; for the second knot, the loop again goes over the needle holder. Further tightening of this knot is possible before it is locked by the use of another overhand knot made in the opposite direction.

Surgeon's Knot. This is the most commonly used knot in implant surgery, used generally with braided suture material and standard mattress suturing: a modified square knot consisting of two overhand knots completed in opposite directions. The first is a double overhand knot, and the second is single. The clinician can prevent the knot from loosening by doubling the first overhand knot.

SUMMARY

Proper understanding of wound healing and surgical suturing techniques is essential for achieving successful tissue healing and favorable long-term implant survival. An understanding of the various types of wounds, how wounds heal, and the complications that can impair wound healing brings into clearer focus the need to apply suturing techniques essential for facilitating the wound healing process.

REFERENCES

1. Moore RL, Hill M: Suturing techniques for periodontal plastic surgery, *Periodontol 2000* 11:103-111, 1996.
2. Gabrielli F, Potenza C, Puddu P, Sera F, Masini C, Abeni D: Suture materials and other factors associated with tissue reactivity, infection, and wound dehiscence among plastic surgery outpatients, *Plast Reconstr Surg* 107(1):38-45, 2001.
3. Kose AA, Karabagli Y, Arici M, Cetin C: Various materials may aid in teaching surgical procedures, *Plast Reconstr Surg* 114(2):611, 2004.
4. Mashadi SA, Imran D, Niranjan N: An application of a rice bag stitch, *Plast Reconstr Surg* 114(2):611-613, 2004.
5. Hurzeler MB, Weng D: Functional and esthetic outcome enhancement of periodontal surgery by application of plastic surgery principles, *Int J Periodontics Restorative Dent* 19(1):36-43, 1999.
6. O'Neal RB, Alleyn CD: Suture materials and techniques, *Curr Opin Periodontol* 4:89-95, 1997.
7. Dunn DL, editor: Ethicon wound closure manual, Somerville, NJ, 2004, Johnson & Johnson (cited 2005 Aug 2). Available at: http://www.jnjgateway.com/public/USENG/Ethicon_WCM_Feb2004.pdf
8. Harrison JW: Healing of surgical wounds in oral mucoperiosteal tissues, *J Endod* 17(8):401-408, 1991.
9. Peters LB, Wesselink PR: Soft tissue management in endodontic surgery, *Dent Clin North Am* 41(3):513-528, 1997.
10. Certosimo FJ, Nicoll BK, Nelson RR, Wolfgang M: Wound healing and repair: a review of the art and science, *Gen Dent* 46(4):362-369, 1998; quiz 370-371.
11. Harrison JW, Jurosky KA: Wound healing in the tissues of the periodontium following periradicular surgery, I. the incisional wound, *J Endod* 17(9):425-435, 1991.
12. Harrison JW, Jurosky KA: Wound healing in the tissues of the periodontium following periradicular surgery, II. the dissectional wound, *J Endod* 17(11):544-552, 1991.
13. Heller AL, Heller RL, Cook G, D'Orazio R, Rutkowski J: Soft tissue management techniques for implant dentistry: a clinical guide, *J Oral Implantol* 26(2):91-103, 2000.
14. Mercandetti M, Cohen AJ: Wound healing, healing and repair, eMedicine, 1996-2005 (cited 2005 Aug 8). Available at: http://www.emedicine.com/plastic/topic411.htm
15. Phillips SJ: Physiology of wound healing and surgical wound care, *ASAIO J* 46(6):S2-S5, 2000.
16. Galko MJ, Krasnow MA: Cellular and genetic analysis of wound healing in *Drosophila* larvae, *PLoS Biol* 2(8):E239, 2004. Epub 2004 Jul 20.
17. Keast D, Orsted H: The basic principles of wound healing, Canadian Association of Wound Care, 2005 (cited 2005 Aug 9). Available at: http://www.cawc.net/open/library/clinical/Principles-of-Wound-Healing.pdf
18. Beanes SR, Dang C, Soo C, Ting K: The phases of cutaneous wound healing: expert reviews in molecular medicine, March 2003 (cited 2005 Aug 8). Available at: http://www.expertreviews.org/03005817h.htm
19. Silverstein LH, Kurtzman GM: A review of dental suturing for optimal soft-tissue management, *Compend Contin Educ Dent* 26(3):163-166, 169-170, 2005; quiz 171, 209.
20. Silverstein LH: *Principles of dental suturing: the complete guide to surgical closure,* Mahwah, NJ, 1999, Montage Media Corporation.
21. Tinti C, Benfenati SP: The ramp mattress suture: a new suturing technique combined with a surgical procedure to obtain papillae between implants in the buccal area, *Int J Periodontics Restorative Dent* 22(1):63-69, 2002.
22. Halfpenny W: Role for sulcus-deepening sutures in reconstructive surgery, *Br J Oral Maxillofac Surg* 38(6):608-609, 2000.

chapter 10

Pharmacological Agents in Implant Dentistry

S URGICAL PROCEDURES TO PLACE ORAL IMPLANTS share with other oral surgery techniques the postoperative sequelae of inflammation and the possibility of infection. Dentists must be skilled in the prevention and treatment of inflammation and infection when performing implant dentistry. To provide the dentist with general criteria for choosing the most appropriate agent for the control and prevention of swelling, pain, and infection in implant dentistry, this chapter reviews the pharmacology of analgesics, opioids, steroids, local anesthetics, anxiolytic medications, and antibiotics (Figure 10-1).

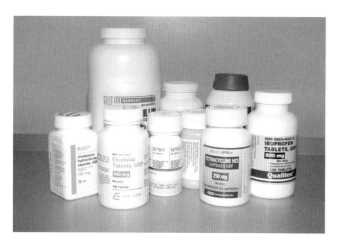

FIGURE 10-1 ■ Many different analgesics (prescription and over-the-counter) are available.

Inflammatory Pain

Appropriate pain management requires an understanding of the physiology and pharmacology of pain.[1-8] The perception of pain is thought to signal the occurrence of tissue damage or the potential for damage. Tissue damage is detected by the terminal endings of two classes of nociceptive (pain-detecting) nerve fibers distributed throughout the oral mucosa and tooth pulp. The A delta fibers are relatively fast-conducting, lightly myelinated fibers. They respond primarily to mechanical or heat stimuli. It is theorized that they mediate the initial (or "first") sensation of pain, which has a sharp or bright quality. The second group of nociceptive fibers, the C fibers, consists of slow-conducting, unmyelinated fibers that respond to heat and mechanical and chemical stimuli. These fibers probably mediate the "second" pain, generally described as having a dull, aching, or burning quality and occurring after the initial "sharp-pricking" pain.

The inflammatory response to tissue damage results in the production of pain, edema, local increased temperature, redness, and loss of function. Tissue trauma or by-products of infection can activate the synthesis of prostaglandins and the release of bradykinins. Because prostaglandins, bradykinins, and histamine (which releases from peripheral mast cells) increase the permeability or vasodilation of local blood vessels, they act synergistically to increase plasma extravasation. Accumulations of extravasated fluid in the tissue spaces produce the clinical signs of edema.

These local factors have two effects on the peripheral nociceptive nerve endings. First, they excite and sensitize the peripheral nerve ending and produce electrophysiological changes. These changes, together with changes occurring in the central nervous system (CNS), result in the clinical presentation of hyperalgesia, which is characterized by spontaneous pain, a decreased pain threshold, and an increased magnitude of perceived pain for any given stimulus.

Second, inflammatory mediators stimulate the release of neuropeptides stored in the peripheral nociceptive nerve ending. These neuropeptides—substance P and calcitonin gene-related peptide (CGRP)—are transported to the CNS and its periphery. In the periphery, substance P and CGRP have proinflammatory properties. They act synergistically with other inflammatory mediators to stimulate histamine release from mast cells and to induce plasma extravasation.

The continued synthesis or release of these mediators explains the prolonged time course of inflammation, which far exceeds the initial stimulation of the implant surgical procedure. The clinical time course of postsurgery pain and edema reflects the prolonged duration of the inflammatory process. Pain reaches moderate to severe intensity by 5 hours, and edema peaks by 48 to 72 hours after the extraction of impacted third molars. In this regard, implant surgery is comparable to the trauma of third molar surgery.[9]

The pharmacological management of pain in the periphery is accomplished by blocking the nociceptive input at the receptor or the nociceptive impulse along the peripheral nerve. Aspirin-like drugs, which include aspirin, acetaminophen, and the nonsteroidal anti-inflammatory drugs (NSAIDs), exert their actions at the nerve endings. These drugs inhibit the generation of the pain signal and the accompanying sensitization at the nerve ending through the blocking of prostaglandin synthesis.[10-14]

Prostaglandins are end products of arachidonic acid and are synthesized as needed. Under the conditions of noxious stimuli, phospholipase A2 and other enzymes liberate arachidonic acid from phospholipids embedded in cell membranes. Because aspirin-like drugs do not inhibit the first step of this cascade (synthesis of arachidonic acid), they can contribute to increased lipoxygenase activity by diverting arachidonic acid metabolism away from the blocked cyclooxygenase pathway. This effect can lead to an increase in leukotriene synthesis, which is known to be a potent mediator of immediate hypersensitivity reactions, which could be responsible in certain susceptible patients for hypersensitivity reactions observed after the administration of aspirin-like drugs.[10-14]

Aspirin-Like Analgesics

Aspirin (acetylsalicylic acid) is the prototype agent of this class of analgesic drugs.[13,15] It is indicated for analgesic, antipyretic, anti-inflammatory, and antirheumatoid effects. Aspirin has numerous side effects, including epigastric distress, ulceration, nausea, vomiting, and increased bleeding times. The acetylsalicylic acid moiety binds irreversibly to platelet cyclooxygenase and prevents the platelet production of prostaglandins and thromboxanes—substances that are essential for platelet aggregation. As a result, bleeding time can be prolonged over the 8- to 11-day period required to replenish circulating platelets. Intolerance to aspirin, a syndrome similar to an allergy but without an immunologic component, occurs frequently but has potentially lethal consequences. Symptoms of intolerance include rhinitis, angioedema, urticaria, bronchospasm, and shock. Patients with chronic urticaria, asthma, and nasal polyps represent a high risk for intolerance. Clinically, aspirin-like drugs have proved to be highly effective for mild to moderate inflammatory pain.[10-14] For the type of pain that occurs after implant surgery, 650 mg of aspirin has been consistently demonstrated to be effective.

Diflunisal is a product derivative of salicylic acid. Its main advantage is prolonged duration of action (8 to 12 hours).[16-18] Three hours, however, is required for a peak effect. Accordingly, an initial loading dose of 1,000 mg is recommended, followed by 500 mg every 12 hours for the treatment of mild to moderate pain. Diflunisal in doses of 250, 500, and 1,000 mg has been shown to be more effective than 650 mg of aspirin.[10]

Ibuprofen, an NSAID and a derivative of propionic acid, is widely used for chronic arthritis and as an analgesic for moderate to acute pain.[10-14] This type of drug exerts its analgesic effect by suppressing prostaglandin-dependent inflammation. However, although it is effective in reducing pain, ibuprofen has less impact on swelling. This effect implies that prostaglandins are not primary factors in the development of postoperative edema since prostaglandins induce vasodilation and mediators, which then increase vascular permeability. Extrapolating to the implant surgery model, the moderate anti-edema effect of NSAIDs is probably due to the limited actions of prostaglandins on increasing blood flow in this tissue and the inability of this drug class to suppress mediators that increase vascular permeability. On the other hand, pretreatment with ibuprofen before implant surgery can significantly delay the onset and decrease the severity of postoperative pain. When used postoperatively, a dose of 400 mg of ibuprofen has been found effective for pain after implant surgery. At present, up to 800 mg of ibuprofen can be administered in a single dose.[19,20] A 2002 study suggests that the enhanced pharmacokinetic characteristics of ibuprofen arginate may provide faster pain relief than standard ibuprofen for patients with acute pain.[21] The 498 randomized patients received ibuprofen arginate (200 mg or 400 mg), ibuprofen (200 mg or 400 mg) or a placebo. Traditional verbal description scales were used to determine pain intensity and relief. Within 1 hour, 77.6% (200 mg) and 83.7% (400 mg) of patients receiving ibuprofen arginate experienced meaningful pain relief versus 61.0% (200 mg) and 63.0% (400 mg) of patients receiving ibuprofen, and 39.8% of patients receiving a placebo. Ibuprofen arginate patients experienced 16 to 24 minutes' faster pain relief than those receiving ibuprofen—this for patients with moderate to severe pain after the extraction of one or more impacted third molars.

Naproxen, another NSAID and propionic acid derivative, has a longer duration of action than ibuprofen.[22] It is available in two formulations, but the sodium salt formulation is absorbed faster. An initial loading dose of 500 mg to 550 mg is used to reach therapeutic blood levels rapidly, with subsequent doses of 250 mg to 275 mg given at 6- to 8-hour intervals.[10] For pain after implant surgery, 550 mg of naproxen sodium is effective.

Acetaminophen, the active metabolite of phenacetin, generally is thought to be equipotent to aspirin, but with fewer side effects. It does not have the anti-inflammatory effects of aspirin. It is only a weak inhibitor of peripheral prostaglandin synthesis and appears to be active in the CNS. It does not inhibit platelet aggregation. Acetaminophen has been shown to be equipotent to aspirin after third molar extraction[10] or implant surgery. To enhance efficacy, this analgesic is commonly combined with centrally acting opiate analgesics, such as codeine or hydrocodone.[23,24] For pain after surgery, 1,000 mg of acetaminophen or 650 mg of acetaminophen plus 60 mg of codeine is recommended.

Opioid Analgesics

The A delta and C fibers from the orofacial region transmit nociceptive information to the nucleus caudalis *(N. caudalis)* of the trigeminal system, which is located in the medulla. Its organization and function in processing pain signals are similar to the organization and function of the site on the dorsal aspect of the spinal cord known as the dorsal horn. The transmission of pain can be modulated in the first few synapses of the *N. caudalis* and spinal dorsal horn by an endogenous pain suppression system.[10-14]

The endogenous opioid peptides (EOPs) are a family of peptides that possess many of the properties of exogenous opiates, such as morphine. Metencephalon, dynorphin, and beta-endorphin all are members of the EOP family. It is important to note that EOPs are found at all three levels of the pain suppression system. This fact underlies the analgesic potency of opioids and exogenous opiates because their administration activates this system at all levels, producing a multiplicative analgesic effect. A site in the gray matter of the brainstem known as the periaqueductal gray (PAG) forms the most effective part of the pain suppression system. The name PAG is descriptive of its location surrounding the aqueduct that carries cerebrospinal fluid from the third to the fourth ventricle. The PAG plays a critical role in the suppression of pain by integrating information from the cortical and brainstem regions together with incoming nociceptive signals.[10-14] The middle level of the pain suppression system includes the nucleus raphe magnus (NRM), nearby medullary reticular nuclei, and the locus coeruleus (LC). The medullary and spinal dorsal horns are the lowest level of the pain suppression system.[10]

At least four types of opiate receptors have been identified, and these are designated mu, kappa, sigma, and delta. The differential binding and activation of the opiate receptor types are thought to account for the variety of pharmacologi-

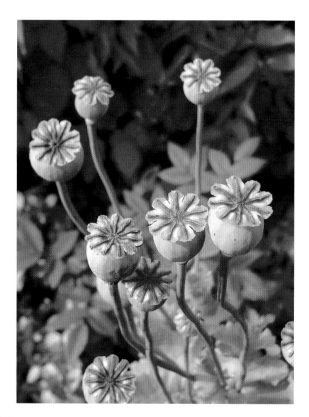

FIGURE 10-2 ■ The seed capsules of the poppy plant provide opium (of which morphine and codeine are alkaloids). These have long been used to treat pain.

cal effects produced by opioid drugs. The binding and activation of mu and kappa receptors results in analgesia, euphoria, and respiratory depression. Sigma receptors are associated with psychotomimetic effects, and delta receptors appear to alter affective behavior and induce analgesia. In addition to receptor binding, another important consideration is activity in the binding site. Opioids can be classified as agonists (morphine, codeine), partial agonists (buprenorphine), agonists-antagonists (pentazocine), and antagonists (naloxone).[10-14]

Morphine and codeine are opium alkaloids. Opium is the dried exudate of the incised unripe seed capsules of the poppy plant (Figure 10-2). These two drugs are considered to be pure opioid agonists because they elicit responses at the opiate receptors to induce analgesia, respiratory depression, euphoria, physical dependence, and sedation. The other agonists include meperidine, fentanyl, oxycodone, dihydrocodeine, hydromorphone, and propoxyphene. These agonists act primarily as mu receptors, but they can have kappa receptor activity.[10-14]

Codeine is the opioid used most frequently in dentistry. It is a pure mu agonist with some additional kappa receptor activity. It has approximately one-sixth the potency of morphine and is highly effective when taken orally. An effective oral dose of codeine is 15 mg to 60 mg, which produces an analgesic effect that lasts from 4 to 6 hours. Increasing doses of codeine above the normal therapeutic range (more than 120 mg orally) increase the effects and respiratory depression.[10-14]

Codeine is the drug of choice when combined with aspirin, acetaminophen, or ibuprofen for moderate to severe postoperative pain after implant surgery. A particularly beneficial combination of NSAIDs and opioids provides a centrally and peripherally acting analgesic and anti-inflammatory effect (Table 10-1).[23]

For implant dentistry, 400 mg to 600 mg ibuprofen or 600 mg ibuprofen plus 60 mg to 90 mg codeine is recommended to curtail moderate to acute postsurgical pain. On the other hand, 600 mg to 1,000 mg acetaminophen plus 60 mg codeine or 600 mg to 1,000 mg acetaminophen plus 5 mg oxycodone will also control pain. Oxycodone and hydrocodone are also used in dentistry. Oxycodone, a semisynthetic derivative of codeine, is approximately 10 to 12 times as potent as codeine. Other opioid agonists, such as dihydrocodeine, propoxyphene, and meperidine, do not offer any advantages over codeine when given orally and can be even less effective (Table 10-2).[10-14]

Opioid partial agonists, such as buprenorphine, bind to opiate receptors to elicit limited analgesia and antagonized morphine effects. Buprenorphine can be used as a potent analgesic in patients who suffer postoperative and chronic pain, particularly pain having a malignant origin. The adverse side effects are similar to those of morphine-like analgesics.[10-14] Opioids with agonist and antagonist effects exert kappa receptor activity to produce analgesia while eliciting antagonist activity or no activity at the mu receptors, thus blocking the actions of morphine. These drugs, such as pentazocine, have a limited analgesic effect and limited respiratory depressant effects.[10-14]

Pure antagonists, such as naloxone, reverse most of the effects of the pure agonists. The drugs bind competitively to the mu and kappa receptors but cannot activate them. They are used parenterally or orally to treat an opioid overdose and are a mainstay in emergency drug kits.[10-14]

Glucocorticosteroids

The earliest published reports of glucocorticosteroids used in dentistry were prepared by Spied et al. in 1952 and Strean and Horton in 1953. The results of these and other studies and the development of more potent synthetic glucocorticosteroids have increased the use of these agents in oral surgery (Figure 10-3).[25-27]

These steroids are but one subdivision within a group of chemically related compounds known as the adrenocorticoids, which are secreted by the adrenal cortex. The primary glucocorticosteroid secreted by the zona fasciculata of the adrenal cortex is cortisol (hydrocortisone), and the primary endogenous mineralocorticoid is aldosterone. Daily secretion of cortisone varies rhythmically and is characterized by peak output in the early morning hours and lowest output in the late afternoon.[9,25,28] Glucocorticosteroids inhibit prostaglandin synthesis and have very potent effects on homeostasis by promoting profound anti-

TABLE 10-1 Composition of Selected Codeine-Containing Analgesic Preparations			
PRODUCT NAME	**AMOUNT OF CODEINE**	**OTHER INGREDIENTS**	**AMOUNT**
Ascription with Codeine (#2, 3)	#2 15 mg	Aspirin	325 mg
	#3 30 mg	Buffering agent	
Empirin with Codeine (#2-4)	#2 15 mg	Aspirin	325 mg
	#3 30 mg		
	#4 60 mg		
Empracet with Codeine (#2-4)	#2 15 mg	Acetaminophen	300 mg
	#3 30 mg		
	#4 60 mg		
Fiorinal with Codeine (#1-3)	#1 7.5 mg	Aspirin	325 mg
	#2 15.0 mg	Butalbital	50 mg
	#3 30.0 mg	Caffeine	40 mg
Phenaphen with Codeine (#2-4)	#2 7.5 mg	Acetaminophen	325 mg
	#3 15.0 mg		
	#4 30.0 mg		
Tylenol with Codeine (#1-4)	#1 7.5 mg	Acetaminophen	300 mg
	#2 15.0 mg		
	#3 30.0 mg		
	#4 60 mg		

TABLE 10-2 Composition of Selected Opioid Analgesic Preparations				
PRODUCT NAME	**OPIOID**	**AMOUNT OF OPIOID**	**OTHER INGREDIENTS**	**AMOUNT**
Darvon Compound-65	Propoxyphene hydrochloride	65 mg	Aspirin, caffeine	389 mg 32 mg
Darvocet N-100	Propoxyphene napsylate	100 mg	Acetaminophen	650 mg
Percocet	Oxycodone	5 mg	Acetaminophen	325 mg
Percodam	Oxycodone	5 mg	Aspirin	325 mg
Synalgos-DC	Dihydrocodeine	16 mg	Aspirin, caffeine	356 mg 30 mg
Tylox	Oxycodone	5 mg	Acetaminophen	500 mg
Vicodin	Hydrocodone	5 mg	Acetaminophen	500 mg

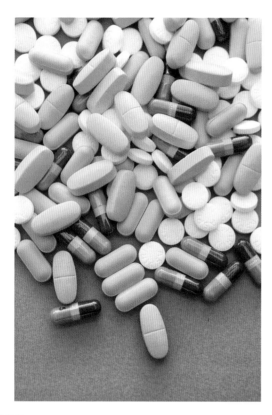

FIGURE 10-3 ■ Corticosteroids can be prescribed to limit edema and postoperative pain.

inflammatory activity. Glucocorticosteroids also inhibit all stages of inflammation, such as capillary dilation, migration of leukocytes, and phagocytosis.

Because of the isolation and early use of hydrocortisone as an anti-inflammatory drug, many synthetic agents have been developed that are more potent, have longer-acting anti-inflammatory activity, and elicit fewer undesirable mineralocorticoid side effects. With regard to the duration of anti-inflammatory action, cortisone, hydrocortisone, prednisone, prednisolone, and methylprednisolone are considered short acting. Triamcinolone is intermediate acting, and betamethasone and dexamethasone are considered long acting. As to the relative potency, 15 mg to 20 mg of hydrocortisone is equivalent to the physiological output of cortisol by the adrenal cortex in an average individual in an average day. Prednisone and prednisolone are about 4 times as potent as hydrocortisone. Methylprednisolone and triamcinolone are about 5 times as potent, whereas betamethasone and dexamethasone are about 20 to 30 times as potent.[25]

Steroids exert many effects on a variety of physiological functions, and their use is accompanied by numerous potential side effects, which are proportional to the duration and intensity of therapy.[25-27] The patient who takes long-term exogenous corticosteroids risks suppression of the hypothalamic-pituitary-adrenal axis. The body then may not adequately respond to the stress of surgery, trauma, or infection. A possible life-threatening symptom complex (acute adrenal insufficiency) may develop. This crisis includes vascular collapse, hypotension, vomiting, and dyspnea. Other associated adverse effects of steroids include fatigue, arthralgia, anorexia, dizziness, nausea, abdominal cramps, abnormal menstruation, and hypoglycemia. In addition, long-term exogenous corticosteroid use can cause alveolar osteoporosis and degeneration of the periodontal fibers, along with an increase in oral infections.[9,28]

Reported contraindications of long-term steroid therapy include acute psychoses, diverticulitis, peptic ulcer, Cushing's syndrome, renal insufficiency, hypertension, thromboembolic tendencies, osteoporosis, myasthenia gravis, intake of anticoagulants, and psychotic tendencies.[25-27] Short-term corticosteroids are contraindicated for patients with a history of tuberculosis or ocular herpes simplex. Steroids are not prescribed for an individual who has existing acute or chronic bacterial, viral, or fungal infection, nor should a patient be vaccinated shortly after steroid administration.[9,28]

Implant surgery is an elective surgery performed primarily on patients who do not have medical conditions listed as contraindications for long-term steroid use.[29-31] The risks associated with long-term steroid use for a healthy patient undergoing implant surgery are minimal. Daily single-dose therapy given in the morning, when natural cortisol peaks, appears to cause less suppression of endogenous production than divided daily doses. Therefore, if the implant surgeon wishes to interfere the least with the adrenal axis system or the positive aspects of inflammation, morning administration of steroids is indicated.[9,28]

The implant surgeon should use short-term glucocorticosteroids to limit edema and postoperative pain when large soft tissue periosteal flaps are reflected. The chosen steroid should have minimal mineralocorticoid effects. Hence, dexamethasone-like drugs are ideal. The drug should be administered before surgery, allowing an optimal decrease in arachidonic acid at the time of the initial tissue trauma, preferably in the morning when cortisol is released naturally in the body. This schedule interferes the least with the adrenal axis system. The prescription should not exceed 5 days because edema peaks in 48 to 72 hours. The dose should not exceed 300 mg of cortisol equivalence on the morning of surgery—the maximum reported amount of natural glucocorticoid released during trauma, surgery, or infection. The dose should be reduced on the second day, and further reduced on the third day because the edema feedback loop decreases daily. The patient should be on an antibiotic, ideally bactericidal if the patient's history permits, to counteract the decreased phagocytosis and the accumulation of leukocytes in the traumatized region and to protect the healing tissue.[25-27]

Local Anesthetics

The first local anesthetic to be described was cocaine. It was reported in the nineteenth century that Indians in the highlands of Peru chewed the leaves of the Erythroxylon coca shrub to stimulate their CNS. Niemann, the German chemist, successfully extracted cocaine from the coca shrub in 1860. In 1884, Hall introduced local cocaine anesthesia to dentistry. One year later, Halstead developed the principles of the nerve block using cocaine.[32-35] Cocaine's untoward properties, such as CNS excitation, mood-altering effects, profound cardiac stimulation, vasoconstriction, and the development of psychological and physical dependence, preclude its use in the routine practice of dentistry today. Safer local anesthetic agents, such as benzocaine, procaine, and lidocaine, have the beneficial local anesthetic properties of cocaine without the unwanted toxicity and potential for abuse.[32-35]

All injectable local anesthetic molecules comprise three structural parts. The aromatic or lipophilic portion of the molecule is necessary for the drug to penetrate lipid-rich nerve sheaths and membranes. The amino terminus confers water solubility on the molecule. The intermediate chain separates the lipophilic and hydrophilic portions of the molecule and divides the local anesthetic into two distinct chemical classes: the esters (−COO−) and the amides (−NHCO−). The esters, represented by drugs such as procaine, tetracaine, and benzocaine, are metabolized primarily by blood pseudocholinesterases. This metabolic route leads to the formation of a by-product, para-aminobenzoic acid, which has been implicated in the development of allergic responses in a small but significant portion of the general population. In contrast, the amides, represented by lidocaine, mepivacaine, prilocaine, bupivacaine, and etidocaine, are metabolized primarily in the liver. These drugs and their metabolites are essentially free of allergy-producing properties. It is mainly for this reason that the amide local anesthetics have gained popularity over the esters in dentistry.[10,32-35]

Clinically useful local anesthetics are all weak bases with a pKa range from 7.6 to 8.9. Therefore, they exist in two states: a free-base and a cationic form. When the environmental pH is below the pKa of the anesthetic, the positively charged cationic form does not actually penetrate the nerve sheaths, and penetration is required if the anesthetic is to reach its site of action, the nerve membrane. This lack of penetration can lead to poor clinical anesthesia.[32-35]

The primary action of local anesthetics involves a reduction in the permeability of the nerve cell membrane to sodium ions, a decreased rate of rise in the depolarization phase of the action potential, and failure of a propagated action potential to develop. Clinically, a sensory blockade and vasodilation appear more rapidly and at a lower anesthetic concentration than does a motor blockade because, generally, the drugs anesthetize small-diameter, slow-conducting, unmyelinated nerve fibers before they anesthetize large-diameter, fast-conducting fibers.[10,32-35] Local anesthetics that possess the greatest potency and the highest lipid solubility also exhibit the longest duration of action. The greater the binding affinity to nerve proteins, the longer is the duration of action[32-35] (Table 10-3).

Most of the vasoconstrictors that are added to local anesthetic solutions are classified as adrenergic or sympathetic amines because they closely resemble the natural mediators of the sympathetic nervous system. They will enhance the duration and effectiveness of anesthesia, decrease system toxicity by lowering the blood concentrations of the anesthetic, and decrease local bleeding at the injection site.

Local anesthetic toxicity is caused most frequently by an overdose of the local anesthetic caused by an inadvertent intravascular injection or an injection administered too rapidly. The toxicity is manifested initially in a variety of CNS symptoms, such as dizziness, ringing in the ears (tinnitus), light-headedness, disorientation, and muscle twitching. If blood levels of the anesthesia increase further, overt CNS stimulation manifested in convulsions can occur. Inadvertent intravascular injections can be avoided by the clinician's using an aspirating syringe and an effective aspiration technique.[10,32-35] A rational approach to the management of anticipated postoperative pain is to combine the preoperative and postoperative administration of a potent NSAID (e.g., ibuprofen) with the use of a long-acting local anesthetic (e.g., etidocaine).

Anxiolytic Medications and Oral Conscious Sedation

Despite incredible achievements in dental care over the past several decades, patients' fears of pain and discomfort keep a significant percentage of the population from seeking proper dental care. In addition to the near universal use of local anesthesia, general dental practitioners—and implant surgeons in particular—should consider using oral sedation as well. Ironically, the number one adverse reaction associated with the use of local anesthetics by dentists is anxiety-induced events.[36] In fact, approximately 30% of Americans avoid dental care altogether because of the anxiety associated with it.[37] The Dental Organization for Conscious Sedation (DOCS) is an international organization dedicated to improving the lives of dentists, dental team members, and patients by advancing the awareness and delivery of conscious sedation dentistry. According to DOCS, almost a third of the patients who avoid dental care need dental implants, representing a significant number of patients whose dental needs are currently unmet.[38]

Two major factors must be considered for sedation implant surgery.[38] The first involves the patient's comfort during treatment and musculature tension. A patient sedated for a surgical visit is less likely to encounter adverse reactions. The second reason to sedate a patient is for postoperative discomfort. When the clinician uses benzodiazepines in oral sedation, prescriptions for postsurgical narcotics are

TABLE 10-3 Duration and Maximal Safe Doses*

LOCAL ANESTHETIC SOLUTION	DURATION PULPAL, MIN	DURATION SOFT TISSUE, MIN	ANESTHETIC DOSE PER CARTRIDGE, MG	BODY WEIGHT	MAXIMUM
2% procaine	0-5	60-90	36	2.7/lb	400
0.4% propoxycaine 2% procaine, and 1:20,000 levonordefrin	30-60	120-180	43.2	3.0/lb	400
2% lidocaine	5-10	60-120	36	2.0/lb	300
2% lidocaine, and 1:100,000 epinephrine	60	180-240	36	2.0/lb	300
2% lidocaine, and 1:50,000 epinephrine	60	180-240	36	2.0/lb	200†
3% mepivacaine	40	120-180	54	2.0/lb	300
2% mepivacaine, and 1:200,000 epinephrine	45-60	180-240	36	2.0/lb	300
4% prilocaine	10-60	90-240	72	2.7/lb	400
4% prilocaine, and 1:200,000 epinephrine	60-90	120-240	72	2.7/lb	400
1.5% etidocaine, and 1:200,000 epinephrine	90-180	240-540	27	3.6/lb	400
0.5% bupivacaine, and 1:200,000 epinephrine	400-500	240-540	9	0.6/lb	90

*Maximal safe dose of anesthetic, mg.
†0.2 mg epinephrine is dose-limiting factor.

extremely uncommon. Several reasons may account for this absence of pain and discomfort after surgery; however, the most likely reason is the level of relaxation for the patient during the visit. Some clinicians note that as long as the patient's medical history is appropriate and he or she meets the requirements for a sedation visit, the patient can be sedated for all oral surgery; the result is that these patients praise the surgical skills of the clinician and refer friends to the dentist because of the lack of fear before surgery and the lack of discomfort afterward.[38]

Although most clinicians are willing to place implants with local anesthesia alone, approximately 96% would be candidates for oral sedation, if required.[38]

Some literature explains that the dental surgeon should consider his or her office a sanctuary for patients who are in physical and emotional pain because of their oral condition.[37] Such patients are considered in need of special care. Although technological miracles such as digital X-rays, titanium implants, bone augmentation, intraoral cameras, laser treatment of hard and soft tissue, computer-aided design (CAD)/computer-aided manufacturing (CAM) impressions and restorations, nickel-titanium rotary endodontic

systems, metal-free restorations, and smile redesigning techniques are available to facilitate implant placement, they are of little use if they are not complemented by patients' feelings of safety and freedom from fear, pain, and discomfort. Many clinicians who have incorporated oral sedation into their practice have created a health care environment that continually expands and improves the quality, quantity, and scope of patients' experience.[38]

Patient-candidates most in need of anxiolytic medications are those patients with high fear, a bad gag reflex, very sensitive teeth, an extremely low pain threshold, a phobia for the smells or sounds of the office, and so on.[38] These are patients who could have their dental care accomplished with no worry about these conditions. Remarkably, fear causes as much as 50% of the population to avoid the implant surgery that dentists can provide, and this statistic indicates that many dentists have, in fact, underserved the people they have been trained to help. Although dentistry has evolved considerably over the past 25 years to an improved state of gentle, almost pain-free care, many dentists' target markets—implant, cosmetic, and reconstruction patients—have the experience of yesterday's techniques, which were less gentle, and these patients' extreme fear of dentists prevents them from seeking the esthetic and functional benefits of modern dentistry. Therefore, the comfort of oral sedation techniques allows dentists to approach these "missing" patients.[38]

Conscious sedation has been defined as "a minimally depressed level of consciousness that retains the patient's ability to independently and continuously maintain an airway and respond appropriately to physical stimulation or verbal command and that is produced by a pharmacological or non-pharmacological method or a combination thereof."[39] Oral or intravenous methods can be used to create this "totally relaxed, yet co-operative patient." The protocols of oral conscious sedation are specific to the level of sedation required.[40] For anxiolysis, the lightest level of sedation—lorazepam or Ativan—is recommended; for oral conscious sedation, triazolam or Halcion should be used.[38] Oral triazolam has long been identified as an alternative to resorting to parenteral sedation or general anesthesia for overly anxious patients, or patients undergoing difficult procedures.[41-43]

The protocols for these drugs can be described in three safety-related categories: documentation, equipment and supplies, and training. The clinician should take a risk management approach to patient selection when considering the use of conscious sedation.[44]

Documentation

A complete oral/medical workup with the doctor is required. If the patient has not seen a physician over the past 2 years, then the dentist should refer the patient for a standard medical workup to rule out any chance of medical conditions that may interfere with the sedation. Typically, it is best to follow the risk assessment method used by the American Society of Anesthesiology (ASA) in creating the safety margins for sedation. The clinician must follow a careful and complete medical history to assess patient ASA status; patients who qualify for such treatment include only ASA I, ASA II, and some ASA III patients.[38] It is important to note that anxiolysis and oral conscious sedation in pediatric dentistry require specific consideration by the clinician; nevertheless, these methods can be safe, cost-effective approaches to providing dental care for children.[45-47]

Equipment and Supplies

An investment of time and money is required to provide sedation dentistry. Equipment and supplies may cost up to several thousand dollars. A pulse oximeter (Figure 10-4) with blood pressure and printer is vital. If a reversal agent is available, it should also be on hand.[48] Positive-pressure oxygen is a must. An automated external defibrillator should be the basic standard of care for any practice, not just a sedation practice. An emergency medical kit should always be available, along with constant patient monitor-

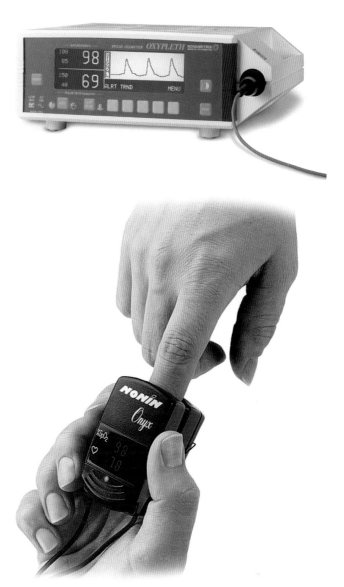

FIGURE 10-4 ■ Pulse oximeter. (From Lewis SL et al: Medical-surgical nursing: assessment and management of clinical problems, ed 7, St Louis, Mosby, 2007.)

ing by a team member who is trained in cardiopulmonary resuscitation (CPR) and is using the appropriate equipment. The only patients who should be treated with this basic technique are adult patients; a pulse oximeter blood pressure monitor is used the moment patients enter the clinical environment, and patients are always accompanied by a trained member of the team throughout treatment.[38] An agonist reversal agent should be available for use on an emergency basis for complete reversal of the sedative effects. With this conscious sedation formula, the practicing clinician can temporarily lighten the level of sedation at any time to obtain X-rays or bite registrations, or when it is time for dismissal. Airway management and emergency medical kits are also available.[38]

Training

In addition to the cost of the equipment, an educational investment may be required, depending on the size of the dental team and the local requirements for certification; for the surgical specialist or the nonsurgical specialist/generalist who is using minimal oral sedation, a 1-day didactic training session for anxiolysis is recommended, but 3 days of didactic training is needed for the more complex oral conscious sedation.[38] For example, the oral sedation formula that is presented in the DOCS seminar "The Essentials of Oral Sedation" is based on a carefully measured system that delivers the appropriately desired effect at the correct time; such a system provides the dental team with the confidence and ability to offer an all-day appointment for extensive care and multiple procedures.[38]

Potential Problems and Complications

A patient who is receiving anxiolytic medications or other forms of conscious oral sedation could develop hiccups for up to 15 minutes during a sedation visit; in such cases, the clinician should just wait and relax. Dry mouth (xerostomia) is another side effect, but one that many clinicians consider a plus, not a complication. Another complication may be that a patient becomes too relaxed and his or her head slumps forward, causing a slight airway closure that would cause a drop in the body's oxygen level and trigger the pulse oximeter to alarm. If this situation arises, one simply commands the patient to reposition his or her head. A third complication that could arise is that before being sedated, the patient may have taken other medications and failed to tell the practitioner. This complication could cause the patient to experience a deeper level of sedation than was intended. This situation occurs in approximately 1 of every 2,000 cases.[38] Under such circumstances, the reversal agent should be administered to reverse the effects of the sedation. A fourth complication may be that a patient is ataxic (unsteady). As a consequence, patients should never drive to or from the office and must be attended at all times by a companion who follows the postoperative instructions carefully. These instructions include maintaining the safety of the patient in a home environment (no steps, no operating heavy/dangerous equipment, no driving, and so on).[38]

The short-term benefits for the "missing" implant patient, of course, are the freedom from fear and discomfort that have kept this patient away from the dentist in the first place.

Cephalosporins are a widely used and expanding family of antibiotics that are relatively nontoxic but, similar to the penicillins, can be inactivated by β-lactamase. First-generation benefits include improved dental esthetics and comfort, amply documented in the literature associated with dental implants. The clinician benefits from the knowledge that he or she has reached a segment of the population statis-tically underserved. The entire dental team benefits from this awareness also, of course. More tangibly, the clinician's total investment of time and money will be recovered through the additional fees that sedation techniques generate. With the economic value of a new sedation patient statistically shown to be 350% higher than that of an average new patient, it is easy to see the bottom-line consequences; the addition of implant and cosmetic care to this statistic means a possible 500% increase in new patient value.[38] Because of their past fear and often prolonged avoidance of dentists, sedation patients realize that their oral neglect cannot be remedied simply and quickly. They understand the monetary investment required of them.

Antibiotics

The prevention of wound infection is a major consideration in implant dentistry. When infection does occur, increased patient morbidity and suffering result, along with additional expense, increased antibiotic usage, delayed recovery, and increased implant failure. Infection occurs when there is a significant quantitative and qualitative bacterial insult. Infection occurs more readily if the patient's host defense mechanisms are reduced, rendering the patient more susceptible to infection. Therefore, prevention of infection can be accomplished first, by reducing the number of bacteria in the surgical wound and second, by enhancing those defenses to prevent the bacteria that inevitably enter the wound from causing clinically evident infection.[9,49-54]

The antibiotic chosen by the surgeon must be effective against the bacteria that are most likely to cause infection after the surgical procedure is completed; it should be the least toxic agent available and should be bactericidal; to be maximally effective, the plasma concentration must be high enough to allow diffusion into tissues contaminated by the bacteria.[9,49-54] Most odontogenic infections involve plaque organisms. Supragingival plaque consists mainly of gram-positive facultative anaerobes, gram-negative rods, and motile forms, including spirochetes. It is now evident that orofacial odontogenic infections usually are polymicrobial, consisting of both anaerobes and aerobes. Indeed, more than 65% of the species isolated are obligate anaerobes; aerobes are also isolated from about one-third of infections. The first choice of prophylactic antibiotic for transoral procedures is amoxicillin or erythromycin. A first-generation cephalosporin is often recommended if the allergic reaction to penicillin is nonanaphylactic.[9,49-54]

Penicillin: Penicillin G and other oral forms such as penicillin V have been widely used for many years; however, increasing resistance to the drug is an ongoing problem. Penicillin V is active against non–penicillinase-producing *Staphylococcus*, most streptococcal species, most gram-positive bacilli *(Actinomyces)*, anaerobic streptococci (peptostreptococci), anaerobic gram-positive rods, spirochetes, and some *Neisseria* species. Aerobic gram-negative bacilli are highly resistant, and *Bacteroides* species are also resistant because of β-lactamase production. Penicillin V is available in 125-mg, 250-mg, and 500-mg tablets, as well as in suspension form. Because of the frequency of bone involvement in odontogenic infection, 1,000 mg every 8 hours is the preferred dosage to maintain therapeutic levels in difficult-to-penetrate bone tissue. Penicillin V is excreted by renal mechanisms.

Amoxicillin has enhanced penetration into gram-negative bacilli and enterococci but, like penicillin V, is inactivated by β-lactamase. It is acid stable with good absorption in the upper gastrointestinal tract and has excellent tissue penetration. The spectrum of activity includes most organisms sensitive to penicillin with the addition of some non–β-lactamase producing gram-negative rods, such as *H. influenzae*. Amoxicillin is marketed in 250-mg and 500-mg capsules, with oral suspension and pediatric drops available. For odontogenic infections in adults, 500 mg every 6 to 8 hours is recommended.

A combination of amoxicillin (250 mg or 500 mg) and clavulanate potassium (125 mg) is available as Augmentin (GlaxoSmithKline, Middlesex, United Kingdom). It has the antimicrobial activity of amoxicillin and is effective against β-lactamase–producing strains of *Bacteroides*, staphylococci (but not methicillin-resistant *S aureus*), and gram-negative bacilli, such as *Haemophilus* and *Moraxella*. The appropriate dose is 500 mg of amoxicillin combined with 125 mg of clavulanate potassium every 6 to 8 hours. Gastrointestinal side effects of diarrhea and nausea may occur, but most patients tolerate them without difficulty. Ampicillin, an extended-spectrum penicillin developed to give coverage against certain cephalosporins, is indicated for surgical prophylaxis and for the treatment of most staphylococcal and streptococcal infections in patients who may be allergic to the penicillins. As the cephalosporins increase from first to third generation, activity against gram-negative bacilli increases, and activity against gram-positive cocci decreases.

Erythromycin is a bacteriostatic macrolide antibiotic. It has activity in vitro against most streptococci: *S aureus, Moraxella, Capnocytophaga*, some anaerobes, and some gram-negative anaerobic bacteria. The common adult dose is 400 mg every 6 hours, or 800 mg every 12 hours. Most patients have some minor adverse gastrointestinal effects, such as nausea, abdominal pain, increased stool volume, and alcohol intolerance. Its main use in implant dentistry is for prophylaxis in the penicillin-allergic patient.

Clindamycin is one of the most reliable antibiotics against serious odontogenic infection. It is bacteriostatic in action, except at high doses, when it becomes bactericidal. It has excellent activity against aerobes and anaerobes. Because of its propensity to cause antibiotic-associated colitis, it has not been widely used for more routine, mild to moderate odontogenic infections.

Vancomycin exerts a bactericidal effect on multiplying microorganisms by inhibiting the biosynthesis of a major structural cell wall polymer. With the introduction of semisynthetic penicillins and the cephalosporins, the role of vancomycin has been relegated to alternate therapy when penicillins or cephalosporins cannot be used.

SUMMARY

Elective procedures such as implant surgery warrant consideration of postoperative edema. Careful manipulation of soft and hard tissues limits the severity of the edema. Postoperative instructions such as elevation of the head, limited activity, and applied pressure are helpful. For pain management, a large body of data has appeared in dental literature over the past decade supporting the use of NSAIDs (ibuprofen) as the agents of choice for moderate pain with a minimal potential for side effects. Additional literature supports the use of a long-acting anesthetic in combination with NSAID pretreatment for preventing the onset and intensity of postoperative pain. Owing to limited oral efficacy and substantial side effects, the use of oral opioids should be limited to those patients whose pain is not relieved by nonopioid therapy. Antibiotic therapy should be provided as a prophylactic measure to prevent infection after implant surgery. If an odontogenic infection is detected after surgery, it should be drained and treated according to the principles of surgical follow-up as a primary mode of therapy, along with adjunctive therapy for pain and infection.

The key to a safe, effective choice of pharmacological agents in implant dentistry depends on the dentist's current knowledge of drug reactions, indications, contraindications, adverse reactions, and interactions with other drugs.[55,56] This chapter presents the dentist with a wide variety of pharmacological agents applicable to implant procedures. Oral implantology today requires a high level of knowledge and expertise. With the judicial application of pharmacological principles to implant dentistry, the dentist can optimize clinical success rates by reducing the variables in the patient's response to surgery and can achieve a success rate comparable to or surpassing rates in other fields of medical treatment.

REFERENCES

1. Park SJ, Chiang CY, Hu JW, Sessle BJ: Neuroplasticity induced by tooth pulp stimulation in trigeminal subnucleus oralis involves NMDA receptor mechanisms, *J Neurophysiol* 85(5):1836-1846, 2001.
2. Dionne RA, Phero JC, Becker DE, editors: *Pain and anxiety control in dentistry*, Philadelphia, 2002, WB Saunders.
3. Chidiac JJ, Rifai K, Hawwa NN, Massaad CA, Jurjus AR, Jabbur SJ, Saade NE: Nociceptive behaviour induced by dental application of irritants to rat incisors: a new model for tooth inflammatory pain, *Eur J Pain* 6(1):55-67, 2002.
4. Motohashi K, Umino M, Fujii Y: An experimental system for a heterotopic pain stimulation study in humans, *Brain Res Brain Res Protoc* 10(1):31-40, 2002.

5. Dussor GO, Helesic G, Hargreaves KM, Flores CM: Cholinergic modulation of nociceptive responses in vivo and neuropeptide release in vitro at the level of the primary sensory neuron, *Pain* 107(1-2):22-32, 2004.

6. Phero JC, Becker DE, Dionne RA: Contemporary trends in acute pain management, *Curr Opin Otolaryngol Head Neck Surg* 12(3):209-216, 2004.

7. Sachs CJ: Oral analgesics for acute nonspecific pain, *Am Fam Physician* 71(5):913-918, 2005.

8. Locher-Claus MT, Erickson TE, Law AS, Johnson WT, Gebhart GF: Effects of pre-emptive morphine, ibuprofen or local anesthetic on fos expression in the spinal trigeminal nucleus following tooth pulp exposure in the rat, *J Endod* 31(8):578-583, 2005.

9. Misch CE, Moore P: Steroids and the reduction of pain, edema and dysfunction in implant dentistry, *Int J Oral Implantol* 6(1):27-31, 1989.

10. Hargreaves KM, Troullos ES, Dionne RA: Pharmacologic rationale for the treatment of acute pain, *Dent Clin North Am* 31(4):675-694, 1987.

11. Dionne RA, Gordon SM: Nonsteroidal anti-inflammatory drugs for acute pain control, *Dent Clin North Am* 38(4):645-667, 1994.

12. Vallerand WP: Pain and principles of effective analgesic use for dental pain control, *J Tenn Dent Assoc* 81(1):10-16, 2001.

13. Haas DA: An update on analgesics for the management of acute postoperative dental pain, *J Can Dent Assoc* 68(8):476-482, 2002.

14. Huynh MP, Yagiela JA: Current concepts in acute pain management, *J Calif Dent Assoc* 31(5):419-427, 2003.

15. Gaciong Z: The real dimension of analgesic activity of aspirin, *Thromb Res* 110(5-6):361-364, 2003.

16. Rodrigo MR, Rosenquist JB: Does midazolam sedation in oral surgery affect the potency or duration of diflunisal analgesia? *Aust Dent J* 35(4):333-337, 1990.

17. Lawton GM, Chapman PJ: Diflunisal—a long-acting non-steroidal anti-inflammatory drug: a review of its pharmacology and effectiveness in management of postoperative dental pain, *Aust Dent J* 38(4):265-271, 1993.

18. Comfort MB, Tse AS, Tsang AC, McGrath C: A study of the comparative efficacy of three common analgesics in the control of pain after third molar surgery under local anaesthesia, *Aust Dent J* 47(4):327-330, 2002.

19. Mehlisch DR, Sollecito WA, Helfrick JF, Leibold DG, Markowitz R, Schow CE Jr, Shultz R, Waite DE: Multicenter clinical trial of ibuprofen and acetaminophen in the treatment of postoperative dental pain, *J Am Dent Assoc* 121(2):257-263, 1990.

20. Mehlisch DR, Jasper RD, Brown P, Korn SH, McCarroll K, Murakami AA: Comparative study of ibuprofen lysine and acetaminophen in patients with postoperative dental pain, *Clin Ther* 17(5):852-860, 1995.

21. Black P, Max MB, Desjardins P, Norwood T, Ardia A, Pallotta T: A randomized, double-blind, placebo-controlled comparison of the analgesic efficacy, onset of action, and tolerability of ibuprofen arginate and ibuprofen in postoperative dental pain, *Clin Ther* 24(7):1072-1089, 2002.

22. Polat O, Karaman AI, Durmus E: Effects of preoperative ibuprofen and naproxen sodium on orthodontic pain, *Angle Orthod* 75(5):791-796, 2005.

23. Phero JC, Becker D: Rational use of analgesic combinations, *Dent Clin North Am* 46(4):691-705, 2002.

24. Litkowski LJ, Christensen SE, Adamson DN, Van Dyke T, Han SH, Newman KB: Analgesic efficacy and tolerability of oxycodone

5 mg/ibuprofen 400 mg compared with those of oxycodone 5 mg/acetaminophen 325 mg and hydrocodone 7.5 mg/acetaminophen 500 mg in patients with moderate to severe postoperative pain: a randomized, double-blind, placebo-controlled, single-dose, parallel-group study in a dental pain model, *Clin Ther* 27(4):418-429, 2005.

25. Montgomery MT, Hogg JP, Roberts DL, Redding SW: The use of glucocorticosteroids to lessen the inflammatory sequelae following third molar surgery, *J Oral Maxillofac Surg* 48(2):179-187, 1990.

26. Devillier P: Pharmacology of glucocorticoids and ENT pathology, *Presse Med* 30(39-40 Pt 2):59-69, 2001. French.

27. Ustun Y, Erdogan O, Esen E, Karsli ED: Comparison of the effects of 2 doses of methylprednisolone on pain, swelling, and trismus after third molar surgery, *Oral Surg Oral Med Oral Pathol Oral Radiol Endod* 96(5):535-539, 2003.

28. Bodnar J: Corticosteroids and oral surgery, *Anesth Prog* 48(4):130-132, 2001.

29. Barbosa F: Patient selection for dental implants, Part 2: contraindications, *J Indiana Dent Assoc* 80(1):10-12, 2001.

30. Sugerman PB, Barber MT: Patient selection for endosseous dental implants: oral and systemic considerations, *Int J Oral Maxillofac Implants* 17(2):191-201, 2002.

31. Marder MZ: Medical conditions affecting the success of dental implants, *Compend Contin Educ Dent* 25(10):739-742, 744, 746, 2004, passim; quiz 772, 795.

32. Haanaes HR: Implants and infections with special reference to oral bacteria, *J Clin Periodontol* 17(7 [Pt 2]):516-524, 1990.

33. Jeske AH: Xylocaine: 50 years of clinical service to dentistry, *Tex Dent J* 115(5):9-13, 1998.

34. Lu DP: Managing patients with local anesthetic complications using alternative methods, *Pa Dent J (Harrisb)* 69(3):22-29, 2002.

35. Calatayud J, Gonzalez A: History of the development and evolution of local anesthesia since the coca leaf, *Anesthesiology* 98(6):1503-1508, 2003.

36. Haas DA: An update on local anesthetics in dentistry, *J Can Dent Assoc* 68(9):546-551, 2002.

37. Silverman MD: The matrix: oral sedation for dentistry, *Int Mag Oral Implantol* 2:453-454, 2001.

38. Silverman MD: Benefits and protocols of oral sedation for implant surgery, *Dent Implantol Update* 14(6):41-45, 2003.

39. American Dental Association: Guidelines for the use of conscious sedation, deep sedation, and general anesthesia for dentists, Online Posting, 2005 Oct. ADA.org (cited 2005 Dec 30). Available at: http://www.ada.org/prof/resources/positions/statements/anesthesia_guidelines.pdf

40. Goodchild JH, Feck AS: Anxiolysis in general dental practice, *Dent Today* 22(3):106-111, 2003.

41. Berthold CW, Schneider A, Dionne RA: Using triazolam to reduce dental anxiety, *J Am Dent Assoc* 124(11):58-64, 1993.

42. Berthold CW, Dionne RA, Corey SE: Comparison of sublingually and orally administered triazolam for premedication before oral surgery, *Oral Surg Oral Med Oral Pathol Oral Radiol Endod* 84(2):119-124, 1997.

43. Quarnstrom FW, Donaldson M: Triazolam use in the dental setting: a report of 270 uses over 15 years, *Gen Dent* 52(6):496-501, 2004.

44. Jackson DL, Johnson BS: Conscious sedation for dentistry: risk management and patient selection, *Dent Clin North Am* 46(4):767-780, 2002.

45. Eid H: Conscious sedation in the 21st century, *J Clin Pediatr Dent* 26(2):179-180, 2002.

46. Webb MD, Moore PA: Sedation for pediatric dental patients, *Dent Clin North Am* 46(4):803-814, xi, 2002.

47. Silegy T, Jacks ST: Pediatric oral conscious sedation, *J Calif Dent Assoc* 31(5):413-418, 2003.

48. Girdler NM, Lyne JP, Wallace R, Neave N, Scholey A, Wesnes KA, Herman C: A randomised, controlled trial of cognitive and psychomotor recovery from midazolam sedation following reversal with oral flumazenil, *Anaesthesia* 57(9):868-876, 2002.

49. Meffert RM: Periodontitis and periimplantitis: one and the same? *Pract Periodontics Aesthet Dent* 5(9):79-80, 82, 1993.

50. Wilson TG Jr: Putting science into practice: the clinical translation of medical approaches, *Compend Contin Educ Dent* 23(5 suppl):22-24, 2002.

51. Heydenrijk K, Meijer HJ, van der Reijden WA, Raghoebar GM, Vissink A, Stegenga B: Microbiota around root-form endosseous implants: a review of the literature, *Int J Oral Maxillofac Implants* 17(6):829-838, 2002.

52. Sanchez-Garces MA, Gay-Escoda C: Periimplantitis, *Med Oral Patol Oral Cir Bucal* 9(suppl):69-74; 63-69, 2004.

53. Binahmed A, Stoykewych A, Peterson L: Single preoperative dose versus long-term prophylactic antibiotic regimens in dental implant surgery, *Int J Oral Maxillofac Implants* 20(1):115-117, 2005.

54. Powell CA, Mealey BL, Deas DE, McDonnell HT, Moritz AJ: Post-surgical infections: prevalence associated with various periodontal surgical procedures, *J Periodontol* 76(3):329-333, 2005.

55. Dresser GK, Bailey DG: A basic conceptual and practical overview of interactions with highly prescribed drugs, *Can J Clin Pharmacol* 9(4):191-198, 2002.

56. Hersh EV, Moore PA: Drug interactions in dentistry: the importance of knowing your CYPs, *J Am Dent Assoc* 135(3):298-311, 2004.

chapter 11

Anterior Single-Tooth Implants in the Esthetic Zone

THE DEVELOPMENT OF ADVANCED SURGICAL and restorative techniques has expanded the application of osseointegrated implants. Implants can be used in partially edentulous patients, for complex combination applications, and for single-tooth restorations, including the anterior esthetic zone.[1-12] However, the clinician must keep a number of extremely important caveats in mind. Implants in the esthetic zone are the most difficult to perform from a number of perspectives, including surgical, bone maintenance/grafting, soft tissue management, and prosthetic esthetics. The general recommendation is that before attempting an implant in the esthetic zone, the clinician should place and restore 100 implants in less challenging areas. Additionally, cases should be categorized to determine the level of difficulty, as well as to assess the procedure(s) required for case completion. Levels range from most optimal for implant success (Level 1) to least optimal (Level 7) and include the following characteristics:

Level 1: Extraction performed by clinician, Good 5-wall bony housing, Great papilla and/or thick-flat periodontal biotype, Low smile line

Level 2: Extraction performed previously and grafted, Good 5-wall bony housing, Great papilla and/or thick-flat periodontal biotype, Low smile line

Level 3: Extraction performed previously and not grafted, Good 5-wall bony housing, Great papilla and/or thick-flat periodontal biotype, Medium smile line

Level 4: Extraction performed previously and not grafted, 4-wall bony housing, Good papilla and/or thick-flat periodontal biotype, Medium smile line

Level 5: Extraction performed previously and not grafted, 4-wall bony housing, Good papilla and/or thick-flat periodontal biotype, High smile line

Level 6: Extraction performed previously and not grafted, 3-wall bony housing, Inadequate papilla mesially or distally, High smile line

Level 7: Extraction performed previously and grafted or not grafted but inadequate bone, 2-wall bony housing, Inadequate papilla mesially and distally, Moderate or high smile line

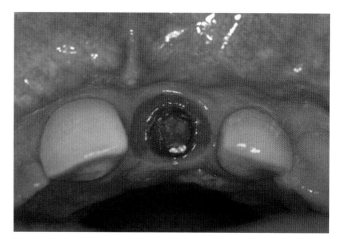

FIGURE 11-1 ■ Buccolingual and incisal-apical implant position is highly important, especially in the esthetic zone.

Single-tooth implants are a viable treatment option for many patients. Although many still regard the fixed partial denture as the standard of care for the replacement of single or multiple missing teeth,[13] the success rate for single-tooth osseointegrated implants is comparable with that of implant-supported prostheses in totally edentulous patients.[1] A success rate of 98.5% has been reported after 3 years in Level 1 cases.[14] Research has noted that given the long-term success of single implants, they are an effective alternative to using teeth as abutments to preserve intact teeth in patients undergoing initial and follow-up prosthodontic therapy.[15] The cosmetic considerations for anterior single-tooth implants are similar or equivalent to those required for an anterior pontic or a single crown on a natural tooth.[16] However, it is frequently more difficult to accommodate the bone and soft tissue architecture when dealing with a single-tooth dental implant. With a natural tooth, the form of an artificial crown is determined by the existing tooth form and periodontal architecture. However, when placing single-tooth implants, the clinician must establish the bone and soft tissue necessary for the implant, and must try to re-create the form of the original tooth and match the porcelain to the adjacent natural teeth (Figure 11-1).

Implant prosthesis treatment planning has become an important element of anterior rehabilitation, because achieving reproducibility is often problematic when a diagnostic wax-up is used as a template for fabricating an implant restoration; consequently, methods have developed for fabrication of a provisional restoration before the implant is placed surgically. A specific method for such fabrication has been described in the literature and involves steps that include determining the mesiodistal inclination of the implant, the buccolingual dimension of the alveolar ridge, and the implant position; fabricating the surgical guide and the provisional restoration; and immediately placing the provisional restoration after implant placement.[17]

Immediate provisionalization of implants when they are placed can give patients restorations that most resemble natural teeth. By fabricating the implant abutment and provisional crown preoperatively, clinicians can provide single-tooth provisionally restored implants based on specific diagnostic criteria. With this method, an implant analog is placed into a diagnostic model preoperatively, and the abutment and the provisional crown are prepared on the model. The provisional crown is fabricated out of occlusion, so that when the implant is placed, the abutment and provisional crown can also be placed. The final restoration is fabricated only after the implant undergoes osseointegration, resulting in success rates comparable with those of two-stage surgery.[18]

A patient's desire for an implant, healthy adjacent teeth with an acceptable form, and a natural diastema within the arch are all indications for single-tooth implants. However, the use of an implant in this situation may be limited by lack of mesiodistal space, deformities of the edentulous crest, an inadequate gingival environment, an abnormal occlusal relationship, or the proximity and angulation of the adjacent roots.[19] Naturally, a number of evaluation criteria, including available bone volume, soft tissue condition, anatomy of the ridge, and the implant components (both surgical and prosthetic), accompany proper treatment planning for placement of the single-tooth implant in the anterior maxilla; consequently, a three-stage approach using an emergence-profile concept can help the clinician choose the type of implant, healing abutment, and provisional prosthesis to be used for optimally esthetic implant placement.[20]

After a discussion of general guidelines, specific guidelines for managing each level of case will be presented.

Pretreatment Guidelines

Before placing anterior single-tooth implants, the clinician must be aware of certain placement criteria, such as the anatomy of the implant, type of periodontium, preexisting tooth form and position, and root morphology.[1-12,16] Additionally, to obtain optimal esthetics, the clinician must consider the soft tissue anatomy, bone dimension, and smile line.[1-12,21] Of particular concern after the loss of an anterior natural tooth is the relatively quick and progressive collapse of the mucogingival complex; the earlier the placement of implants, the more likely it is that such collapse can be prevented or minimized.[22] Additionally, changes in soft tissue margins can cause titanium at the gingival crevice to become visible. As a result, all-ceramic restorations have become more popular in recent years to meet patients' esthetic demands.[23]

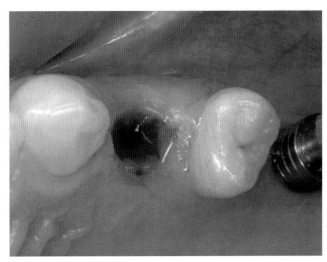

FIGURE 11-2 ■ Collapsing soft tissue during impression taking will compromise the outcome of the final restoration.

Soft Tissue Considerations

To achieve an esthetically pleasing final result, the clinician must consider the anatomy of the soft tissue. The underlying contours of the bone determine the soft tissue contours.[21] Not treating soft tissue properly could result in a gingival appearance dissimilar to that of adjacent teeth.[9] Generally speaking, when an anterior single-tooth implant is placed in a site without tissue deficiencies, treatment outcomes and esthetics are predictable, mainly because of the tissue support from adjacent teeth; however, when multiple adjacent teeth in the anterior maxilla are missing, fixed implant restorations are not as reliably treated, especially with regard to the contours of the interimplant soft tissue.[5]

Patients can present with two types of periodontium: thin and scalloped or thick and flat. Thin, scalloped periodontium is characterized by a small amount of attached gingiva, delicate soft tissue, and a scalloped underlying osseous form. Thick, flat periodontium is characterized by denser and more fibrotic soft tissue, an underlying osseous form that is flatter and thicker, and a larger amount of attached gingiva.[16]

The tooth form varies depending on the type of periodontium present. With thick, flat periodontium, the anatomic crowns are essentially square, the contact areas of adjacent teeth are located more apically and are greater incisogingivally and faciolingually, and more bulbous convexities are located in the cervical thirds. With thin, scalloped periodontium, the anatomic crowns are essentially triangular, the contact areas of adjacent teeth are located more incisally and occlusally and are smaller faciolingually and incisogingivally, and small, more subtle convexities are located in the cervical thirds of the facial areas.[16]

Facial and interproximal gingival recession is more likely to occur in patients with thin, scalloped periodontium.[14,16] Gingival recession on adjacent teeth may occur when implants are placed immediately after tooth extraction. It has been shown that the use of conservative flap designs (in other words, labial flap extension of 3 mm or less beyond the alveolar crest) may eliminate gingival recession of teeth adjacent to implant sites.[14] Onlay, subepithelial, and interpositional grafts can be used to correct mucogingival deficiencies that occur after tooth extraction[1] (Figure 11-2).

Predictable esthetic results can be complicated if two or more implants are placed in adjacent sites in the anterior maxilla. The presence of interdental papillae can be adversely affected by inadequate maintenance of the distance from the interproximal crest of bone to the contact point. The design of the coronal portion of the implant, as well as the contour of the implant-abutment junction, can also influence the maintenance of the interdental papilla between adjacent implants.[24] When several adjacent teeth in the anterior maxilla are removed at the same time, the labial bony plate can collapse, and the interproximal bony scallop can become flattened, resulting in missing interimplant papillae and requiring the use of long implants for restoration. As a result, papilla preservation techniques, including alternate immediate implant placement and provisionalization as a series of implants heal/osseointegrate one after the other, have been developed.[25] Because of this interimplant bone flattening and soft tissue position changing, which take place during the establishment of biological width around adjacent implants, the loss of the usual support of papillae provided by natural teeth can lead to the requirement for additional techniques, including the use of scalloped implant designs to maintain the interdental bony peaks and interimplant papillae.[26]

Bone Dimension

In the anterior maxilla, the emergence profile and fixture position are determined by the height and width of the remaining bone.[21] Because of the occurrence of ridge

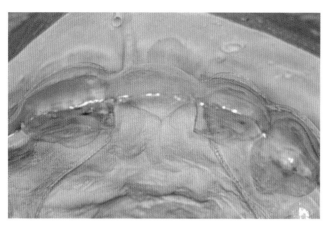

FIGURE 11-3 ■ In the anterior maxilla, the emergence profile of the crown is determined by the implant position, which is determined by the height and width of the remaining bone. The area can and should be grafted as necessary for optimal implant.

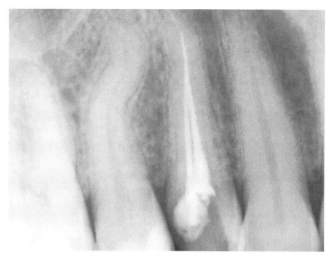

FIGURE 11-4 ■ Evaluate the radiograph of the tooth prior to extraction to avoid complications.

resorption after tooth extraction, grafting of the extraction socket and placement of an ovate pontic bonded to adjacent teeth will assist in site preparation. Implants should be placed soon after initial socket healing to maintain internal stimulation of the bone and prevent collapse of the facial plate.[21] If traumatic tooth loss is a factor in the anterior maxilla, the clinician should be prepared for alveolar ridge resorption, especially in the sagittal direction, due mainly to avulsion of bone, which occurred as a result of the accident, or subsequent resorption of the alveolar crest.[27] Regardless, proper implant positioning requires that the bone volume be increased for both esthetic and functional purposes. Documented treatment options in such cases in the anterior maxilla include bone grafting, bone substitutes, guided bone regeneration, osteocompression, and distraction; additional options include crestal split osteotomy (with chisels and osteotomes) to widen the ridge[27] (Figure 11-3).

Placing implants too close to natural teeth can cause bone loss adjacent to the tooth. Adequate osseous and restorative dimensions are essential when single-tooth implants are placed. There must be a balance between the restorative dimension and the existing bone dimension—one may be adequate, whereas the other may not. Clinicians must be familiar with the anatomy of the implant and implant components to adequately evaluate these dimensions.[16]

On the facial and lingual areas of the implant, a minimum of 1 mm of bone is required around the implant. To place a standard-size implant, a 6-mm bone bed is necessary buccolingually.[16] In areas where there is reduced bone, smaller-diameter implants can be placed, or bone grafting or guided bone regeneration can be used.

For implant placement, the clinician must consider the implant angulation. In esthetic areas, primary closure must be obtained to allow optimal soft tissue height for esthetics.

Root Morphology

Before an implant is placed, the root form must be evaluated (Figure 11-4). Evaluating radiographs of the tooth before it was lost as well as the remaining teeth may be beneficial. In patients with thin, scalloped periodontium, the roots are narrow and more tapered. In the interproximal areas between adjacent roots, a wide mesiodistal area of bone is observed, as the result of significant tapering of the roots. In patients with thick, flat periodontium, the roots are wider and less tapered. A smaller area of mesiodistal bone is noted in the interproximal areas between the roots, because the roots are similar in width to the crowns. When a standard-diameter implant is placed, a minimum of 6.5 mm of space is needed between the roots of the teeth.[16]

Site Preparation Using Osteotomes

In the standard method for preparing the bone site for implant placement, drills are used to remove bone. However, drilling in the maxilla may be difficult because of anatomical and bone quality limitations. An alternative technique using osteotomes can be applied in sites that cannot be sufficiently developed using standard drilling techniques. Instead of removing bone, osteotomes compress the bone laterally, allowing for bone preservation, condensation, and expansion; osteotomes can used to widen thin ridges to facilitate implant placement.[28-34]

Elements that characterize the osteotome technique include the absence of drilling, conservation of osseous tissue, improvement of bone density, and proper selection of implant type and design. Under normal circumstances, the osteotomy for an endosseous implant is created by removing bone from the site through the use of progressively larger drill bits, the last of which is approximately the same diameter and length as the implant. Where bone types D1 (dense compacta, composed of almost all cortical bone, typically found in the anterior mandible and corresponding to the basal bone of the symphysis; able to support great loads because of its highly mineralized matrix) and D2 (thick, porous compacta and coarse trabecular bone; commonly located in the posterior mandible and sometimes in the anterior maxilla) predominate, a traditional drilling approach generally is appropriate. However, when bone type D3 (porous compacta and fine trabecular bone; found primarily in the anterior maxilla, with the tactile sensation when drilled similar to balsa wood) or D4 (fine trabecular bone; most commonly found in the long-term edentulous posterior maxilla) dominates at the proposed implant site, a different approach often is needed. Generally, the more posterior the location of the implant site in the maxilla, the less dense is the bone quality.

An additional advantage of osteotomes over drilling in the maxilla and other bone-compromised sites is increased tactile sensitivity for the clinician. Types of bone (including elements of both texture and density) are assessed more easily by probing with an osteotome than by drilling. Furthermore, sound can be an assessment feature for the clinician using osteotomes. Also, damage to existing osseous tissue is less likely through the use of an osteotome, as the clinician redirects the instrument to find the bone location best suited for the axis of implant placement.

The tips of most osteotomes (intended to provide more bone height) are not pointed; rather, they are concave and have sharp edges, effectively shaving and then pushing bone in front of them as they are pushed or malleted into position (Figure 11-5). The effect is conservation of osseous tissues. Laser lines on the osteotomes mark insertion depths for threaded or cylinder implant lengths. For bone compaction (to provide increased width of bone), most clinicians favor round-tipped osteotomes to blunt or convex ones. Such preferences are based on evidence that the bone is entered with

less resistance with round-tipped osteotomes, thus reducing the risk of fracturing the buccal or lingual plate of bone.

When osteotomes are used to create an osteotomy for implant placement, the bone surrounding the future osteotomy is compacted as osteotomes of progressively larger diameters are pushed or malleted into the alveolar ridge. The less dense bone at the implant site chosen for the osteotomy is relocated, not removed as it would be through drilling. This preserves the bone at the site and, ideally, makes it denser, increasing the chances of implant survival once the implant is in place. Additionally, because minimal heat is created by using osteotomes, there is no compromise of the osseointegration process in the short term, unlike with drilling, which does create heat.

When the selection of implant type and design is discussed, the pioneering work by Summers must be addressed; Summers indicates that when osteotomes are used in spongy bone, an implant with a neck that is wider than the shaft often allows better implant fixation initially.[28-31,33] Although both screw-shape and press-fit implants have been used after osteotome preparation of a site (whether hydroxyapatite-coated or titanium plasma spray–coated), press-fit implants appear to be a superior choice.

A pilot drill, such as a #1701 or Lindeman bur in a straight handpiece, should be used to start the initial pilot hole to the predetermined depth. The pilot hole is then enlarged, starting with the smallest osteotome and followed by a series of larger osteotomes as needed, depending on the type and size of the implant being placed.[32]

Implant Placement

An optimum emergence profile in the single-tooth implant crown has become increasingly important, particularly in the anterior esthetic zone, as the routine nature of the practice has grown. Many healing abutments and transfer

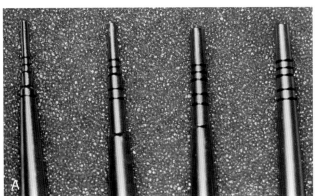
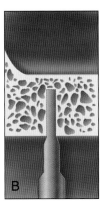
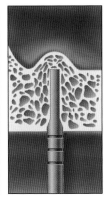
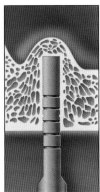

FIGURE 11-5 ■ **A,** Osteotomes of increasing diameter have a concave tip, thereby advancing and condensing the bone in an apical and lateral direction. **B,** Diagram showing how the osteotome technique increases the bone density of type IV bone by condensing the bone laterally. (From Rose LF, Mealey BL: *Periodontics: medicine, surgery, and implants,* St. Louis, Mosby, 2004.)

copings are round (and do not resemble the cross section normally seen in the anterior maxilla), resulting in restorations that can be less than natural looking, specifically, unnatural sulcular form around implant abutments.[35] Some researchers have developed specific implant protocols for placement of implants in the anterior maxilla to optimize emergence profile, believing that such planning promotes precise criteria evaluation involving bone volume, soft tissues, dental anatomy, and surgical and prosthetic components. For example, a three-stage approach to the emergence profile concept can guide the selection of implant, healing abutment, and provisional prosthesis.[20] Accurate place-

ment of single-tooth implants is very important because it determines the tooth form, emergence profile, location of the screw hole, and dimensions of the interproximal papillae.[36] A thorough preoperative radiographic and clinical examination and the use of a surgical template are necessary to develop space for the interproximal papillae mesially and distally. The development of this space is necessary to achieve anatomical flow of the gingival tissues and good crown contours (Figure 11-6, *A*).[6,36]

Several guidelines have been developed for the placement of anterior single-tooth implants. For cement-retained restorations, the implant should be angled buccally, which

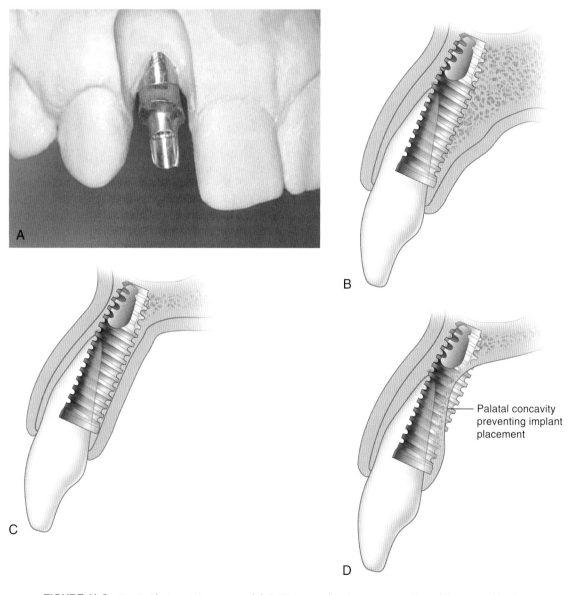

FIGURE 11-6 ■ **A,** Abutment in cast model. **B,** Diagram showing cross section of the central incisor site with excellent palatal bone thickness. In this situation, the implant can be placed immediately after the tooth extraction, with assurance of its stability. **C,** Diagram showing cross section of a central incisor site with narrow palatal bone thickness. In this clinical situation, immediate implant placement may not be stable because of lack of bone availability, and a delayed approach may be appropriate. **D,** Diagram depicting the palatal concavity problem, where the implant would have a palatal dehiscence if the crest were sufficiently wide for placement of the implant.

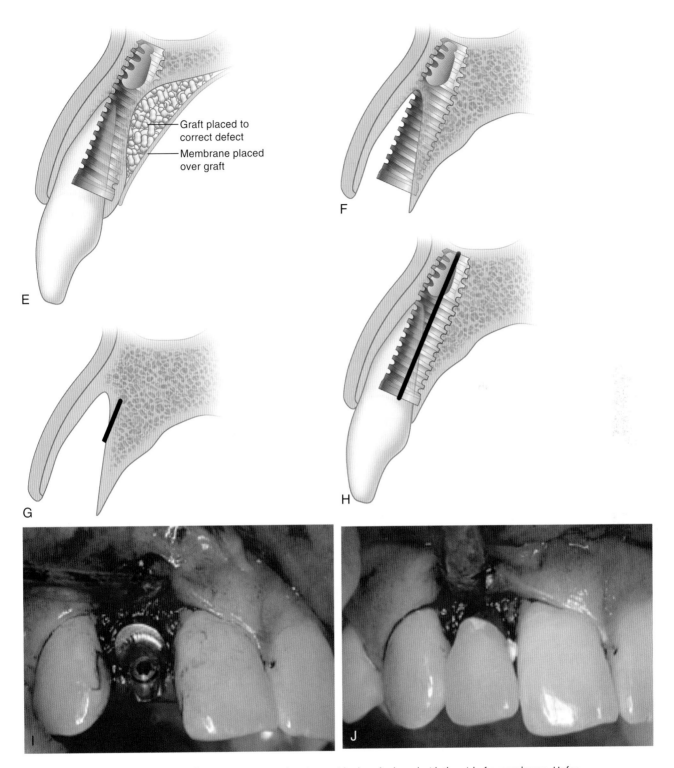

FIGURE 11-6, cont'd ■ **E,** Diagram showing an ideal graft placed with the aid of a membrane. Unfortunately, the success rate with grafting palatal defects is low. **F,** When implants are placed simultaneously with tooth extraction in the anterior esthetic zone, it is important to place the implant slightly palatal to the apex of the extracted tooth. **G,** The initial osteotomy should be approximately 3 mm up the palatal slope from the apex. **H,** This allows for optimal positioning for maintaining the facial bone and for esthetic prosthetics. **I, J,** To optimize esthetics, an abutment and temporary should be placed at the time of stage II surgery. (From Block MS: *Color atlas of dental implant surgery*, ed 2, St. Louis, Saunders, 2007.)

provides a good emergence profile for the final restoration, because the occlusal aspect of the implant is brought toward the labial aspect. This angulation also provides optimal positioning for the prosthesis, ensuring that the cingulum will not be overbuilt[36] (Figure 11-6, F, G).

The position of the implant apically and occlusally should also be considered. A line is drawn between the gingival margins of adjacent natural teeth, and the implant should be countersunk approximately 3 mm apical to the line.[36] Single-tooth restorations also should be evaluated to ensure that they have only centric contacts, because loosening of the final prosthetic restoration can occur with noncentric contacts[36] (Figure 11-6, D and E).

When the sulcular depth is greater than 4 mm, an intermediary abutment should be used, which raises the prosthetic working surface to within 2 mm to 3 mm of the soft tissue margins. Soft tissue collapse can occur with greater tissue depths, causing problems with try-ins, seating the impression coping, and seating of the final restoration.[36] Placement of the final abutment at the time of second-stage surgery can result in exposure of the underlying titanium abutment due to soft tissue recession and dimensional changes.[37] A temporary healing abutment that is the same size as the tooth being replaced can be placed after second-stage surgery, allowing the soft tissue to heal along the borders of the abutment. This approach results in a space for the crown that more closely resembles that of the missing natural tooth and a more natural appearance along the gingival margin[37] (Figure 11-6, F through H).

Tapering healing abutments can also be used to create a good emergence profile. When tapered healing caps are used, the soft tissue heals to the size of the tooth that is being replaced, instead of the 4.5-mm diameter of the implant abutment, which eliminates ridge lapping of the final restoration (Figure 11-6, I, J).[36] A restoration with a flat emergence profile is favorable; ridge lapping may cause problems with hygiene.[3,9] The soft tissue should be given sufficient time to mature (approximately 8 weeks) before the final impression is taken and the final abutment is selected.[36,37]

Flap Design

Incision design within the attached keratinized gingiva can prevent excessive bleeding, facilitate implant placement and flap closure, limit swelling and postsurgical discomfort, and achieve faster access to the alveolar bone.[19] It is important to preserve the hard and soft tissues around the teeth adjacent to the edentulous space. Minimal incisions should be made for single-tooth implants to limit flap extension and elevation. Black triangles can occur between the mesial and distal aspects of the restoration if attachment of the interproximal papillae on the adjacent teeth is not maintained as a result of shrinkage during healing. It is difficult to regenerate and augment interproximal papillae once they are lost.[36]

In patients with resorbed ridges, adequate flap coverage of the implant and maintenance of the mucogingival junction may be difficult. When regenerative materials are placed to correct ridge resorption, substantial releasing and coronal positioning of the labial flap are necessary to achieve primary coverage.[38] Of course, the need to augment the anterior maxilla often can best be determined by diagnostic imaging, including spiral tomography.[39] The anterior maxilla is an especially difficult area to diagnose for bone volume adequacy because of variations in the amount of residual alveolar bone, so implant position becomes crucial as a result of the high esthetic results needed in this area. Spiral tomography provides a means for more precise planning and placement of endosseous implants. Initial spiral tomographic radiographs can be used for planning and then for surgical guide fabrication; after implant placement, tomography can be used to evaluate implant position and inclination.[39]

As described in the literature, the clinician can choose from an assortment of techniques, which have been developed over the years regarding augmentation of the anterior maxilla, both vertically and horizontally, to optimize implant placement. For example, the resorbed anterior maxilla can be augmented through the use of autogenous bone grafts harvested from the patient's mandibular symphysis, followed by implant placement and restoration after adequate healing.[40,41] Some studies suggest that an excellent complement to particulated autogenous bone can be autogenous platelet gel in conjunction with a titanium mesh for alveolar bone reconstruction of the anterior maxilla before implant placement.[42] A relatively recent report describes a surgical preservation technique that uses maxillary bone from the surgical site and a soft tissue rotated palatal flap; in the cases reported, the procedure began with maxillary lateral incisor extraction and periapical surgery of the central incisors.[43] Dual bone cores harvested from the neighboring buccal vestibular region were placed in the sockets of the lateral maxillary incisors, followed by implant placement after 3 months and prosthetic restoration cementing after 12 weeks.[43]

One very effective type of flap design allows for the placement of regenerative materials without coronal displacement of the labial flap.[38] On the palatal aspect of the ridge crest, a horizontal releasing incision is made that does not penetrate down to the bone. Perpendicular to the ridge crest, two beveled labial vertical releasing incisions are extended apically and then flared mesially and distally beyond the mucogingival junction. Flaring of the incisions in the mucosal tissue provides enhanced access and positioning ability on reflection and improves the blood supply to the flap, as well as preserving the tissue of teeth adjacent to the edentulous space.[38]

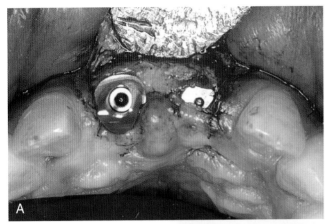

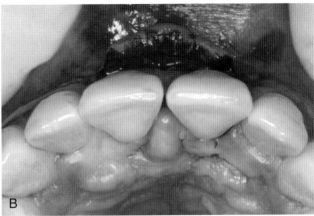

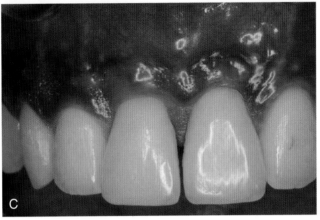

FIGURE 11-7 ■ **A,** The incision is slightly palatal to the midcrest. The flap is rotated buccally, the implant cover screws removed, and implant abutments placed. **B,** Temporaries are placed on the abutments. The flap is then incised, positioned, and sutured as needed to optimize papillae formation and soft tissue contours. **C,** After the papillae formation and soft tissue maturation at 6 weeks, as shown, the temporaries can be removed and an impression taken for the definitive restorations.

A split-thickness labial flap design is used to the labial line angle of the ridge crest, where it becomes full thickness to the most apical extent. Connective tissue is left covering the osseous crest. Reflection of the palatal flap incorporates the tissues left overlying the ridge from the labial flap reflection, beginning at the point where the labial flap was scored. After the point of the original horizontal crestal incision, the palatal flap becomes full thickness.[38]

Using a split-thickness labial flap and a full-thickness palatal flap maintains the position of the labial mucogingival junction, while displacing palatal tissues. After the regeneration materials have been placed, an incision is made on the internal aspect of the base of the palatal flap that is approximately half of its thickness. Tissue forceps are used to split the tissue internally toward the most coronal aspect and are rotated occlusally, leaving the flap attached. This secondary flap increases the length of the palatal flap, and primary closure is achieved.[38]

Prosthetic Considerations

Achieving esthetically pleasing single-tooth implant restorations depends on specific anatomical and surgical parameters (Figures 11-7, *A* and *B*). To avoid visible cervical metal or margins, the implant shoulder should be located subgingivally in the anterior region. To obtain symmetry between the emergence profile of the implant and the natural tooth, the restoration profile can be developed gradually using an acrylic temporary with appropriate contours at the time of second-stage surgery. The implant should be placed as far to the labial aspect as possible and more apically because of the difference between the diameter of a natural maxillary incisor and that of most implants.[3] It is also important to achieve adequate three-dimensional positioning of implants because in a buccal palatal direction, this position significantly influences the axial profile of the restoration. At the time of abutment connection, an excess of vertical and orofacial keratinized soft tissue is desirable to create an emergence profile that matches that of the adjacent natural tooth.[3] If the implant crown is too far facial, gingival recession occurs in the area, and if the implant crown is too far palatal, excess gingival tissue forms in the area. During the temporary crown phase, the facial contours of the crown should be slightly palatal as compared with adjacent teeth, to avoid the possibility of gingival recession. It will be easier to remove excess tissue in the future as compared with trying to grow back tissue that has receded because of a bulky temporary crown.

Final Restoration

Single-tooth restorations use an all-ceramic or ceramometal crown. The location of the implant determines which restoration should be used. All-ceramic crowns can generally be used only in the premolar and incisor areas because of the lesser strength of the crown (Figure 11-7, C).

The final restoration is constructed on a cast with the implant position recorded. Because most single-tooth restorations require modification of the abutment to accommodate clearance for porcelain or metal or to develop the interproximal tooth contour, abutment selection in the laboratory is necessary. A metal casting to accept the porcelain is constructed on the final modified abutment. The porcelain is applied; particular attention should be given to the subgingival contours because they require a smooth polish and high glaze.[19]

Two-Stage vs. One-Stage Protocols in the Anterior Maxilla

Many of the implantation techniques that were used in the relatively early days of implants have been forgotten because of adherence to the dogmatic approaches that have become mainstream in contemporary implant dentistry, including the two-stage implantation techniques generally discussed previously.[44] Therefore, a discussion of the two-stage technique for restoration in the anterior maxilla is in order, to be followed by a discussion of the rationale for a single-stage approach, particularly after immediate extraction.

Current Two-Stage Approach to Single-Tooth Implants in the Anterior Maxilla

Some implant clinicians believe that the best policy for restoring a single tooth implant or multiple tooth implants on the same arch is to always provide a provisional restoration first (Figure 11-8)—to allow the tissues to heal on two levels (around the coronal aspect of the crown, which can be augmented if necessary, and around the bone interface, which involves proper osseointegration of the implant). Osseointegration is particularly important in a patient who presents with poor quality bone, because implants placed in such alveolar bone can be loaded progressively while a provisional crown is in place.[45]

Implant patients' expectations for function, comfort, and esthetics have increased, along with the reliability of endosseous implants. Implant dentistry has never been more restoration driven. In addition to hard and soft tissue enhancements, as well as precise implant placement, impression and indexing techniques are becoming increasingly reliable. Impression and implant indexing techniques performed at stage 1 or 2 implant surgery are essential for satisfying patient expectations, for decreasing chair time, and for enhancing implant function and esthetics. These techniques accomplish these goals because, ultimately, they provide optimal fitting of the abutment and finished restoration.

Single-tooth restorations for implants in the anterior maxilla may be complicated by improper crown shape, emergence profile, and soft tissue contours. The shape of the alveolar ridge as well as insufficient alveolar bone height and width can further complicate cases. Crown position can suffer as a result of these latter complications. Accordingly, methods for selecting and producing properly fitting abutments and crowns are included in crucial implantation steps.[45] Sometimes the clinician must angle the implant to obtain proper anchorage in compromised bone; the angle of the implant could complicate the seating of the abutment for proper orientation with existing dentition. When abutments are placed at second-stage surgery, gingival tissues could collapse, making the fitting of a crown problematic. Radiography can be used to confirm abutment placement and seating. The need for a custom abutment, then, becomes even more important.[45]

Implant-level indexing and impression systems facilitate the cost-effective laboratory selection of an abutment (Figure 11-9). Clinicians may prefer a closed-tray impression system or an open-tray system. In either case, the impression system should provide master casts to be used for production and selection of the abutment and final restorations. The clinician must always bear in mind the functional and esthetic needs of patients.[45]

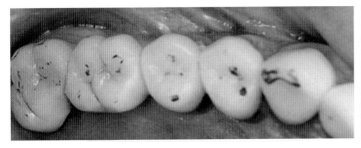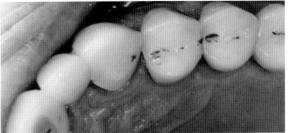

FIGURE 11-8 ■ Make sure to check the bite when providing a provisional restoration during stage II implant surgery.

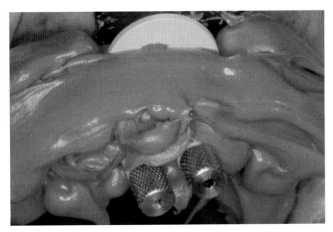

FIGURE 11-9 ■ Appropriate impression systems facilitate the cost-effective laboratory selection.

The traditional approach for providing restorations after stage 2 surgery is to first take impressions for the fabrication of a provisional crown. The clinician must note that at stage 2 surgery impressions, gingival contours and esthetics may have changed during the bone/implant healing process. Once the provisional crown is in place, the soft tissue adapts to the crown's surface, which has been fabricated on the basis of the indexing and impression information given to the laboratory.

As noted, either a closed-tray (indirect) or an open-tray (direct) procedure can be used at stage 2 surgery to make a master cast impression of the patient's dentition. Along with soft tissue casts, these impressions provide information for the laboratory to use when fabricating the abutments and crowns for the restoration. Accurate records of the implant-abutment positions and gingival contours are essential. Once the crown—which matches the height and buccal/lingual contours of the implant area—is manufactured, the restoration can be cemented into place using conventional crown and bridge procedures. Furthermore,

modified impression techniques can be used to register soft tissues around the implant.[46] The purpose of such an impression is to enable the laboratory to fabricate a restoration with a superior emergence profile. When a final impression is taken, an interim restoration is used as an abutment, thus providing a more precise record of soft tissues. Only when the clinician considers the soft tissue contours for each patient can the best function and esthetics of the final restoration become possible.

The usual sequence for the restoration begins during or after stage 2 surgery; an impression is taken when the implant is exposed, or approximately 10 days later, when stitches are removed. The clinician can remove the healing collar and put on the transfer coping, often using a closed tray, and then can send the impression to the laboratory for the fabrication of a custom abutment and a provisional plastic crown.[45] A provisional plastic crown can give the patient a chance to provide the clinician with feedback about the shape, size, color, phonetics, and esthetics of the crown, and the provisional crown can give hard and soft tissues the opportunity to heal.[45] Research indicates that the clinician should wait approximately 2 to 3 months to ensure that there is no contraction or change of dimension of the coronal tissues.[45] The clinician can allow the provisional plastic crown to be loaded progressively and can provide the patient with a regimen of postsurgical diet control to offer the implant the best chance of survival, particularly in cases of poor quality bone.[47] The laboratory can perform an additional procedure that actually produces the metalwork for the eventual definitive, or bonded, crown.

When the final impressions are taken, the provisional plastic crown is removed and the screw of the implant is topped off. In situations with poor quality bone, however, the clinician should only tighten the abutment by hand, then after 3 months should tighten it up mechanically, then try on the metal abutment again to make sure it is placed just below the tissues. At this stage, an impression can be taken with the abutment in place, allowing the laboratory technician to provide the optimal crown. At the time that the custom abutment is delivered, the clinician tries on the metal casting. Assuming that it fits well, he or she moves to the final crown. With fewer problems arising today with anterior implants, implant restoration increasingly resembles conventional dentistry. Even though esthetics are generally more important in anterior than in posterior restorations, both types of restorations follow similar procedures, although a greater number of impressions are usually taken for anterior restoration procedures.[45]

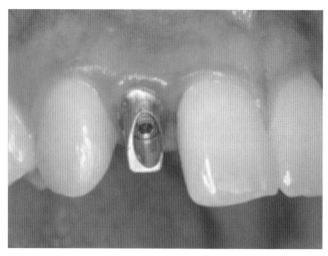

FIGURE 11-10 ■ An abutment in place. This can be modified, if needed, for a definitive crown.

Original Techniques and New Technologies for Implant Placement and Restoration

Many of the dental implant techniques and practices followed in the past had a good rationale for success, and if those techniques and practices—particularly immediate provisionalization and immediate restoration of implants—were incorporated using today's technology, clinicians could actually shorten treatment plans and treatment times, as well as significantly improve patients' function and esthetics.[44]

When clinicians started to do more crown and bridge and routine cases and two-stage implants became very popular, many of those concepts involving immediate load disappeared as practices seemed dominated by a two-stage process, allowing the implants to heal and integrate before being loaded. The negative side to a two-stage approach is that much of the soft tissue support, time, and patient expectations were lost.[44]

Today, the clinician's understanding of proper bioacceptable materials, proper surgical techniques, and proper prosthetic techniques allows immediate placement of implants in numerous situations, in conjunction with extractions or in areas that are edentulous, followed by immediate loading with a high degree of success, not only for bar overdentures but also for fixed crown and bridge. Not every case lends itself to one-stage/multitasked procedures—there are limits for cases best suited to such procedures, but numerous indications and patients present the opportunity for such procedures.

Even if immediate provisional loading or immediate loading of implants is not feasible, clinicians should take primary bone-level impressions at the time of implant placement, because many believe that starting the process of restoration at the time of implant placement is very important. Taking a primary impression allows the restorative dentist the opportunity to start the treatment

before the case is exposed or completed. Abutments can be selected, temporaries can be fabricated, and final castings can be made, all while the patient is going through a standard procedure. Subsequently, abutments can be placed, temporaries can be placed, and emergence profiles can be developed (Figure 11-10). This kind of planning allows the laboratory to view the level of bone so that the contact points can be made in such a way that the clinician can support and regenerate interdental soft tissue and papilla. In a number of distinct ways, even a two-stage process can benefit from one-stage techniques. In some cases, a one-stage process of implant placement and immediate provisionalization and loading can include the use of transfer copings after implant placement, along with customized fabrication of abutment and final restoration.[44]

Some patients can be treated relatively quickly, even aggressively, with extractions, implants, and restorations, or just with implants and restorations. However, for those cases that are more involved or that present medical compromises, clinicians may have to follow a standard two-stage conventional approach. In any event, the decision resides with the individual implant practitioner based on his or her ability to understand how implant dentistry works and how his or her patients can best be treated, always keeping in mind that a high percentage of success—regarding both esthetics and function—must be kept as the highest priority.

In some dental practices, approximately 60% of all implants have some type of initial provisional restoration placed, if not immediately loaded. In fact, a great percentage of them are placed by a one-stage procedure.[44] Such procedures may seem totally different from those followed just 15 or 20 years ago, but they were very common pro-

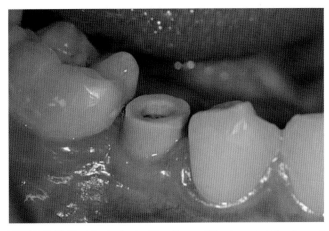

FIGURE 11-11 ■ A gingival healing cuff is placed at the time of implant placement.

cedures in the pioneering days of implants. When implant dentistry was first started, taking an impression at the time of implant placement was part of the procedure, because whether a one-stage screw, a blade, or a subperiosteal implant was used, restorations had to be made almost immediately to help stabilize the implant. However, when two-stage implants became the accepted protocol, clinicians routinely abandoned taking an impression or diagnostic images at the time of implant placement. In fact, many clinicians realize now that not following such procedures can be detrimental to achieving the best esthetic and functional results for some patients.[44]

The complicated nature of implant dentistry may have caused many practitioners to wholeheartedly adopt dogmatic protocols. However, with standardization often comes a lack of innovation and vision required for some cases. Sophisticated implantologists very often can provisionalize an implant at the time of placement, but the novice, following a systematic two-stage approach, typically performs immediate loads only with full arch cases until he or she feels proficient enough to progress to immediate loading of single implants[44] (Figure 11-11).

Today's clinician can incorporate a lot of two-stage implants with one-stage techniques, placing abutments at the time of implant placement or utilizing new types of implants that are specifically designed to be prepared for certain types of situations and certain types of crown and bridge.[44] Several systems now make themselves available as immediate load implants. Some still happen to have a two-stage design, with placement of abutments and so forth at the time of implant placement; others consist of new one-piece implants that eliminate the abutment component. It is up to the practitioner to decide which implant system is best suited for the restoration, and which implant system or implant surface and which implant design are best suited for the type of bone that that patient may have.[44]

Immediate Placement and Loading of Implants in Extraction Sites in the Esthetic Zone

Several advantages are associated with extraction and immediate implant placement and loading in the anterior maxilla.[48,49] Of course, patients receive faster restoration with minimally invasive surgery and minimum pain. Procedural advantages include that after the tooth extraction, a natural healing process is mobilized in the maxilla. The extraction site wants to "feel" growth in the extraction cavity; this reaction causes the bone to grow toward the implant.[48] A second advantage is the absence of bone loss, which reduces the need for traditional augmentation procedures. Drilling, which sometimes destroys or damages the bone around the implant, is reduced because the immediate implant must be approximately 5 mm longer than the natural root. So, drilling is done 5 mm into the natural bone. A third advantage is that the number of surgical stages is reduced to a minimum. The patient comes to the office for an initial visit and receives the exact information about the procedure. When he or she comes to the next appointment, the local anesthesia is applied to the tooth or teeth to be removed, and a perfect insertion of the implant is accomplished owing to a surgical index that preceded the appointment. After the implant has been inserted, the clinician judges the parameters for immediate loading or immediate restoration, including a minimum of 10 mm length of the implant, 3.7 diameter, 1.5 mm bone around the implant, and, most important, the likelihood for primary stability.[48]

A fourth advantage of immediate implantation and loading involves simplified maintenance of the natural design and contour of the gingiva. The dentist knows exactly where the papillae are, and the vestibular position of the implant is exact. The clinician must remain 2 mm below and behind the vestibulary line of adjacent teeth to finalize a large esthetic zone.[48] A fifth advantage, considered the most important, is the positive, immediate psychological effect on the patient.

The literature generally supports the practice of immediate implanting and loading after tooth extraction.[50-57] The literature strongly suggests that immediate placement with immediate restoration or loading can be an accurate and predictable method.

Typically, an impression of the patient's mouth is taken approximately a week before the surgical intervention. The clinician decides which tooth will be extracted and provides the surgical index for the ideal implant position. With the aid of the surgical index, he removes the tooth. After the implant is inserted in the exact position, a dual impression is taken and is transferred to the fixed mount in the laboratory. An analog is prepared for a stone mortar impression of the patient's mouth. This procedure takes ½ to ¾ of an hour. After the implant analog is fixed into the stone mortar, a temporary abutment is made of titanium or acrylic material, and the natural tooth is cut approximately 3 mm below the line. The instrument is sandblasted to remove any organic particles from the inner part of the tooth. Now there is a ceramic analog with a dental crown. The inner part of this crown will be adapted to the temporary abutment with acrylic. A composite with 50% ceramic is used to provide perfect stability. This adapted crown will be cemented in the mouth of the patient, taking approximately 1.5 hours to finalize.[48] The clinician is then provided with the customized abutment along with the custom-prepared natural tooth, which should be out of occlusion and protrusive around movement. Controlling the occlusion may be necessary for 8 to 14 days after the intervention.[48] The abutment is placed, the natural tooth cemented, and the bone augmented before suturing. Leaving this tooth in place undisturbed for 3 to 6 months gives the bone the possibility to regenerate to replace the augmentation with natural bone before the final restoration is started.

The surgical technique begins with one of the most important aspects of immediate implant placement, which is opening a minimal flap; essentially, this approach means that no incision is made. The tooth is removed gently and with minimal trauma to the alveolar bone, to avoid breaking the buccal plate and in many cases the vestibulary wall. After a gentle extraction, the next step is to clean around the surface of the bone, removing soft tissue and other infected tissue. After the thickness of the flap is measured, probing into the extraction socket is performed to ensure that there is no perforation of the vestibulary wall. Next, a round bur is used to help determine exactly the access of the implant, which sometimes is different from that of the natural tooth. A round bur is used to fix the position of the implant. Afterward, the length and the access of the future implant are finalized, and then the access and the occlusion are controlled to enable correction of the implant access. If a second drill is used, the correction will be very difficult and bone loss will be produced. If the position is perfect, this again involves controlled occlusion in the vestibule, allowing three-dimensional control with the second drill and the last drill for the implant diameters. In the upper jaw, the osteotome technique can be used to compress the bone for better stability.[48]

The implant must be 2 mm to 3 mm smaller than the diameter of the natural tooth. Producing a space between the implant and the vestibulary plate in many cases allows filling it with an augmenting material with a particle dimension of 100 to 300 microns, mixed with blood. After the material is set and the implant is inserted, closing is performed with the insertion of a temporary titanium or plastic abutment on the top of the implant. This temporizing of the implant abutment is a critical step for getting the esthetics and the occlusion correct, including a temporary acrylic crown.[48]

If at 20 Ncm there is no movement, an immediate load can proceed. If there is movement, then loading is delayed; 20 Ncm is needed at the reverse to control the primary stability. This is the most predictable method. With a temporary abutment, it is very important to cement after removing any occlusion points. This single tooth must be completely out of occlusion. A temporary crown that contacts adjacent teeth should never be used. The chisel level must be short, half a millimeter, to avoid any contact. The crown must be cemented before final augmentation, which means delaying the close of the flap. The clinician then cements the crown and the temporary abutment, and finalizes the augmentation around the implant in terms of the depth between implant and vestibular bone for the papillae and adjacent teeth; after the cemented crown has been perfectly cleaned, the case is closed with sutures. The provision of the implants is always 1.5 mm palatal or lingual from the vestibulary plate, and the neck of the implant is 2 mm to 3 mm below the suture line of the natural tooth. The clinician should assume a resorption of 0.5 mm to 1 mm from the height of the existing bone, and this resorption must be considered before the implant is inserted, so the optimal esthetic outcome is achieved. The literature boasts a success rate of 97.6% for this protocol, which is, essentially, not immediate loading on single implants but immediate restoration: The crown has to function as a healing abutment without any occlusal forces; furthermore, the protocol calls for the patient to consume only soft foods for 4 to 6 weeks after the procedure.[48]

Discussion

Single-tooth implants, when chosen as the appropriate treatment modality for restoring a single tooth in the anterior maxillary region, can have the distinct advantage of completely preserving the enamel and dentinal tissue because the adjacent teeth are fully preserved.[58,59] Before implant placement, certain criteria must be evaluated, including the type of periodontium, preexisting tooth form and position, and root morphology. Soft tissue anatomy, bone dimension, and the smile line also must be considered for the clinician to obtain an esthetically pleasing implant restoration.[1-12] Esthetically unacceptable restorations that may be difficult to correct are often the result of soft tissue mismanagement.[9,60] Surgical correction may be necessary if the resting position and normal activity of the lip are unsatisfactory.[21]

A one-piece screw-retained restoration for single-tooth replacement provides good esthetics, is easy to retrieve, and does not require the use of cement. A one-piece screw-retained prosthesis is recommended in situations where the anatomy of the alveolar ridge allows the implant axis to pass through the occlusal or lingual surface of the planned restoration.[61-65]

Correct abutment selection is necessary when single-tooth implants are placed, to avoid phonetic problems from a bulky palatal side.[58] To avoid overload of the implant, clinicians should carefully check the occlusion of the implant. To compensate for the reduced axial mobility of single-tooth implants, the occlusal clearance on the implant should be approximately 20 μm greater than the clearance of adjacent natural teeth.[58]

To ensure lasting esthetics with implant restorations, the clinician must be concerned with the stability of the gingival margin and the crown dimensions and its contours as it emerges from the soft tissue. The soft tissue must be allowed to heal and mature properly after second-stage surgery (approximately 6 to 8 weeks). A temporary or tapering healing abutment can be placed after second-stage surgery, allowing for a more natural emergence profile. The emergence profile of the single-tooth restoration should match that of the adjacent and contralateral tooth.[1]

There is a difference of opinion regarding implant placement following tooth extraction. The need for an additional surgical procedure is eliminated with immediate implant placement. With delayed implant placement, clinicians can determine the final position of the soft tissue. A "compromise" between these two situations has also been suggested for root-canaled teeth. Instead of the tooth being extracted, the crown is reduced to 2 mm to 3 mm below the free gingival margin. After 3 to 4 weeks, the root is removed and the implant is placed. This 3-week to 4-week delay allows for proliferation of soft tissue over the residual root. Grafting procedures can be performed, if needed, and the flap is covered with the newly formed tissue.[16]

Restoring a missing lower incisor with an implant can be challenging because the delicate crown form of the lower incisor needs to be duplicated while room for the fixation screw is provided. The final result should be retrievable and antirotational to prevent loosening or breakage of the screw, and it should be esthetically pleasing.[54,66-69]

Certain complications—such as abutment screw loosening and fractures, periodontal abscesses, gingival inflammation, fistula formation, and retention of screw and implant fractures—have been reported to occur more frequently in patients with single-tooth implants than in partially and completely edentulous patients.[16] Most of the problems associated with the survival of single-tooth implants appear to be related to loose abutment screws.[70] With the use of single-tooth restorations, the crown can be connected to the abutment using a screw or cement. Cementation may provide better esthetics, whereas screw retention provides retrievability.[70-74]

Several advantages and disadvantages are associated with the use of single-tooth implants. Retrievability and complete preservation of the tooth structure of adjacent natural teeth are some of the advantages of these implants. Disadvantages include longer treatment time, the necessity for additional surgical procedures (such as bone aug-

mentation and soft tissue surgery), increased costs, and an esthetic result that may be more technically difficult to achieve.[1-12,58]

Case Management

- **Level 1: Extraction performed by clinician, good 5-wall bony housing, great papilla and/or thick-flat periodontal biotype, low smile line.** This level generally requires extraction, curettage of the tooth socket with hand and rotary instruments, placement of the implant tip 3 mm palatal to the root apex with grafting on the facial aspect of the socket. An additional requirement is placement of an anatomical abutment fabricated by a laboratory or manufactured chairside to create a one-stage implant situation and thereby maintain the soft tissue architecture at the time of extraction and implant placement.[48,75,76] There is also the need for placement of an Essix appliance as a provisional over the anatomical abutment but with some spacing, ensuring no pressure from the provisional onto the anatomical abutment.

- **Level 2: Extraction performed previously and grafted, good 5-wall bony housing, great papilla and/or thick-flat periodontal biotype, low smile line.** Requirements in these cases include placement of the implant with grafting if required as a two-stage procedure and possible indexing for a custom abutment. Stage II surgery includes placement of a stock-angled abutment or placement of an anatomical abutment, fabricated and temporary, with soft tissue surgery to maintain/create soft tissue architecture.

- **Level 3: Extraction performed previously and not grafted, good 5-wall bony housing, great papilla and/or thick-flat periodontal biotype, medium smile line.** Requirements here include placement of an implant with grafting, if required, as a two-stage procedure and indexing for a custom abutment. At stage II surgery, placement of an anatomical milled abutment and temporary is required, with soft tissue surgery to maintain/create soft tissue architecture.

- **Level 4: Extraction performed previously and not grafted, 4-wall bony housing, good papilla and/or thick-flat periodontal biotype, medium smile line.** This level requires particulate grafting with a membrane and a connective tissue graft or flap advancement at a subsequent surgery. There is the further requirement of placement of the implant with additional grafting, if necessary, as a two-stage procedure and indexing for a custom abutment; stage II surgery includes placement of an anatomical milled abutment and temporary with soft tissue surgery to maintain/create soft tissue architecture.

- Level 5: Extraction performed previously and not grafted, 4-wall bony housing, good papilla and/or thick-flat periodontal biotype, high smile line. Requirements here include block grafting with an autogenous chin block or allogenic block graft and a connective tissue graft. A subsequent surgery includes placement of the implant with additional grafting, if required, as a two-stage procedure and indexing for a custom abutment. Stage II surgery commences placement of an anatomical abutment (Atlantis Abutment) and temporary with soft tissue surgery to maintain/create soft tissue architecture.
- Level 6: Extraction performed previously and not grafted, 3-wall bony housing, inadequate papilla mesially or distally, high smile line. Requirements here include possible extraction of an adjacent tooth with simultaneous socket grafting; afterward commences block grafting with autogenous chin block and a connective tissue graft. A subsequent surgery includes placement of the implant (or possibly two implants if an adjacent tooth was extracted) with additional grafting, if required, as a two-stage procedure and indexing for a custom abutment. Then, at stage II surgery, an anatomical abutment and temporary are placed with soft tissue surgery to maintain/create soft tissue architecture. Soft tissue can be manipulated to create papillae using the Palacci techniques.
- Level 7: Extraction performed previously and grafted or not grafted but inadequate bone, 2-wall bony housing, inadequate papilla mesially and distally, moderate or high smile line. This level generally requires extraction of adjacent teeth with socket grafting, then block grafting with autogenous chin block[77-80] and a vascularized interpositional connective tissue graft.[81-84] Subsequently, there is placement of two implants and restoration as a 3-unit bridge, or possibly three implants placed with three individual crowns and stage I indexing for computer-shaped and -milled abutments. Computer-milled abutments and a temporary are placed at stage II surgery, and soft tissue manipulation is performed to create papillae using the Palacci techniques.

SUMMARY

A single-tooth implant in the anterior esthetic zone is a viable treatment option for many patients, but it is complex and requires the clinician to follow specific guidelines for the pretreatment phase, implant placement, flap design, bone grafting and bone maintenance, and soft tissue manipulation; the clinician also must consider certain anatomical and surgical parameters. With proper planning and technique, moderately experienced clinicians can successfully place and restore single-tooth implants.

REFERENCES

1. Hurzeler MB, Quinones CR, Strub JR: Advanced surgical and prosthetic management of the anterior single tooth osseointegrated implant: a case presentation, *Pract Periodontics Aesthet Dent* 6(1):13-21, 1994; quiz 23.
2. Binon PP: The spline implant: design, engineering, and evaluation, *Int J Prosthodont* 9(5):419-433, 1996.
3. Belser UC, Bernard JP, Buser D: Implant-supported restorations in the anterior region: prosthetic considerations, *Pract Periodontics Aesthet Dent* 8(9):875-883, 1996; quiz 884.
4. Schincaglia GP, Nowzari H: Surgical treatment planning for the single-unit implant in aesthetic areas, *Periodontol* 2000 27:162-182, 2001. Review.
5. Belser UC, Schmid B, Higginbottom F, Buser D: Outcome analysis of implant restorations located in the anterior maxilla: a review of the recent literature, *Int J Oral Maxillofac Implants* 19(suppl):30-42, 2004. Review.
6. Buser D, Martin W, Belser UC: Optimizing esthetics for implant restorations in the anterior maxilla: anatomic and surgical considerations, *Int J Oral Maxillofac Implants* 19(suppl):43-61, 2004. Review.
7. Sclar AG: Strategies for management of single-tooth extraction sites in aesthetic implant therapy, *J Oral Maxillofac Surg* 62(9 suppl 2):90-105, 2004. Erratum in *J Oral Maxillofac Surg* 63(1):158, 2005.
8. Tischler M: Dental implant placement in the maxillary anterior region: guidelines for aesthetic success, *Dent Today* 24(3):72, 74, 76, 2005, passim; quiz 78, 61.
9. Carrion JB, Barbosa IR: Single implant-supported restorations in the anterior maxilla, *Int J Periodontics Restorative Dent* 25(2):149-155, 2005.
10. Levin L, Pathael S, Dolev E, Schwartz-Arad D: Aesthetic versus surgical success of single dental implants: 1- to 9-year follow-up, *Pract Proced Aesthet Dent* 17(8):533-538, 2005; quiz 540, 566.
11. Hakimi NM: Anterior single-tooth dental implant: current concepts for enhanced aesthetics, *J West Soc Periodontol Periodontal Abstr* 53(1):5-10, 2005.
12. Holst S, Blatz MB, Hegenbarth E, Wichmann M, Eitner S: Prosthodontic considerations for predictable single-implant esthetics in the anterior maxilla, *J Oral Maxillofac Surg* 63(9 suppl 2):89-96, 2005.
13. Salinas TJ, Block MS, Sadan A: Fixed partial denture or single-tooth implant restoration? Statistical considerations for sequencing and treatment, *J Oral Maxillofac Surg* 62(9 suppl 2):2-16, 2004.
14. Becker W, Becker BE: Flap designs for minimization of recession adjacent to maxillary anterior implant sites: a clinical study, *Int J Oral Maxillofac Implants* 11(1):46-54, 1996.
15. Gunne J, Astrand P, Lindh T, Borg K, Olsson M: Tooth-implant and implant supported fixed partial dentures: a 10-year report, *Int J Prosthodont* 12(3):216-221, 1999.
16. Jansen CE, Weisgold A: Presurgical treatment planning for the anterior single-tooth implant restoration, *Compend Contin Educ Dent* 16(8):746, 748-752, 754, 1995, passim; quiz 764.
17. Di Sario F: A system for the diagnosis, placement, and prosthetic restoration of root form implants (U.S. Patent #5,769,636), *J Prosthodont* 12(1):2-7, 2003.

18. Block M, Finger I, Castellon P, Lirettle D: Single tooth immediate provisional restoration of dental implants: technique and early results, *J Oral Maxillofac Surg* 62(9):1131-1138, 2004.

19. Saadoun AP, Sullivan DY, Krischek M, Le Gall M: Single tooth implant—management for success, *Pract Periodontics Aesthet Dent* 6(3):73-80, 1994; quiz 82.

20. Davarpanah M, Martinez H, Celletti R, Tecucianu JF: Three-stage approach to aesthetic implant restoration: emergence profile concept, *Pract Proced Aesthet Dent* 13(9):761-767, 2001; quiz 768, 721-722.

21. Trushkowsky RD: Esthetic restoration of a single-tooth implant using a precision ceramic coping, *Compend Contin Educ Dent* 17(4):394, 398, 400, 1996, passim.

22. Doring K, Eisenmann E, Stiller M: Functional and esthetic considerations for single-tooth Ankylos implant-crowns: 8 years of clinical performance, *J Oral Implantol* 30(3):198-209, 2004.

23. Schiroli G: Single-tooth implant restorations in the esthetic zone with PureForm ceramic crowns: 3 case reports, *J Oral Implantol* 30(6):358-363, 2004.

24. Elian N, Jalbout ZN, Cho SC, Froum S, Tarnow DP: Realities and limitations in the management of the interdental papilla between implants: three case reports, *Pract Proced Aesthet Dent* 15(10):737-744, 2003; quiz 746. Review.

25. Kan JY, Rungcharassaeng K: Interimplant papilla preservation in the esthetic zone: a report of six consecutive cases, *Int J Periodontics Restorative Dent* 23(3):249-259, 2003.

26. Leziy SS, Miller BA: Replacement of adjacent missing anterior teeth with scalloped implants: a case report, *Pract Proced Aesthet Dent* 17(5):331-338, 2005; quiz 340.

27. Oikarinen KS, Sandor GK, Kainulainen VT, Salonen-Kemppi M: Augmentation of the narrow traumatized anterior alveolar ridge to facilitate dental implant placement, *Dent Traumatol* 19(1):19-29, 2003. Review.

28. Summers RB: A new concept in maxillary implant surgery: the osteotome technique, *Compendium* 15(2):152, 154-156, 158, 1994, passim; quiz 162.

29. Summers RB: The osteotome technique: Part 2—the ridge expansion osteotomy (REO) procedure, *Compendium* 15(4):422, 424, 426, 1994, passim; quiz 436.

30. Summers RB: The osteotome technique: Part 3—less invasive methods of elevating the sinus floor, *Compendium* 15(6):698, 700, 702-704, 1994, passim; quiz 710.

31. Summers RB: The osteotome technique: Part 4—future site development, *Compend Contin Educ Dent* 16(11):1080, 1092, 1995, passim; quiz 1099.

32. Saadoun AP, Le Gall MG: Implant site preparation with osteotomes: principles and clinical application, *Pract Periodontics Aesthet Dent* 8(5):453-463, 1996.

33. Summers RB: Sinus floor elevation with osteotomes, *J Esthet Dent* 10(3):164-171, 1998.

34. Garg AK: Osteotomes vs. traditional drilling for implant placement, *Dent Implantol Update* 16(5):33-39, 2005.

35. Bain CA, Weisgold AS: Customized emergence profile in the implant crown—a new technique, *Compend Contin Educ Dent* 18(1):41-45, 1997; quiz 46.

36. Lazzara RJ: Achieving critical emergence profile for the anterior single tooth implant, *Dent Implantol Update* 4(11):88-92, 1993.

37. Lazzara RJ: Managing the soft tissue margin: the key to implant aesthetics, *Pract Periodontics Aesthet Dent* 5(5):81-88, 1993.

38. Fugazzotto PA, DePaoli S, Parma-Benfenati S: Flap design considerations in the placement of single maxillary anterior implants: clinical report, *Implant Dent* 2(2):93-96, 1993.

39. Dixon DR, Morgan R, Hollender LG, Roberts FA, O'Neal RB: Clinical application of spiral tomography in anterior implant placement: case report, *J Periodontol* 73(10):1202-1209, 2002.

40. John V, Gossweiler M: Implant treatment planning and rehabilitation of the anterior maxilla, Part 2: the role of autogenous grafts, *J Indiana Dent Assoc* 81(1):33-38, 2002.

41. Balaji SM: Management of deficient anterior maxillary alveolus with mandibular parasymphyseal bone graft for implants, *Implant Dent* 11(4):363-369, 2002.

42. Thor A: Reconstruction of the anterior maxilla with platelet gel, autogenous bone, and titanium mesh: a case report, *Clin Implant Dent Relat Res* 4(3):150-155, 2002.

43. Penarrocha M, Garcia-Mira B, Martinez O: Localized vertical maxillary ridge preservation using bone cores and a rotated palatal flap, *Int J Oral Maxillofac Implants* 20(1):131-134, 2005.

44. Rosenlicht JL: History of immediate load in implant dentistry: interview, *Dent Implantol Update* 15(10):73-79, 2004.

45. Scher EL: Single- or multiple-tooth implant restoration on the same arch, *Dent Implantol Update* 15(7):49-53, 2004.

46. Attard N, Barzilay I: A modified impression technique for accurate registration of peri-implant soft tissues, *J Can Dent Assoc* 69(2):80-83, 2003.

47. Misch C: Progressive bone loading, *Dent Today* 14(1):80-83, 1995.

48. Palti A: Immediate placement and loading of implants in extraction sites: procedures in the aesthetic zone, *Dent Implantol Update* 15(6):41-47, 2004.

49. Nuzzolese E: Immediate loading of two single tooth implants in the maxilla: preliminary results after one year, *J Contemp Dent Pract* 6(3):148-157, 2005.

50. Cooper LF, Rahman A, Moriarty J, Chaffee N, Sacco D: Immediate mandibular rehabilitation with endosseous implants: simultaneous extraction, implant placement, and loading, *Int J Oral Maxillofac Implants* 17(4):517-525, 2002.

51. Schiroli G: Immediate tooth extraction, placement of a Tapered Screw-Vent implant, and provisionalization in the esthetic zone: a case report, *Implant Dent* 12(2):123-131, 2003.

52. Petropoulos VC, Balshi TJ, Balshi SF, Wolfinger GJ: Extractions, implant placement, and immediate loading of mandibular implants: a case report of a functional fixed prosthesis in 5 hours, *Implant Dent* 12(4):283-290, 2003.

53. Castellon P, Block MS, Smith M, Finger IM: Immediate implant placement and provisionalization using implants with an internal connection, *Pract Proced Aesthet Dent* 16(1):35-43, 2004.

54. Norton MR: A short-term clinical evaluation of immediately restored maxillary TiOblast single-tooth implants, *Int J Oral Maxillofac Implants* 19(2):274-281, 2004.

55. Jivraj S, Reshad M, Chee WW: Critical appraisal: immediate loading of implants in the esthetic zone, *J Esthet Restor Dent* 17(5):320-325, 2005.

56. Attard NJ, Zarb GA: Immediate and early implant loading protocols: a literature review of clinical studies, *J Prosthet Dent* 94(3):242-258, 2005. Review.

57. Lindeboom JA, Frenken JW, Dubois L, Frank M, Abbink I, Kroon FH: Immediate loading versus immediate provisionalization of maxillary single-tooth replacements: a prospective randomized study with BioComp implants, *J Oral Maxillofac Surg* 64(6):936-942, 2006.

58. Studer S, Pietrobon N, Wohlwend A: Maxillary anterior single-tooth replacement: comparison of three treatment modalities, *Pract Periodontics Aesthet Dent* 6(1):51-60, 1994; quiz 62. Review.

59. Meyenberg KH, Imoberdorf MJ: The aesthetic challenges of single tooth replacement: a comparison of treatment alternatives, *Pract Periodontics Aesthet Dent* 9(7):727-735, 1997; quiz 737.

60. Grunder U, Spielman HP, Gaberthuel T: Implant-supported single tooth replacement in the aesthetic region: a complex challenge, *Pract Periodontics Aesthet Dent* 8(9):835-842, 1996; quiz 844.

61. Khayat P, Nader N, Exbrayat P: Single tooth replacement using a one-piece screw-retained restoration, *Pract Periodontics Aesthet Dent* 7(9):61-69, 1995; quiz 70.

62. Clausen GF: The lingual locking screw for implant-retained restorations—aesthetics and retrievability, *Aust Prosthodont J* 9:17-20, 1995.

63. Chee WW, Torbati A, Albouy JP: Retrievable cemented implant restorations, *J Prosthodont* 7(2):120-125, 1998.

64. Cho SC, Small PN, Elian N, Tarnow D: Screw loosening for standard and wide diameter implants in partially edentulous cases: 3- to 7-year longitudinal data, *Implant Dent* 13(3):245-250, 2004.

65. Sadan A, Blatz MB, Bellerino M, Block M: Prosthetic design considerations for anterior single-implant restorations, *J Esthet Restor Dent* 16(3):165-175, 2004; discussion 175.

66. Marlin GM, Baraban D: Restoring the single lower incisor implant with esthetics, antirotation, and retrievability, *Compendium* 15(5):624, 626, 628-629, 1994; quiz 630.

67. Aboyoussef H, Weiner S, Ehrenberg D: Effect of an antirotation resistance form on screw loosening for single implant-supported crowns, *J Prosthet Dent* 83(4):450-455, 2000.

68. Malo P, Friberg B, Polizzi G, Gualini F, Vighagen T, Rangert B: Immediate and early function of Branemark System implants placed in the esthetic zone: a 1-year prospective clinical multicenter study, *Clin Implant Dent Relat Res* (5 suppl 1):37-46, 2003.

69. Schwedhelm ER, Raigrodski AJ: A technique for locating implant abutment screws of posterior cement-retained metal-ceramic restorations with ceramic occlusal surfaces, *J Prosthet Dent* 95(2):165-167, 2006.

70. Andersson B, Odman P, Lindvall AM, Lithner B: Single-tooth restorations supported by osseointegrated implants: results and experiences from a prospective study after 2 to 3 years, *Int J Oral Maxillofac Implants* 10(6):702-711, 1995.

71. Scheller H, Urgell JP, Kultje C, Klineberg I, Goldberg PV, Stevenson-Moore P, Alonso JM, Schaller M, Corria RM, Engquist B, Toreskog S, Kastenbaum F, Smith CR: A 5-year multicenter study on implant-supported single crown restorations, *Int J Oral Maxillofac Implants* 13(2):212-218, 1998.

72. Andersson B, Taylor A, Lang BR, Scheller H, Scharer P, Sorensen JA, Tarnow D: Alumina ceramic implant abutments used for single-tooth replacement: a prospective 1- to 3-year multicenter study, *Int J Prosthodont* 14(5):432-438, 2001.

73. Vigolo P, Givani A, Majzoub Z, Cordioli G: Cemented versus screw-retained implant-supported single-tooth crowns: a 4-year prospective clinical study, *Int J Oral Maxillofac Implants* 19(2):260-265, 2004.

74. Gotfredsen K: A 5-year prospective study of single-tooth replacements supported by the Astra Tech implant: a pilot study, *Clin Implant Dent Relat Res* 6(1):1-8, 2004.

75. Mankoo T: Contemporary implant concepts in aesthetic dentistry—part 3: adjacent immediate implants in the aesthetic zone, *Pract Proced Aesthet Dent* 16(4):327-334, 2004; quiz 336. Review.

76. Casellini RC: Achieving implant success through prosthetic design: interview, *Dent Implantol Update* 15(11):81-85, 2004.

77. Garg AK, Morales MJ, Navarro I, Duarte F: Autogenous mandibular bone grafts in the treatment of the resorbed maxillary anterior alveolar ridge: rationale and approach, *Implant Dent* 7(3):169-176, 1998.

78. Yeung R: Simultaneous placement of implant and bone graft in the anterior maxilla: a case report, *Int J Oral Maxillofac Implants* 19(6):892-895, 2004.

79. Schwartz-Arad D, Levin L: Intraoral autogenous block onlay bone grafting for extensive reconstruction of atrophic maxillary alveolar ridges, *J Periodontol* 76(4):636-641, 2005.

80. Jemt T, Lekholm U: Single implants and buccal bone grafts in the anterior maxilla: measurements of buccal crestal contours in a 6-year prospective clinical study, *Clin Implant Dent Relat Res* 7(3):127-135, 2005.

81. Wang PD, Pitman DP, Jans HH: Ridge augmentation using a subepithelial connective tissue pedicle graft, *Pract Periodontics Aesthet Dent* 5(2):47-51, 1993; quiz 52.

82. Nemcovsky CE, Artzi Z, Moses O: Rotated split palatal flap for soft tissue primary coverage over extraction sites with immediate implant placement: description of the surgical procedure and clinical results, *J Periodontol* 70(8):926-934, 1999.

83. Khoury F, Happe A: The palatal subepithelial connective tissue flap method for soft tissue management to cover maxillary defects: a clinical report, *Int J Oral Maxillofac Implants* 15(3):415-418, 2000.

84. Mathews DP: The pediculated connective tissue graft: a technique for improving unaesthetic implant restorations, *Pract Proced Aesthet Dent* 14(9):719-724, 2002; quiz 726.

chapter 12

Implant Exposure Techniques at Second-Stage Surgery

A NUMBER OF CONSIDERATIONS are touted in the literature as essential and often-overlooked aspects of dental implant surgery, which, when ignored by the clinician, can mean the difference between successful and failed implants. These considerations run the preoperative, perioperative, and postoperative gamut—from proper filling out of patient information forms and patient interviews to regular office evaluations and patient home care. Certainly an essential element of the perioperative category must include exposure techniques at second-stage surgery. This crucial middle moment in dental implantology can determine how well the dental implant and its restorative components suit the biological, functional, and esthetic needs of the individual patient. This chapter discusses issues of peri-implant tissue health, its preservation, its reconstruction, and its long-term "relationship" with implant components, all of which hinge on successful second-stage surgical techniques for exposing the implant (Figure 12-1).

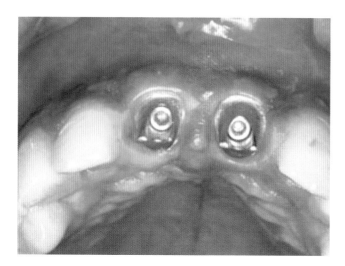

FIGURE 12-1 ■ Peri-implant soft tissue after second-stage implant surgery.

General Considerations for Second-Stage Surgery

Dental implant surgery can be performed as a one-stage or two-stage procedure, as comparative studies frequently remind us.[1-5] In one-stage surgery, the implant is immediately exposed to the oral cavity by means of a gingival healing device or abutment at the time of implant placement. In the two-stage modality, the implant is left dormant underneath the mucosa for the period of its osseointegration until a second surgery is performed to uncover and expose the implant after the healing period (Figure 12-2). At the time of implant uncovering, the surgeon encounters the challenge of maintaining or improving the condition of the peri-implant tissues and the implant that was placed months before.[6] Techniques chosen for uncovering the implant will depend on the characteristics of the tissue that overlies the implant. The amount of attached gingiva, the thickness of the overlying mucosa, and the presence or the absence of interdental papillae are some of the issues to be considered before uncovering an implant.

Peri-implant health and implant longevity depend greatly on the attached gingiva, which is needed to reduce the probability of gingival recession in areas of esthetic margin placement, to facilitate impressions, and, in some cases, to increase patient comfort.[7] In fact, for gingival tissues to attach to a natural tooth (and, by extension, to the implant abutment and restoration), a minimal biological width (2 mm to 3 mm of supra-alveolar tooth surface) is required; furthermore, in the absence of this minimal width, soft tissue surgery may be needed before final restorations are provided.[7-9] Studies in the canine mandible have shown that biological width dimensions resemble natural teeth around one-piece non-submerged implants.[10] Additionally, sufficiently attached gingiva enhances plaque removal around the gingival margin and reduces inflammation around restored teeth.[11]

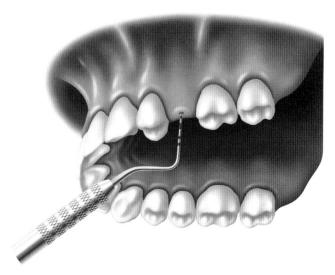

FIGURE 12-2 ■ The clinician must be exactly sure of the implant position before uncovering the implant. This can be determined by using the original surgical template from stage 1 surgery and probing through the soft tissue, once the patient is anesthetized. (Courtesy of Zimmer Dental. All rights reserved.)

The characteristics of peri-implant soft tissue are similar to those of soft tissue around the teeth.[12-16] A 2003 study that evaluated the status of teeth adjacent to single-tooth implants in the anterior and posterior jaw concluded that the periodontal status of teeth adjacent to implant restorations was excellent, suggesting a strong similarity in the biological and functional aspects of peri-implant structures.[17] Although differences in approaches to peri-implant and periodontal probing have been recommended owing to anatomical disparities,[18-20] nonetheless, a recent study concluded that the soft tissue seal around osseointegrated implants appears not to be adversely affected by clinical probing, so long-term survival of implants is not affected; the study also concluded that epithelial attachment healing occurs to be complete 5 days after such probing.[21] Questions surrounding probing are important, because the mucosal seal between the implant surface and the surrounding gingiva acts as a barrier to the entrance of toxins produced by plaque that could later jeopardize treatment if it progresses into bone loss.[20,22-24]

The biological seal around oral implants consists of two principal layers: the epithelial attachment (which forms a cuff-like barrier adherent to the surface of the abutment via hemidesmosomes) and the underlying connective tissue barrier (which is organized in bundles, presenting a constant spatial arrangement of circular fibers, observed in transversal sections 200 μm to 800 μm from the titanium surface; longitudinal fibers, observed in longitudinal sections in the first 200 μm from the abutment surface; and oblique fibers, in small separate bundles, which can be observed externally to the above systems, with variable orientation and connecting the inner fibers with the submucosa and periosteum).[25] Properly performed second-stage surgery can help control the presence of connective tissue around the implant. One study has determined that the fibroblast-rich barrier tissue adjacent to the titanium surface of an implant helps maintain a suitable seal between the bone surrounding the implant and the oral environment surrounding the bone.[26]

Before various techniques for uncovering the implant are described, it is important to mention that in some situations, the cover screw will expose itself completely or partially to the oral cavity (Figure 12-3). In such cases, second-stage surgery might not be necessary; nevertheless, special care should be used. If the cover screw is not kept plaque free during this healing period, the implant eventually could be lost owing to inflammation, mucosal damage, and bone loss related to untreated plaque accumulation.[27-29] Studies have concluded that as a result of the relationship between degree of exposure and amount of peri-implant bone loss, implants that are exposed prematurely should be exposed as quickly as possible after such perforation.[30] In some cases, depending on the size of the exposure, if any additional attached gingiva or a change in contours is desired, there is no other option but to consider a soft tissue graft at a later stage.[31,32]

An additional consideration involves a modified surgical procedure for implant restoration that can be undertaken at second-stage surgery. During implant placement, an impression can be taken so the clinician can have an abutment and temporary ready for second-stage surgery performed by using computer-aided design (CAD)/computer-aided manufacturing (CAM) technology.[33,34] This procedure is recommended to achieve better healing of the soft tissues around the implant after second-stage surgery is performed, so that the resulting contour of the gingiva will strongly resemble the contour present around a natural tooth. This result can be obtained by placing the abutment and temporary, instead of a regular healing abutment, at the second-stage surgery. Such a procedure not only improves tissue health and esthetics, it also provides greater patient satisfaction, in that the patient will receive a tooth instead of the regular healing abutment. This method can also be used for multiple implant restorations. In fact, many practitioners believe that the precision, cost-effectiveness, and relative ease of this method for producing implant impressions that eventually yield technologically "personalized" healing abutments will lead to the continued popularity of implant procedures by replacing traditional implant restorative procedures.[35]

Second-Stage Surgery Techniques

Implant exposure techniques for second-stage surgery can be divided into excisional and incisional techniques, the former considered "destructive" and the latter "reconstructive," because excisional techniques reduce the width of the fixed mucosa, and incisional techniques do so to a lesser extent.[36] Incisional techniques preserve the soft tissues at the implant site, and they can be classified into two categories: those without tissue transference and those with tissue transference (rotation, displacement). Additionally,

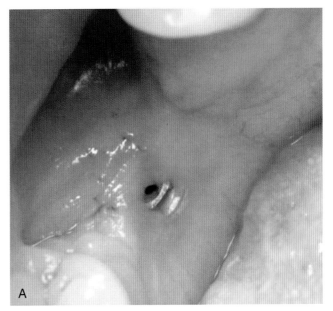

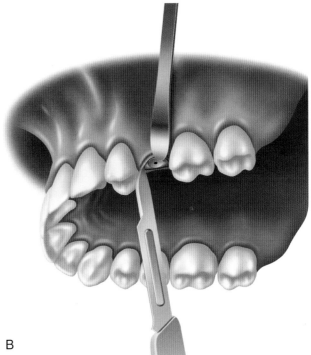

FIGURE 12-3 ■ **A,** Sometimes it is not necessary to surgically expose the cover screws, as they eventually will become exposed to the oral cavity on their own. **B,** Incisional technique to perform stage II implant surgery. (Courtesy of Zimmer Dental. All rights reserved.)

the amount of preoperative fixed gingiva can help clinicians determine which technique to employ, if at all: excisional techniques for fixed mucosa greater than 4 mm; incisional techniques for fixed mucosa between 1 mm and 4 mm; or a free-gingival graft preceding incisional techniques for patients with too little mucosa.[36]

The literature notes that minimally invasive procedures during second-stage implant surgery are especially important for single-tooth implants, particularly in the esthetic zone; in addition to yielding an esthetically appealing result, simple and effective exposure techniques facilitate healing of the site.[37-41] Distinguishing between esthetic and nonesthetic implantation sites can help clinicians determine the degree of surgical finesse required for each patient's circumstance, and so can reduce unnecessary chairtime and cost.[42] Additionally, as a way to meet increasing patient demand for esthetic zone "perfection," fibrin sealants can be used as a complement to, or replacement for, the traditional needle-and-suture armamentarium, to facilitate minimally invasive surgery.[43]

Excisional Techniques

Excisional techniques include all situations in which gingival tissue over the implant will be removed and discarded. For this type of technique, the tissues over the cover screw can be removed using a scalpel blade or a punch instrument. Electrosurgery instruments and high-speed motors should be avoided, because the implant can be harmed with these difficult-to-control methods[36] (Figure 12-4).

Excisional techniques are ideal only if sufficient attached gingival tissue is present around the head of the implant. In some cases, the implant head can be seen or palpated throughout the soft tissues; if this is not possible, there is always the help of X-ray films and remaining teeth or other

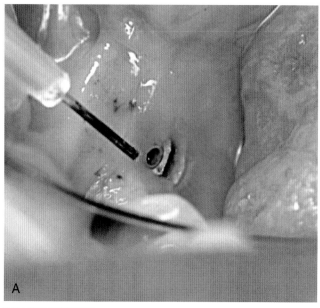

A

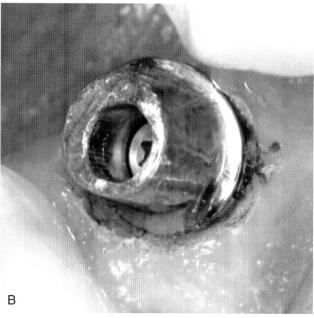

B

FIGURE 12-4 ■ **A, B,** Laser techniques are an excellent excisional method to uncover dental implants in areas of thin tissue.

anatomical sites that can be used as references for locating the implant. At times, the excisional method can be preferred even if the attached gingiva is insufficient, as is the case with mandibular implants, with which there is no other choice but to perform a connective tissue graft taken from the palate at a later time. A variation of this technique, with removal of minimal tissue, has been described in a procedure that begins with a vertical incision and then proceeds with a round incision from 1 mm to 3 mm around the tissue that will be removed and then utilizes a blunt instrument to stretch the tissues, to remove the cover screw and then insert the healing abutment.[37]

Incisional Techniques Without Tissue Transference

The midcrestal incision is very useful, especially when multiple implants are placed one next to the other, because they can be located as the incision progresses. This incision must be performed when the attached gingiva is sufficient, or when there is no area from which to take donor tissue, as is the case with mandibular implants. After the implants have been located and the cover screws replaced by healing abutments, interrupted sutures are placed between the implants to approximate the buccal and lingual flaps (Figure 12-3).

The "+" or "X" incision technique is a simple technique that should be performed when the attached gingiva is sufficient. There are two ways to start this incision. The first involves a small crestal incision that will later give place to a cross-type incision ("+"). This first incision can be extended and the technique modified to a midcrestal incision if the exact position of the implant is not well targeted. The second way is to use diagonal incisions ("X"); this type of incision should be used if the position of the implant is accurate, because there is less chance of switching to another technique without mistreating the tissues with excess incisions. Once the two overlying incisions are made, a periosteal elevator can be used to elevate the edges outward, which allows the appropriate driver to take the cover screw out. After this step, the healing abutment is screwed in part of the way to give it enough stabilization to permit the corners of the incised tissue to be elevated with a thin, blunt instrument.

Preservation of the papillae can be accomplished via another type of incision, which is midcrestal or a few millimeters toward the palate with a U shape, open toward the buccal aspect of the implant site with slightly divergent arms. Sometimes the releasing incisions are made more mesial and distal in the apical portion of the mucoperiosteal flap to create a wider reflection of the flap.[24]

The papillae of the proximal teeth remain adhered. A full-thickness flap is then raised and a de-epithelization of the outer edges of the incision and the proximal papillae is performed.[44] The surgical cover screw is now changed for a healing abutment. Once the healing abutment is placed, the flap should be split in whole thickness through its center, separating it into mesial and distal parts. Each of these parts of the buccal flap is positioned over the de-epithelized papillae and is secured to the palate with vertical mattress sutures.

Incisional Techniques With Tissue Transference

These methods include tissue displacement (rotation) toward the buccal area to achieve more fixed mucosa and/or the fabrication of papillae if needed. Such a technique is simple and predictable, and the result is an increased zone of keratinized gingiva in the buccal aspect of the future restoration site.[45] The incision for this technique is not performed in the middle of the ridge but a few millimeters toward the palate. Where it will start will depend on how much attached gingiva is desired. This first incision will now be connected to vertical incisions mesial and distal to the implant, or mesial and distal to the first and last implant if it is a multiple case. Now the mucosa can be corrugated toward the buccal, gaining fixed gingiva; in any of these cases, the flap can be a full-thickness flap, or it can be modified as a split-thickness flap (Figure 12-5).[46-49]

The advantage of a split-thickness flap is that it will not create an area of exposed bone in the palatal area or between the implants that will need to granulate by second intention, resulting in bone loss in the interproximal area and causing considerable pain and discomfort for the patient. Once the buccal portion of the implant(s) is reached, when the flap is elevated, the incision should continue in a full-thickness fashion. The above technique can be modified to create papillae and therefore a natural architecture of the mucosa around the implants.[24]

The unilateral semilunar incision is another technique available to the clinician. Once the incision is made and a full-thickness or split-thickness flap is reflected, allowing the exchange of the surgical cover screw(s) for the healing abutment(s), a semilunar bevel incision is made in the reflected flap in relation to each implant. The first incision is made at the distal area of the most mesially placed implant. This incision should be extended far enough to allow the pedicle that is formed to be rotated 90 degrees toward the mesial aspect of the healing abutment. This procedure is repeated for each implant.[24] After the interproximal areas are occupied by the rotated pedicles, sutures can be placed to attach them to the adjacent soft tissue.

The bilateral semilunar bevel incision allows yet another approach. Once the flap is elevated and the healing abutment is placed, a semilunar incision is made distal to mesial, and the pedicle is rotated 90 degrees. After placing the pedicle in a mesial position, the clinician performs a second semilunar incision from mesial to distal, and the pedicle is also rotated 90 degrees to fill the space between the healing abutment and the distal tooth.[24]

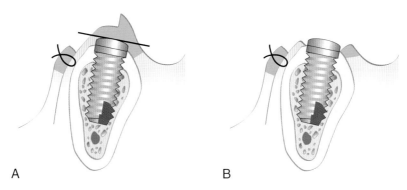

A   B

FIGURE 12-5   ■   **A,** Partial-thickness flap is apically sutured to the periosteum, and excess connective tissue coronal to the cover screw is excised by gingivectomy. **B,** Sharp blade used to eliminate all tissue coronal to the cover screw. (Care should be taken to avoid removing keratinized tissue from the lingual aspect of the implant.) (From Newman MG, Takei HH, Klokkevold PR, Carranza FA: *Carranza's clinical periodontology*, ed 10, St. Louis, 2006, Saunders.)

When restoring more than one implant, the clinician can use this technique to create a central papillae-like formation between two implants, besides the formation of papillae between the healing abutments and adjacent teeth.

The T-shaped incision can also be performed. After reflecting the flap, the clinician can make a T-shaped incision on the buccal aspect, allowing both sides of the flap to slide laterally to fill the spaces between healing abutments and adjacent teeth.[24] Preservation and reconstruction of papillae between adjacent implants are often necessary for esthetic reasons, so a similar technique could be used between implants, as well as between the implant and the teeth; in such cases, clinical photographs taken before the operation can be used to draw a line of reference between the highest point of the gingiva and the target site of the surgery involving soft tissue preservation or reconstruction.[50]

The literature frequently contains examples of innovative methods for promoting and preserving such formation of papillae.[51,52]

SUMMARY

Implant exposure during second-stage surgery is the crucial middle moment in dental implantology that can determine how well the dental implant and restorative components "fit" the individual patient biologically, functionally, and esthetically. The health of peri-implant tissue, as well as its preservation and reconstruction, is critical to the long-term "relationship" that the tissue has with implant components. When the implant is uncovered, the clinician must rise to the challenge of optimizing the condition of the peri-implant tissues; therefore, a thorough knowledge of implant exposure techniques at second-stage surgery is necessary for the clinician to match excisional or incisional techniques with characteristics of tissue overlying the implant, based on the amount of attached gingiva, the thickness of the overlying mucosa, and the presence or absence of interdental papillae.

REFERENCES

1. Barber HD, Seckinger RJ, Silverstein K, Abughazaleh K: Comparison of soft tissue healing and osseointegration of IMZ implants placed in one-stage and two-stage techniques: a pilot study, *Implant Dent* 5(1):11-14, 1996.
2. Heydenrijk K, Raghoebar GM, Meijer HJ, van der Reijden WA, van Winkelhoff AJ, Stegenga B: Two-stage IMZ implants and ITI implants inserted in a single-stage procedure: a prospective comparative study, *Clin Oral Implants Res* 13(4):371-380, 2002.
3. Cooper LF: A modular approach to dental implant therapy: the appropriate selection of one- and two-stage surgeries, *Compend Contin Educ Dent* 23(9 suppl 2):4-12, 2002.
4. Heydenrijk K, Raghoebar GM, Meijer HJ, Stegenga B: Clinical and radiologic evaluation of 2-stage IMZ implants placed in a single-stage procedure: 2-year results of a prospective comparative study, *Int J Oral Maxillofac Implants* 18(3):424-432, 2003.
5. Cecchinato D, Olsson C, Lindhe J: Submerged or non-submerged healing of endosseous implants to be used in the rehabilitation of partially dentate patients, *J Clin Periodontol* 31(4):299-308, 2004.
6. Saadoun AP: Periimplant tissue considerations for optimal implant results, *Pract Periodontics Aesthet Dent* 7(3):53-60, 1995.
7. Goldberg PV, Higginbottom FL, Wilson TG: Periodontal considerations in restorative and implant therapy, *Periodontol 2000* 25:100-109, 2001.
8. Lanning SK, Waldrop TC, Gunsolley JC, Maynard JG: Surgical crown lengthening: evaluation of the biological width, *J Periodontol* 74(4):468-474, 2003.
9. Mankoo T: Contemporary implant concepts in aesthetic dentistry—part 1: biologic width, *Pract Proced Aesthet Dent* 15(8):609-616, 2003.
10. Hermann JS, Buser D, Schenk RK, Schoolfield JD, Cochran DL: Biologic width around one- and two-piece titanium implants, *Clin Oral Implants Res* 12(6):559-571, 2001.
11. Takei HH, Azzi RR: Chapter 66: Periodontal plastic and esthetic surgery. In: Newman, MG, Takei HH, Carranza FA, editors: *Carranza's clinical periodontology*, ed 9, New York, 2002, Elsevier.
12. Bragger U, Burgin WB, Hammerle CH, Lang NP: Associations between clinical parameters assessed around implants and teeth, *Clin Oral Implants Res* 8(5):412-421, 1997.

13. Weber HP, Cochran DL: The soft tissue response to osseointegrated dental implants, *J Prosthet Dent* 79(1):79-89, 1998.

14. Fritz ME: Two-stage implant systems, *Adv Dent Res* 13:162-169, 1999.

15. Karoussis IK, Muller S, Salvi GE, Heitz-Mayfield LJ, Bragger U, Lang NP: Association between periodontal and peri-implant conditions: a 10-year prospective study, *Clin Oral Implants Res* 15(1):1-7, 2004.

16. Cardaropoli D, Re S, Corrente G: The Papilla Presence Index (PPI): a new system to assess interproximal papillary levels, *Int J Periodontics Restorative Dent* 24(5):488-492, 2004.

17. Krennmair G, Piehslinger E, Wagner H: Status of teeth adjacent to single-tooth implants, *Int J Prosthodont* 16(5):524-528, 2003.

18. Hunter F: Periodontal probes and probing, *Int Dent J* 44(5 suppl 1):577-583, 1994.

19. Mombelli A, Muhle T, Bragger U, Lang NP, Burgin WB: Comparison of periodontal and peri-implant probing by depth-force pattern analysis, *Clin Oral Implants Res* 8(6):448-454, 1997.

20. Atassi F: Peri-implant probing: positives and negatives, *Implant Dent* 11(4):356-362, 2002.

21. Etter TH, Hakanson I, Lang NP, Trejo PM, Caffesse RG: Healing after standardized clinical probing of the periimplant soft tissue seal: a histomorphometric study in dogs, *Clin Oral Implants Res* 13(6):571-580, 2002.

22. James RA, McKinney RV Jr: Tissues surrounding dental implants. In: Misch CE, editor: *Contemporary implant dentistry*, Chicago, 1999, Mosby.

23. Garg AK: Practical implant dentistry, Dallas, 2001, Taylor.

24. Palacci P, Ericsson I: Esthetic implant dentistry: soft and hard tissue management, Chicago, 2001, Quintessence.

25. Schierano G, Ramieri G, Cortese M, Aimetti M, Preti G: Organization of the connective tissue barrier around long-term loaded implant abutments in man, *Clin Oral Implants Res* 13(5):460-464, 2002.

26. Moon IS, Berglundh T, Abrahamsson I, Linder E, Lindhe J: The barrier between the keratinized mucosa and the dental implant: an experimental study in the dog, *J Clin Periodontol* 26(10):658-663, 1999.

27. Tal H: Spontaneous early exposure of submerged implants: I. classification and clinical observations, *J Periodontol* 70(2):213-219, 1999.

28. Tal H, Dayan D: Spontaneous early exposure of submerged implants: II. histopathology and histomorphometry of non-perforated mucosa covering submerged implants, *J Periodontol* 71(8):1224-1230, 2000.

29. Barboza EP, Caula AL: Diagnoses, clinical classification, and proposed treatment of spontaneous early exposure of submerged implants, *Implant Dent* 11(4):331-337, 2002.

30. Tal H, Artzi Z, Moses O, Nemcovsky CE, Kozlovsky A: Spontaneous early exposure of submerged endosseous implants resulting in crestal bone loss: a clinical evaluation between stage I and stage II surgery, *Int J Oral Maxillofac Implants* 16(4):514-521, 2001.

31. Landi L, Sabatucci D: Plastic surgery at the time of membrane removal around mandibular endosseous implants: a modified technique for implant uncovering, *Int J Periodontics Restorative Dent* 21(3):280-287, 2001.

32. Nemcovsky CE: Interproximal papilla augmentation procedure: a novel surgical approach and clinical evaluation of 10 consecutive procedures, *Int J Periodontics Restorative Dent* 21(6):553-559, 2001.

33. Schneider A, Kurtzman GM: Computerized milled solid implant abutments utilized at second stage surgery, *Gen Dent* 49(4):416-420, 2001.

34. Garg AK: The Atlantis Components Abutment: simplifying the tooth implant procedure, *Dent Implantol Update* 13(9):65-70, 2002.

35. Priest G: Virtual-designed and computer-milled implant abutments, *J Oral Maxillofac Surg* 63(9 suppl 2):22-32, 2005.

36. Hertel RC, Blijdorp PA, Kalk W, Baker DL: Stage II surgical techniques in endosseous implantation, *Int J Oral Maxillofac Implants* 9:273-278, 1994.

37. Bernhart T, Haas R, Mailath G, Watzek G: A minimally invasive second-stage procedure for single-tooth implants, *J Prosthet Dent* 79(2):217-219, 1998.

38. Adriaenssens P, Hermans M, Ingber A, Prestipino V, Daelemans P, Malevez C: Palatal sliding strip flap: soft tissue management to restore maxillary anterior esthetics at stage 2 surgery: a clinical report, *Int J Oral Maxillofac Implants* 14(1):30-36, 1999.

39. Vogel RE, Wheeler SL: Tissue preservation for single-tooth anterior esthetics, *Compend Contin Educ Dent* 22(8):657-662, 2001.

40. Smukler H, Castellucci F, Capri D: The role of the implant housing in obtaining aesthetics: generation of peri-implant gingivae and papillae—part 1, *Pract Proced Aesthet Dent* 15(2):141-149, 2003.

41. Zadeh HH, Daftary F: Minimally invasive surgery: an alternative approach for periodontal and implant reconstruction, *J Calif Dent Assoc* 32(12):1022-1030, 2004.

42. Buser D, von Arx T: Surgical procedures in partially edentulous patients with ITI implants, *Clin Oral Implants Res* (11 suppl 1):83-100, 2000.

43. Becker W: Fibrin sealants in implant and periodontal treatment: case presentations, *Compend Contin Educ Dent* 26(8):539-544, 2005.

44. Nemcovsky CE, Moses O, Artzi Z: Interproximal papillae reconstruction in maxillary implants, *J Periodontol* 71(2):308-314, 2000.

45. Nemcovsky CE, Moses O: Rotated palatal flap: a surgical approach to increase keratinized tissue width in maxillary implant uncovering: technique and clinical evaluation, *Int J Periodontics Restorative Dent* 22(6):607-612, 2002.

46. Michaelides PL, Wilson SG: A comparison of papillary retention versus full-thickness flaps with internal mattress sutures in anterior periodontal surgery, *Int J Periodontics Restorative Dent* 16(4):388-397, 1996.

47. Fugazzotto PA: Flap designs and suturing techniques related to anterior single-tooth implant placement, *Dent Implantol Update* 9(2):13-16, 1998.

48. el Askary A el-S: Esthetic considerations in anterior single-tooth replacement, *Implant Dent* 8(1):61-67, 1999.

49. Velvart P, Ebner-Zimmermann U, Ebner JP: Comparison of long-term papilla healing following sulcular full thickness flap and papilla base flap in endodontic surgery, *Int Endod J* 37(10):687-693, 2004.

50. Grossberg DE: Interimplant papilla reconstruction: assessment of soft tissue changes and results of 12 consecutive cases, *J Periodontol* 72(7):958-962, 2001.

51. Misch CE, Al-Shammari KF, Wang HL: Creation of interimplant papillae through a split-finger technique, *Implant Dent* 13(1):20-27, 2004.

52. Zetu L, Wang HL: Management of inter-dental/inter-implant papilla, *J Clin Periodontol* 32(7):831-839, 2005.

chapter 13

Impression Materials, Concepts, and Techniques for Dental Implants

THE ART AND SCIENCE OF IMPRESSION MAKING is an ancient endeavor, with the earliest dentures carved from ivory by hand. The fit was essentially determined by sight and palpation, with some results considered works of art. However, historical accounts described the discomfort and suffering that the average patient had to endure. Later, waxes, plaster, and other compounds were used with varying degrees of success.

With the development of new instrumentations and new techniques, the availability of better quality impression materials became imperative. For example, although it was possible to produce extremely fine detail as well as maintain good dimensional stability with plaster, the fact that it was inelastic limited its use in impression making. Thus, the goal of researchers and clinicians was to develop materials that had elastic properties, were easy to handle, and still retained good accuracy and dimensional stability.[1-10]

Today's advancements in the science of dental materials and the development of modern impression materials are generally considered to have had their origins in the mid-1920s, coinciding with the inception of the American Dental Association (ADA) Council on Dental Materials and Devices. Over time, the ADA directly and indirectly improved the quality of dental technology and materials, which had previously been left in the hands of any individual or company who had the means of developing and marketing such to highly receptive dental professionals, whose field was experiencing significant growth, both scientifically and intellectually.

Today's dentist has a number of different choices of impression materials, including agar-agar, alginates, polysulfides, silicones, and polyethers. Each has its advantages and disadvantages. The correct choice is dictated by the particular prosthodontic case and depends on a number of different factors, such as accuracy (immediate and time-dependent), dimensional stability, handling properties, hardness, elasticity, working time, esthetic appearance, odor, shelf life, cost, and acceptance by the dentist and patient (Figure 13-1).

Classification of Impression Materials

Although impression materials can be classified by a number of different criteria, such as by their generic chemical name, a more general method involves consideration of the properties of the materials before or after setting.

Before setting, the property most often used to characterize impression materials is viscosity. The viscosity of the material can affect the time that the detail can be recorded in hard tissue impressions and can influence the extent to which tissue compression or displacement can be achieved in impressions of soft tissue. Viscosity often varies, however, with the applied stress. Material that appears viscous under low stress conditions may become more fluid during the recording of the impression, when it is placed under greater stress. When a substance reacts in this manner, the reaction is often due to the spacing of the impression tray. A relatively fluid impression mate-

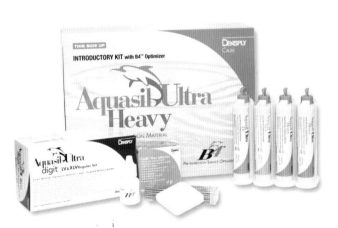

FIGURE 13-1 ■ The correct choice of an impression material is dictated by the particular situation and depends on a number of different factors. (Courtesy of Dentsply.)

rial confined in a close-fitting tray will be compressed to a greater degree than the same material in a loose-fitting tray. Thus, classifying impression materials by their viscosity is more difficult than it may seem at first.

A more widely used classification system uses the properties associated with impression materials after setting. Of these, the two most significant are elasticity and rigidity. Impression materials that are elastic possess the ability to change their shape in direct response to a force (such as compression) and to recover their original form to a measurable degree after removal of the force. Nonelastic impression materials may clearly be plastic, or they may be very rigid but show little evidence of plastic deformation (e.g., waxes, impression plasters). The degree of elasticity and rigidity is important because it determines whether the material can be used to record undercuts. When elastic impression materials are removed from the undercut areas, they often are put under significant tensile stress. If a patient has deep soft tissue undercuts, the set impression material must be flexible enough to pass the undercut and must have enough elasticity to allow for proper recovery and to provide an accurate impression.

Requirements for Implant Prosthetics

Accuracy: To record the fine detail of hard or soft tissue, the impression material should be fluid when inserted into the patient's mouth. This requires the material to have a low viscosity and a degree of pseudoelasticity. The manner in which the material interacts with moisture and saliva also affects fine detail reproduction. Some impression materials are compatible with moisture and saliva and require no special precautions. Others, however, are hydrophobic and may be repelled by moisture and saliva in a critical area of the impression, causing formation of a "blow-hole" in the material.

Dimensional changes that generally occur during the setting of impression material (which sometimes involves a chemical reaction or simply a physical change of state) can also affect accuracy. These dimensional changes can involve contraction or expansion. Materials that contract during setting are firmly attached to the impression tray, resulting in expansion of the impression space and oversized dies or casts, whereas materials that expand during setting produce undersized dies or casts. How this affects the fit of the resultant restoration depends on the type of restoration being made. In the case of implants, excessive space results in loose fitting of the impression plate and subsequent incorrect construction of the framework.

Thermal contraction occurs because of the difference in temperature between the patient's mouth (32°C to 37°C) and the operating area (23°C), and is a result of the value of the coefficient of thermal expansion of the impression material and the tray to which it is attached. Thus, it is crucial that the impression material stays attached to the tray while the impression is being recorded. Impression trays are often provided with adhesives to enhance bonding.

Dimensional Stability: Dimensional stability, defined as the change in accuracy with respect to time, is an important factor when a particular impression material is chosen. For most impression materials, accuracy is best maintained by pouring the cast as soon as possible after recording the impression. However, when it is not convenient for the dentist to cast the model, the impression has to be sent to a dental laboratory. If the laboratory is not on the same premises or is a long distance from the dentist's office, the delay between recording the impression and fabricating the cast can be several hours or even days (Figure 13-2).

The "ideal" impression material would have perfect dimensional stability, such that the impression would keep its original accuracy indefinitely. Various factors can contribute to dimensional changes during storage or transformation of impressions. When elastomers are bound with adhesive to a custom tray, the dimensional stability of the impression materials is significantly improved. Continuation of the setting reaction past the expected setting time can result in dimensional changes. When viscoelastic materials exhibit continued elastic recovery for some time after the impression has been taken, the dimensional changes result in a more accurate impression. However, many impression materials contain volatile substances, which may be primary components or by-products of the setting reaction. When these volatile materials are lost during storage, the impression material shrinks, with a resultant decrease in accuracy.

Manipulative Variables: Impression materials can be dispensed in a number of different ways. Some do not require any mixing, whereas others involve the mixing of powder and water, paste and liquid, or paste and paste. When materials need to be mixed, the two-paste system (usually supplied in toothpaste-like tubes) makes proportioning easier. One simply squeezes out equal lengths of paste from each tube onto a paper mixing pad or a glass plate. In contrast, the point at which mixing has been satisfactorily completed with the paste/liquid or powder/water systems is not as clearly defined.

Impression materials that soften when warmed and set when cooled are sometimes difficult to control. The setting characteristics are completely out of the control of the operator because they depend on the temperature at which the material is heated and the time at which it is maintained at that temperature before the impression is recorded. For impression materials that set through a chemical reaction, the working time for the material extends from the beginning of mixing until the material is no longer suitable to record the impression. This time period is usually defined as how long it takes for the materials' viscosity to increase by a given amount above that of the freshly mixed material.

Whereas the working time of the impression material is determined at room temperature, the setting time is usually determined at mouth temperature. The setting time of an impression material can be defined as the time required to complete the setting reaction. For the convenience and comfort of both the operator and the patient, the ideal handling properties of an impression material are, naturally, short working and setting times. This can be realized with materials that set through chemical reactions, provided that the reaction rate is much faster at mouth temperature than at room temperature.

Other Variables: Impression materials should be nontoxic, nonirritating, clean, easy to use, and esthetic, and should have an acceptable odor and taste. It also should be possible to decontaminate the material to make it safe for further handling.

Nonelastomeric Impression Materials

Before the development and availability of complex polymer impression materials, nonelastomeric impression materials, such as gypsum, impression compounds, and zinc oxide/eugenol-based impression materials, were used by the dentist. Although these materials enabled the dentist to reproduce oral structures with greater accuracy and detail, they have their limitations.

Gypsum: The setting expansion, setting time, and consistency of gypsum are well controlled. The material

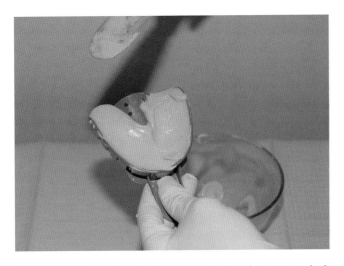

FIGURE 13-2 ■ One disadvantage of using alginate is its lack of stability.

assumes an early set, is easily read, and, in general, makes a good mucostatic impression that does not disturb loose or fibrous oral tissue. In addition, it is relatively esthetic in appearance and has a satisfactory taste for the patient. However, as an impression material, gypsum has many characteristics that make it undesirable and limit its use, such as difficulty separating it from a working cast. Thus, when it is used in the preparation of fixed or removable partial dentures, it is used mainly as an indexing material that can be mixed with starch to provide an index that dissolves in hot water.

Impression Compound: Impression compound, composed mostly of natural products (e.g., resin, copal resins, carnauba wax, stearic acid), is usually limited to primary impressions for edentulous patients. Although the impression compound can sometimes be removed from the undercuts, it usually distorts when removed. In addition, the material can be unesthetic and may have a disagreeable taste. Impression compound can be used in individualized copper bands for single-tooth impressions; however, when used in this manner, it demonstrates undesirable temperature-related expansion and contraction, as well as deleterious flow and distortion after hardening. Thus, similar to gypsum, impression compound has limited use in fixed partial dentures.

Zinc Oxide/Eugenol Pastes: Zinc oxide/eugenol (ZOE) pastes, developed for making impressions of the tissues of edentulous patients, are good as a secondary or wash impression. Like plaster, they are capable of producing fine detail and maintaining excellent dimensional stability, and they have a reasonable setting time. Zinc oxide/eugenol paste is usually used for a final impression in full denture construction. The material can also be used as corrective lining in preparatory impressions, as a liner for full denture bases to create a tissue-based contact, and as an interocclusal recorder in conjunction with a bite registration tray. However, because ZOE is brittle, it cannot be used where undercuts are present. It also has an unesthetic appearance, has a bad odor and taste, and, in some patients, causes tissue reactions due to sensitivity.

Hydrocolloids

Two types of hydrocolloids (a colloid with water as a dispersion medium) can be used to make direct impressions. One is the agar-agar type of material, which is reversible from liquid to solid and from solid to liquid, and the other is alginate, which is irreversible.

Agar-Agar: Agar-agar, a complex polysaccharide extracted from seaweed, was the first elastic impression material that could be removed from undercut areas without fracturing. Despite some drawbacks, the material was con-

sidered to represent an important development in removable prosthodontics. Two initial limitations—a retarding effect on gypsum products that resulted in casts with chalky or soft surfaces, and rapid shrinkage of the impression after removal from the patient's mouth—have essentially been overcome, the first by adding strong gypsum-product accelerators, and the second by promptly filling the impression with the cast material.

The steps involved in making an impression with agar require a team effort and should not be attempted by a single individual. The materials are usually supplied as a gel in a flexible, toothpaste-like tube or syringe. The gel is composed primarily of a 15% colloidal suspension of agar-agar in water, with small quantities of borax and potassium sulfate present. Agar-agar sets at a temperature at or greater than mouth temperature. Three baths (i.e., boiling, storage, and tempering) are needed to prepare the material. The impression material first is liquefied in boiling water, in a syringe or a tube, and then is stored in a chamber at 145°F to 150°F until it is used. Before the material is placed in a tray, it is tempered in a third bath at a temperature between 102°F and 105°F to avoid burning any soft tissue bordering the bridge. The agar-agar is then injected into the gingival crevice, and the tray is seated over the area to be impressioned.

It is important that definite stops be made in the tray before it is filled with the impression material and placed in the storage chamber, so that the tray always seats itself properly in the same position. All bleeding or seepage in the patient's mouth must be stopped before the impression material is applied. After the tray has been placed over the impression area, water (at room temperature first, then colder and colder) is circulated through the impression tray until the material has set. This usually takes about 5 to 6 minutes. To maintain accuracy, the cast is poured immediately after the tray is removed.

In general, agar-agar has a high degree of immediate accuracy, is able to reproduce fine detail well, is esthetic in appearance, has an acceptable taste and agreeable smell, and is low in cost.[11-16] The most obvious drawback of agar is that the material has to be poured immediately.

Alginate: Alginates, like agar, are elastic impression materials that can be removed from the undercut areas. Instead of through a syringe, the material is usually applied to the impression area with a wiping motion of the finger. When placed in the tray without stops, the material should be carefully seated over the area to be impressioned, to prevent the material from becoming perforated. The dimensional stability of an alginate and its effect on gypsum casts are similar to those of agar, and the materials are easier to use than agar, require simpler equipment, and can be handled by one person (although an assistant makes the preparation easier). Alginates can be measured easily, are esthetic in appearance, have a pleasant odor, are easy to handle, and are low in cost (Figure 13-3).

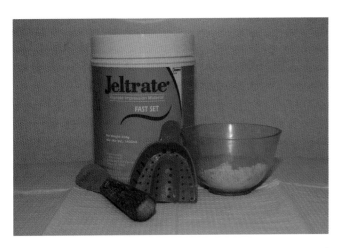

FIGURE 13-3 ■ For dental implant surgery, alginate is used only for opposing arch models.

For these reasons, alginates have been considered reasonable satisfactory substitutes for agar that are better than waxes and compounds.[13,17-20] However, they have definite disadvantages that make them less desirable than agar. The materials are not as accurate and do not reproduce the fine detail seen with agar.[21] They produce cases that frequently are not suitable as bases for casting. Alginates also have poor time-dependent dimensional stability and thus should not be used in fixed prosthodontics. Although these materials can be used as opposing models and templates for restoration, they usually are used in fashioning removable partial dentures. Alginates can also be used as impressions for fabricating individual trays for plant-supported prostheses.

Elastomeric Impression Materials

Because many dentists are not able to pour their own impressions immediately, the impressions must be stable enough over an extended period of time that they can continue to be used to produce accurate casts. This need led to the development of more stable and accurate elastomeric impression materials. These materials, also known as elastomers, are soft and rubber-like and easily stretched, and are able to return to a relaxed state when the stress is removed.

Polysulfide Rubbers: Polysulfides are synthetic materials that have elasticity similar to that of the hydrocolloids, but they do not have the same deleterious effect on gypsum casts. Polysulfides are regarded by some dentists as more convenient than agar (e.g., the gypsum cast does not have to be poured immediately), and the material has significantly better dimensional stability than either agar-agar or alginates. However, polysulfides do undergo dimensional changes over time. Although polysulfides are not quite as accurate as agar, they are capable of very fine reproduction and very good immediate accuracy. However, polysulfides have an unesthetic appearance and a bad odor.

Lead peroxide, organic hydroperoxide, and copper hydroxide can be used as accelerators in the system. Custom impression trays are necessary to provide uniform thickness of the impression material, so that distortion is minimized and accuracy is enhanced. Although historically, these custom trays have been made from acrylic resin, other materials, such as polycaprolaitone, are being evaluated.[22]

The impression materials, usually supplied as paste dispensed from tubes, consist of a base and a catalyst. After the base and catalyst pastes are mixed together, a condensation polymerization reaction is induced with the lead dioxide, resulting in a rapidly polymerizing or vulcanizing elastic polymer. As polymerization proceeds, the viscosity of the material increases, and when the degree of cross-linking attains a certain level, the material develops elastic properties. The setting is characterized by a gradual increase in viscosity and slow development of elasticity. Polysulfides have very good tear resistance. As viscoelastics, they recover slowly and incompletely after being compressed or stretched. To optimize elastic recovery, the impression should be removed with a single, rapid pull.

Silicone Polymers (Condensation Rubber): Silicone synthetic polymers are capable of very fine reproduction and very good immediate accuracy. The materials also have a better esthetic appearance and a more agreeable odor and taste than polysulfides. The initial drawbacks of a short shelf life and dimensional instability have been reduced to some extent. However, silicones still suffer from dimensional changes over time (even more so than polysulfides) and tend to separate in tubes when standing because of their relatively short shelf life. Both silicone polymers and polysulfides have a notable degree of acceptability and accuracy as long as their limitations are taken into account.

The materials are supplied either as two pastes or as a paste and a liquid. The liquid component of the paste/liquid system can be hazardous if not handled carefully. The ingredients required for this reaction are reflected in the composition of a typical paste and liquid material. Light, regular, heavy-bodied, and putty materials are available; the latter is a paste of very high viscosity that is not available in polysulfides (Figure 13-4).

On mixing the two pastes or the paste and the liquid, an immediate reaction begins in which the catalyst reacts with the cross-linking agent. Although the catalyst is a heavy metal, silicone polymers are considered essentially nontoxic. The principle of the setting reaction is similar for the two systems. Each setting reaction stage also produces one molecule of ethyl alcohol as a by-product. Cross-linking results in an increase in viscosity and the rapid development of elastic properties.

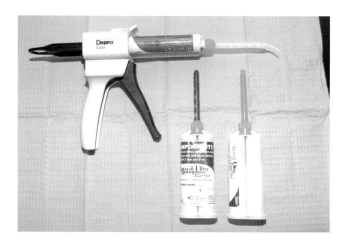

FIGURE 13-4 ■ Silicone polymers should be selected when impressions are taken for crowns and bridges over dental implants.

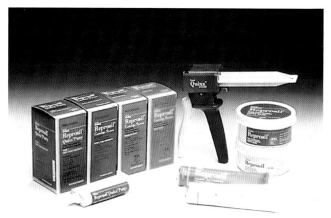

FIGURE 13-5 ■ Addition reaction silicone rubbers, also known as polyvinyl siloxane impression materials, are available in a variety of viscosities and have a high elastic modulus. Their stiffness makes them an ideal material for implant prostheses. (Courtesy of Dentsply.)

Silicone impression materials are very hydrophobic, and thus are readily repelled by water or saliva. Because of this characteristic, the material is kept in the patient's mouth for only a few minutes. The set material has adequate tear resistance for most purposes. Although a regular-bodied silicone is able to undergo only about a 300% extension before fracturing, most of this strain is recoverable. Dimensional changes after setting, such as condensation, may be due to the continued slow setting or to the loss of alcohol by-products from the setting reaction. To obtain optimum accuracy, the models should be cast as soon as possible after the impression is recorded.

Silicone polymers are used frequently for crowns and bridges and sometimes for partial dentures. They are used more often with a stock tray. The availability of the putty material increases accuracy and stability. The use of silicone polymers in implant dentistry is limited because the material has to be poured immediately.

Addition Reaction Silicone Rubbers: Addition reaction silicone rubbers, also known as polyvinyl siloxane impression materials, have excellent physical properties, dimensional stability, and handling characteristics[23,24] (Figure 13-5). The materials have outstanding accuracy, the capability to record fine detail, and the best elastic recovery of all available impression materials.[25] They are clean, odorless, and tasteless. Because of its exceptional dimensional stability, addition reaction silicone rubber can be poured at the convenience of the operator.[26] The handling characteristics of these materials are enhanced by the fact that the silicones are available in viscosities ranging from very low (for use with a syringe or wash material) to very high. All of these features have made addition reaction silicone rubbers the impression material of choice for many (even though they are among the most expensive) and allow them to be applied in a wide variety of clinical situations in operative dentistry, fixed and removable prosthodontics, and implant dentistry.

These silicone materials are supplied by many manufacturers in a convenient auto-mix system that provides a consistent mix and is cost-effective.[27] The materials polymerize rapidly, with practically no by-product from the polymerization reaction. When a custom tray is used, the bulk of the material can be minimized.

Polyvinyl siloxanes have a relatively short working time; however, in general, the time is sufficient, particularly when the auto-mix system is used.[28] If working time needs to be increased, refrigerating the syringe material has been reported to extend it by about 1 minute without adversely affecting the accuracy or handling characteristics of the material.[1] Because addition reaction silicone rubbers can be sensitive to technique, a completely dry field is necessary when the impressions are made, an acrylic resin custom tray should be used, and contact with critical oral structures should be avoided when wearing latex gloves, because polymerization of these materials can be inhibited by latex (the use of nonlatex gloves is recommended).[23]

The materials are supplied as two pastes. When the two parts are mixed, a platinum-catalyzed addition reaction takes place, resulting in a cross-linkage between the two types of siloxane pre-polymers. Some manufacturers recommend that pouring of the cast be delayed until the evolution of hydrogen is achieved so that the cast surface does not become pitted. Although the exact process of hydrogen release is not clear, it may involve reaction of the platinum catalyst with moisture. Cross-linkage increases the viscosity of the material, in conjunction with the development of elastic properties. It is important, of course, to use a tray of correct size. If necessary, an adhesive should be applied to make sure that separation of the tray and impression material does not occur, because this can cause gross distortion in the impression. The rigidity of the tray

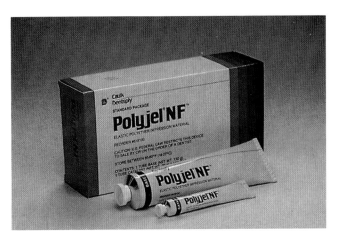

FIGURE 13-6 ■ This popular impression material has a fast setup time, easy cleanup, and good patient acceptance. (Courtesy of Dentsply.)

can also affect the accuracy of the impression, especially when viscous materials are used, because the tray may come under substantial stress during the reaction time of the impression.

Polyethers: Polyether impression materials are the most accurate and dimensionally stable of the elastomeric impression materials.[29-31] The excellent accuracy of the material, along with its dimensional stability, ease of handling, extended shelf life, acceptable odor, and patient acceptance are very attractive features for the clinician (Figure 13-6).

Polyethers make the most accurate casts, and because of the rate and degree of polymerization, they do not undergo continued polymerization after removal from the patient's mouth (as is seen with other elastomers). Thus, the dimensions of the impression are not affected by shrinkage. In addition, no by-products (e.g., water, alcohol, other volatiles) are formed during polymerization, as can be seen with silicone and polysulfide materials. Evaporation of these by-products can cause small, variable stresses that result in a slowly changing shape of the impression. The accuracy of the impressions is usually long-lasting.

Because of the material's high degree of dimensional stability, polyethers do not have to be poured immediately after mixing, and they can be sent safely to a laboratory without fear of time-dependent dimensional change, thus eliminating the main cause of ill-fitting cast metal restorations. After the polyether material has set in the mouth, there is little if any subsequent change in its shape. It is also possible to store polyethers for a long time before the materials are mixed and poured. However, because of their hydrophilic properties, polyethers should not be stored in any type of solution. In general, polyethers will displace tissue fluids and saliva to a slight degree.

Although the polyethers have a relatively short working time (typically less than 2 minutes), this factor can usually

be overcome with experience. Polyether materials mix easily, but because they are not as elastic as polysulfides or silicones, they are somewhat more rigid when set. The stiffness of the set material can be a drawback and can limit the use of polyethers in complicated periodontal cases that take a long time to complete, when severe undercuts are present (proximal tears can occur when the impression is remolded), and in cases of previously placed fixed bridges (unless the undercuts were removed before the impression was made). However, its stiffness is a major advantage for impressions of implant components, as it allows for more accurate seating of parts into the set material after removal from the mouth. A custom tray should be used when impressions are made from polyethers.

Impression Technique for Osseointegrated Implants

Conventional fixed prosthodontics uses elastic impression materials for replicating prepared and unprepared tooth surfaces and for accurately relating these surfaces within the complete dental arch.[32] Studies of the accuracy of different materials and techniques in an individual die and the entire arch have provided information regarding the possible directions and magnitudes of local (die) and regional (arch) distortion likely to occur with the various procedures used to transfer intraoral shapes and relationships to a working cast for indirect prosthesis construction.[33-37]

Impression techniques and materials for osseointegrated implants have largely been borrowed from conventional prosthodontic impression methods,[38-40] with modifications made to address situations specific to implants and to enable the dentist to fabricate the prostheses more quickly.[41-45] The same material characteristics that are important for conventional impression making, accuracy, dimensional stability, elasticity, and so forth, are also important with implants. In cases of completely edentulous patients, it appears that current clinical techniques, in which restoration is accomplished with a conventional maxillary complete denture and a mandibular implant-supported prosthesis, are effective.[46-48] The fabrication of prostheses supported by rigid implants is apparently comparable with that of conventional fixed prostheses. In cases of nonparallel implants, various options are available to accurately transfer these relationships to a working cast. When working casts for implants are fabricated, the primary goal of current prosthodontic techniques is to correlate implant analogs in a similar manner, as the implants or abutments are related intraorally[32] (Figures 13-7). Construction of the required passively fitting (tension-free) prosthesis demands precise interimplant dimension transfer.[38-40,49,50] An inability to meet this requirement can result

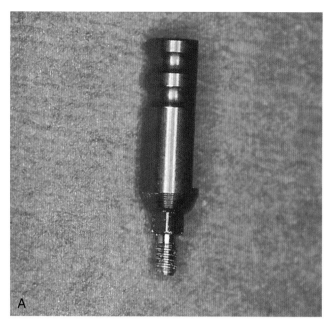

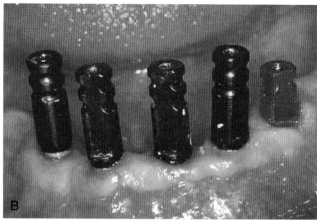

FIGURE 13-7 ■ **A,** Thread transfers are screwed into the implants. These components transfer orientation of the implant's internal thread pattern to the implant analog in the working cast. **B,** Thread transfers are color-coded to match the corresponding implant analog.

in loss of fixture integration and subsequent treatment failure.[51] Forced tightening of the superstructure can cause microfractures of bone, create a zone of marginal ischemia, and result in healing with a nonmineralized attachment to the implant fixture.

Two techniques have been developed to transfer implant positions from the patient's mouth to the working cast.[32] In the indirect method, a one-piece transfer coping is fastened to the implant to make the impression. When setting of the impression material is completed, the impression is removed, with the transfer coping left fastened in place. The impression coping is then removed and attached to an appropriate analog, and is placed in its respective impression space. In the direct method, the fastening screw projects above the height of the coping. The impression is made with a window in the top of the tray. After the impression material has completely set, the screw is loosened and the tray is removed in a manner that allows the impression to retain the transfer coping. After the impression is removed, the transfer coping (while still in the impression material) should be fastened to an appropriate analog (Figure 13-8).

Both techniques offer advantages and disadvantages.[32] The main advantages of the indirect method are that the technique is more similar to conventional crown and bridge impression making than is the direct method, and fastening of the analog can be accomplished visually. However, it is more difficult to recover from nonparallel implants, and multiple deformations can occur in the impression material. Both of these factors can contribute to the inaccuracy seen with the indirect method. In addition, the coping needs

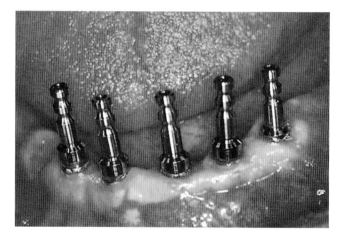

FIGURE 13-8 ■ After the appropriate abutments have been selected and placed into the implant, impression posts can be placed into the abutment, and a final impression can be obtained using rigid impression material.

to be placed into the impression material at the respective positions. With the direct method, there are more parts to manipulate during fastening, and fastening of the analog is done blindingly, leading to possible inaccuracies. However, the impression material is not deformed when removed from the patient's mouth, the coping remains in the impression and does not need to be replaced into respective positions, and angulation of the implant is not a factor. Overall, the correct method for each practitioner has been found to be the one that provides the most accurate outcome in his or her hands.

SUMMARY

Taking accurate impressions with accurate impression materials is the single-most important step in effective and long-lasting prosthetics for the patient.

REFERENCES

1. Asgar K: Elastic impression materials, *Dent Clin North Am* 15:18-21, 1971.
2. Bell JW, Davies EH, von Fraunhofer JA: The dimensional changes of elastomeric impression materials under conditions of humidity, *J Dent* 4:73-77, 1976.
3. Braden M: Viscosity and consistency of impression rubbers, *J Dent Res* 46:429-432, 1976.
4. Davis GB, Moser JB, Brinsden GI: The bonding properties of elastomer tray adhesives, *J Prosthet Dent* 36:278-281, 1976.
5. Hembree JH: Comparative accuracy of elastomer impression materials, *J Tenn Dent Assoc* 54:164-166, 1974.
6. Kaloyannides TM, Christidou I: Elasticity of impression materials: IV. permanent deformation as a function of time, *J Dent Res* 54:168-173, 1975.
7. Mansfield MA, Wilson HJ: Elastomeric impression materials: a method for determining dimensional stability, *Br Dent J* 139:267-271, 1975.
8. Philipps RW: *Science of dental materials*, ed 7, St. Louis, 1973, CV Mosby, pp 136-156.
9. Sawyer HF, Birtles JT, Nieman R: Accuracy of casts produced from five mercaptan rubber impression materials, *Int Assoc Dent Res Prog* 62, 1972. Abstract
10. Schwindling R: Thermal correction of the volume changes of a silicone impression, *Quintessence Int* 10:35-37, 1971.
11. Tylman SD: Reversible and irreversible hydrocolloid impression materials, *Dent Clin North Am* 713-717, 1958.
12. Skinner EW, Hoblit NE: A study of the accuracy of hydrocolloid impression, *J Prosthet Dent* 6:80-84, 1956.
13. Schwartz JR: The use of the hydrocolloids or alginates as impression materials for indirect or indirect-direct inlay construction procedure, *Dent Items Interest* 379-384, 1951.
14. Phillips RW, Ito BY: Factors influencing the accuracy of reversible hydrocolloid impressions, *J Am Dent Assoc* 43:1-4, 1951.
15. Lewis J: The hydrocolloid impression materials, *Northwest Dent* 273-276, 1975.
16. Kendrick ZV: The physical properties of agar type hydrocolloid impression material, *J Am Dent Assoc* 40:575-577, 1950.
17. Rapuano JA, Marra RR, Tuffo SD: Irreversible hydrocolloid (alginate) in fixed prosthodontics, *J Acad Gen Dent* 29-33, 1973.
18. Zuckerman GR: Irreversible hydrocolloid for fixed partial denture impressions, *J Prosthet Dent* 32:657-660, 1974.
19. Skinner EW, Pomes CE: Alginate impression materials: technique for manipulation and criteria for selection, *J Am Dent Assoc* 35:245-249, 1947.
20. Fusayama T: Indirect inlay and crown techniques using alginate, *J Am Dent Assoc* 54:74-77, 1957.
21. Sawyer HF, Sandrick JL, Nieman R: Accuracy of casts produced from alginate and hydrocolloid impression materials, *J Am Dent Assoc* 93:806-809, 1976.
22. Pilcher ES, Draughn RA: Evaluation of polycaprolaitone custom tray material, *J Prosthodont* 2:174-177, 1993.
23. Chee WWL, Donovan TE: Polyvinyl silicone impression materials: a review of properties and techniques, *J Prosthet Dent* 68:728-732, 1992.
24. Johnson GH, Graig RG: Accuracy of additional silicones as a function of technique, *J Prosthet Dent* 55:197-203, 1986.
25. Phillips RW: *Skinner's science of dental materials*, ed 9, Philadelphia, 1991, WB Saunders, pp 145-147.
26. Lacy AM, Fukui H, Bellman T, et al: Time dependent accuracy of elastomeric impression materials: part II: polyether, polysulfides, and polyvinylsiloxane, *J Prosthet Dent* 45:329-333, 1981.
27. Graig RG: Evaluation of an auto-mix mixing system for an addition silicon impression material, *J Am Dent Assoc* 110:213-215, 1985.
28. Sy JT, Munoz CA, Schnell RJ, et al: Some effects of cooling and chemical retarders on five elastomeric impression materials, *Int J Prosthodont* 1:252-258, 1988.
29. Hanah C, Pearson SL: Some observations of the clinical handling and stability of elastomeric impression materials, *J Baltimore College Dent Surg* 24:5-9, 1969.
30. Sawyer H, Birtles JT, Nieman R: Accuracy of casts produced from seven rubber impression materials, *J Am Dent Assoc* 87:126-130, 1973.
31. Sawyer HR, Dilts WE, Aubrey ME, et al: Accuracy of casts produced from three classes of elastomer impression materials, *J Am Dent Assoc* 89:644-647, 1974.
32. Carr AB: A comparison of impression techniques for a five-implant mandibular model, *Int J Oral Maxillofac Implants* 6:448-455, 1991.
33. Reisbick MH, Matyeas J: The accuracy of highly filled elastomer impression materials, *J Prosthet Dent* 33:67-72, 1975.
34. Augsburger RM, Sodberg KB, Pelzner RB, et al: Accuracy of casts from three impression materials and effect of a gypsum hardener, *Oper Dent* 6:70-74, 1981.
35. Finger W, Ohsawa M: Accuracy of stone casts produced from selected addition type silicone impressions, *Scand J Dent Res* 91:61-65, 1983.
36. Linke BA, Nicholls JI, Faucher RR: Distortion analysis of stone casts made from impression materials, *J Prosthet Dent* 54:794-802, 1985.
37. Lewinstein I, Graig RG: Accuracy of impression materials measured with a vertical height gauge, *J Oral Rehabil* 17:303-310, 1990.
38. Zarb GA, Jansson T: Laboratory procedures and protocol. In: Brånemark P-I, Zarb GA, Albrektsson T, editors: *Tissue-integrated prostheses: osseointegration in clinical dentistry*, Chicago, 1985, Quintessence, pp 117-128.
39. Proceedings of a Consensus Conference on Implantology, October 18, 1989, Mainz, West Germany, *Int J Oral Maxillofac Implants* 5:182-187, 1990.
40. Zarb GA, Schmidt A: The longitudinal clinical effectiveness of osseointegrated dental implants: the Toronto study, part II: the prosthetic results. *J Prosthet Dent* 64:53-61, 1990.
41. Loos L: A fixed prosthodontic technique for mandibular osseointegrated titanium implants, *J Prosthet Dent* 55:232-242, 1986.
42. Tautin FS: Impression making for osseointegrated dentures, *J Prosthet Dent* 54:250-251, 1985.
43. Rasmussen EJ: Alternative prosthodontics technique for tissue integrated prostheses, *J Prosthet Dent* 57:198-204, 1987.
44. Ivanhoe JR, Adrian ED, Krantz WA, et al: An impression technique for osseointegrated implants, *J Prosthet Dent* 66:410-411, 1991.

45. Spector MR, Donovan TE, Nicholls JI: An evaluation of impression techniques for osseointegrated implants, *J Prosthet Dent* 63:444-447, 1990.

46. Cox JF, Zarb GA: The longitudinal clinical efficacy of osseointegrated dental implants: a three-year report, *Int J Oral Maxillofac Implants* 2:91-100, 1987.

47. Adell R, Lekholm D, Rockier B, et al: A 15 year study of osseointegrated implants in the treatment of the edentulous jaw, *Int J Oral Burg* 10:387-416, 1981.

48. Laney WR, Tolman DE, Keller EE, et al: Dental implants: tissue integrated prosthesis utilizing the osseointegration concept, *Mayo Clin Proc* 61:91-97, 1986.

49. Adell R, Andersson C, Brånemark P-I, et al: *Manual for treatment with jawbone anchored bridges according to the osseointegrated method*, Goteborg, 1981, Sweden Faculty of Dentistry Goteborg, and the Institute for Applied Biotechnology.

50. Zarb GA, Zarb FL: Tissue integrated dental prostheses, *Quintessence Int* 1:39-42, 1985.

51. Skalak R: Biomechanical considerations in osseointegrated prostheses, *J Prosthet Dent* 49:843-848, 1983.

chapter 14

Principles of Occlusion in Implant Dentistry

LTHOUGH THE CLINICIAN'S UNDERSTANDING OF THE ROLE OF OCCLUSION is important to successful osseointegrated prostheses, its importance is not always taken under proper consideration during routine prosthetic procedures. Numerous factors are involved in the neuromuscular reflex action in the natural dentition where periodontal ligament receptors protect the teeth and periodontium from excessive occlusal forces that can cause trauma to the supporting bone (Figure 14-1). However, no specific defense mechanisms can combat adverse occlusal forces in osseointegrated implants. Thus, the overall long-term success of osseointegrated implants depends not only on adherence to fundamental prosthodontic principles to produce proper restorations, but also on a clear understanding of the potential effects that occlusal stresses can have on the implants.

Because osseointegrated implants have demonstrated high rates of success due to improved surgical protocols since the early 1990s, restoration-related complications have increasingly become the focus of dental clinicians who wish to extend success rates even further; therefore, the biomechanical elements associated with occlusion have been an increasing focus of treatment planning and coordination among clinicians.[1-3] The inherent differences between teeth (with their associated periodontal ligaments) and implants require systematic evaluation and evidence-based research to arrive at what has been described

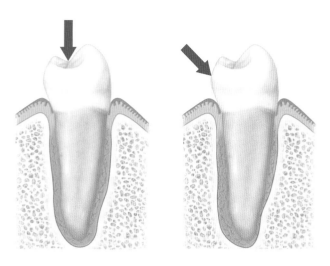

FIGURE 14-1 ■ In the natural dentition, the periodontal ligament protects the teeth and the periodontium from excessive occlusal forces that can cause trauma to supporting bone.

as an implant-specific concept of occlusion.[4,5] Patients who present with occlusal dysfunction and other indications for occlusal reconstruction are in particular need of implant management techniques that focus on prosthodontics, including lack of distal abutment, long span segment, and compromised natural abutments.[6]

Although opinions differ about the superiority of a particular form of occlusion, the anatomic, mechanical, physiologic, and esthetic limits presented by each patient will control the dentist's choice of occlusal schemes. Consideration of one factor alone (such as anatomy, oral tissue conditions, and so on) is not an adequate basis for choosing a specific pattern of occlusion, although emphasis on one factor over another will vary with each patient. For example, understanding occlusal forces is particularly important with patients who exhibit conditions consistent with bruxism.[7-9] The dentist should select a plan for occlusion based on factors such as age of the patient, condition of the alveolar ridge, quality of the mucosa, position and direction of the implants, condition of the remaining teeth, esthetic interests, oral dexterity, and oral awareness.

Ideal Occlusion

The "ideal occlusion" has been generally defined as the existence of intermaxillary relationships compatible with the stomatognathic system, resulting in functional mastication and good patient esthetics without causing physiologic abnormalities.[10] Although no ideal occlusal pattern exists for all persons, a suitable model can be made by incorporating factors that reduce vertical and horizontal stresses,

provide maximum intercuspation during centric relation, and load horizontal forces produced during eccentric excursions on those teeth or implants that are most capable of bearing these stresses.[11] Four primary patterns of ideal occlusion have been developed on the basis of these criteria: balanced occlusion, lingualized occlusion, mutually protected occlusion, and group function occlusion.

Balanced Occlusion

Balanced occlusion is based on three classic theories—Bonwill's three points of occlusal balance, Spee's curve of Spee, and Monson's spherical theory.[12-15] In balanced occlusion (also known as "fully balanced" or "bilateral balanced" occlusion), all of the patient's teeth simultaneously contact during both maximum intercuspation and eccentric mandibular masticatory movements.[16]

The lateral occlusal forces that are produced during eccentric movements are distributed evenly to all teeth and temporomandibular joints.[17-19] Horizontal (rather than vertical) forces are produced during masticatory movements. Destructive lateral forces then are transmitted from the teeth to the periodontal ligaments, where they are absorbed. To compensate physiologically for these lateral stresses, the occlusal load must be widely distributed, thus the necessity for maximum contact area during intercuspation and all eccentric movements. Predicting masticatory jaw movements continues to be the subject of research.[20-23] For example, a recent study that attempted to correlate chin and jaw movements concluded that jaw and chin movements were qualitatively similar, and that at least 74% of the variation in jaw movement could be accounted for by multivariate linear models of chin movement[22].

A balanced occlusion is considered ideal for edentulous patients for whom complete dentures are the treatment of choice (Figure 14-2).[24] However, a balanced occlusion is difficult to achieve on the natural dentition with a normal periodontium.[25,26] A recent prospective clinical trial comparing lingualized occlusion versus bilateral balanced occlusion in complete dentures found that edentulous patients fitted with complete dentures with lingualized occlusion experienced and expressed greater satisfaction with their denture retention. In addition, it was observed that a higher alveolar ridge resulted in greater masticatory performance.[27] When seen in the natural dentition, a balanced occlusion is usually the result of advanced attrition. A balanced occlusion has been used in fully bone-anchored prostheses, but the use of this occlusal pattern for osseointegrated prostheses has been debated[25,26,28] (Figure 14-3).

In a 20-year longitudinal study of balanced occlusion used over a 12-year period in both dentate and fully edentulous patients, a few patients experienced treatment failure 5 to 10 years later and developed discrepancies between the centric relation position and maximum intercuspation.[29] The primary cause of failure was believed to be occlusal surface wear secondary to excess contact area. Factors that led to failure included the following: (1) a cusp-to-fossa relationship in only a portion of the molar contacts, with the bicuspids working only as an embrasure, making wedging and tooth drifting possible; (2) extensive areas of tooth contact and broad occlusal surfaces; (3) slight changes resulting in a readily perceptible discrepancy occurring in "tight" occlusion; (4) errors in full-mouth balance as a result of commission, rather than omission; and (5) the necessity sometimes to increase the vertical dimension to a risky degree to achieve full balance.

Lingualized Occlusion

In 1927, Gysi introduced the concept of lingualized occlusal schemes. Lingualized occlusion might be considered a form of organic occlusion because the concept emphasizes that teeth are in effect blocks of resin or porcelain that need to be modified to fit the requirements of the patient. The shape of the occlusal surfaces can be altered to accommodate each patient's individual needs, chewing patterns, condylar guidance, and incisal guidance.[30] Although this occlusion concept provides a useful combination of several occlusal methods, and even though the clinician can retain many advantages of anatomical and nonanatomical occlusions (for example, adjustment to compensate for minor changes in vertical and centric relation, satisfactory balanced occlusion), some believe that this concept should not be used in isolation to obtain optimal occlusion[30-32] (Figure 14-4).

Lingualized occlusion can be defined as an occlusal scheme that uses the maxillary lingual cusps as the major

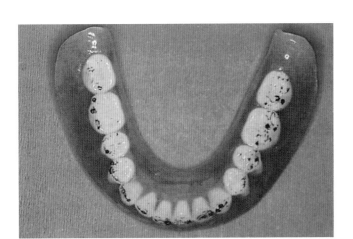

FIGURE 14-2 ■ The balanced occlusion is considered ideal for edentulous patients.

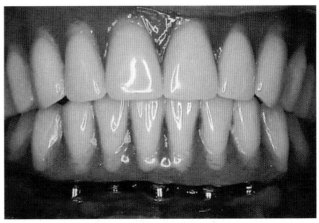

FIGURE 14-4 ■ In the lingualized type of occlusion, contact of the lingual cusps of the uppers against the semianatomic teeth on the lowers will be seen in lateral, protrusive, and eccentric movements.

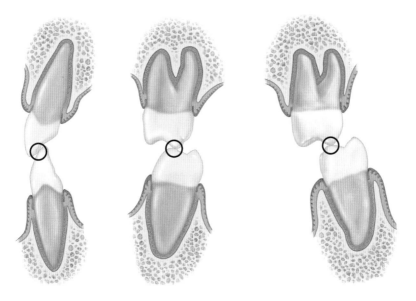

FIGURE 14-3 ■ In balanced occlusion, all the patient's teeth simultaneously contact in maximum intercuspation and eccentric mandibular masticatory movements.

functional occlusive element. These cusps oppose the mandibular zero degree or shallow, cusp teeth. Lingualized integration calls for anteroposterior and mediolateral compensating curves to be arranged in the mandibular arch, permitting balanced articulation between the maxillary lingual cusps and the mandibular teeth during jaw movements.

Too high or too low placement of occlusion can destroy the smooth functioning coordination of these structures. Teeth positioned too far buccally or lingually can result in forces loaded axially or laterally on the implants. The central fossae of the mandibular posterior teeth are positioned on a line that extends from the distal portion of the canine to the middle of the retromolar pad. During arrangement of the teeth, a premolar is eliminated and the first molar will assume a more anterior position. Because this arrangement can contribute to crowding of the tongue, the two molars should be positioned slightly to the buccal side of the reference line to increase the space available for the tongue.

An anteroposterior curve is established to enhance balanced articulation along the protrusive pathway. In addition, a mediolateral compensating curve is established to provide balanced articulation during lateral movements. Lingualized occlusion represents an occlusal scheme that uses specific tooth molds designed (1) to improve the likelihood of maximum intercuspation with an absence of deflective occlusal contacts, (2) to provide cusp height for selective occlusal reshaping, and (3) to achieve a natural and esthetically pleasing appearance for the patient.

Lingualized occlusion offers several advantages. A decrease in the vertical forces occurs, along with a reduction in the lateral forces directed against the ridges. Furthermore, stability is maintained during parafunctional movements. This pattern can be used for all types of maxillary relationships and is easily adjustable. Finally, lingualized occlusion is particularly helpful in maintaining good esthetics.[30,33]

Mutually Protected Occlusion

In a 1960 study of the occlusion of patients over the age of 60 without attrition, it was noted that their molars did not contact during eccentric movements. However, in maximum intercuspation, the molars contacted but the anterior teeth did not.[34] Clearly, the molars were responsible for supporting the occlusal loads. In 1974, Dawson established the criteria for ideal occlusion that defined the mutually protected occlusion scheme.[35] For this pattern, there has to be (1) stable stops on all teeth when the condyles are in their most superior-posterior position (centric relation), (2) an anterior guidance in accord with border movements of the envelope of function, (3) disclusion of all posterior teeth in protrusive movements and on the balancing side, and (4) noninterference of all posterior teeth on the working side with lateroanterior guidance or with border movements of the condyles.

As the pattern name indicates, mutually protected occlusion is based on the anterior teeth protecting the posterior teeth, and the posterior teeth protecting the anterior teeth. The posterior teeth protect the anterior teeth in centric position, with centric stops on posterior teeth also deterring excess loading from being transferred to the temporomandibular joints.[36-39] During protrusive movement, the canine and posterior teeth are protected by the incisors, and during lateral movement, the incisors and posterior teeth are protected by the canines.[10,29,40-43]

The canine plays a key role in this type of intermaxillary relationship.[44] The mandible is positioned into maximum intercuspation by canine guidance, mandibular eccentric movements are controlled by the canines (except during protrusive movement), and the canine controls lateral stresses by directing vertical masticatory movements. The canine provides a good crown-to-root ratio, adequate hard compact bone encompassing the tooth, less stress because of its distance from the temporomandibular joint, and numerous receptors in the periodontal ligament. When canine guidance cannot be established, the anterior teeth on the working side must help guide posterior disclusion during lateral movement (known as anterior group function).[35] When the anterior teeth cannot guide mandibular movement, all working side teeth need to be used for guidance during lateral movement.[45]

Mutually protected occlusion is believed to be the best occlusal pattern for the natural dentition, with the vertical dimension maintained by the posterior teeth.[36] The cusp-to-fossa relationship results in interlocking of the upper and lower components, providing maximum support in centric relation in all directions.[29] In addition, forces are closer to the long axis of each tooth. Mutually protected occlusion has been contraindicated when a horizontal masticatory cycle and compromised periodontium are present, and when the patient has a missing canine or a prosthetic canine. However, with the advent of osseointegrated implant treatment, few contraindications to this pattern of occlusion remain.[46]

Group Function Occlusion

The concept of group function occlusion was introduced by Schuyler, who questioned whether the canine should bear all occlusal loads during lateral movement.[47,48] Group function occlusion occurs when all facial cusps on the working side contact the opposing dentition, with no contact on the nonworking side. In this occlusal pattern, the teeth should receive stress along the long axis of the tooth. In lateral movement, the total stress should be transmitted among the tooth segment, there should be no interferences during closure into the intercuspal position, proper interocclusal clearance should be maintained, and the teeth should contact in lateral movement without interferences[49] (Figure 14-5).

The need for group function occlusion depends on various requirements regarding the distribution of lateral

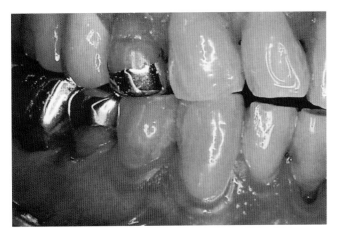

FIGURE 14-5 ■ All occlusal loads are shared by more than one tooth during lateral movement to prevent stress in a single tooth while at the same time stabilizing the mandible.

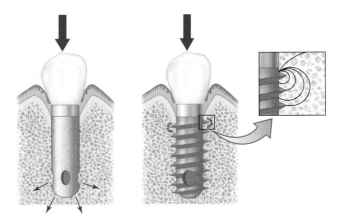

FIGURE 14-6 ■ In cylindrical implants, or in implants with microthreads near the crest the occlusal forces are concentrated at the apex, while in screw-shaped implants (without microthreads), the force is concentrated at the outside edges of the screw threads. Microthreads on the implant near the bone crest help dissipate forces apically.

pressure. In group function occlusion, lateral stresses are distributed to all working side teeth, whereas in mutually protected occlusion, lateral stresses are directed to the working side canine only. No tooth contacts are present on the nonworking side. Also, when the mandible is closed, the mandibular buccal cusps contact the facial ridges of the maxillary lingual cusps, and the cusps are not maintained in a stable position. Because group function occlusion does not result in the detrimental effects sometimes seen with lingualized and balanced occlusion and is easier to create than mutually protected occlusion, this occlusal pattern is believed to be the most appropriate for occlusal adjustments and short-span prosthetic treatment.[50-53]

Different Types of Occlusal Loads

Crucial parameters to consider when one is evaluating acceptable loading of bone as part of the overall accommodation of occlusal forces include bone quality, fixture length, fixture-anchorage healing time, and fixture loading.[54-58] The literature generally reveals that the flexibility of natural teeth allows for certain occlusal irregularities, but the implantologist must be precise in his or her diagnosis of occlusal properties, and corrections or compensations must be made to complete the proper design of prostheses, particularly regarding implant-supported prosthodontics adjacent to teeth.[58] "Therapeutic biomechanics" promotes such corrective procedures to reduce implant loading.[56] Under such procedures, the clinician positions the head of the implant as close as possible to the midline of the restoration; subsequently, angulated abutments provide necessary access or parallelism. A significant reduction in the posterior cusp inclination occurs. For anterior vertical overlap, the clinician uses a horizontal stop on the maxillary lingual surface

to redirect lateral force, making it vertical and toward the implant and bone.[56]

Animal studies have revealed important results concerning the breakdown of bone surrounding oral implants after occlusal overload or plaque accumulation. A study with monkeys, for example, revealed that, after occlusal overloading, six of eight implants became loose, but only two were lost.[54] Another study with monkeys examined the influence of controlled occlusal overload, with results showing implants remaining integrated with bone; in this study, none of the subjects showed gross bone loss after excessive occlusal force for 1 to 4 weeks. Researchers concluded that these overload conditions left peri-implant tissues unharmed.[55]

The two types of loading that are of primary interest in oral implantology are axial forces and bending movement.[59-61] Axial forces are considered to be more favorable because they distribute stress more evenly throughout the implant, whereas bending movement exerts pressure gradients in both the implant and the bone.

Although mastication primarily creates vertical forces in the dentition, transfer forces are also induced by the horizontal motion of the mandible and the inclination of the tooth cusps. These forces are transferred to the osseointegrated prosthesis, where they are transmitted into the fixture and, finally, distributed into the bone. During this force flow, occlusal force will create different patterns of stress and strain, which depend on the particular geometric configuration of the prosthesis[62-64] (Figure 14-6).

A sudden force, referred to as impact force, occurs when the mandible closes with high velocity and power. This type of force can have destructive effects on the osseointegrated prosthesis (for example, on implant components such as the abutment, fixtures, and connecting screws) as well as on the supporting bone. To help lessen potential damage secondary to the impact forces, the teeth should contact simultaneously when the mandible goes to maximum intercuspation.

Occlusal Factors Specific to Osseointegrated Implants

Because osseointegrated implant systems connect the prosthesis firmly to the supporting fixtures and there is no cushioning effect between the fixtures and the bone, occlusal stresses (from both masticatory and impact forces) are distributed directly to the surrounding bone through the prosthesis.[62] The occlusal pattern chosen (whether it is balanced, lingualized, mutually protected, or group function) should provide dynamic elements for each prosthesis.

Masticatory efficiency can be improved by cusp height; however, exaggerated cuspal inclinations can result in interference with mastication.[65-68] In cases of low cuspal inclinations, the lateral elements of mastication are increased, whereas with steep cuspal inclinations, the vertical elements are increased.[69-71] During normal masticatory movements, the mandible moves vertically, with occlusal forces transmitted in the same direction. Force vectors on the mandibular cusps are divided into vertical and horizontal elements, with vertical pressure equal to the forces on the opposing dentition (such as grinding force during mastication) and the horizontal component equivalent to pressures applied to the opposing maxillary molars (such as shearing force during mastication) (Figure 14-7).

If the implant is cylindrical, the occlusal forces are concentrated at the apex; if the implant has a screw-like configuration, the force is concentrated at the outside edges of the screw threads. Vertical component force on the cantilever, however, will tend to cause apically directed forces to the

distal fixture and occlusally directed forces to the prosthesis anterior to it. This force distribution is created by micromovement between the prosthesis, abutment, and implant, resulting in elongation and potential fatigue of the retaining screw, rather than movement of the implant within the bone.

No force distribution to multiple implants in the same prosthesis is effective, because the prosthesis is rigid, and the implants and the bone have no movement (nonetheless, some researchers talk about micromovement),[62] which effectively distributes forces to all of the implants. However, multiple-fixture force transmission can take place because of deformation of the retaining screws and possible overload caused by a poor interface fit between prosthesis and abutments.

Different factors have to be considered when the clinician is attempting to reduce occlusal problems in an implant-prosthesis situation, such as the location of the impact area. In the posterior maxillary area, the implant is placed most often lingually and slightly inclined because of bone topography. In these cases, the use of a crossbite relationship is recommended because forces are exerted on the same cuspal inclination, which produces a resultant line of force that falls much closer to the crestal bone and in an axial direction, thus reducing the torque.

Shear forces, which act horizontally on a surface, produce a cutting action. Shear forces are increased between the maxillary and mandibular molars when grinding forces are applied and with steeper cusps and vertical occlusal forces. With flatter cusps, shear forces are absent, and a more prominent horizontal force is created during mastication. Thus, sharper cusps will increase the shear forces in a prosthesis.

It has been reported that when osseointegrated implants are used over a short span, with fixed partial dentures and in single-tooth replacement, the occlusion should be distributed in maximum intercuspation, and all cusp interference should be eliminated in eccentric position.[72-75] This accepted concept for the natural dentition can be applied to osseointegrated implant treatments. In occlusion for a fully bone-anchored prosthesis, the fixtures are interconnected by the framework, and stresses are distributed to all fixtures located in the anterior region. These forces then are transferred through the prosthesis, into the fixture, and finally into the bone. During this force flow, a given occlusal force creates different patterns of strain and stress based on the geometric configuration of the particular prosthesis.[62,76-81]

When lateral loads are applied to posterior areas during eccentric movement, there is a tendency to overstress the fixture. This result is why some disclusion of the posterior region is preferred to a fully balanced occlusion in prosthetic restoration of posterior osseointegrated implants. Fully bone-anchored prostheses are designed to have cantilever extensions that can resist fulcrum forces through a lever effect. With this type of restoration, the anterior fixture absorbs a tension force proportional to the lever arm

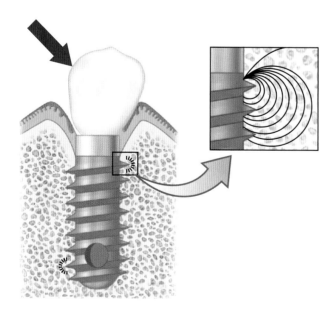

FIGURE 14-7 ■ When excessive off-axis forces are applied to the restoration, bending movements can cause loosening of the retaining screw or breakage of the abutment.

ratio, and the posterior fixture is subjected to compressive forces that are the sum of the applied occlusal force and the compensating tension forces.[65] To avoid destructive forces in lateral movement, the occlusal forces should be shared by the anterior teeth (the occlusal force on a canine is approximately one-eighth less than that on a second molar).[29]

Bruxism and Occlusion

Implant predictability regarding occlusion for the bruxing patient is at its lowest because bruxism in its pure form is uncontrolled increased contact time between the teeth with the potential to overload the prosthesis and the implant interface. At least seven differences have been noted between implants and teeth, differences that represent Nature's built-in, protective mechanisms: an alarm system that helps teeth survive in the mouth under load and in function. Differences include issues involving the periodontal ligament (which can act as a shock absorber), pulpal tissue (which provides thermal and pain feedback), the neck (which can reduce stress on the ridge), a tapered root (which directs forces apically), the size and number of roots (which help to provide surface area and support), the lamina dura (which pertains to cortical bone issues), and the structural composition (which pertains to flexing dentin). So, understanding all the elements of occlusion relative to implant dentistry is crucial.[7-9]

Signs of Unstable Occlusion

There are five basic issues regarding unstable occlusion: joint pain, muscle pain, broken teeth, worn teeth, and mobile teeth. The clinician must carefully approach diagnosis and treatment planning for such occlusal issues. All occlusal evaluation must begin with an evaluation of the temporomandibular joint (TMJ), using the proper armamentarium.

Additionally, to diagnose occlusal pathology properly, the clinician needs to employ a semiadjustable articulator and a facebow in order to take a centric relation bite record, which is important to understand in terms of diagnosis and restorative issues. The significance of this process is that, first and foremost, centric relation involves bone-brace positioning at the border position: The mandible hinges, which rotate from this position to the back of the bone bridge, reveal that the condylar assembly can go no higher up the eminent ostoses, which means that the clinician has the ability to control all tooth contact from this position. A second important concern is the reproducible position; when the clinician hears that position, it does not mean he or she can take a profile or multiple profiles and verify the position of the jaw in the mouth. What "reproducibility" means is that the clinician can take a centric relation profile from the mouth, transfer it to the articulator in the labo-

ratory, fabricate a prosthesis in the laboratory, and, with these specific occlusal schemes in mind, transfer it to the mouth and have it function in the mouth the way it was designed to do.

Finally, the only crucial position is the centric relation position, which shuts off the inferior head of the lateral pterygoid muscle, which has a superior head and an inferior head.[9] These two muscles have to work in opposition. The superior head is a disc-stabilizing muscle, which is primarily active during closure; the inferior head is inactive. These two muscles begin to act antagonistically when the teeth make contact before the condylar assembly reaches that fully seated position; this antagonism creates centric interference. The teeth touching before the condyle fully seats itself during closure causes the inferior head of the lateral pterygoid muscle to fire and then creates an antagonistic relationship between the superior muscle and the inferior muscle. The most common trigger for pain is centric interference—tooth interference that occurs before the condyle has reached that fully seated position. The forward position is the only position from which all tooth contact can be controlled. Therefore, it is the only position from which an occlusion can be properly analyzed.

Trial Therapy for the Bruxing Patient

Trial therapy enables a clinician to determine whether a bruxing habit is occlusal (treatable) or central nervous system (CNS) based (essentially, untreatable). Trial therapy means altering or correcting the occlusion and then monitoring the response. The easiest way to accomplish this goal is through appliance therapy. To fashion a properly made appliance, the clinician must have a model mounted on a semiadjustable articulator with a facebow transfer of the upper arch in order to take a centric relation profile.

Assuming that the patient's habit is an occlusal one, the clinician can create an ideal occlusion on the appliance and then can see what the patient's response to the appliance is; the response will dictate which types of diagnoses are made. The appliance should be rigid and flat with an anterior discluding ledge. The patient wears the appliance for about 3 months, and then it is checked for the reproduction wear present; the teeth then are checked to see if any symptoms (muscle pain, joint, and so on) are present. If no wear is present on the appliance after 3 months based on the type of wear seen in the mouth, then the diagnosis is that of an occlusal bruxer.

Occlusal Triggers to Bruxing Habits

The first occlusal trigger to bruxism is joint pain, which, potentially, has at least three sources. Joint pain can cause patients to brux when they have pain. The next trigger for an occlusal bruxing habit is a centric premature tooth contact, which occurs before the condyle fully seats itself; this is the number one potent trigger to an occlusal muscle habit—a tooth contact that blocks a condyle from fully seating itself. Finally, there is an eccentric prematurity, when the teeth touch where they are not supposed to at the back of the mouth, in other words, the muscles contract inappropriately.

Triggers of occlusal bruxing habits involve issues regarding the joint, the centric relation, and the occlusion. When diagnosing and treating occlusal issues, the clinician must consider the keystone muscles in the joint. The next thing needed to treat this patient is to identify the envelope of parafunction and incorporate it into the occlusal treatment plan. The patient will have one habit or the other because the brain is telling the jaw to move a certain way every time. CNS-based habits may be horizontal or vertical.

Horizontal bruxers reveal wear facets that traverse across the buccal cusp of the posterior teeth, across the cusp tips of the canine, or across the incisal edges of an anterior tooth. They display a decrease in the overbite and a broad range of mandibular motion—left and right lateral excursions are very broad. These types of bruxers are difficult to treat because the clinician must account for the left side of the lower jaw and its potential contact on the right side of the upper and vice versa. Central nervous system horizontal bruxers need a permissive occlusal scheme—an occlusal scheme of shallow contact angles and shallow guidance that allows mechanical freedom for the bruxing habit. Such an occlusal scheme allows the teeth to survive the habit.

The other type of CNS bruxer is the vertical bruxer. In this group, the wear facets are linguals of maxillary anterior teeth and facials of lower anterior teeth. An increase in overbite is seen, along with a narrow range of mandibular motion. This type of bruxer is easy to treat with a special occlusal scheme. Central nervous system vertical bruxers require a lingual maxillary vertical stop 90 degrees to the lower incisal edges and with enough overjet for the mandible to move when they brux, with no incline centric stops. By providing a centric stop 90 degrees to the central incisors on the lower, the clinician can keep these bruxers from wearing the centric stop down.

Bruxism and Contraindications for Implants

Certain patients should not be treated with implants: A CNS horizontal bruxer should not be treated with implants. In this type of patient, occlusal forces indicate an inability to keep lateral forces off posterior teeth. In such cases, the dentist's only alternative is to treat the caries and any other biological problems, while just maintaining existing dentition.

SUMMARY

No one specific occlusal pattern has been developed that is ideal for oral implantology; however, research does provide us with some general criteria for deciding on a particular occlusal pattern that will help reduce cuspal interferences and lessen horizontal or lateral forces on the fixtures. Anticipated occlusal and chewing forces need to be taken under consideration with any implant-supported prosthesis. In addition, opposing dentition, as well as potential parafunctional mandibular movements, should be noted.

When combining natural teeth and implants, the clinician must remember that implants support teeth, not vice versa. In addition, attaching or splinting natural teeth to an implant creates a supported cantilever that increases the load on the implant, rather than supporting it. Thus, when an implant-supported prosthesis is used with natural teeth, the lever arm on the implant-supported portion should be reduced as much as possible; it should be even shorter than if it is a free-standing prosthesis using only implants.

For edentulous patients who need a fully bone-anchored prosthesis, a mutually protected occlusion should be attempted to attain posterior disclusion. For edentulous patients who need an overdenture prosthesis, a lingualized or balanced occlusion should be used. Because the anterior teeth are supported by overdenture attachments and the posterior teeth by tissues, a modified mutually protected occlusion may be possible if a slight molar disclusion is present.

For partially edentulous patients (Kennedy Class III or IV) who need a free-standing fixed partial denture for the anterior region (including the canine), a group function occlusion is best, because horizontal loads during lateral movements are shared between the prosthesis and the natural teeth. For partially edentulous patients whose natural anterior teeth are still present (Kennedy Class I or II in the posterior region) and who need a free-standing fixed partial denture for the posterior teeth, a mutually protected occlusion with posterior disclusion is recommended.

It has long been maintained that one of the essential reconstruction goals for the implant patient is to obtain the least stress possible on abutments, whether the abutments are natural or artificial; an additional axiom has been that stress can be lowered by using larger implants, by using additional implants, and by reducing and managing the force application.[82] Clinicians should strive for a minimum of three fixtures, offset slightly (approximately 5 degrees from each other) for posterior restorations, to provide for maximum axial loading and minimal torque. However, some believe that more important factors than the number of implants on stress distribution are the superstructure design and the related direction of forces.[83] Adequate precision of the fit between the prosthesis and abutments and appropriate tightening of the screw joints are important factors for obtaining full mechanical strength of the implant components. The use of posterior fixtures to avoid cantilevers should be considered. The presence of broken retaining screws, loose or fractured abutment screws, or bone resorption should be evaluated immediately and the cause of the complication should be corrected to avoid redistributing the load onto the other implants.

REFERENCES

1. Dario LJ: How occlusal forces change in implant patients: a clinical research report, *J Am Dent Assoc* 126(8):1130-1133, 1995.
2. Curtis DA, Sharma A, Finzen FC, Kao RT: Occlusal considerations for implant restorations in the partially edentulous patient, *J Calif Dent Assoc* 28(10):771-779, 2000.
3. Jackson BJ: Occlusal principles and clinical applications for endosseous implants, *J Oral Implantol* 29(5):230-234, 2003. Erratum in *J Oral Implantol* 29(6):314, 2003.
4. Kim Y, Oh TJ, Misch CE, Wang HL: Occlusal considerations in implant therapy: clinical guidelines with biomechanical rationale. *Clin Oral Implants Res* 16(1):26-35, 2005.
5. Stanford CM: Issues and considerations in dental implant occlusion: what do we know, and what do we need to find out? *J Calif Dent Assoc* 33:329-336, 2005.
6. Phillips K, Mitrani R: Implant management for comprehensive occlusal reconstruction. *Compend Contin Educ Dent* 22(3):235-238, 240, 242-246, 2001.
7. Gittelson GL: Vertical dimension of occlusion in implant dentistry: significance and approach, *Implant Dent* 11(1):33-40, 2002.
8. Misch CE: The effect of bruxism on treatment planning for dental implants, *Dent Today* 21(9):76-81, 2002.
9. Gittelson G: Occlusion, bruxism, and dental implants: diagnosis and treatment for success, *Dent Implantol Update* 16(3):17-24, 2005.
10. Hobo S: *Encyclopedia of occlusion*, Tokyo, 1978, Shorin Ltd.
11. Guichet NF: *Principles of occlusion*, Anaheim, Calif, 1970, Denar.
12. Bonwill WGA: The science of the articulation of artificial dentures, *Dent Cosmos* 20:321, 1858.
13. Spee FG: The condylar path of the mandible along the skull, *Arch Anat Physiol* 16:285-294, 1890 (in German); *J Am Dent Assoc* 100:670-675, 1980 (in English).
14. Monson GS: Some important factors which influence occlusion, *J Am Dent Assoc* 9:498-503, 1922.
15. Monson GS: Applied mechanics to the theory of mandibular movements, *Dent Cosmos* 74:1039-1053, 1932.
16. Scaife RR Jr, Holt JE, Natural occurrence of cuspid guidance, *J Prosthet Dent* 22(2):225-229, 1969.
17. Granger ER: Functional relations of the stomatognathic system, *J Am Dent Assoc* 48(6):638-647, 1954.
18. Granger ER: *Practical procedures in oral rehabilitation*, Philadelphia, 1962, JB Lippincott.
19. Kaplan RL: Gnathology as a basis for a concept of occlusion, *Dent Clin North Am* Nov:577-590, 1963.
20. Gallo LM: Modeling of temporomandibular joint function using MRI and jaw-tracking technologies—mechanics, *Cells Tissues Organs* 180(1):54-68, 2005.
21. van Essen NL, Anderson IA, Hunter PJ, Carman J, Clarke RD, Pullan AJ: Anatomically based modelling of the human skull and jaw, *Cells Tissues Organs* 180(1):44-53, 2005.
22. Gerstner GE, Lafia C, Lin D: Predicting masticatory jaw movements from chin movements using multivariate linear methods, *J Biomech* 38(10):1991-1999, 2005.
23. Yashiro K, Takada K: Model-based analysis of jaw-movement kinematics using jerk-optimal criterion: simulation of human chewing cycles, *J Electromyogr Kinesiol* 15(5):516-526, 2005. Epub 2005 Feb 1.
24. Grubwieser G, Flatz A, Grunert I, Kofler M, Ulmer H, Gausch K, Kulmer S: Quantitative analysis of masseter and temporalis EMGs: a comparison of anterior guided versus balanced occlusal concepts in patients wearing complete dentures, *J Oral Rehabil* 26(9):731-736, 1999.
25. Ramfjord SP, Ash MM: *Occlusion*, Philadelphia, 1966, WB Saunders.
26. Posselt U: *Physiology of occlusion and rehabilitation*, Oxford and Edinburgh, 1962, Blackwell Scientific Publishing.
27. Kimoto S, Gunji A, Yamakawa A, Ajiro H, Kanno K, Shinomiya M, Kawai Y, Kawara M, Kobayashi K: Prospective clinical trial comparing lingualized occlusion to bilateral balanced occlusion in complete dentures: a pilot study, *Int J Prosthodont* 19(1):103-109, 2006.
28. Stallard H, Stuart CE: What kind of occlusion should recusped teeth be given? *Dent Clin North Am* Nov:591-606, 1963.
29. Lucia VO: *Modern gnathological concepts*, St. Louis, 1961, CV Mosby.
30. Becker CM, Swoope CC, Guckes AD: Lingualized occlusion for removable prosthodontics, *J Prosthet Dent* 38(6):601-608, 1977.
31. Parr GR, Ivanhoe JR: Lingualized occlusion: an occlusion for all reasons, *Dent Clin North Am* 40(1):103-112, 1996.
32. Garcia LT, Bohnenkamp DM: Lingualized occlusion: an occlusal solution for edentulous patients, *Pract Proced Aesthet Dent* 17(9):628, 2005.
33. Smith DE: The simplification of occlusion in complete denture practice: posterior tooth form and clinical procedures, *Dent Clin North Am* 14(3):493-517, 1970.
34. Stuart CE: Why dental restorations should have cusps, *J Prosthet Dent* 10:553-555, 1960.
35. Dawson PE: *Evaluation, diagnosis, and treatment of occlusal problems*, St. Louis, 1974, CV Mosby.
36. Ito T, Gibbs CH, Marguelles-Bonnet R, Lupkiewicz SM, Young HM, Lundeen HC, Mahan PE: Loading on the temporomandibular joints with five occlusal conditions, *J Prosthet Dent* 56(4):478-484, 1986.
37. Milosevic A: Occlusion: 1. Terms, mandibular movement and the factors of occlusion, *Dent Update* 30(7):359-361, 2003.
38. Milosevic A: Occlusion: 2. Occlusal splints, analysis and adjustment, *Dent Update* 30(8):416-422, 2003.
39. Milosevic A: Occlusion: 3. Articulators and related instruments, *Dent Update* 30(9):511-515, 2003.
40. Thomas PK: *Full mouth waxing technique for rehabilitation: tooth-to-tooth cusp-fossa concept of organic occlusion*, San Francisco, 1967, University of California School of Dentistry.
41. Shupe RJ, Mohamed SE, Christensen LV, Finger IM, Weinberg R: Effects of occlusal guidance on jaw muscle activity, *J Prosthet Dent* 51(6):811-818, 1984.
42. Fitins D, Sheikholeslam A: Effect of canine guidance of maxillary occlusal splint on level of activation of masticatory muscles, *Swed Dent J* 17(6):235-241, 1993.
43. Kimoto K, Tamaki K, Yoshino T, Toyoda M, Celar AG: Correlation between elevator muscle activity and direction of sagittal closing pathway during unilateral chewing, *J Oral Rehabil* 29(5):430-434, 2002.
44. D'Amico A: The canine teeth: normal functional relation of the natural teeth of man, *J South Calif Dent Assoc* 26:1-7, 1958.
45. Schuyler CHP: Fundamental principles in the correction of occlusal disharmony, natural and artificial, *J Am Dent Assoc* 22:1193-1202, 1935.

46. Lucia VO: The fine points in the reconstruction of osseointegrated fixtures, *J Gnathology* 6:3-21, 1987.
47. Schuyler CH: Principles employed in full denture prosthesis which may be applied in other fields of dentistry, *J Am Dent Assoc* 16:2045-2054, 1929.
48. Schuyler CH: Factors contributing to traumatic occlusion, *J Prosthet Dent* 11:708-715, 1961.
49. Beyron HL: Characteristics of functionally optimal occlusion and principles of occlusal rehabilitation, *J Am Dent Assoc* 48(6):648-656, 1954.
50. Beyron HL: Optimal occlusion, *Dent Clin North Am* 3:537-554, 1969.
51. Wang MQ, Zhang M, Zhang JH: Photoelastic study of the effects of occlusal surface morphology on tooth apical stress from vertical bite forces, *J Contemp Dent Pract* 5(1):74-93, 2004.
52. Christensen GJ: Is occlusion becoming more confusing? A plea for simplicity, *J Am Dent Assoc* 135(6):767-768, 770, 2004.
53. Lang BR: Complete denture occlusion, *Dent Clin North Am* 48(3):641-665, vi, 2004.
54. Isidor F: Histological evaluation of peri-implant bone at implants subjected to occlusal overload or plaque accumulation, *Clin Oral Implants Res* 8(1):1-9, 1997.
55. Miyata T, Kobayashi Y, Araki H, Motomura Y, Shin K: The influence of controlled occlusal overload on peri-implant tissue: a histologic study in monkeys, *Int J Oral Maxillofac Implants* 13(5):677-683, 1998.
56. Weinberg LA: Reduction of implant loading with therapeutic biomechanics, *Implant Dent* 7(4):277-285, 1998.
57. Miyata T, Kobayashi Y, Araki H, Ohto T, Shin K: The influence of controlled occlusal overload on peri-implant tissue. Part 3: A histologic study in monkeys, *Int J Oral Maxillofac Implants* 15(3):425-431, 2000.
58. Saba S: Occlusal stability in implant prosthodontics—clinical factors to consider before implant placement, *J Can Dent Assoc* 67(9):522-526, 2001.
59. Rangert B, Jemt T, Jorneus L: Forces and moments on Branemark implants, *Int J Oral Maxillofac Implants* 4(3):241-247, 1989.
60. Porter JA Jr, Petropoulos VC, Brunski JB: Comparison of load distribution for implant overdenture attachments, *Int J Oral Maxillofac Implants* 17(5):651-662, 2002.
61. Alkan I, Sertgoz A, Ekici B: Influence of occlusal forces on stress distribution in preloaded dental implant screws, *J Prosthet Dent* 91(4):319-325, 2004.
62. Weinberg LA: The biomechanics of force distribution in implant-supported prostheses, *Int J Oral Maxillofac Implants* 8(1):19-31, 1993.
63. Weinberg LA: Therapeutic biomechanics concepts and clinical procedures to reduce implant loading, Part I, *J Oral Implantol* 27(6):293-301, 2001.
64. Weinberg LA: Therapeutic biomechanics concepts and clinical procedures to reduce implant loading, Part II, therapeutic differential loading, *J Oral Implantol* 27(6):302-310, 2001.
65. Belser UC, Hannam AG: The influence of altered working-side occlusal guidance on masticatory muscles and related jaw movement, *J Prosthet Dent* 53(3):406-413, 1985.
66. Baba K, Akishige S, Yaka T, Ai M: Influence of alteration of occlusal relationship on activity of jaw closing muscles and mandibular movement during submaximal clenching, *J Oral Rehabil* 27(9):793-801, 2000.
67. Baba K, Yugami K, Yaka T, Ai M: Impact of balancing-side tooth contact on clenching induced mandibular displacements in humans, *J Oral Rehabil* 28(8):721-727, 2001.
68. Okano N, Baba K, Ohyama T: The influence of altered occlusal guidance on condylar displacement during submaximal clenching, *J Oral Rehabil* 32(10):714-719, 2005.
69. Ai M, Ishiwara T: A study of masticatory movement at the incision inferius, *Bull Tokyo Med Dent Univ* 15(4):371-386, 1968.
70. Sohn BW, Miyawaki S, Noguchi H, Takada K: Changes in jaw movement and jaw closing muscle activity after orthodontic correction of incisor crossbite, *Am J Orthod Dentofacial Orthop* 112(4):403-409, 1997.
71. Kimoto K, Fushima K, Tamaki K, Toyoda M, Sato S, Uchimura N: Asymmetry of masticatory muscle activity during the closing phase of mastication, *Cranio* 18(4):257-263, 2000.
72. Jemt T, Carlsson L, Boss A, Jorneus L: In vivo load measurements on osseointegrated implants supporting fixed or removable prostheses: a comparative pilot study, *Int J Oral Maxillofac Implants* 6(4):413-417, 1991.
73. Mericske-Stern R, Venetz E, Fahrlander F, Burgin W: In vivo force measurements on maxillary implants supporting a fixed prosthesis or an overdenture: a pilot study, *J Prosthet Dent* 84(5):535-547, 2000.
74. Chiapasco M, Gatti C: Implant-retained mandibular overdentures with immediate loading: a 3- to 8-year prospective study on 328 implants, *Clin Implant Dent Relat Res* 5(1):29-38, 2003.
75. Ochiai KT, Ozawa S, Caputo AA, Nishimura RD: Photoelastic stress analysis of implant-tooth connected prostheses with segmented and nonsegmented abutments, *J Prosthet Dent* 89(5):495-502, 2003.
76. van Rossen IP, Braak LH, de Putter C, de Groot K: Stress-absorbing elements in dental implants, *J Prosthet Dent* 64(2):198-205, 1990.
77. Holmes DC, Grigsby WR, Goel VK, Keller JC: Comparison of stress transmission in the IMZ implant system with polyoxymethylene or titanium intramobile element: a finite element stress analysis, *Int J Oral Maxillofac Implants* 7(4):450-458, 1992.
78. Hedia HS: Stress and strain distribution behavior in the bone due to the effect of cancellous bone, dental implant material and the bone height, *Biomed Mater Eng* 12(2):111-119, 2002.
79. Tada S, Stegaroiu R, Kitamura E, Miyakawa O, Kusakari H: Influence of implant design and bone quality on stress/strain distribution in bone around implants: a 3-dimensional finite element analysis, *Int J Oral Maxillofac Implants* 18(3):357-368, 2003.
80. Mellal A, Wiskott HW, Botsis J, Scherrer SS, Belser UC: Stimulating effect of implant loading on surrounding bone: comparison of three numerical models and validation by in vivo data, *Clin Oral Implants Res* 15(2):239-248, 2004.
81. Kitagawa T, Tanimoto Y, Nemoto K, Aida M: Influence of cortical bone quality on stress distribution in bone around dental implant, *Dent Mater J* 24(2):219-224, 2005.
82. McCoy G: Recognizing and managing parafunction in the reconstruction and maintenance of the oral implant patient, *Implant Dent* 11(1):19-27, 2002.
83. Chao YL, Meijer HJ, Van Oort RP, Versteegh PA: The incomprehensible success of the implant stabilised overdenture in the edentulous mandible: a literature review on transfer of chewing forces to bone surrounding implants, *Eur J Prosthodont Restor Dent* 3(6):255-261, 1995.

chapter 15

Immediate Loading of Implants in the Edentulous Patient

SINCE THE 1970S, one of the major guidelines for successful osseointegration of dental implants has been a nonloaded healing period of 3 months for implants placed in the mandible and 6 months for those placed in the maxilla.[1,2]

With the availability of new types of implants and a growing understanding of the biological principles of osseointegration, however, the necessity of this tenet in all cases of implant surgery has been challenged. In recent years, histologic and histomorphometric studies in both animals and humans have shown that more rapid and greater bone-to-implant contact can be achieved with implants that incorporate certain surface characteristics compared with the original machined-surface implants.[3-6] For instance, Lazzara et al. reported unloaded 6-month average bone-to-implant contact amounts of 72% with threaded commercially pure (CP)-titanium implants versus 34% for machined-surface implants, all placed in the posterior maxilla. Such findings are significant in that these types of implants may allow an implant to sufficiently resist functional loading sooner than was originally thought.

Indeed, a number of clinical and case studies have reported that immediate loading of implants with a provisional prosthesis following stage 1 surgery can be a very successful treatment alternative[7-15] (Figure 15-1).

The benefit of immediate loading, of course, is that it significantly shortens the treatment duration for patients, eliminating one of the surgeries and allowing patients to wear a fixed interim restoration immediately following implant placement. In addition, it may reduce the risk for trauma to the implant-bone interface, which can be caused by a removable transitional complete denture worn during the usual interim. However, because some studies indicate that immediate loading is still somewhat less predictable than allowing the traditional 3- to 6-month healing period,[8,9] patients must be informed about the possibility of losing some implants before their consent is accepted (Figure 15-2).

Introduction

The high cost of dental implant surgery requires predictable and permanent procedures whenever possible. Primary stability and minimal micromovement are essential for osseointegration. Frequently, a two-stage procedure has been followed to help guarantee primary stability and the absence of micromovement; the clinician waits from 3 to 6 months after implant placement before beginning stage 2 surgery and subsequent loading. However, the demands of time, comfort, and esthetics have required that clinicians accelerate the loading of implants by placing and loading

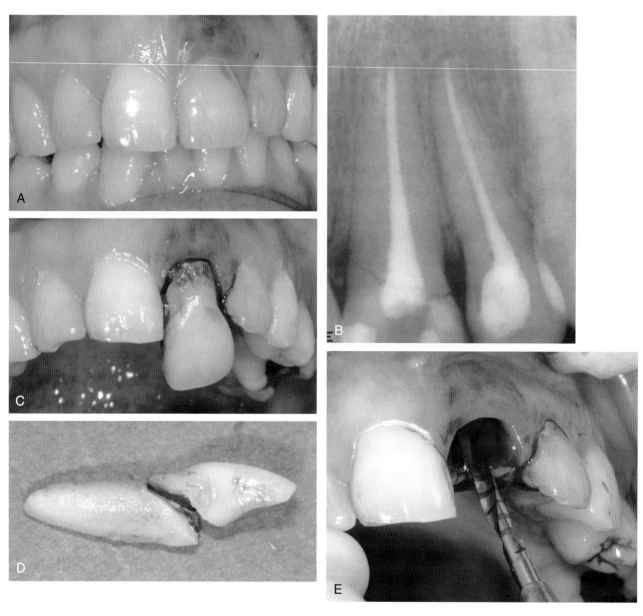

FIGURE 15-1 ■ A-I, Clinical case showing step-by-step procedure of an extraction, immediate implant placement, and temporary crown.

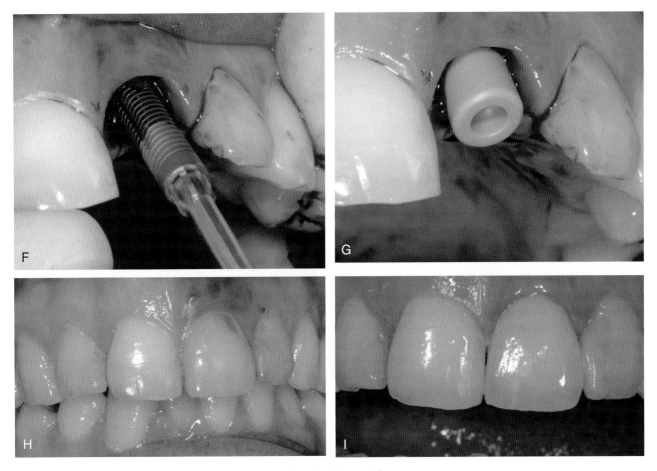

FIGURE 15-1, cont'd.

them in a one-stage procedure, yet keeping the criteria of predictability and permanence always in mind. Our protocols used in well-defined cases have yielded excellent results, even when we were dealing with extraction sites or other sites requiring simultaneous bone grafting, in addition to implant placement and immediate loading.

The appliance shown in Figure 15-3 could be used to measure primary stabilization of the implant in order to determine whether immediate loading could be done at the time of implant placement.

Whether in edentulous sites or in fresh extraction sites in the mandible or maxilla, loading implants immediately with temporary restorations requires precise and predictable surgical and restorative techniques. Because this approach involves immediate minimally traumatic extraction, precise implant placement, grafting with appropriate materials, the effective use of barrier membranes, and immediate restoration with a temporary prosthesis with good retention and occlusion, it requires state of the art procedures, understanding, and skills for the clinician, particularly in the esthetic zone. To understand the proper materials and procedures needed for such an enterprise, the clinician must understand not only the statistical evidence in the literature,

but also the wound healing and tissue augmenting elements (such as platelet-rich plasma, bone grafts, and guided bone regeneration), as well as essential implant loading protocols (including abutment types and rationale for different implant designs and occlusal forces and loading forces) (Figure 15-4).

Immediate Extractions, Implant Placement, Grafting, and Loading

Many different types of extraction sockets are available. They can be categorized as follows:

- Grade I—Obliterated by implant
- Grade II—Ovoid or triangular void
  - Grade IIb—Large volume—No vertical loss
- Grade III—Facial plate loss—Horizontal
- Grade IV—Horizontal and vertical loss

Then the following is suggested:

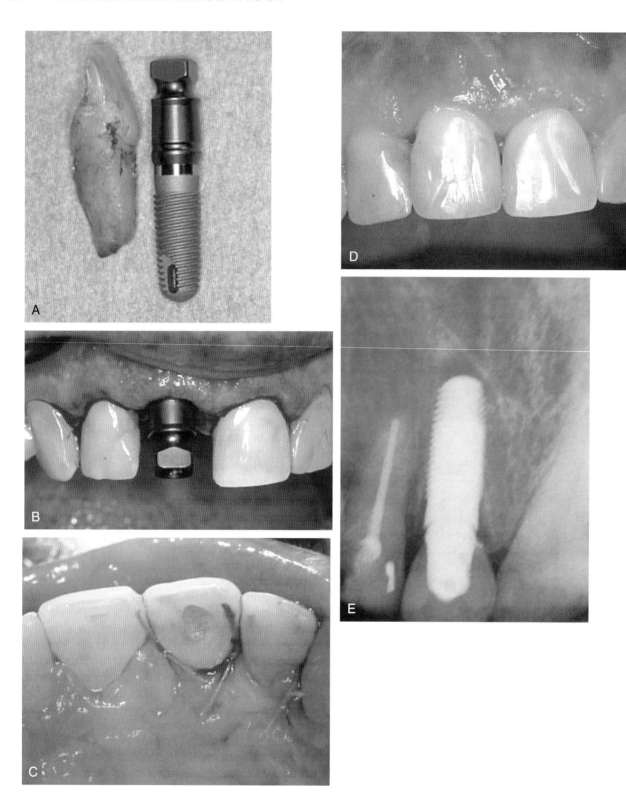

FIGURE 15-2 ■ **A-E,** Immediate loading implant placement reduces the necessity for second surgery. The temporary needs to be out of occlusion.

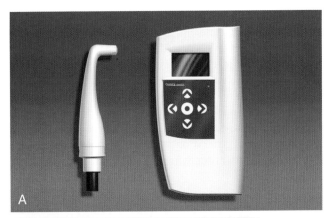

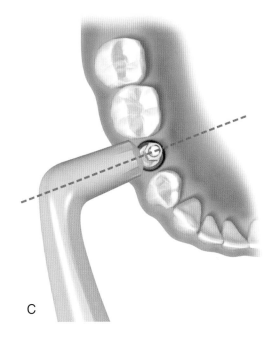

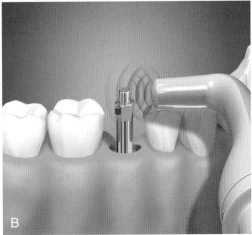

FIGURE 15-3 ■ This device can be used to measure the primary stabilization of the implant to determine whether immediate loading can be done at the same time as the implant placement. (Courtesy of Osstell.)

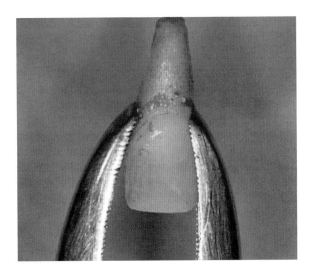

FIGURE 15-4 ■ The length of the root of the extracted tooth can be used to verify the length of the implant to be placed.

- Grade I and II can be simultaneous extraction and implant placement.
- Some grade III situations can be simultaneous, whereas some grade III are staged placement.
- Grade IIb and IV should be extraction, graft, and staged placement.

Nonintegration rates in these categories are shown in Table 15-1.

When the tooth is extracted, this should be done with a minimal amount of bone removal and minimal expansion of the adjacent bone. When the implant is placed into this graft socket, it should be torqued to 35 Newton-centimeters (Ncm) to ensure stability. If it torques down and feels tight while it is being torqued down, then it is safe for immediate loading. If it has mobility while it is torqued down, then it should not be loaded immediately. On occasion, transitional implants should be used to immediate load as opposed to immediate loading of conventional implants. The criteria are as follows in those cases in which the extraction sockets are grade III or IV and/or the implants are not stable in bone when being torqued down to 35 Ncm.

TABLE 15-1	Nonintegration Rates of this Classification System	
	MANDIBLE	**MAXILLA**
Grade I (simultaneous)	0.25%	0.46%
Grade IIa (simultaneous)	1.04%	1.12%
Grade III (simultaneous)	6.56%	7.75%
Grade III (delayed)	2.18%	2.46%
Grade IIb (delayed)	2.67%	3.86%
Grade IV (delayed)	4.77%	5.86%

Although several studies have documented failure rates for implants immediately placed into extraction sockets,[1-5] other studies have shown comparable failure rates for immediate loading and delayed loading of implants. Most studies agree that immediately loaded implants are successful when certain criteria are met, even rivaling the two-stage approach; these criteria include the distribution of an adequate number of implants, primary stability, rigid splinting, and screw-type implants with a rough surface, regardless of the implant system used. A thorough understanding of the subject requires an investigation into the gamut of literature-supported procedures and protocols ranging from immediate and early loading of implants in fresh extraction sites, to immediate and early loading of implants in bone graft sites.

Immediate Implants in Extraction Sites

Immediate implantation after tooth extraction can provide many benefits over delayed implantation, including less bone resorption, shorter treatment times (as well as fewer office visits), and facilitated implant positioning.[7-11] Even in the esthetic zone of the maxilla that requires augmentation, immediate implants may be the option of choice[12,13] (Figure 15-5).

Autogenous bone chips or allogeneic bone putties can be used successfully as the only grafting material during immediate implant placement to fill any openings left by the extraction.[14,15] Other cases may require more extensive use of bone graft materials to fill defects surrounding implants placed immediately after extraction.[16-19] For example, in the maxillary sinus area, bone grafting often is required when implants are placed immediately into extraction sites.[20] In addition, guided bone regeneration via barrier membranes has been used along with bone graft materials to augment the bone in immediate implantation extraction cases,[21-26] and it has even been suggested that no barrier membranes or grafting materials are necessarily required for implants placed immediately after tooth extraction; bone remodeling around implants can proceed with little resorption and good bone apposition around the implant neck, leaving no peri-implant bone defects.[27] Other studies show that the use of guided bone regeneration and pedicle flaps can facilitate healing of defects around immediately placed implants in extraction sites.[28]

Immediate Loading of Implants in Extraction Sites

Immediate loading of implants placed in edentulous and fresh extraction sites with sufficient bone quality is well documented in the literature for both the mandible and the maxilla, including the use of "expendable" and "transitional" implants to assist healing during the provisional restoration phase, and the use of platelet-rich plasma to facilitate healing.[29-40] Some studies have revealed a relatively high risk of failure (as much as 20%) when a single-tooth implant placed in a fresh extraction site is loaded immediately; however, similarly loaded single-tooth implants placed in healed sites appear to represent a viable treatment option.[41] Nevertheless, immediate loading in the esthetic zone immediately after tooth extraction can be a predictable therapy, especially when the clinician is aware of the soft and hard tissue criteria essential for temporization in extraction and healing sites.[42-44] In fact, some studies have revealed no significant difference in the success rates of implants immediately loaded in extraction sites and those loaded in edentulous sites.[45]

Immediate Loading in Extraction, Implantation, and Augmented Sites

To satisfy the esthetic needs of the patient in as timely and cost-effective a fashion as possible, the clinician increasingly is faced with cases calling for simultaneous surgical/restorative procedures such as extraction, bone augmentation, implant placement, and restoration. Studies have shown a remarkable number of successfully accomplished procedures covering the gamut of surgical and restorative procedures, including the use of growth factors to enhance healing.[46] It is interesting to note that cases involving craniofacial trauma may hold the key to an understanding of cases in which esthetics and timeliness drive patient satisfaction. Such cases involving the use of implants often have involved surgery that includes immediate bone grafting and internal rigid fixation.[47,48]

Restoring a single tooth in the esthetic zone often forces the clinician to meet extensive patient demands, which

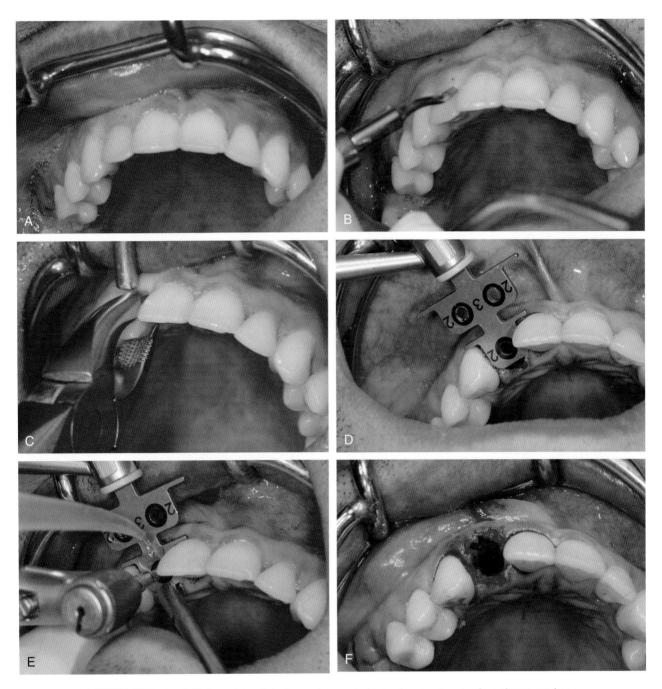

FIGURE 15-5 ■ **A-Q,** Complete clinical case from anterior tooth extraction, implant placement, bone graft, and membrane placement to temporary placement.

may include immediate implantation in extraction sites and augmenting sites, which requires improvement of bone quality followed by provisionalization; as long as only minor grafting is required, the clinician can proceed with relative confidence that the patient will be satisfied with the results.[49] Provisionalization of an implant placed in a fresh extraction site, which includes bone graft, can present a number of advantages for facilitating final tooth replacement, including retention of papillae and lack of preparation of adjacent teeth.[50]

The Mandible: Immediate and Early Loading Protocols

In the mandible, immediate loading of implants connected by a U-shaped bar often produces results similar to those seen with the two-stage approach. Other studies have shown comparable success rates for immediately loaded implants in extraction sites versus edentulous sites. The

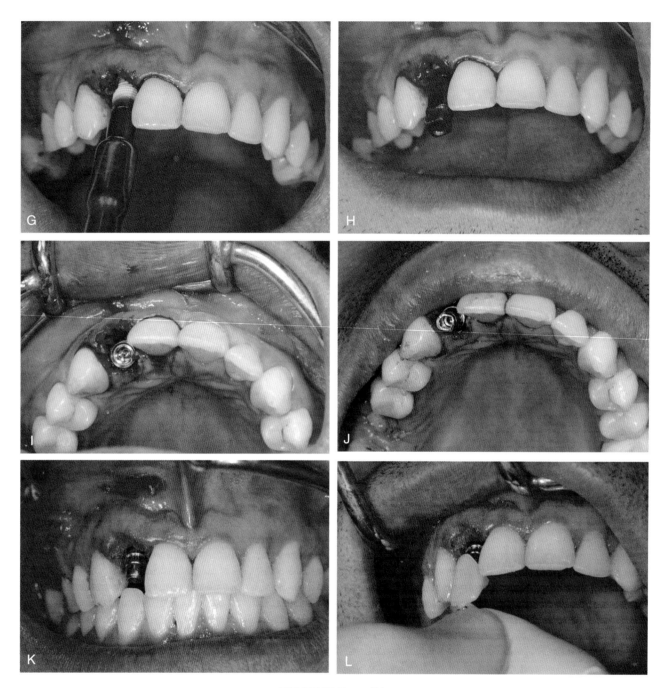

FIGURE 15-5, cont'd.

edentulous anterior mandible often lends itself to immediate or delayed loading of implants in a one-stage protocol, allowing the clinician and the patient the benefits of a considerably shortened implant-to-restoration timeline, including greater patient comfort and less anxiety, as well as less expense and greater convenience for both patient and clinician.[37,51-54] Of course, successful immediate loading or early loading procedures in the mandible require attention to a number of factors, including hard tissue (e.g., predictable

osseointegration, bone loss) and soft tissue (e.g., esthetics, peri-implant health) concerns[57] (Figure 15-6).

The literature supports the assumption that immediate or early loading of implant-supported overdentures and fixed bridges in the mandible is a highly successful procedure, especially when the clinician exercises proper caution, with results sometimes rivaling those of traditional two-stage protocols.[41,58-67] In fact, even in cases in which a patient's condition may seem to contraindicate or otherwise preclude

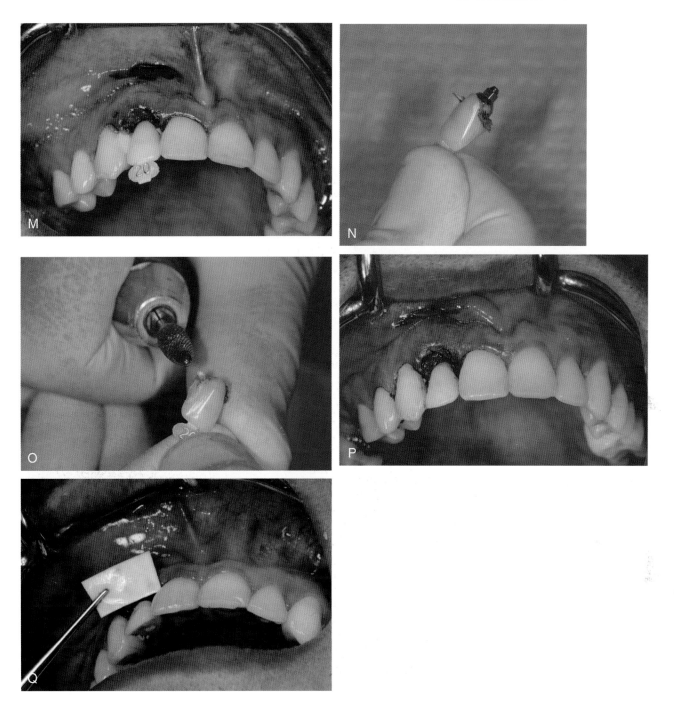

FIGURE 15-5, cont'd.

the use of implants and their immediate or early loading, the anterior mandible still may offer the clinician and the patient attractive alternatives for prosthetic rehabilitation. Under certain circumstances, the clinician may decide to remove any few remaining mandibular teeth if they are no longer salvageable, and cases of severe bone resorption in the mandible may call for special sophisticated procedures that cannot be performed simultaneously.[68]

A number of studies have shown comparable success rates in overdenture retention and overall implant osseointegration, even when different implant designs or implant systems were used in the mandible.[60,69-73] Adequate ridge size is an essential criterion for the clinical decision to load implants immediately; other criteria involve implant location and placement, implant coating, and implant length.[67,74-76] It should be noted that numerous studies have

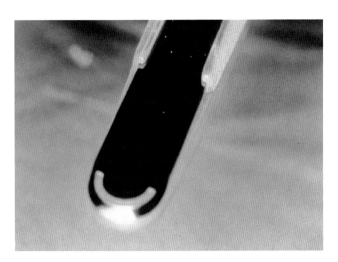

FIGURE 15-6 ■ During immediate-loading implant surgery, bone scrapers are useful for providing autogenous graft material to increase the success rate.

used a variety of patient criteria for measuring the performance and outcomes of procedures involving immediate loading of the anterior mandible.[70]

Similarly, "expendable" implants have been used to support both maxillary and mandibular provisional fixed restorations during the healing phase of submerged fixtures.[29] Such precautions reflect the importance of the clinician's considering the possible need for rescue procedures, given the less than ideal predictability of immediately loaded and early loaded implants, even in the anterior mandible. Considerations should include the possible choice of implant systems designed for such an eventuality.[77]

The Maxilla: Immediate and Early Loading Protocols

A single tooth extracted from the anterior maxilla can be replaced successfully with an immediate implant, even without primary closure, and the use of only autogenous bone chips as a grafting material to fill any extraction.[15] Some studies have revealed no significant difference between the success rates of implants immediately loaded in extraction sites and those loaded in edentulous sites, including sites in the maxilla.[45] At times, such immediately loaded implants in extraction sites require the use of a temporary bridge, which, after a period of osseointegration, can be removed and replaced with individual crowns for permanent restorations.[78]

One of the essential factors for success in early and immediately loaded implants in fresh extraction sites and edentulous sites in the maxilla and mandible very well may be the type of implant used; suggestions from studies are that roughened surfaces increase the chances for success.[30,79-82] Immediate provisionalization of immediately placed implants in extraction sites in the maxilla can provide the distinct advantage of preserving gingival topography and thickness. Gradual loading of implants in the maxilla is another method used to achieve the many clinical and patient advantages associated with this procedure.[83-84]

Wound Healing and Tissue Augmentation

Because the "wild card" in the immediate-implant/immediate-to-early loading game is augmenting sites otherwise unsuitable for such procedures, discussion of wound healing and tissue augmentation protocols is warranted. Such discussion requires an understanding of platelet-rich plasma as well as of proper bone grafting and membrane barrier techniques.

Platelet-Rich Plasma

Platelet-rich plasma (PRP) results from the sequestration and concentration of platelets and therefore the many growth factors (more than 30 to date) that they contain. Platelets exert a hemostatic effect while initiating the wound healing process.[85] The strategy behind PRP is to amplify and accelerate the effects of growth factors contained in platelets—the universal initiators of almost all wound healing.

Platelet-rich plasma can be prepared for office procedures with small volumes of autologous blood. The blood is separated into three components as a function of density: platelet-poor plasma (PPP), the least dense; platelet-rich plasma (PRP); and red blood cells (RBCs), the most dense. Approximately two-thirds of the PPP is removed and can be saved for hemostatic applications. The platelet concentrate then is resuspended in the remaining PPP, thereby creating a very concentrated PRP solution. PRP application requires initiation of the coagulation process with a mixture of 5 ml of 10% calcium chloride mixed with 5,000 units of topical bovine thrombin (Gen Trac, Bristol, TN). The activator is drawn into a 1-ml syringe, and 10-ml of PRP is drawn into a 10-ml syringe. The two syringes are attached to a 20G dual cannula applicator tip (Micromedics Inc., Eagan, MN), where the contents are mixed as they are applied to the bone graft, wound, or incision (Figure 15-7).

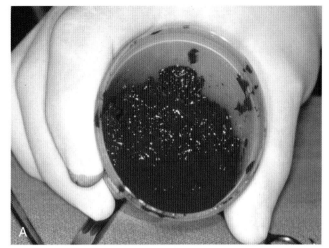

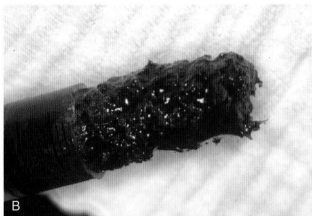

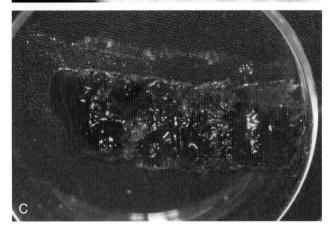

FIGURE 15-7 ■ **A-C,** Platelet-rich plasma (PRP) can be mixed with autogenous bone. When used with the bone graft or on the flap, it increases its adhesion, in addition to the added growth factors.

When PRP (now a gel) is added to a bone graft, for example, the fibrin formation binds the otherwise loose graft material together to assist the surgeon in sculpting the graft material. When used on incisions, PRP initially increases adhesion of the flaps to the undersurface, thereby eliminating dead space and improving hemostasis.[85]

Many of the assumptions about the efficacy of using PRP to treat periodontal defects in humans come from dental studies in which PRP was used in a variety of ways to promote wound healing. Early animal studies, as well as more recent ones, indicate that growth factors promote periodontal regeneration by increasing cell migration and proliferation.[86-91] Other animal studies have shown promising results with the use of PRP as a facilitator in healing and regenerative therapies.[92-99]

Human studies on the use of PRP in periodontal therapy suggest that platelet attachment and activation could be used to indicate tooth root surface thrombogenicity and fibrous attachment,[100] to enhance cancellous bone grafts in the mandible after tumor excision,[101] to facilitate the hard tissue mineralization rate of the grafted sinus,[102] to enhance tissue generation in connective and gingival tissues, and to facilitate surgical technique through the easy handling of PRP. Additionally, PRP can be effective when used in conjunction with deproteinated bovine bone to augment the maxillary sinus, even when resorption of the posterior maxillae is severe.[103] Favorable reports have described numerous cases involving the immediate restoration of dental implants after tooth removal when growth factors are used to enhance wound healing.[104] One study has shown the efficacy of using PRP with autologous bone for soft tissue repair and bone regeneration after tooth extraction to treat periodontal disease and to prepare the alveolar bone for later implant placement.[105] Several case reports demonstrate the efficacy of using PRP in a variety of periodontal procedures involving osseous defects. For example, some studies have shown the effectiveness of PRP, along with guided tissue regeneration and bone allografts, in treating intrabony and infrabony defects.[106-110] Treating osseous defects with the combination of PRP and demineralized freeze-dried bone allografts significantly increased wound healing rates in those cases with deep probing and severe bone loss; probing depths were markedly reduced, and new bone growth was detected radiographically as early as 2 months after surgery.[106]

Other studies have focused on determining the potential benefit of using PRP with allografts, alloplasts, and soft tissue grafts, for implants or for periodontal surgery.[111-113] Their results, together with those of other reported cases, suggest that the use of PRP facilitates clinical handling of the graft material, decreases the incidence of postoperative bleeding and pain, aids in initial stabilization of the graft, promotes more rapid revascularization and healing, and enhances cell adhesion.

Bone Grafting Materials

Lost alveolar bone can cause numerous complications for dental surgeons who wish to place dental implants in extraction sites (Table 15-2). In such cases, bone grafting

TABLE 15-2   Potential Complications

COMPLICATION	CAUSE	PREVENTIVE MEASURES
Unstable implant at time of placement	Receptor site for implant is too large, inadequate host bone, poor bone density, too much of space contains graft material	If the implant requires less than 25 Ncm of torque at the time of placement, consider a nonfunctional load period.
Limitation of autogenous graft material available for grafting	Hesitation to harvest due to inexperience with the procedure or inadequate sedation, patient with poor quality/quantity bone available for harvested bone	Consider use of commercial graft materials to supplement the autogenous graft. If an adequate quantity is unobtainable for a particular patient, consider adding volume expanders to harvested bone.
Unstable implant within 3 weeks of implant placement	Possibility of occlusion is high; overload; graft material washed out, or infected	Ensure that the prosthesis is in lighter/less occlusion than adjacent natural teeth for partially edentulous areas. Ensure that for fully edentulous areas, the prosthesis is in one piece and a definitive cement was used to provide for rigid splinting during osseointegration phase. Be sure soft tissue flaps were closed primarily and passively to minimize flap opening and washout of graft material.
Inadequate soft tissue or inappropriate soft tissue esthetics	Soft tissue was inadequate in the area and/or the immediate prosthesis design had a bulky facial contour or inadequate embrasure spaces	Ensure that there is appropriate soft tissue preoperatively, or consider preoperative, intraoperative, or postoperative soft tissue grafting. Prosthesis should have minimal bulk facial to prevent recession and minimal contact area interproximally to allow for soft tissue maintenance in embrasure areas.
Postoperative infection or edema	Intraoperative soft tissue trauma. Introduction of bacteria into surgical site intraoperatively or postoperatively	Minimize stripping of the flap beyond the area required for bone harvest, implant, and graft placement and passive primary closure. Use ice packs and antiinflammatory drugs and consider corticosteroids postoperatively to minimize edema. Consider the use of postoperative antibiotics prophylactically.

can provide the structural or functional support necessary. The clinician must have a thorough understanding of bone remodeling and of different types of bone, and must realize how these factors can affect the integration of osseous dental implants.[114] Grafting can provide filling for extraction sites. Purely from a perspective of bone growth, autogenous bone remains the best grafting material because of its osteogenic properties, which allow bone to form more rapidly in conditions that require significant bone augmentation or repair. The primary allografts used for restoring osseous defects are freeze-dried bone allograft (FDBA) and demineralized freeze-dried bone allograft (DFDBA). The primary alloplasts are hydroxyapatite (HA), bioactive glasses, tricalcium phosphate (TCP) particulates, and synthetic polymers.[123-127] The primary xenograft material consists of purified anorganic bone, either alone or enhanced with tissue-engineered molecules. Any of these augmentation materials can be incorporated into the modeling, remodeling, or healing process of bone to assist or to stimulate bone growth in areas where resorption has occurred and where implants are needed, depending on a variety of clinical factors.[115-119] Determination of what type of graft material to use, alone or in combination, can be based on the char-

acteristics of the bony defect to be restored.[120] Soft tissue ingrowth can be a complication during augmenting procedures with any grafting materials, so bone regeneration often is guided through the use of resorbable or nonresorbable membranes.[121,122]

Membrane Barriers for Guided Tissue Regeneration

The purpose of membrane barrier procedures is selective cell repopulation: to guide proliferation of different tissues during healing after therapy.[128] Placement of a physical barrier between the gingival flap and the defect before flap repositioning and suturing prevents gingival epithelium and connective tissue (undesirable cells) from contacting the space created by the barrier. Placement also facilitates repopulation of the defect by regenerative cells[129-132] (Figure 15-8).

Although most early studies were concerned with the treatment of patients with periodontal defects, the principal objectives of membrane barrier techniques are to

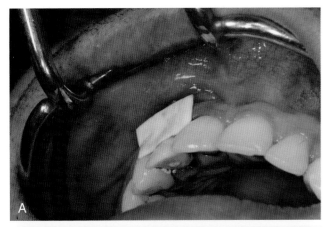

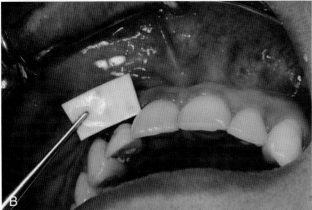

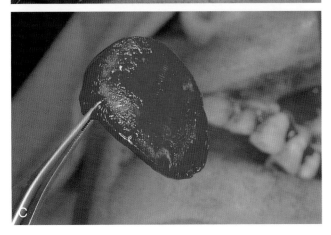

FIGURE 15-8 ■ **A-C,** Membrane barriers help bone graft material stay in the desired place. They can be soaked in platelet-rich plasma (PRP) to speed up the healing time.

facilitate augmentation of alveolar ridge defects, improve bone healing around dental implants, induce complete bone regeneration, improve bone grafting results, and treat failing implants.[24,133-138] Membrane barrier techniques, or osteopromotion procedures, use a barrier to prevent other tissues, especially connective tissue, from entering the intended site of bone reformation and from interfacing with osteogenesis and direct bone formation.[134]

The final goal of membrane barrier technologies is the restitution of supporting tissues (e.g., bone) that were lost as a consequence of inflammatory disease or trauma.[139,140] Several treatment modalities have been used in an attempt to reach this goal, with or without the placement of bone grafts or bone substitutes.[139,141] Generally, membrane barrier technologies can be described in two categories: nonresorbable and resorbable.

To date, most studies related to membrane barriers have used expanded polytetrafluoroethylene (ePTFE) membranes. Widely used in many animal and human studies, these membranes have been considered the gold standard against which other types of membranes are compared.[128,142] In some situations, nonresorbable membranes provide a more predictable performance, with less risk for long-term complications and simplified clinical management.[143] Use of ePTFE membranes may be advantageous in situations in which soft tissue management problems are anticipated and those in which complete flap closure cannot be achieved. If premature removal of the membrane is required, this can be accomplished without interfering with regenerated tissues.[142] The main advantage of using resorbable membranes is the avoidance of a second surgical procedure, thus reducing patient morbidity and expense.[144] A disadvantage of using bioresorbable membranes is that material exposure or flap dehiscence can cause postoperative tissue management problems. Material exposure after surgery can lead to bacterial growth, alteration of fibroblast morphology, and migration, all of which may jeopardize the success of the regeneration process. Another common problem is the difficulty of preventing membrane collapse into the defect, which can result in inadequate space making.[145-154]

Immediate Loading: Abutment Types and Rationale for Different Implant Designs

Whether it is the single-tooth implant or multiple teeth or an entire arch that is immediately restored after placement, numerous studies suggest that the primary factor for success in immediate and delayed loading cases is the type of implant system used, whether because of the general implant design of the system or its specific manufacture for the mandible.

General Implant Designs

Because primary stability is one of the key conditions for the immediate and early loading of implants, much of implant design is concentrated on this factor. When implants help to promote primary stability, other conditions are complemented to facilitate immediate and early loading (including sufficient bone quality and elimination of micromovement), leading to greater chances for successful osseointegration.[155] For example, studies have revealed that an acid-etched surface resulted in osseointegration of implants with a significantly higher bone-to-implant contact than is seen in machined implants, including implants placed in augmented sites and in sites that were loaded sooner than traditional protocols normally allowed.[81,82] Following the criteria of primary stability enhances immediate loading of implants placed not only in cases of individual tooth replacement but also in edentulous arches. An excellent choice of implant system for immediate load is the tapered screw design implant because of its shape, surface texture, internal connection, and precision manufacturing.[13]

Implant Designs: Mandible

The traditional approach to loading an implant has required two stages: An impression of the implant is made at the abutment connection during a second appointment, so that a temporary abutment and crown could be fabricated to help support the healing of soft tissues surrounding the abutment and crown. By contrast, immediate-loading procedures require that a healing abutment and temporary crown be placed at the first stage of surgery, after the implant has been placed; so, impressions are made at the time of placement, and a quick turnaround fabrication is required.

Final impressions of the arches can be made and working models cast before surgery begins. An articulator, a facebow, and bite registration on occlusal rims can establish the relation of implants to existing structures, and patients can confirm the settings. The setting data are duplicated to create an acrylic surgical template for placing implants in the correct buccal-lingual position.

SUMMARY

Successful osseointegration of dental implants traditionally has meant that the clinician allows a stress-free healing period for implants. This two-stage protocol initially calls for the submerging of several implants, which remain load-free for 3 to 6 months to ensure implant integration with alveolar bone. However, the edentulous mandible and maxilla, as well as fresh extraction sites in the arches of the alveolar ridge, often lend themselves to immediate or delayed loading of implants through a one-stage protocol; this often includes bone augmentation, which allows the clinician and the patient the benefits of a considerably shortened implant-to-restoration timeline, including greater patient comfort, reduced anxiety, and

improved convenience, although generally it also means greater expense.

REFERENCES

1. Gelb DA: Immediate implant surgery: three-year retrospective evaluation of 50 consecutive cases, *Int J Oral Maxillofac Implants* 8:388-399, 1993.
2. Becker W, Becker BE, Polizzi G, et al: Autogenous bone grafting of bone defects adjacent to implants placed in immediate extraction sockets in patients: a prospective study, *Int J Oral Maxillofac Implants* 9:389-396, 1994.
3. Becker W, Dahlin C, Becker BE, et al: The use of e-PTFE barrier membranes for bone promotion around titanium implants placed into extraction sockets: a prospective multicenter study, *Int J Oral Maxillofac Implants* 9:31-40, 1994.
4. Haas R, Mensdorff N, Mailath G, et al: Brånemark single tooth implants: a preliminary report of 76 implants, *J Prosthet Dent* 73:274-279, 1995.
5. Rosenquist B, Grenthe B: Immediate placement of implants into extraction sockets: implant survival, *Int J Oral Maxillofac Implants* 11:205-209, 1996.
6. Grunder U, Polizzi G, Goené R, et al: A 3-year prospective multicenter follow-up report on immediate and delayed immediate placement of implants, *Int J Oral Maxillofac Implants* 14:210-216, 1999.
7. Tsai ES, Crohin CC, Weber HP: A five-year evaluation of implants placed in extraction sockets, *J West Soc Periodontol Periodontal Abstr* 48(2):37-47, 2000.
8. Douglass GL, Merin RL: The immediate dental implant, *J Calif Dent Assoc* 30(5):362-365, 368-374, 2002.
9. Fugazzotto PA: Implant placement in maxillary first premolar fresh extraction sockets: description of technique and report of preliminary results, *J Periodontol* 73(6):669-674, 2002.
10. Simsek B, Simsek S: Evaluation of success rates of immediate and delayed implants after tooth extraction, *Chin Med J (Engl)* 116(8):1216-1219, 2003.
11. Schropp L, Isidor F, Kostopoulos L, Wenzel A: Patient experience of, and satisfaction with, delayed-immediate vs. delayed single-tooth implant placement, *Clin Oral Implants Res* 15(4):498-503, 2004.
12. Tipps WE, Carden ZF Jr: Complicated comprehensive reconstruction: report of a case, *J Tenn Dent Assoc* 84(2):28-30, 2004.
13. Palti A: Immediate placement and loading of implants in extraction sites: procedures in the aesthetic zone, *Dent Implantol Update* 15(6):41-47, 2004.
14. Schwartz-Arad D, Chaushu G: Placement of implants into fresh extraction sites: 4 to 7 years retrospective evaluation of 95 immediate implants, *J Periodontol* 68(11):1110-1116, 1997.
15. Schwartz-Arad D, Chaushu G: Immediate implant placement: a procedure without incisions, *J Periodontol* 69(7):743-750, 1998.
16. van Steenberghe D, Callens A, Geers L, Jacobs R: The clinical use of deproteinized bovine bone mineral on bone regeneration in conjunction with immediate implant installation, *Clin Oral Implants Res* 11(3):210-216, 2000.

17. Huys LW: Replacement therapy and the immediate post-extraction dental implant, *Implant Dent* 10(2):93-102, 2001.
18. Glickman RS, Bae R, Karlis V: A model to evaluate bone substitutes for immediate implant placement, *Implant Dent* 10(3):209-215, 2001.
19. Rebaudi A, Silvestrini P, Trisi P: Use of a resorbable hydroxy-apatite-collagen chondroitin sulfate material on immediate postextraction sites: a clinical and histologic study, *Int J Periodontics Restorative Dent* 23(4):371-379, 2003.
20. Vergara JA, Caffesse RG: Immediate replacement of single upper posterior teeth: a report of cases, *Clin Implant Dent Relat Res* 5(2):130-136, 2003.
21. Nemcovsky CE, Moses O, Artzi Z, Gelernter I: Clinical coverage of dehiscence defects in immediate implant procedures: three surgical modalities to achieve primary soft tissue closure, *Int J Oral Maxillofac Implants* 15(6):843-852, 2000.
22. Maksoud MA: Immediate implants in fresh posterior extraction sockets: report of two cases, *J Oral Implantol* 27(3):123-126, 2001.
23. Novaes Junior AB, Papalexiou V, Luczyszyn SM, Muglia VA, Souza SL, Taba Junior M: Immediate implant in extraction socket with acellular dermal matrix graft and bioactive glass: a case report, *Implant Dent* 11(4):343-348, 2002.
24. Nemcovsky CE, Artzi Z: Comparative study of buccal dehiscence defects in immediate, delayed, and late maxillary implant placement with collagen membranes: clinical healing between placement and second-stage surgery, *J Periodontol* 73(7):754-761, 2002.
25. Nemcovsky CE, Artzi Z, Moses O, Gelernter I: Healing of marginal defects at implants placed in fresh extraction sockets or after 4-6 weeks of healing: a comparative study, *Clin Oral Implants Res* 13(4):410-419, 2002.
26. Hoexter DL: Osseous regeneration in compromised extraction sites: a ten-year case study, *J Oral Implantol* 28(1):19-24, 2002.
27. Covani U, Cornelini R, Barone A: Bucco-lingual bone remodeling around implants placed into immediate extraction sockets: a case series, *J Periodontol* 74(2):268-273, 2003.
28. Goldstein M, Boyan BD, Schwartz Z: The palatal advanced flap: a pedicle flap for primary coverage of immediately placed implants, *Clin Oral Implants Res* 13(6):644-650, 2002.
29. Salama H, Rose LF, Salama M, Betts NJ: Immediate loading of bilaterally splinted titanium root-form implants in fixed prosthodontics—a technique reexamined: two case reports, *Int J Periodontics Restorative Dent* 15(4):344-361, 1995.
30. Calvo MP, Muller E, Garg AK: Immediate loading of titanium hexed screw-type implants in the edentulous patient: case report, *Implant Dent* 9(4):351-357, 2000.
31. Petrungaro PS, Windmiller N: Using transitional implants during the healing phase of implant reconstruction, *Gen Dent* 49(1):46-51, 2001.
32. Clausen GF, Chen ST: Immediate restoration of an immediate single-tooth implant, *Aust Dent J* 47(2):178-181, 2002.
33. Petrungaro PS: Immediate restoration of multiple tooth implants for aesthetic implant restorations, *Implant Dent* 11(2):118-127, 2002.
34. Balshi TJ, Wolfinger GJ: Teeth in a day for the maxilla and mandible: case report, *Clin Implant Dent Relat Res* 5(1):11-16, 2003.
35. Leary JC, Hirayama M: Extraction, immediate-load implants, impressions and final restorations in two patient visits, *J Am Dent Assoc* 134(6):715-720, 2003.
36. Schiroli G: Immediate tooth extraction, placement of a Tapered Screw-Vent implant, and provisionalization in the esthetic zone: a case report, *Implant Dent* 12(2):123-131, 2003.
37. Petropoulos VC, Balshi TJ, Balshi SF, Wolfinger GJ: Extractions, implant placement, and immediate loading of mandibular implants: a case report of a functional fixed prosthesis in 5 hours, *Implant Dent* 12(4):283-290, 2003.
38. Tupac RG: When is an implant ready for a tooth? *J Calif Dent Assoc* 31(12):911-915, 2003.
39. Ormianer Z, Garg AK, Palti A: Immediate loading of implant-supported overdentures with ball attachment connection using modified loading protocol for reduction of initial occlusal forces, *Implant Dent* 13(4):265-272, 2005.
40. Castellon P, Block MS, Smith M, Finger IM: Immediate implant placement and provisionalization using implants with an internal connection, *Pract Proced Aesthet Dent* 16(1):35-43, 2004.
41. Chaushu G, Chaushu S, Tzohar A, Dayan D: Immediate loading of single-tooth implants: immediate versus non-immediate implantation. A clinical report, *Int J Oral Maxillofac Implants* 16(2):267-272, 2001.
42. Salama H, Salama MA, Li TF, Garber DA, Adar P: Treatment planning 2000: an esthetically oriented revision of the original implant protocol, *J Esthet Dent* 9(2):55-67, 1997.
43. Garber DA, Salama MA, Salama H: Immediate total tooth replacement, *Compend Contin Educ Dent* 22(3):210-216, 218, 2001.
44. Saadoun AP: Immediate implant placement and temporization in extraction and healing sites, *Compend Contin Educ Dent* 23(4):309-312, 314-316, 2002.
45. Aires I, Berger J: Immediate placement in extraction sites followed by immediate loading: a pilot study and case presentation, *Implant Dent* 11(1):87-94, 2002.
46. Petrungaro PS: Immediate implant placement and provisionalization in edentulous, extraction, and sinus grafted sites, *Compend Contin Educ Dent* 24(2):95-100, 103-104, 106, 2003.
47. Garg AK, Reiche O: Mandibular reconstruction after a gunshot wound: a case report, *Implant Soc* 1(3):10-21, 1990.
48. Stevens MR, Heit JM, Kline SN, Marx RE, Garg AK: The use of osseointegrated implants in craniofacial trauma, *J Craniomaxillofac Trauma* 4(1):27-34, 1998.
49. Hui E, Chow J, Li D, Liu J, Wat P, Law H: Immediate provisional for single-tooth implant replacement with Branemark system: preliminary report, *Clin Implant Dent Relat Res* 3(2):79-86, 2001.
50. Misch CM: The extracted tooth pontic—provisional replacement during bone graft and implant healing, *Pract Periodontics Aesthet Dent* 10(6):711-718, 1998.
51. Ledermann PD: Stegprothetische Versorgung des zahnlosen Unterkiefers mit Hilfe plasmabeschichteten Titanschraubimplantaten, *Deutsche Zahnartzlische Zeitung* 34:907-911, 1979.
52. Babbusch CA, Kent J, Misiek D: Titanium plasma-sprayed (TPS) screw implants for the reconstruction of the edentulous mandible, *J Oral Maxillofac Surg* 44:274-282, 1986.
53. Chee W, Jivraj S: Efficiency of immediately loaded mandibular full-arch implant restorations, *Clin Implant Dent Relat Res* 5(1):52-56, 2003.
54. Testori T, Meltzer A, Del Fabbro M, Zuffetti F, Troiano M, Francetti L, Weinstein RL: Immediate occlusal loading of Osseotite

implants in the lower edentulous jaw: a multicenter prospective study, *Clin Oral Implants Res* 15(3):278-284, 2004.

55. Schnitman PA, Wohrle PS, Rubenstein JE, DaSilva JD, Wang NH: Ten-year results for Branemark implants immediately loaded with fixed prostheses at implant placement, *Int J Oral Maxillofac Implants* 12(4):495-503, 1997.

56. van Steenberghe D, Molly L, Jacobs R, Vandekerckhove B, Quirynen M, Naert I: The immediate rehabilitation by means of a ready-made final fixed prosthesis in the edentulous mandible: a 1-year follow-up study on 50 consecutive patients, *Clin Oral Implants Res* 15(3):360-365, 2004.

57. Raghoebar GM, Friberg B, Grunert I, Hobkirk JA, Tepper G, Wendelhag I: 3-Year prospective multicenter study on one-stage implant surgery and early loading in the edentulous mandible, *Clin Implant Dent Relat Res* 5(1):39-46, 2003.

58. Testori T, Del Fabbro M, Szmukler-Moncler S, Francetti L, Weinstein RL: Immediate occlusal loading of Osseotite implants in the completely edentulous mandible, *Int J Oral Maxillofac Implants* 18(4):544-551, 2003.

59. Schnitman PA, Wohrle PS, Rubenstein JE: Immediate fixed interim prostheses supported by two-stage threaded implants: methodology and results, *J Oral Implantol* 16(2):96-105, 1990.

60. Chiapasco M, Gatti C, Rossi E, Haefliger W, Markwalder TH: Implant-retained mandibular overdentures with immediate loading: a retrospective multicenter study on 226 consecutive cases, *Clin Oral Implants Res* 8(1):48-57, 1997.

61. Ericsson I, Nilson H, Lindh T, Nilner K, Randow K: Immediate functional loading of Branemark single tooth implants: an 18 months' clinical pilot follow-up study, *Clin Oral Implants Res* 11(1):26-33, 2000.

62. Gatti C, Haefliger W, Chiapasco M: Implant-retained mandibular overdentures with immediate loading: a prospective study of ITI implants, *Int J Oral Maxillofac Implants* 15(3):383-388, 2000.

63. Porter JM: Same-day restoration of mandibular single-stage implants, *J Indiana Dent Assoc* 81(3):22-25, 2002.

64. Romeo E, Chiapasco M, Lazza A, Casentini P, Ghisolfi M, Iorio M, Vogel G: Implant-retained mandibular overdentures with ITI implants, *Clin Oral Implants Res* 13(5):495-501, 2002.

65. Engstrand P, Grondahl K, Ohrnell LO, Nilsson P, Nannmark U, Branemark PI: Prospective follow-up study of 95 patients with edentulous mandibles treated according to the Branemark Novum concept, *Clin Implant Dent Relat Res* 5(1):3-10, 2003.

66. Lorenzoni M, Pertl C, Zhang K, Wegscheider WA: In-patient comparison of immediately loaded and non-loaded implants within 6 months, *Clin Oral Implants Res* 14(3):273-279, 2003.

67. Gapski R, Wang HL, Mascarenhas P, Lang NP: Critical review of immediate implant loading, *Clin Oral Implants Res* 14(5):515-527, 2003.

68. Peleg M, Mazor Z, Chaushu G, Garg AK: Lateralization of the inferior alveolar nerve with simultaneous implant placement: a modified technique, *Int J Oral Maxillofac Implants* 17(1):101-106, 2002.

69. Spiekermann H, Jansen VK, Richter EJ: A 10-year follow-up study of IMZ and TPS implants in the edentulous mandible using bar-retained overdentures, *Int J Oral Maxillofac Implants* 10(2):231-243, 1995.

70. Gatti C, Chiapasco M: Immediate loading of Branemark implants: a 24-month follow-up of a comparative prospective pilot study between mandibular overdentures supported by conical transmucosal and standard MK II implants, *Clin Implant Dent Relat Res* 4(4):190-199, 2002.

71. Chiapasco M, Gatti C: Implant-retained mandibular overdentures with immediate loading: a 3- to 8-year prospective study on 328 implants, *Clin Implant Dent Relat Res* 5(1):29-38, 2003.

72. Mau J, Behneke A, Behneke N, Fritzemeier CU, Gomez-Roman G, d'Hoedt B, Spiekermann H, Strunz V, Yong M: Randomized multicenter comparison of 2 IMZ and 4 TPS screw implants supporting bar-retained overdentures in 425 edentulous mandibles, *Int J Oral Maxillofac Implants* 18(6):835-847, 2003.

73. Meijer HJ, Batenburg RH, Raghoebar GM, Vissink A: Mandibular overdentures supported by two Branemark, IMZ or ITI implants: a 5-year prospective study, *J Clin Periodontol* 31(7):522-526, 2004.

74. Tarnow DP, Emtiaz S, Classi A: Immediate loading of threaded implants at stage 1 surgery in edentulous arches: ten consecutive case reports with 1- to 5-year data, *Int J Oral Maxillofac Implants* 12(3):319-324, 1997.

75. Schwartz-Arad D, Yaniv Y, Levin L, Kaffe I: A radiographic evaluation of cervical bone loss associated with immediate and delayed implants placed for fixed restorations in edentulous jaws, *J Periodontol* 75(5):652-657, 2004.

76. Tarnow D, Elian N, Fletcher P, Froum S, Magner A, Cho SC, Salama M, Salama H, Garber DA: Vertical distance from the crest of bone to the height of the interproximal papilla between adjacent implants, *J Periodontol* 74(12):1785-1788, 2003.

77. Parel SM, Triplett RG: Rescue procedure for the Branemark Novum protocol, *Int J Oral Maxillofac Implants* 19(3):421-424, 2004.

78. Kosinski TE, Skowronski R Jr: Immediate implant loading: a case report, *J Oral Implantol* 28(2):87-91, 2002.

79. Iamoni F, Rasperini G, Trisi P, Simion M: Histomorphometric analysis of a half hydroxyapatite-coated implant in humans: a pilot study, *Int J Oral Maxillofac Implants* 14(5):729-735, 1999.

80. Testori T, Szmukler-Moncler S, Francetti L, Del Fabbro M, Trisi P, Weinstein RL: Healing of Osseotite implants under submerged and immediate loading conditions in a single patient: a case report and interface analysis after 2 months, *Int J Periodontics Restorative Dent* 22(4):345-353, 2002.

81. Trisi P, Lazzara R, Rebaudi A, Rao W, Testori T, Porter SS: Bone-implant contact on machined and dual acid-etched surfaces after 2 months of healing in the human maxilla, *J Periodontol* 74(7):945-956, 2003.

82. Veis AA, Trisi P, Papadimitriou S, Tsirlis AT, Parissis NA, Desiris AK, Lazzara RJ: Osseointegration of Osseotite and machined titanium implants in autogenous bone graft: a histologic and histomorphometric study in dogs, *Clin Oral Implants Res* 15(1):54-61, 2004.

83. Kan JY, Rungcharassaeng K: Immediate placement and provisionalization of maxillary anterior single implants: a surgical and prosthodontic rationale, *Pract Periodontics Aesthet Dent* 12(9):817-824, 2000.

84. Scher E: Single- or multiple-tooth implant restoration in the same arch, *Dent Implantol Update* 15(7):49-53, 2004.

85. Adler SC: Autologous platelet gel with growth factors in facial plastic surgery, Submitted for Journal Review.

86. Lynch SE, Williams RC, Polson AM, et al: A combination of platelet-derived and insulin-like growth factors enhances periodontal regeneration, *J Clin Periodontol* 16:545-548, 1989.

87. Lynch SE, Ruiz de Castilla G, Williams RC, et al: The effects of short-term application of a combination of platelet-derived and insulin-like growth factors on periodontal wound healing, *J Periodontol* 62:458-467, 1991.

88. Matsuda N, Lin WL, Kumar NM, Cho MI, Genco RJ: Mitogenic, chemotactic, and synthetic responses of rat periodontal ligament fibroblastic cells to polypeptide growth factors in vitro, *J Periodontol* 63(6):515-525, 1992.

89. Rutherford RB, Niekrash CE, Kennedy JE, Charette ME: Platelet derived and insulin-like growth factors stimulate regeneration of periodontal attachment in monkeys, *J Periodont Res* 27:285-290, 1992.

90. Di Genio M, Barone A, Ramaglia L, Sbordone L: [Periodontal regeneration: the use of polypeptide growth factors]. *Minerva Stomatol* 43(10):437-443, 1994. Review. Italian.

91. Giannobile WV, Finkelman RD, Lynch SE: Comparison of canine and non-human primate animal models for periodontal regenerative therapy: results following a single administration of PDGF/IGF-I, *J Periodontol* 65(12):1158-1168, 1994.

92. Siebrecht MA, De Rooij PP, Arm DM, Olsson ML, Aspenberg P: Platelet concentrate increases bone ingrowth into porous hydroxyapatite, *Orthopedics* 25(2):169-172, 2002.

93. Kim SG, Kim WK, Park JC, Kim HJ: A comparative study of osseo-integration of Avana implants in a demineralized freeze-dried bone alone or with platelet-rich plasma, *J Oral Maxillofac Surg* 60(9):1018-1025, 2002.

94. Saito Y, Okuda K, Suzuki H, Nakasone N, Yoshie H: The effect of platelet-rich plasma and atelo-collagen on calcification and proliferation of rat osteoblast and periodontal ligament-derived cells. Abstract, *J Periodontol* 74(11):1710, 2003.

95. Fuerst G, Gruber R, Tangl S, Sanroman F, Watzek G: Enhanced bone-to-implant contact by platelet-released growth factors in mandibular cortical bone: a histomorphometric study in minipigs, *Int J Oral Maxillofac Implants* 18(5):685-690, 2003.

96. Fennis JP, Stoelinga PJ, Jansen JA: Mandibular reconstruction: a histological and histomorphometric study on the use of autogenous scaffolds, particulate cortico-cancellous bone grafts and platelet rich plasma in goats, *Int J Oral Maxillofac Surg* 33(1):48-55, 2004.

97. Fukazawa M, Kobayashi Y, Takeda H, Ohashi T, Omura H, Shin K: Effect of platelet-rich plasma on regeneration of periodontal tissue. Abstract, *J Periodontol* 74(11):1707, 2003.

98. Choi BH, Im CJ, Huh JY, Suh JJ, Lee SH: Effect of platelet-rich plasma on bone regeneration in autogenous bone graft, *Int J Oral Maxillofac Surg* 33(1):56-59, 2004.

99. Arpornmaeklong P, Kochel M, Depprich R, Kubler NR, Wurzler KK: Influence of platelet-rich plasma (PRP) on osteogenic differentiation of rat bone marrow stromal cells: an in vitro study, *Int J Oral Maxillofac Surg* 33(1):60-70, 2004.

100. Steinberg AD, LeBreton G, Willey R, Mukherjee S, Lipowski J: Extravascular clot formation and platelet activation on variously treated root surfaces, *J Periodontol* 57(8):516-522, 1986.

101. Marx RE, Carlson ER, Eichstaedt RM, Schimmele SR, Strauss JE, Georgeff KR: Platelet-rich plasma: growth factor enhancement for bone grafts, *Oral Surg Oral Med Oral Pathol Oral Radiol Endod* 85(6):638-646, 1998.

102. Petrungaro PS: The use of platelet-rich plasma with growth factors (autologous platelet gel) to enhance hard and soft tissue healing and maturation in the reconstruction of the maxillary pneumatized sinus, February-March 2001. Available at: http://www.harvesttech.com/bone_publications.htm.

103. Rodriguez A, Anastassov GE, Lee H, Buchbinder D, Wettan H: Maxillary sinus augmentation with deproteinated bovine bone and platelet rich plasma with simultaneous insertion of endosseous implants, *J Oral Maxillofac Surg* 61(2):157-163, 2003.

104. Petrungaro PS: Immediate restoration of dental implants after tooth removal: a new technique to provide esthetic replacement of the natural tooth system, *International Magazine of Oral Implantology* 2:5-16, 2001.

105. Anitua E: Plasma rich in growth factors: preliminary results of use in the preparation of future sites for implants, *Int J Oral Maxillofac Implants* 14(4):529-535, 1999.

106. de Obarrio JJ, Aruz-Dutari JI, Chamberlain TM, Croston A: The use of autologous growth factors in periodontal surgical therapy: platelet gel biotechnology—case reports, *Int J Periodontics Restorative Dent* 20(5):487-497, 2000.

107. Camargo PM, Lekovic V, Weinlaender M, Vasilic N, Madzarevic M, Kenney EB: Platelet-rich plasma and bovine porous bone mineral combined with guided tissue regeneration in the treatment of intrabony defects in humans, *J Periodontal Res* 37(4):300-306, 2002.

108. Lekovic V, Camargo PM, Weinlaender M, Vasilic N, Kenney EB: Comparison of platelet-rich plasma, bovine porous bone mineral, and guided tissue regeneration versus platelet-rich plasma and bovine porous bone mineral in the treatment of intrabony defects: a reentry study, *J Periodontol* 73(2):198-205, 2002.

109. Lekovic V, Camargo PM, Weinlaender M, Vasilic N, Aleksic Z, Kenney EB: Effectiveness of a combination of platelet-rich plasma, bovine porous bone mineral and guided tissue regeneration in the treatment of mandibular grade II molar furcations in humans, *J Clin Periodontol* 30(8):746-751, 2003.

110. Lekovic V, Aleksic Z, Vasilic N: The use of platelet-rich plasma in the treatment of periodontal osseous defects. Abstract, *J Periodontol* 74(11):1708-1709, 2003.

111. Petrungaro PS: Using platelet-rich plasma to accelerate soft tissue maturation in esthetic periodontal surgery, *Compend Contin Educ Dent* 22(9):729-732, 734, 736, 2001.

112. Kassolis JD, Rosen PS, Reynolds MA: Alveolar ridge and sinus augmentation utilizing platelet-rich plasma in combination with freeze-dried bone allograft: case series, *J Periodontol* 71(10):1654-1661, 2000.

113. Kim SG, Chung CH, Kim YK, et al: Use of particulate dentin-plaster of Paris combination with/without platelet-rich plasma in the treatment of bone defects around implants, *Int J Oral Maxillofac Implants* 17:86-94, 2002.

114. Marx RE, Garg AK: Bone structure, metabolism, and physiology: its impact on dental implantology, *Implant Dent* 7(4):267-276, 1998.

115. Boyne PJ: Advances in preprosthetic surgery and implantation, *Curr Opin Dent* 1(3):277-281, 1991.

116. Kraut RA: Composite graft for mandibular alveolar ridge augmentation: a preliminary report, *J Oral Maxillofac Surg* 43(11):856-859, 1985.

117. Kent JN, Finger IM, Quinn JH, Guerra LR: Hydroxylapatite alveolar ridge reconstruction: clinical experiences, complications, and technical modifications, *J Oral Maxillofac Surg* 44(1):37-49, 1986.

118. Valen M, Ganz SD: A synthetic bioactive resorbable graft for predictable implant reconstruction: part one, *J Oral Implantol* 28(4):167-177, 2002.

119. Ganz SD, Valen M: Predictable synthetic bone grafting procedures for implant reconstruction: part two, *J Oral Implantol* 28(4):178-183, 2002.

120. Misch CE, Dietsh F: Bone-grafting materials in implant dentistry, *Implant Dent* 2(3):158-167, 1993.

121. Schopper C, Goriwoda W, Moser D, Spassova E, Watzinger F, Ewers R: Long-term results after guided bone regeneration with resorbable and microporous titanium membranes, *Oral Maxillofac Surg Clin North Am* 13(3):449-457, 2001.

122. Meffert RA: Current usage of bone fill as an adjunct in implant dentistry, *Dent Implantol Update* 9:9, 1998.

123. Ashman A: The use of synthetic bone materials in dentistry, *Compendium* 13(11):1020, 1022, 1024-1026, 1992, passim.

124. Ashman A: Clinical applications of synthetic bone in dentistry. Part 1, *Gen Dent* 40(6):481-487, 1992.

125. Ashman A: Clinical applications of synthetic bone in dentistry. Part II: Periodontal and bony defects in conjunction with dental implants, *Gen Dent* 41(1):37-44, 1993.

126. Yukna RA, Saenz AM, Shannon M, Mayer ET: Use of HTR synthetic bone as an augmentation material in conjunction with immediate implant placement: a case report, *J Oral Implantol* 29(1):24-28, 2003.

127. Kirsh ER, Garg AK: Postextraction ridge maintenance using the endosseous ridge maintenance implant (ERMI), *Compendium* 15(2):234, 236, 238, 1994, passim; quiz 244.

128. Gottlow J: Guided tissue regeneration using bioresorbable and non-resorbable devices: initial healing and long-term results, *J Periodontol* 64(11 suppl):1157-1165, 1993.

129. Rowe DJ, Leung WW, Del Carlo DL: Osteoclast inhibition by factors from cells associated with regenerative tissue, *J Periodontol* 67(4):414-421, 1996.

130. Pecora G, Baek SH, Rethnam S, Kim S: Barrier membrane techniques in endodontic microsurgery, *Dent Clin North Am* 41(3):585-602, 1997.

131. Caffesse RG: Regeneration of soft and hard tissue defects. Medicine meets millennium: World congress on medicine and health, 21 July-31 August 2000. Hanover, Denmark, 2000 (cited 2003 Aug 6). Available at: http://www.mh-hannover.de/aktuelles/projekte/mmm/englishversion/fs_programme/speech/Caffesse_V.html

132. Froum SJ, Gomez C, Breault MR: Current concepts of periodontal regeneration: a review of the literature, *N Y State Dent J* 68(9):14-22, 2002.

133. Payne JM, Cobb CM, Rapley JW, Killoy WJ, Spencer P: Migration of human gingival fibroblasts over guided tissue regeneration barrier materials, *J Periodontol* 67(3):236-244, 1996.

134. Linde A, Alberius P, Dahlin C, Bjurstam K, Sundin Y: Osteopromotion: a soft-tissue exclusion principle using a membrane for bone healing and bone neogenesis, *J Periodontol* 64(11 suppl):1116-1128, 1993.

135. Assenza B, Piattelli M, Scarano A, Lezzi G, Petrone G, Piattelli A: Localized ridge augmentation using titanium micromesh, *J Oral Implantol* 27(6):287-292, 2001.

136. Hammerle CH, Jung RE, Feloutzis A: A systematic review of the survival of implants in bone sites augmented with barrier membranes (guided bone regeneration) in partially edentulous patients, *J Clin Periodontol* 29(suppl 3):226-231, 2002; discussion 232-233.

137. Lorenzoni M, Pertl C, Polansky RA, Jakse N, Wegscheider WA: Evaluation of implants placed with barrier membranes: a retrospective follow-up study up to five years, *Clin Oral Implants Res* 13(3):274-280, 2002.

138. Kohal RJ, Hurzeler MB: Bioresorbable barrier membranes for guided bone regeneration around dental implants, *Schweiz Monatsschr Zahnmed* 112(12):1222-1229, 2002.

139. Karring T, Nyman S, Gottlow J, Laurell L: Development of the biological concept of guided tissue regeneration—animal and human studies, *Periodontol 2000* 1:26-35, 1993.

140. Caffesse RG, Quinones CR: Guided tissue regeneration: biologic rationale, surgical technique, and clinical results, *Compendium* 13(3):166, 168, 170, 1992, passim.

141. Lang NP, Karring T, editors: Proceedings of the 1st European Workshop on Periodontology, Berlin, 1994, Quintessence.

142. Becker W, Becker BE, Mellonig J, Caffesse RG, Warrer K, Caton JG, Reid T: A prospective multi-center study evaluating periodontal regeneration for Class II furcation invasions and intrabony defects after treatment with a bioabsorbable barrier membrane: 1-year results, *J Periodontol* 67(7):641-649, 1996.

143. Hardwick R, Hayes BK, Flynn C: Devices for dentoalveolar regeneration: an up-to-date literature review, *J Periodontol* 66(6):495-505, 1995.

144. Yukna CN, Yukna RA: Multi-center evaluation of bioabsorbable collagen membrane for guided tissue regeneration in human Class II furcations, *J Periodontol* 67(7):650-657, 1996.

145. Anson D: Calcium sulfate: a 4-year observation of its use as a resorbable barrier in guided tissue regeneration of periodontal defects, *Compend Contin Educ Dent* 17(9):895-899, 1996.

146. Juodzbalys G: Instrument for extraction socket measurement in immediate implant installation, *Clin Oral Implants Res* 14(2):144-149, 2003.

147. Oh TJ, Meraw SJ, Lee EJ, Giannobile WV, Wang HL: Comparative analysis of collagen membranes for the treatment of implant dehiscence defects, *Clin Oral Implants Res* 14(1):80-90, 2003.

148. Zitzmann NU, Naef R, Scharer P: Resorbable versus nonresorbable membranes in combination with Bio-Oss for guided bone regeneration, *Int J Oral Maxillofac Implants* 12(6):844-852, 1997. Erratum in *Int J Oral Maxillofac Implants* 13(4):576, 1998.

149. Camelo M, Nevins ML, Schenk RK, Simion M, Rasperini G, Lynch SE, Nevins M: Clinical, radiographic, and histologic evaluation of human periodontal defects treated with Bio-Oss and Bio-Gide, *Int J Periodontics Restorative Dent* 18(4):321-331, 1998.

150. Hockers T, Abensur D, Valentini P, Legrand R, Hammerle CH: The combined use of bioresorbable membranes and xenografts or autografts in the treatment of bone defects around implants: a study in beagle dogs, *Clin Oral Implants Res* 10(6):487-498, 1999.

151. Camelo M, Nevins ML, Lynch SE, Schenk RK, Simion M, Nevins M: Periodontal regeneration with an autogenous bone-Bio-Oss composite graft and a Bio-Gide membrane, *Int J Periodontics Restorative Dent* 21(2):109-119, 2001.

152. Tawil G, El-Ghoule G, Mawla M: Clinical evaluation of a bilayered collagen membrane (Bio-Gide) supported by autografts in the treatment of bone defects around implants, *Int J Oral Maxillofac Implants* 16(6):857-863, 2001.

153. Carmagnola D, Adriaens P, Berglundh T: Healing of human extraction sockets filled with Bio-Oss, *Clin Oral Implants Res* 14(2):137-143, 2003.

154. Dietrich T, Zunker P, Dietrich D, Bernimoulin JP: Periapical and periodontal healing after osseous grafting and guided tissue regeneration treatment of apicomarginal defects in periradicular surgery: results after 12 months, *Oral Surg Oral Med Oral Pathol Oral Radiol Endod* 95(4):474-482, 2003.

155. Romanos GE: Present status of immediate loading of oral implants, *J Oral Implantol* 30(3):189-197, 2004.

chapter 16

Bone Biology, Osseointegration, and Bone Grafting

ONE is a living tissue that serves two primary functions—structural support and calcium metabolism.[1] It has a collagen protein matrix that is impregnated with mineral salts, including calcium phosphate (85%), calcium carbonate (10%), and small quantities of calcium fluoride and magnesium fluoride.[2] The collagen protein fibers that form the bone matrix are extremely complex. To maintain normal bone structure, there must be a sufficient quantity of both proteins and minerals. The minerals found in bone are present primarily in the form of hydroxyapatites. Bone mass is an important concept because bone is a mass-efficient structure in which maximal strength is achieved with minimal mass owing to its architecture. Unnecessary bone is lost (e.g., atrophy and bone loss seen in paraplegic patients) through a net loss effect as bone remodeling occurs. Bone also contains small quantities of noncollagen proteins embedded in its mineral matrix. The important family of bone morphogenetic proteins (BMPs) is part of this group.

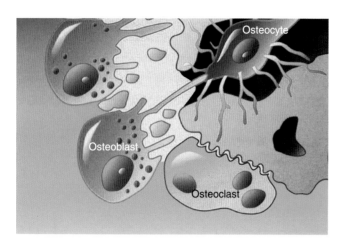

FIGURE 16-1 ■ Osteoclasts resorb bone as it ages, while osteoblasts deposit new bone simultaneously and adjacently. Once the osteoblasts deposit bone and become encapsulated, they are known as osteocytes.

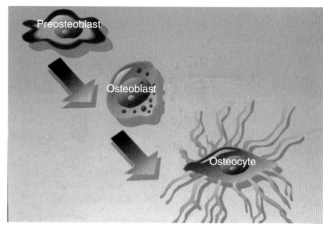

FIGURE 16-2 ■ Pre-osteoblasts mature into osteoblasts, which then mature into osteocytes.

Bone Biology

A study of bone biology includes elements related to bone cells, metabolism, structure, and repair.

Bone Cells

Three different types of cells—osteoblasts, osteocytes, and osteoclasts—are related to bone metabolism and physiology. The three are closely related to each other and are derived from similar precursors (Figure 16-1).

Osteoblasts, which are associated with the process of osteogenesis, are located in two general areas next to the bone surfaces where they deposit bone matrix. Therefore, they frequently are referred to as endosteal osteoblasts or periosteal osteoblasts. The cytoplasm of osteoblasts is intensely basophilic, which suggests the presence of ribonucleoproteins related to bone matrix protein component synthesis. Fine granules, which can be observed in the cytoplasm, are closely related to the site of active matrix deposit (Figure 16-2).

When osteoblasts become embedded in the bone matrix, they transform into osteocytes, which have a slightly basophilic cytoplasm. Prolongations of this cytoplasm extend from the osteocyte, through a network of fine canaliculi that emerge from the lacunae, to a specific distance. During bone formation, these prolongations extend beyond their normal limit, and a direct contiguity, or continuity, with adjacent osteocytes is evident. In mature bone, almost no extension of these prolongations is seen, but the canaliculi continue to function as a means of metabolic and biochemical messenger exchange between the blood system and the osteocytes.

The system of canaliculi connects the osteocyte lacunae with each other and the tissue spaces. Tissue fluid in these spaces mixes with fluid from the canaliculi, allowing a metabolic and biochemical messenger exchange between the bloodstream and the osteocytes. This mechanism allows the osteocytes to remain alive, regardless of the calcified intercellular substance that surrounds them. However, this duct system is not functional if it is located more than 0.5 mm from a capillary, which is why such an abundant blood supply is found in bone through capillaries that run through Haversian systems and Volkmann's canals.

Osteoclasts are fused monocytes that appear histologically as multinucleated giant cells located in shallow excavations (Howship's lacunae) along the mineralized surface.[3] The cytoplasm of osteoclasts is slightly basophilic and granular, with characteristic vacuoles. Osteoclasts are responsible for bone resorption and form in response to parathyroid hormone. After the process of local bone resorption is complete, osteoclasts disappear, probably by degeneration.

Bone Metabolism

Bone, the primary reservoir of calcium, has a tremendous turnover capability for responding to the metabolic needs of the body and is critical for maintaining a stable serum calcium level.[1,2] Because calcium participates in many reactions, it has an essential life support function. It works in conjunction with the lungs and kidneys to help maintain the pH balance of the body through the production of additional phosphates and carbonates, as well as by electrical charge conduction in nerve and muscle, including cardiac muscle. In addition, the metabolic environment is an extremely important component of the biomechanical structure of bone. Bone undergoes continuous turnover in response to metabolic reactions, with the skull and jaws unquestionably affected by this turnover.

The structural integrity of bone may be compromised in times of normal metabolic calcium need and in disease states, thus altering bone structure and mass. This phenomenon can be noted in the bone structure of postmenopausal women, who experience a decrease in estrogen hormones. As bone mass is lost, the interconnections between bone trabeculae also are lost. Because normal interconnections play an important role in making bone a biomechanically rigid structure, this decrease leads to fragility.

Metabolic/hormonal interactions play an important role in the maintenance of bone structure, the most important of which is the linkage of bone resorption to new bone apposition through BMP in normal daily remodeling of bone. Approximately 0.7% of a human skeleton is resorbed daily and is replaced by new, healthy bone. Therefore, a turnover in the entire skeleton occurs approximately every 142 days. When osteoblasts lay down bone, they also secrete BMP into the mineral matrix. This acid-insoluble protein resides there until it is released by osteoclastic resorption. This acid insolubility is an evolutionary mechanism by which the pH of 1 created by osteoclasts is able to dissolve bone mineral without affecting BMP.[4] Released BMP then is bound to the cell surface of undifferentiated mesenchymal stem cells, where it causes a membrane signal protein to become activated with high-energy phosphate bonds. This activation, in turn, affects the gene sequence in the nucleus, causing expression of osteoblast differentiation and stimulation of new bone production. A disturbance in this linkage may be the center point of osteoporosis.

Aging and metabolic disease states may reduce the normal turnover process, causing an increase in the mean age of the present bone. This increase may lead to fatigue, bone damage, compromised bone healing, failure to integrate implants, or loss of integration with an implant.[5] Thus, it becomes very important for surgeons to realize that a compromised status may not be recognized until the clinician attempts to place implants, or until the implants have been in place for some time.

Bone Structure

The macroscopic structure of bone is a continuum from dense cortical tissue to fine trabecular tissue (Figure 16-3). Between the two ends of this spectrum, no histological difference is seen in the type of bone, only in the relative amount of solid substance present and the geometrical fashion in which it is laid down (the size and number of spaces within it). In most cases, both cortical and trabecular tissues are found at every bone site, but the quantity and distribution of each may vary.

Cortical or compact bone is found in the diaphysis of long bones and on the external surface of flat bones (Figure 16-4). This tissue is organized in bony cylinders consolidated around a central blood vessel (referred to as a Haversian system). Trabecular, spongy, cancellous bone occupies substantial space within the bony tissue that constitutes the medullary cavity of the bone (Figure 16-5). The medullary cavities are filled with marrow: red marrow when there is

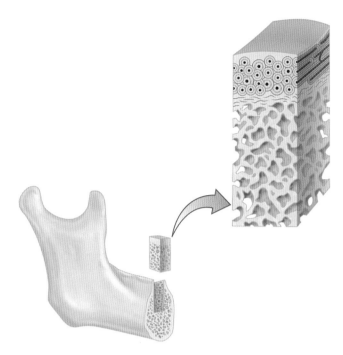

FIGURE 16-3 ■ The inner cancellous bone is surrounded with an outer layer of cortical bone.

active production of blood cells or a reserve population of mesenchymal stem cells, and yellow marrow when the cavity has been converted into a site for fat storage with age (Figures 16-6, 16-7).

Except for the articular surfaces, the bone surface is covered with periosteum, which is composed of two layers of specialized connective tissue. The outer fibrous layers provide toughness to the periosteum because of its configuration of mainly dense collagenous fibers and fibroblasts. This layer is rich in nerve fibers and blood supply. The inner cellular layer, which is in direct contact with the bone, contains functioning osteoblasts and often is referred to as the cambium layer. The medullary cavities and spaces are covered by endosteum, which consists of a single layer of osteoblasts that form a very thin, delicate membrane. The endosteum is architecturally similar to the cellular cambium layer of the periosteum because of the presence of osteoprogenitor cells, osteoblasts, and osteoclasts.

At the microscopic level, four types of bone are present: woven, composite, lamellar, and bundle. Woven bone plays a principal role during healing. The ability of woven bone to form quickly (at a rate of approximately 30 to 60 m per day) is its main property. However, because woven bone is formed so rapidly, it develops in a disorganized fashion without lamellar architecture or Haversian systems and therefore is soft. As a result, woven bone has low biomechanical strength. Although it often is referred to in the literature as "embryonic bone," this term is somewhat misleading because all adults have the ability to form this type of bone. Instead, woven bone is referred to as phase I bone

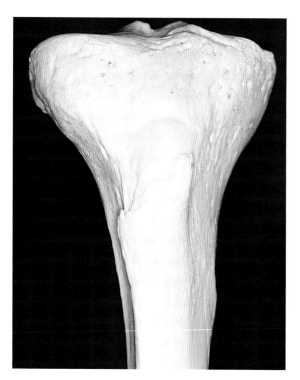

FIGURE 16-4 ■ Cortical bone is found on the external sur-faces of bone. The tibia has a wide plateau region with a bump (Gerdy's tubercle), which is the site of entry into the cancellous portion of the tibia. The bone is harvested across the wide portion of the tibia and inferiorly, avoiding thinning of the superior weight-bearing portion of the tibia.

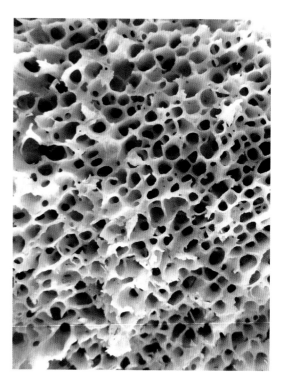

FIGURE 16-5 ■ Cancellous bone is found internally in bone. The cancellous bone structure is generally extremely porous.

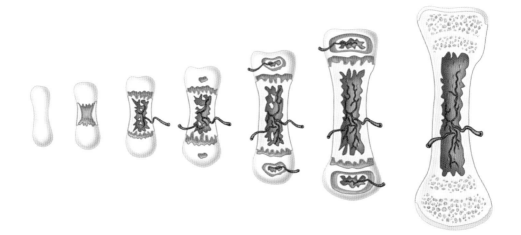

FIGURE 16-6 ■ Different stages of endochondreal ossification, from all cartilage to all bone with a minimal cartilage layer.

during bone healing.[6] Although woven bone (phase I bone) is laid down quickly, it normally does not last very long because it is not biomechanically sound. Obligatory resorp-tion and replacement with more mature bone, termed phase II or lamellar bone, occurs.[6-8] The term "composite bone" is used to describe the transitional state between woven bone (phase I bone) and lamellar bone (phase II bone). It is a woven bone lattice that is filled with lamellar bone.

Lamellar bone (phase II bone) is the principal, mature, load-bearing bone in the body, and this bone is extremely strong. Because it forms very slowly (at a rate of approxi-mately 0.6 to 1.0 μm per day), it is well organized in its collagen structure and, thus, in its mineralized structure. Lamellar bone consists of multiple, oriented layers. Bundle bone is the principal bone found around ligaments and joints and consists of striated interconnections with ligaments.

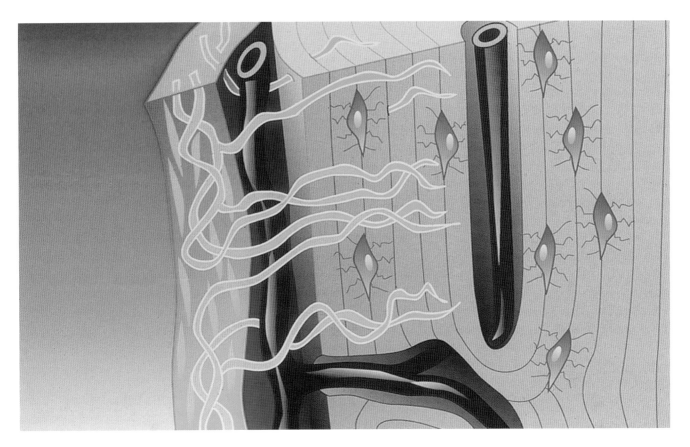

FIGURE 16-7 ■ The periosteum, a connective tissue membrane surrounding cortical bone, should be repositioned carefully, so that its osteogenic potential after surgery can nurture the graft and/or underlying bone.

At the molecular level, bone is a composite material. It is a cross-linked collagen matrix that consists of a three-dimensional multiple arrangement of matrix fibers. The orientation of collagen fibers determines the mineralization pattern. In this way, bone adapts to its biomechanical environment and projects maximal strength in the direction that is being loaded; this is the primary role of collagen fibers.

Intercellular bone substance has the homogenous aspect of an organized structure. The organic portion occupies 35% of the matrix and is formed primarily by osteocollagenous fibers, which are similar to collagen fibers in connective tissue. These fibers are joined by a cement-like substance, consisting mainly of glucosaminoglycan (protein-polysaccharide).

Sixty-five percent of bone weight corresponds to its inorganic component, localized only in the interfibrinous cement. Minerals are found predominantly in the form of calcium phosphate crystals with an apatite structure that corresponds to hydroxylapatite. These minerals form deposits of dense particles along the osteocollagenous fibers. The lacunae and ducts are covered by a thin layer of special organic cement that differs from the rest of the intercellular substance by its lack of fibers.

Calcified bone protein matrix consists of mineral components (65%), mainly hydroxylapatite, and nonmineral components (collagen [35%] and other proteins and peptides [5%]). These other proteins and peptides, such as BMP, regulate how bone is laid down and maintained. Bone matrix has the characteristic aspect of sequential layers that vary in thickness from 300 to 700 μm. These layers are the result of a rhythmical and uniform deposition of matrix. The fibers within each layer are parallel, with a spiral orientation that changes between layers, so that the fibers in one layer run perpendicular to those in the adjacent layer. This alternate disposition in fiber directions explains the division that occurs between layers.

Osseous Repair (Bone Modeling and Remodeling)

Bone modeling is defined as any change in the form, size, or shape of bone. It can be an anabolic process with apposition of bone on the surface, or it can be a catabolic process with resorption of the surface. Because these two processes can occur separately on different surfaces, bone modeling is a surface-specific phenomenon that occurs during growth, as part of wound healing (e.g., during stabilization of an endosseous implant), and in response to bone loading. Modeling is an uncoupled process in which formation does not have to be preceded by resorption. Activation of cells to resorb or form bone can occur within the same bone on different surfaces. An example of this phenomenon is the orthodontic movement of a tooth, wherein the force applied results in bone resorption on the tooth surface and bone formation on the opposite surface, resulting in tooth movement with surrounding bone and not through the alveolus.

Bone modeling may be controlled by mechanical factors, as is the case with orthodontic tooth movement, or by growth factors, as is the case with bone healing, bone grafting, and osseointegration. Microstrain (ME) is a method of measuring the load applied to bone as percent deformation of tissue. For example, a load of 200 ME produces a deformation of 0.2% of the tissue. Between the range of 200 and 2,500 ME, there is normal functional response, in which strong bone is produced that is effective in facing increased loads. Atrophy occurs in cases in which the force is low (i.e., less than 200 ME). When the load is between 2,500 and 4,000 ME (i.e., a deformation of 0.25% to 0.4%), hypertrophy occurs, and there is a change in the size of the bone segment.[9] The modeling that occurs during hypertrophy is lamellar bone formation. If the load exceeds 4,000 ME, there is a pathological overload, and the modeling that occurs is woven bone formation. In this situation, the bone responds as quickly as possible to meet the excessive load by producing the tissue that can be formed the fastest (i.e., woven bone, which has limited load-bearing capacity).[9]

The effects of biochemical control and growth factor influences can be seen in the two respective models of bone graft healing and osseointegration. For the purpose of a clear-cut understanding of the intricacies of bone formation and remodeling, the bone graft healing model will be discussed first.

Placement of a graft that consists of endosteal osteoblasts and stem cells (from a donor site such as the ileum or tibial head), and that is surrounded by a vascular and cellular tissue bed, creates a recipient site with a biochemistry that is hypoxic (O_2 tensions, 3 to 10 mm Hg), acidic (pH 4.0 to 6.0), and rich in lactate.[10] The graft itself contains the osteocompetent cell populations, as well as islands of mineralized cancellous bone, fibrin from blood clotting, and platelets within the clot (Figure 16-8).

The endosteal osteoblasts and marrow stem cells survive the first 3 to 5 days largely because of their surface position and ability to absorb nutrients from recipient tissues. Osteocytes within the mineralized cancellous bone die as a result of their encasement in mineral, which serves as a nutritional barrier. Because the graft is inherently hypoxic (5 to 10 mm Hg) and the surrounding tissue is normoxic (50 to 55 mm Hg), an oxygen gradient that is greater than the 20 mm Hg (usually 35 to 50 mm Hg) required to stimulate macrophage chemotaxis is set up, and, in turn, the macrophages are stimulated to secrete macrophage-derived angio-

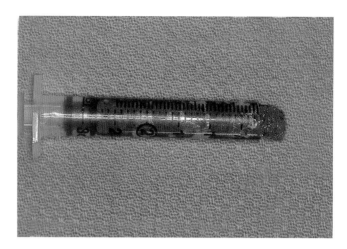

FIGURE 16-8 ■ Bone graft material mixed with platelet rich plasma (PRP) in a syringe to be carried to the graft recipient site.

genesis factor (MDAF) and macrophage-derived growth factor (MDGF).

Within the graft, the platelets entrapped within the clot degranulate within hours of graft placement, releasing platelet-derived growth factor (PDGF). Therefore, the inherent properties of the wound, particularly the oxygen gradient phenomenon and PDGF, initiate early angiogenesis from surrounding capillaries and mitogenesis of transferred osteocompetent cells[11].

By day 3, capillary buds from existing capillaries outside of the graft can be seen. They penetrate the graft and proliferate within the cancellous bone network to form a complete network by day 10 to 14. As these capillaries respond to the oxygen gradient, MDAF messengers effectively reduce the oxygen gradient as they perfuse the graft, thus creating a shut-off mechanism to prevent over-angiogenesis.

Although PDGF seems to be the earliest messenger to stimulate early osteoid formation, PDGF probably is replaced by MDGF and other mesenchymal tissue stimulators from the transforming growth factor-beta family. During the first 3 to 7 days, stem cell populations and endosteal osteoblasts produce only a small amount of osteoid. After the vascular network has been established, osteoid production accelerates, presumably as a result of oxygen and nutrient availability. The initial osteoid that forms develops on the surface of the mineralized cancellous trabeculae from the endosteal osteoblasts. Shortly thereafter, individual osteoid islands develop between cancellous bone trabeculae, presumably from stem cells transferred within the graft. A third source of osteoid production develops from circulating stem cells, which also are attracted to the biochemical environment of the wound.[12] These stem cells are postulated to seed the graft and proliferate, thereby contributing to osteoid production.

Throughout the first 3 to 4 weeks, this biochemical and cellular phase of bone regeneration proceeds to coalesce individual osteoid islands, surface osteoid on cancellous trabeculae, and host bone to clinically consolidate the graft. This process uses the fibrin network of the graft as a framework. Normally nonmotile cells, such as osteoblasts, may be somewhat motile via the process of endocytosis along a scaffold such as fibrin. The process of endocytosis is merely the transfer of the cell membrane from the retreating edge of the cell through the cytoplasm as a vesicle to the advancing edge to re-form a cell membrane. This process slowly advances the cell and allows it to secrete its product in the process. In this case, the product is osteoid on the fibrin network. This cellular regeneration phase often is referred to as phase I bone regeneration.[6] By the time regeneration is nearly complete (4 to 6 weeks), sufficient osteoid production and mineralization have occurred to permit graft function. Bone at this stage has formed without going through a chondroblastic phase and histologically appears as random cellular bone, which a pathologist would refer to as woven bone.[13]

Because the amount of bone formed during phase I depends on osteocompetent cell density, donor sites with the highest cancellous trabecular bone areas are chosen. In rank order, it has been shown that the posterior and anterior ileum, tibial plateau, femoral head, and mandibular symphysis are potential donor sites with greater availability of cancellous bone than the calvarium, rib, or fibula.[14] In addition, enhanced phase I bone yields are achieved by compacting the graft material. Technically, this enhancement often is accomplished with the use of a bone mill, followed by compaction in a syringe and then further compaction into the graft site using bone-packing instruments.

As was previously stated, the biochemistry of the recipient tissue and the graft itself is largely inherent. However, studies and experience with platelet-rich plasma (PRP)

additions to the graft have shown early consolidation and graft mineralization in half the time, with a 15% to 30% improvement in trabecular bone density.[12] The concept is that PRP, which is a fibrin clot (also called fibrin glue), is rich in platelets, which, in turn, release PDGF. It has been theorized that this enhanced quantity of PDGF initiates the osteocompetent cell activity more completely than what will inherently occur in the graft and clot milieu alone. Additionally, the enhanced fibrin network created by PRP is believed to enhance osteoconduction throughout the graft, supporting graft consolidation.

The cellular bone regeneration that occurs during phase I is disorganized woven bone that is structurally sound but is not structurally on par with mature bone. The random organization and hypercellular nature of this bone are similar to those seen in a fracture callus. This bone will undergo obligatory resorption and replacement remodeling. Eventually, it will be replaced by phase II bone, which is less cellular, more mineralized, and more structurally organized (Figure 16-9).[6,13]

As occurs with all bone remodeling, the replacement of phase I bone by phase II bone is initiated by osteoclasts, which are fused mononuclear cells that arrive at the graft site though the newly developed vascular network.[3] It has been postulated that these osteoclasts resorb phase I bone in a normal remodeling-replacement cycle. BMP is released during resorption of both the newly formed phase I bone and the nonviable original cancellous trabecular bone. As with normal bone turnover, BMP acts as the link or couple between bone resorption and new bone apposition. Stem cells in the graft from the original transplantation and newly arrived stem cells from local tissues and the circulation respond by osteoblast differentiation and new bone formation. New bone forms as the jaw and graft function, developing in response to the demands placed on it. This bone develops into mature Haversian systems and lamellar

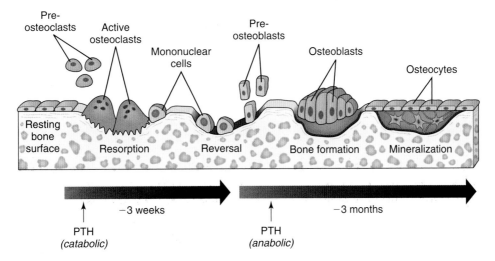

Bone Remodeling Cycle

FIGURE 16-9 ■ There is a sequence of events that takes place over time for bone remodeling/formation.

bone that is capable of withstanding the normal shear forces placed on the jaw through opening and closing functions, and it tolerates impact compressive forces that are typical of denture-borne and implant-borne prosthetic functions. Histologically, such grafts are involved in long-term remodeling that is consistent with normal skeletal turnover. A periosteum and an endosteum develop as part of this long-term remodeling cycle. Radiographically, the graft takes on the morphology and cortical outlines of the mandible or maxilla over several years.

Osseointegration

Studies of roughened titanium implants indicate a three-phase process of osseointegration: osteophyllic phase, osteoconductive phase, and osteoadaptive phase[12].

Osteophyllic Phase

When a roughened surface implant is placed into the cancellous marrow space of the mandible or maxilla, only a small amount of bone from the trabecular bone within the marrow is in contact with the metal surface of the implant. The remaining surface of the implant is exposed to the fibrofatty marrow space. The initial response seen is a migration of osteoblasts and osteoid production to the implant surface. The source of these osteoblasts is surface endosteal osteoblasts of the trabecular bone and the inner surface of the buccal and lingual cortex. It is probable that these cells are responding to the release of BMP from surgical placement of the implant and the initial resorption of bone crushed against the metal surface. The osteophyllic phase lasts for approximately 1 month (Figure 16-10).

Osteoconductive Phase

After contact, the bone cells spread along the metal surface (osteoconduction), laying down osteoid. The bone that is deposited is often a thin layer. This phase continues over the next 3 months as more bone is added to the total surface area of the implant. At this time (4 months after initial placement), the maximum surface area is covered by bone, and after this, no further increase in bone to the surface area is observed.

Osteoadaptive Phase

The final phase, the osteoadaptive phase, begins approximately 4 months after implant placement, at the same time that the osteoconductive phase ends. It is associated with a steady state (no gain or loss of bone against metal) resorption remodeling sequence that continues even after the implants are exposed and loaded (Figure 16-11).

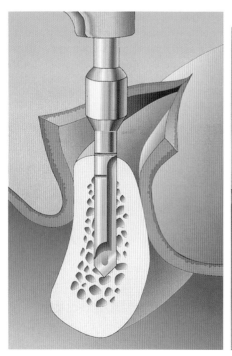
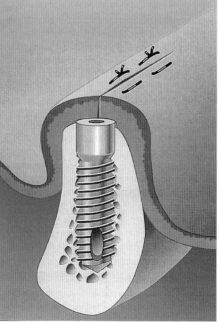

FIGURE 16-10 ■ Placing an implant traumatizes the bone, stimulating a response to repair and remodel.

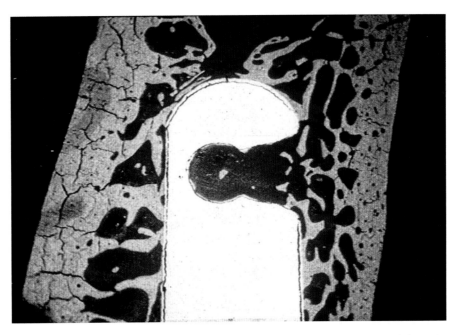

FIGURE 16-11 ■ Bone grows from host bone out to the surface of the implant and then along the implant surface.

Biological Factors Related to Failure of Osseointegrated Oral Implants

One of the first definitions of osseointegration was a "direct functional and structural connection between living bone and the surface of a load-bearing implant." However, perspectives on what constitutes osseointegration may vary.

From the perspective of the patient, an implant fixture is osseointegrated if it provides stable and apparently immobile support of a prosthesis under functional loads, without pain, inflammation, or loosening. From a biological and medical point of view, osseointegration of a fixture in bone is defined as the close apposition of new and re-formed bone in congruence with the fixture, including surface irregularities, so that at the light microscopic level, no interpositioned connective or fibrous tissue is seen, and so that a direct structural and functional connection is established, which is capable of carrying normal physiological loads without excessive deformation and without initiation of rejection reactions.

From a biomechanical point of view, a fixture is osseointegrated if there is no progressive relative motion between the fixture and surrounding living bone and marrow under functional loading for the entire life of the patient, and if the fixture exhibits deformations of the same order of magni-

tude as when the same loads are applied directly to the bone. From a biophysical point of view, osseointegration implies that at light microscopic and electron microscopic levels, the components of tissue within a thin zone of a fixture surface are identifiable as normal bone and marrow constituents, which continuously grade into a normal bone structure surrounding the fixture: Mineralized tissue is found to be in contact with the fixture surface within nanometers so that no functionally significant intervening material exists at the interface. From a clinical point of view, osseointegration is the approximation of viable bone to the implant surface and into the surface irregularities; the bone is stable, capable of carrying normal physiological loads, and free of infection, pain, pathology, or long-term bone loss.

Obviously, every single implant has to fulfill and be tested for all the defined success criteria, otherwise it should be considered as surviving. This term applies to those implants that are still in function, but that have not been tested with respect to success criteria, or for which neither the criteria for success nor those for failure are met[15,16].

Consensus seems to be unanimous that progressive marginal bone loss is a pathological sign that can lead to implant failure. However, to what extent marginal bone resorption should progress in order to advocate treatment and which is the most appropriate treatment procedure remain to be decided. One of the most commonly used success criteria suggests the use of less than 1.5 mm of marginal bone loss during the first year of loading, and thereafter, less than 0.2 mm yearly.[17] It is interesting to observe that despite the fact that most clinical follow-up studies refer to this success criterion, few authors or clinicians actually apply this bone loss criterion to individual implants or implant cases.

Systemic Factors

Age and Genetics

With aging, changes occur in the mineral composition, collagen, BMP content, and conformation of bone.[18] Furthermore, fracture healing tends to be delayed.[19] An experimental study that evaluated bone healing around hydroxylapatite-coated implants in rats of different ages yielded a decreased rate and quantity of regenerated bone with increased age.[20] Therefore, it is conceivable that in older patients, bone healing may be slower and failure rates may be slightly increased; recent findings suggest this to be the case.

General Health

The nutritional status[21,22] and general diseases such as bone metabolic disease (e.g., osteoporosis, osteomalacia, hyperparathyroidism, Paget's disease), rheumatic disease (e.g., rheumatoid arthritis, Sjögren's syndrome, systemic lupus erythematosus), hormonal disease (e.g., diabetes, Cushing's syndrome, hyperparathyroidism), lichen planus, anomalies of neutrophil granulocytes, delayed hypersensitivity, immunological disorders, and malabsorption syndromes have been suggested to influence the outcomes of implant treatment.[22-24]

Diabetes mellitus is a metabolic disease that may influence wound healing as the typical vascular alterations associated with this condition could disturb the circulation at the implanted site. Further, chemotactic and phagocytic functions of neutrophils are reported to be reduced, resulting in increased susceptibility to infection and lower survival rates. Osteoporosis, head and neck radiation, and chemotherapy all have been found to decrease survival rates of implants.

Smoking

Smoking is one of the factors often discussed in relation to implant failure. Several studies have shown that smoking can be associated with higher failure rates, complications, and altered peri-implant tissue conditions.[25-30]

Local Factors

Bone Quality, Quantity, and Anatomical Location

The characteristics of the bone at the implantation site and the anatomical locations are among those factors that seem to profoundly influence implant failure rates, independently of whether implants are loaded or not.[31,32] In general, higher failure rates have been reported for implants placed in maxillae[31-35] and in posterior segments of both jaws. These rates may be explained in part by different types of bone quality and loading conditions in these locations. In fact, mandibles generally have a denser and thicker cortical layer than do maxillae, and the cortical layer of both jaws tends to become thinner and more porous posteriorly. Also, the trabecular bone component is denser in mandibles than in maxillae and in anterior areas than in posterior locations,[32,36-39] although an extreme range of variation has been observed in mandibles.[40] In addition, distal implants have to withstand the heaviest loading[41,42] and in general are short owing to an insufficient quantity of available bone in this region. The presence of anatomical structures, such as the maxillary sinus and the inferior alveolar nerve, frequently limits the amount of bone available for implants in posterior locations. However, higher success rates can be obtained in areas of poor bone density when surface-enhanced implants are used.

Based on extrapolations from patients affected by severe periodontitis, it is advisable to avoid placement of implants in individuals with diseases frequently associated with functional defects of polymorphonuclear leukocytes (PMNs) (for example, Chédiak-Higashi syndrome, Down's syndrome, cyclical neutropenia, benign chronic neutropenia, secondary agranulocytosis, and diabetes mellitus type I).[43]

Radiation Therapy

Radiation therapy provokes early and late alterations in tissues and has profound effects on bone cells and blood vessels.[44] In fact, not only are tumor cells affected, but the entire cell population is affected as well. The tissue response to radiation is bimodal, with an acute and a chronic phase. Early (acute) changes include mucositis, dermatitis, and xerostomia, which affect mainly soft tissue structures.[45,46] Among late (chronic) changes affecting bone are cell death, increased susceptibility to infection, and delayed and impaired bone healing.[47-50] In addition, a decrease in bone-to-implant contact,[50-52] bone resorption,[51] fibrosis,[51,53] and avascular necrosis (osteoradionecrosis)[54-56] has been reported. The end result is often a hypocellular, hypovascular, and hypoxic tissue, which does not tolerate traumatic or surgical insult.[54] The extent of cellular damage seems to be dose dependent[47,48,51] and is influenced by delivery protocol. In particular, for total radiation doses below 48 Gy (1 Gy = 100 rad), complications are rarely seen, whereas increased complication rates have been observed for doses exceeding 64 Gy.[55,56]

The use of hyperbaric oxygen (HBO) therapy prior to implant placement to provide support to areas with compromised blood flow is recommended. Experimental data of increased bone mineralization[57,58] and of increased biomechanical forces needed to unscrew Ti implants[59] after HBO treatment have supported this hypothesis. Clinical studies on craniofacial implants in radiated patients have shown higher implant survival rates in patients treated with HBO than in those who had not received HBO therapy.[60,61]

In conclusion, radiation therapy should not be considered an absolute contraindication for implant therapy, particularly in the mandible. However, implant treatment to radiated patients should be delivered exclusively by experienced teams, with an appropriate HBO protocol. When performed under these conditions, implant-retained prostheses are an excellent treatment option for this severely disabled patient category.

Operator-Related Factors

Operator Experience
Early failure rates for surgeons who have placed fewer than 50 implants are almost twice as high as for those who have placed 50 or more implants.[62,63] Early failure rates for the first nine implant surgeries were found to be approximately twice as high as those that occurred afterward.

It has been suggested that the high success rates reported by experienced clinical centers may be difficult to reproduce by beginning clinicians under ordinary practice conditions.[31,64] On the other hand, it has been shown that noncomplicated cases (single restorations) can be treated successfully with high success rates by general practitioners who have undergone 8 days of training.[65]

Operator Technique (surgical trauma, bacterial contamination)
Surgical preparation of the implant site may produce a zone of necrotic bone surrounding the inserted implant.[66] The extent of this zone is likely to be influenced by the degree of surgical trauma.[66] To achieve osseointegration, the dead bone has to be resorbed and new bone formed. In addition, when a sufficient bone-to-implant fit cannot be achieved, avoiding micromotion of the implant may be difficult, and this could act as an additional negative factor. Bone overheating at the implant site and the absence of primary implant stability, together with reduced healing ability of the host, can lead to soft tissue encapsulation (repair) rather than osseointegration (regeneration). Microorganisms preferentially adhere to implant surfaces and then may form a glycocalyx (biofilm or slime) to protect themselves from the host.[67-70] For instance, dental plaque is a typical example of biofilm in the oral environment. Among the slime-producing bacterial species often encountered and well characterized in biomaterial-centered infections are *Staphylococcus epidermidis, Staphylococcus aureus,* and *Pseudomonas aeruginosa.* The glycocalyx itself has been found to have anti-immune properties in vitro.[71,72] Such biofilms have been shown to protect the enclosed bacteria from antibiotics in vitro.[73,74] Also, adherent non–slime-producing bacteria have demonstrated enhanced resistance to antibiotics in vitro.[73] It is interesting to note that this phenomenon does not seem to be related to a barrier effect of the biofilm, as a sufficient concentration of antibiotics may reach bacteria and biomaterial surfaces,[75] according to mathematical models. Conversely, bacterial antibiotic resistance has been attributed to a decreased metabolic rate and phenotypic transformation.[73,75] Therefore, microorganisms on surfaces and in

microcolonies are probably physiologically different from free-floating bacteria.

Operator Policy
In some situations, to reduce treatment time for the patient, to preserve as much crestal bone as possible, and to insert implants in the most ideal position, implants are placed immediately after tooth extraction.[76] Early data indicate that a predictable outcome seems achievable with the use of a one-stage placement modality, along with early loading.[77]

The number of supporting implants, the choice of prosthetic design, the precision of the superstructure, the type of restorative materials used, and so on, are factors that influence implant osseointegration. With the low failure rates generally reported, a large number of patients have to be included in long-term clinical trials to establish clinically and statistically significant associations between osseointegration and potential contributing factors.[64] In addition, the tendency of failures to cluster in a few individuals may affect failure rates considerably.

Finally, the clinician should be aware that even though several factors are associated with less osseointegration and higher risks for implant losses, these factors do not mean that potential patients not fulfilling such requirements should not receive the benefit of implant therapy. However, patients should be informed correctly that they may have a reduced chance for implant osseointegration.

Autogenous Bone Graft Techniques

Our bone grafting considerations include sinus augmentation procedures, anatomy, materials, techniques, and complications.

Sinus Augmentation Procedures

Dental implant placement in patients who are edentulous in the posterior maxilla can be difficult for many reasons, including inadequate posterior alveolar height and increased pneumatization of the maxillary sinus, and therefore close approximation of the maxillary sinus to crestal bone (Figure 16-12). The size of the maxillary sinus correlates with the degree of pneumatization. If appropriate graft materials are being used (i.e., at least 50% autogenous bone with good cellular density) and principles to maximize bone are followed, bone grafting and implant placement can be performed at the same time (i.e., in a one-step method) in ridges with as little as 1 to 5 mm residual crestal bone.[78]

Maxillary Sinus Anatomy

Maxillary bone is primarily medullary (or spongy) in character and finely trabecular. It generally has less osseous

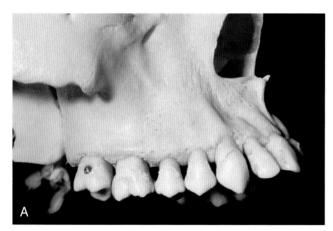

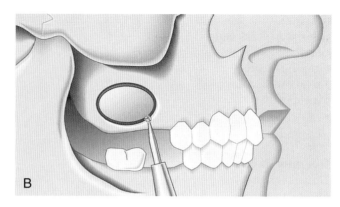

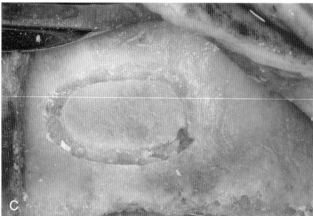

FIGURE 16-12 ■ **A-C,** An outline being created in posterior maxilla for sinus augmentation of the maxillary sinus.

density when compared with premaxillary or mandibular bone. Adjacent cortices consist of compact bone. However, they generally are very thin, providing minimal strength compared with the cortices surrounding the mandible. Because of its spongy nature, medullary bone must establish a stress-bearing surface next to an endosteal implant, so the functioning implant can remain stable and able to transmit physiological load to the supporting bone[79,80].

The maxillary sinus is lined with pseudostratified columnar epithelium, which is called the Schneiderian membrane. Beneath the surface epithelium is a loosely cellular but highly vascular, thin tissue. Beneath this, and adjacent to the bony surface in all areas, is a periosteum.

The blood supply to the maxilla normally emanates from three parent arteries—superior labial, anterior ethmoidal, and internal maxillary. The area of sinus lift surgery is supplied mainly by branches from the internal maxillary artery. The sinus floor derives some of its blood flow from the greater and lesser palatine vessels, as well as from the incisal artery, which is a terminal branch of the spheno-palatine artery (which is yet another portion of the internal maxillary artery). These vessels penetrate the bony palate and ramify within the sinus floor and its medial and lateral walls. Another vascular contribution arises from the pos-terosuperior alveolar artery, which enters the maxilla in the

superior tuberosity area to supply most of the posterior and lateral walls. The infraorbital branch of the internal maxillary artery helps supply blood to the superolateral sinus area. The anterior ethmoidal artery, which is a terminal branch of the internal carotid system (via the ophthalmic artery), supplies the superomedial sinus area.[81]

Bone Grafting Materials

To date, no consensus has been reached regarding which graft material or combination of materials is best for augmenting the sinus antral void created by the sinus lift operation.[82] Grafting materials that are being used currently for antral floor augmentation include autogenous bone,[81,83-89] bone allografts,[9,90-94] and alloplasts such as tricalcium phosphate (TCP), bioactive glass, and resorbable and nonresorbable hydroxylapatite (HA)[9,95,96].

Autogenous bone has long been considered the "gold standard" and remains the best grafting material because of its highly osteogenic, osteoinductive, and osteoconductive properties. These properties allow bone to form more rapidly and in conditions where significant bone augmentation or repair is required. Autogenous bone can be harvested from the iliac crest or from intraoral sites such as the mandibular symphysis (Figure 16-13A-C), maxillary tuberosity, ramus, exostoses, and extraneous bone from an implant osteotomy.[9,85,97-99] Resorption after transplantation of mandibular bone grafts has been reported to be less when compared with iliac crest grafts.[85,99] In addition, intraorally obtained bone grafts result in less morbidity than is associated with iliac crest grafts. The procedure can be accomplished easily in an office setting with the patient under parenteral sedation and local anesthesia, so that no postoperative hospitalization is required, resulting in lower costs. A disadvantage is that intraoral donor sites provide a smaller volume of bone than is provided by the iliac crest. The donor site usually is chosen depending on the volume and type of bone desired (Figure 16-14).

Bone allografts, which may be cortical or trabecular, may form bone by osteoinduction or osteoconduction. They are obtained from cadavers—living related persons and living unrelated persons—and are processed under complete sterility and stored in bone banks. Transplanted bone induces a host-immune response, with fresh allografts the most antigenic. However, this response can be reduced considerably by first freezing or freeze-drying the bone.[100] Freeze-dried bone allograft (FDBA) can be used in mineralized or demineralized form. We recommend FDBA for grafting purposes over demineralized FDBA for the following reasons: (1) We maintain the mineral component and provide a localized bone mineral source for bone formation, and (2) we avoid the destruction of some BMPs and growth factors that occur in demineralized bone as the result of processing procedures (Figure 16-15).

A pilot study was conducted in monkeys to examine the effects of recombinant human bone morphogenetic protein-2 (rhBMP-2) on bone regeneration following bilat-

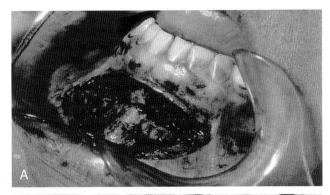

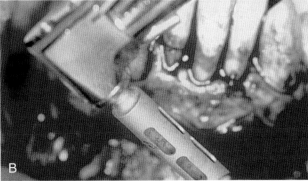

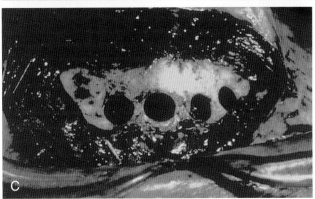

FIGURE 16-13   ■   **A-C,** Autogenous bone graft taken from the anterior mandible.

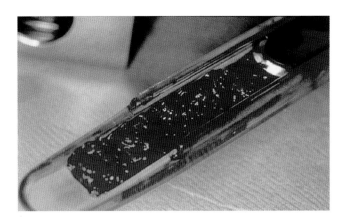

FIGURE 16-14   ■   Bone scrapers can be utilized to quickly and efficiently harvest small quantities of autogenous bone.

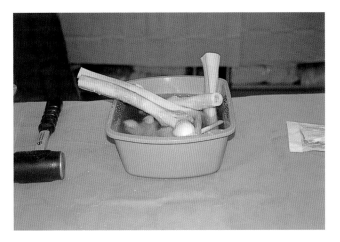

FIGURE 16-15   ■   Bone allografts obtained from cadavers undergo strict screening and processing by tissue banks before they are made available to surgeons. Large pieces of bone are cleaned and are placed in separate containers.

eral hemimandibulectomy.[103] In three monkeys, a dose of 0.8 mg rhBMP-2 per cc in a collagen I sponge was applied to a single mandibulectomy site, and 0.2 mg rhBMP-2 per cc was applied to the contralateral side. In four other monkeys, a dose of 0.4 mg rhBMP-2 per cc was applied to a single site, and an autogenous bone graft was used on the contralateral side. Complete regeneration was observed in all seven monkeys. Histomorphometric analysis showed excellent calcified bone matrix-to-marrow space ratios in animals sacrificed at 5 months.

Surgical Techniques

Antibiotics that are effective against both aerobic and anaerobic bacteria should be prescribed preoperatively and postoperatively. The patient's oral-facial area should be prepared and draped. Surgery can be performed with the patient sedated with intravenous medication unless the graft material is procured from the iliac crest, in which case general anesthesia is used. A local anesthetic, with a vasoconstrictor for hemostasis, is infiltrated into the maxillary surgical site and the maxillary or mandibular donor sites (if autogenous bone will be harvested from an intraoral site). The lateral wall of the maxilla is exposed by reflecting a mucoperiosteal flap superiorly to the level of the malar buttress. After the lateral maxillary wall has been completely exposed, a No. 8 round diamond bur should be used at low speed (100 rpm) to make an oval osteotomy in the lateral wall of the maxillary sinus. An oval osteotomy is recommended as opposed to a rectangular or trapezoidal osteotomy, to minimize sharp edges of the bony window, which can cause tears in the underlying Schneiderian membrane.[81]

The sinus floor septa (convolutions) are not altered. A variable number of septa divide the floor of the maxillary sinus into several recesses and may complicate sinus lift procedures.[104,105] Most of the septa are located in the region between the second premolar and the first molar.

Intraoperative Bleeding

Because no major vascular structures are present in the area of the sinus lift surgery, any intraoperative bleeding that does occur usually comes from capillary soft tissue or bony ooze. No doubt, all of the interconnecting vascular contributions to the maxilla and the maxillary sinus account for the "forgiving" nature and rapid healing of maxillary sinus surgery. However, the vascular system can produce brisk intraoperative oozing, which usually is related to the patient's systemic blood pressure and/or the presence of local inflammation. Only rarely is it due to a bleeding disorder or coagulopathy. Most hemostatic disorders are already known by the time a patient reaches the age at which he or she requires a sinus lift operation, or they are noted when a good preoperative history is obtained. For those patients who claim to be "bleeders," or who have a suspicious history of "bleeding problems," a simple battery of screening blood tests will identify 98.5% of bleeding disorders. This series of tests includes a complete blood count (CBC)

with a platelet count and differential, a bleeding time test, a prothrombin time (PT), and a partial prothrombin time (PTT).

If brisk intraoperative oozing develops, the patient's systemic blood pressure should be checked. Hypertension control usually is established by reinforcing local anesthesia, verbally reassuring the patient, and using additional sedation if necessary. It is rare, but possible, that a procedure may have to be stopped because of uncontrollable hypertension. Locally, a brisk ooze is best controlled by temporarily packing the wound. Sometimes, saturating the packing with 1:100,000 epinephrine or 4% cocaine will assist hemostasis, particularly if the oozing is coming from soft tissue. If the oozing is coming from bone, and a temporary packing will not control it, pressing bone wax into the area usually will be effective.

Grafting Procedure

Autogenous bone is harvested from the predetermined site and is mixed with reconstituted freeze-dried bone in a 1:2 ratio. This mixture then is packed into 1-cc tuberculin syringes and is set aside. The mixture is used to densely fill the sinus. After completely filling the maxillary sinus with the desired level of bone mixture, as above, the clinician repositions the mucoperiosteal flap, and the incisions are closed with interrupted nonresorbable sutures.

After the bone has matured, it is evaluated to ensure that there is sufficient quantity for implant placement. Implants then can be placed in the mature graft material according to the surgical protocol for the particular implant system and can be allowed to integrate.

Postoperative considerations are similar to those for most oral surgery and sinus manipulation procedures.

Nasal Floor and Block Grafts for Premaxilla Augmentation

Anterior tooth loss usually compromises ideal bone volume and position for proper implant placement[106]. Patients can present with an array of conditions that limit or prevent ideal endosteal implant placement. The facial cortical plate over the roots of the maxillary teeth is very thin and porous. It may be resorbed from periodontal disease and often is fractured during extraction of teeth.[106] One of the primary reasons for compromised osseointegration is inadequate primary stabilization of the maxillary implants at the time of placement.[107] Several long-term studies indicate reduced survival rates for osseointegrated implants in the maxilla compared with the mandible.[86,87,108]

Augmentation procedures can be used to increase the amount of bone in the maxillary alveolar ridge. The crown-to-implant ratio and the incisal edge position in relation to the implant body are factors that need to be considered when one is selecting an augmentation procedure. Nasal floor elevation, bone spreading with the use of osteotomes, corticocancellous block bone grafting, guided tissue regeneration, and a combination of these are all ridge augmentation techniques used for implant placement in the anterior maxilla. When selecting a ridge augmentation technique, the clinician must consider the morphology of the osseous defect.

Cortical membranous grafts revascularize more quickly than do endochondral bone grafts and have been shown to have less resorption (Figure 16-16). This difference may explain why chin grafts, which consist primarily of cortical bone with few osteogenic cells, show less volume loss and good incorporation, and have a shorter healing time. Bone from the mandibular symphysis is biochemically similar to bone in the maxillofacial region, and this similarity may promote better incorporation.[109] Disadvantages of using the mandibular symphysis at a donor site include a limited amount of available bone and the risk for damage to the mandibular tooth roots or mental nerve.[109]

When the anterior maxillary residual crest is less than 10 mm in height, subnasal elevation, in conjunction with bone graft augmentation, can be used to provide adequate bone quantity and quality for implant placement. With subnasal elevation, the nasal mucosa can be elevated pre-

dictably 3 to 5 mm; elevation is followed by placement of particulate bone graft material to augment the ridge. The periosteum of the labial aspect of the anterior maxilla is reflected to expose the inferior and/or lateral piriform rim. A nasal undercut region typically is present in the area of the lateral inferior piriform rim. In this region, the nasal mucosa may be elevated with a curette similar to that used to elevate the membrane during maxillary sinus grafting procedures. Because the nasal mucosa generally is much thicker and more tear resistant, it is easier to elevate. However, because of the presence of an elastic fiber that causes the nasal mucosa to adhere more firmly to underlying bone, greater pressure is required than is necessary for membrane elevation during maxillary sinus procedures.[110]

A highly resorbed maxilla, which often presents with reverse architecture in the anterior maxilla, where retained or supererupted mandibular incisor teeth have accelerated bone resorption into the basal bone, may leave only a few millimeters or complete dehiscence of the anterior nasal floor. In these situations, a 5- to 7-mm block graft is placed after nasal mucosal elevation and inferior septoplasty are performed. When used in conjunction with alveolar augmentation grafting, this procedure provides additional stability and vertical dimension for the implants[111] (Figures 16-17, 16-18).

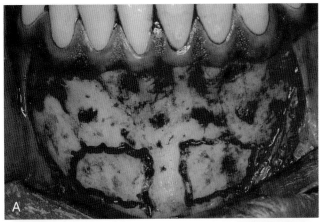

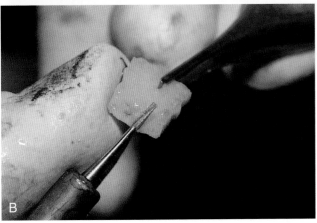

FIGURE 16-16 ■ **A, B,** Autogenous bone graft taken from anterior mandible.

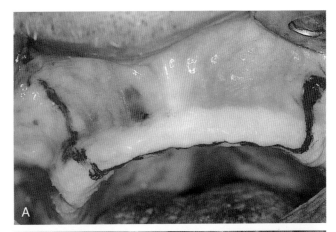

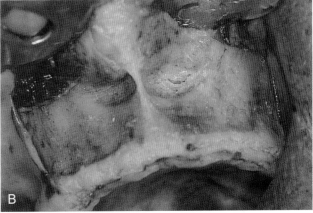

FIGURE 16-17 ■ **A, B,** In the anterior maxilla, a nasal lift procedure can be performed to elevate the floor and graft bone in order to allow for longer implants to be placed.

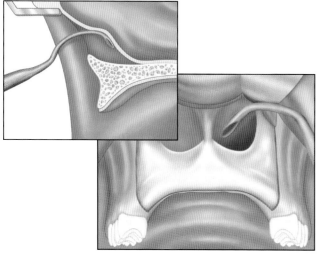

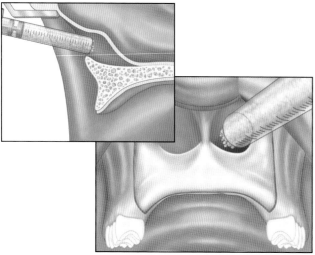

FIGURE 16-18 ■ A maximum of 5 mm of additional height is possible with the nasal lift procedure. Beyond this can affect air inspiration for the patient.

Autogenous bone is the bone-grafting material recommended for use in the nasal fossa. This material allows bone to form more rapidly and can be used where significant bone augmentation or repair is required. Alloplasts and allografts may be used to expand the autogenous graft. However, alloplasts or allografts are not recommended for subnasal grafting by themselves until evidence of their effectiveness has been established.[110]

SUMMARY

It is important for the dental surgeon to understand bone biology and osseointegration. Therefore, the surgeon must understand the important interrelated subjects of physiology of bone growth, biology of bone and bone grafting, causes of success and failure in the bone-to-implant bond, and clinical bone grafting techniques and principles.

Without this understanding, today's surgeon is little more than a technician in a modern operating room. However, proper understanding allows the surgeon to optimize the benefits of osseointegration for patients.

REFERENCES

1. Roberts WE, Turley PK, Brezniak N, Fielder PJ: Implants: bone physiology and metabolism, *CDA J* 15(10):54-61, 1987.
2. Dalén N, Olsson KE: Bone mineral content and physical activity, *Acta Orthop Scand* 45:170-176, 1974.
3. Bonucci E: New knowledge on the origin, function and fate of osteoclasts, *Clin Orthop Relat Res* (158):252-269, 1981.
4. Urist MR: Bone morphogenetic protein. In: Hdd MB, Reddi AR, editors: Bone graft and bone substitute, Philadelphia, 1992, WB Saunders, pp 70-82.
5. Marx RE, Ehler WJ, Peleg M: "Mandibular and facial reconstruction" rehabilitation of the head and neck cancer patient, *Bone* 19(1 suppl):59S-82S, 1996.
6. Axhausen W: The osteogenetic phases of regeneration of bone: a historical and experimental study, *J Bone Joint Surg Am* 38(3):593-600, 1956.
7. Gray JC, Elves MW: Donor cells' contribution to osteogenesis in experimental cancellous bone grafts, *Clin Orthop Relat Res* (163):261-271, 1982.
8. Burwell RG: Studies in the transplantation of bone. VII. The fresh composite homograft-autograft of cancellous bone: an analysis of factors leading to osteogenesis in marrow transplants and in marrow-containing bone grafts, *J Bone Joint Surg Br* 46:110-140, 1964.
9. Misch CE, Dietsh F: Bone-grafting materials in implant dentistry, *Implant Dent* 2(3):158-167, 1993.
10. Knighton DR, Halliday B, Hunt TK: Oxygen as an antibiotic: the effect of inspired oxygen on infection, *Arch Surg* 119(2):199-204, 1984.
11. Marx RE, Garg AK: Bone graft physiology with use of platelet-rich plasma and hyperbaric oxygen. In: Jensen O, editor: The sinus bone graft, Chicago, 1998, Quintessence, pp 183-190.
12. Marx RE, Garg AK: Bone structure, metabolism, and physiology: its impact on dental implantology, *Implant Dent* 7(4):267-276, 1998.
13. Marx RE: Clinical application of bone biology to mandibular and maxillary reconstruction, *Clin Plast Surg* 21(3):377-392, 1994.
14. Marx RE: Philosophy and particulars of autogenous bone grafting, *Oral Maxillofac Surg Clin North Am* 5(4):599-612, 1993.
15. Albrektsson T, Zarb GA: Current interpretations of the osseointegrated response: clinical significance, *Int J Prosthodont* 6(2):95-105, 1993.
16. Albrektsson and Isidor 1994.
17. Albrektsson T, Zarb GA, Worthington P, Eriksson AR: The long-term efficacy of currently used dental implants: a review and proposed criteria of success, *Int J Oral Maxillofac Implants* 1:11-25, 1986.
18. Syftestad GT, Urist MR: Bone aging, *Clin Orthop Relat Res* (162):288-297, 1982.
19. Ekeland A, Engesaeter LB, Langeland N: Influence of age on mechanical properties of healing fractures and intact bone in rats, *Acta Orthop Scand* 53:527-534, 1982.

20. Shirota T, Ohno K, Suzuki K, Michi K: The effect of aging on the healing of hydroxylapatite implants, *J Oral Maxillofac Surg* 51(1):51-56, 1993.

21. Matukas VJ: Medical risks associated with dental implants, *J Dent Educ* 52:745-747, 1988.

22. Zoldos J, Kent JN: Healing of endosseous implants. In: Block MS, Kent JN, editors: Endosseous implants for maxillofacial reconstructions, Philadelphia, 1995, WB Saunders, pp 40-69.

23. Adell R: The surgical principles of osseointegration. In: Worthington P, Branemark PI, editors: Advanced osseointegration surgery: applications in the maxillofacial region, Chicago, 1992, Quintessence, pp 94-107.

24. Garg AK, Winkler S, Bakaeen LG, Mekayarajjananonth T: Dental implants and the geriatric patient, *Implant Dent* 6(3):168-173, 1997.

25. Smith RA, Berger R, Dodson TB: Risk factors associated with dental implants in healthy and medically compromised patients, *Int J Oral Maxillofac Implants* 7(3):367-372, 1992.

26. Bain CA, Moy PK: The association between the failure of dental implants and cigarette smoking, *Int J Oral Maxillofac Implants* 8(6):609-615, 1983.

27. Gorman LM, Lambert PM, Morris HF, Ochi S, Winkler S: The effect of smoking on implant survival at second-stage surgery: DICRG Interim Report No. 5, Dental Implant Clinical Research Group, *Implant Dent* 3(3):165-168, 1994.

28. Bain CA: Smoking and implant failure—benefits of a smoking cessation protocol, *Int J Oral Maxillofac Implants* 11(6):756-759, 1996.

29. Lindquist LW, Carlsson GE, Jemt T: A prospective 15-year follow-up study of mandibular fixed prostheses supported by osseointegrated implants: clinical results and marginal bone loss, *Clin Oral Implants Res* 7(4):329-336, 1996. Erratum in *Clin Oral Implants Res* 8(4):342, 1997.

30. Lemons JE, Laskin DM, Roberts WE, Tarnow DP, Shipman C Jr, Paczkowski C, Lorey RE, English C: Changes in patient screening for a clinical study of dental implants after increased awareness of tobacco use as a risk factor, *J Oral Maxillofac Surg* 55(12 suppl 5):72-75, 1997.

31. Esposito M, Thomsen P, Molne J, Gretzer C, Ericson LE, Lekholm U: Immunohistochemistry of soft tissues surrounding late failures of Branemark implants, *Clin Oral Implants Res* 8(5):352-366, 1997.

32. Friberg B, Jemt T, Lekholm U: Early failures in 4,641 consecutively placed Branemark dental implants: a study from stage 1 surgery to the connection of completed prostheses, *Int J Oral Maxillofac Implants* 6(2):142-146, 1991.

33. Drago CJ: Rates of osseointegration of dental implants with regard to anatomical location, *J Prosthodont* 1(1):29-31, 1992.

34. Buser D, Mericske-Stern R, Bernard JP, Behneke A, Behneke N, Hirt HP, Belser UC, Lang NP: Long-term evaluation of non-submerged ITI implants. Part 1: 8-year life table analysis of a prospective multi-center study with 2359 implants, *Clin Oral Implants Res* 8(3):161-172, 1997.

35. Friberg B, Nilson H, Olsson M, Palmquist C: Mk II: the self-tapping Branemark implant: 5-year results of a prospective 3-center study, *Clin Oral Implants Res* 8(4):279-285, 1997.

36. von Wowern N: Variations in bone mass within the cortices of the mandible, *Scand J Dent Res* 85(6):444-455, 1977.

37. Friberg B, Sennerby L, Roos J, Lekholm U: Identification of bone quality in conjunction with insertion of titanium implants: a pilot study in jaw autopsy specimens, *Clin Oral Implants Res* 6(4):213-219, 1995.

38. Truhlar RS, Orenstein IH, Morris HF, Ochi S: Distribution of bone quality in patients receiving endosseous dental implants, *J Oral Maxillofac Surg* 55(12 suppl 5):38-45, 1997.

39. Truhlar RS, Farish SE, Scheitler LE, Morris HF, Ochi S: Bone quality and implant design-related outcomes through stage II surgical uncovering of Spectra-System root form implants, *J Oral Maxillofac Surg* 55(12 suppl 5):46-54, 1997.

40. Ulm CW, Kneissel M, Hahn M, Solar P, Matejka M, Donath K: Characteristics of the cancellous bone of edentulous mandibles, *Clin Oral Implants Res* 8(2):125-130, 1997.

41. Rangert B, Jemt T, Jorneus L: Forces and moments on Branemark implants, *Int J Oral Maxillofac Implants* 4(3):241-247, 1989.

42. Rangert BR, Sullivan RM, Jemt TM: Load factor control for implants in the posterior partially edentulous segment, *Int J Oral Maxillofac Implants* 12(3):360-370, 1997.

43. Newman MG, Flemmig TF: Bacteria-host interactions. In: Worthington P, Branemark PI, editors: Advanced osseointegration surgery: applications in the maxillofacial region, Chicago, 1992, Quintessence, pp 67-79.

44. Granstrom G: The use of hyperbaric oxygen to prevent implant loss in the irradiated patient. In: Worthington P, Branemark PI, editors: Advanced osseointegration surgery: applications in the maxillofacial region, Chicago, 1992, Quintessence, pp 336-345.

45. Shafer WG, Hine MK, Levy BM: Physical and chemical injuries of the oral cavity. In: Shafer WG, Hine MK, Levy BM, editors: A textbook of oral pathology, Philadelphia, 1983, WB Saunders, pp 528-593.

46. Cooper JS, Fu K, Marks J, Silverman S: Late effects of radiation therapy in the head and neck region, *Int J Radiat Oncol Biol Phys* 31(5):1141-1164, 1995.

47. Jacobsson M, Jonsson A, Albrektsson T, Turesson I: Dose-response for bone regeneration after single doses of 60Co irradiation, *Int J Radiat Oncol Biol Phys* 11(11):1963-1969, 1985.

48. Jacobsson MG, Jonsson AK, Albrektsson TO, Turesson IE: Short- and long-term effects of irradiation on bone regeneration, *Plast Reconstr Surg* 76(6):841-850, 1985.

49. Jacobsson M, Albrektsson T: Integration of bone implants in a previously irradiated bed. In: Van Steenberghe D, Albrektsson T, Branemark PI, Henry PJ, Holt R, Liden G, editors: Tissue integration in oral and maxillo-facial reconstruction, Amsterdam, 1986, Excerpta Medica, pp 110-117.

50. Schon R, Ohno K, Kudo M, Michi K: Peri-implant tissue reaction in bone irradiated the fifth day after implantation in rabbits: histologic and histomorphometric measurements, *Int J Oral Maxillofac Implants* 11(2):228-238, 1996.

51. Ohrnell LO, Branemark R, Nyman J, Nilsson P, Thomsen P: Effects of irradiation on the biomechanics of osseointegration: an experimental in vivo study in rats, *Scand J Plast Reconstr Surg Hand Surg* 31(4):281-293, 1997.

52. Hum SA, Larsen PE: The effect of radiation at the titanium/bone interface. In: Laney WR, Tolman DE, editors: Tissue integration in oral, orthopedic and maxillofacial reconstruction, Proceedings of the Second International Congress in oral, orthopedic and maxillofacial reconstruction, Chicago, 1992, Quintessence, pp 234-239.

53. Jisander S, Grenthe B, Alberius P: Dental implant survival in the irradiated jaw: a preliminary report, *Int J Oral Maxillofac Implants* 12(5):643-648, 1997.

54. Marx RE: Osteoradionecrosis: a new concept of its pathophysiology, *J Oral Maxillofac Surg* 41(5):283-288, 1983.

55. Murray CG, Herson J, Daly TE, Zimmerman S: Radiation necrosis of the mandible: a 10 year study. Part I. Factors influencing the onset of necrosis, *Int J Radiat Oncol Biol Phys* 6(5):543-548, 1980.

56. Beumer J 3rd, Harrison R, Sanders B, Kurrasch M: Preradiation dental extractions and the incidence of bone necrosis, *Head Neck Surg* 5(6):514-521, 1983.

57. Nilsson P, Albrektsson T, Granstrom G, Rockert HO: The effect of hyperbaric oxygen treatment on bone regeneration: an experimental study using the bone harvest chamber in the rabbit, *Int J Oral Maxillofac Implants* 3(1):43-48, 1988.

58. Larsen PE, Stronczek MJ, Beck FM, Rohrer M: Osteointegration of implants in radiated bone with and without adjunctive hyperbaric oxygen, *J Oral Maxillofac Surg* 51(3):280-287, 1993.

59. Johnsson K, Hansson A, Granstrom G, Jacobsson M, Turesson I: The effects of hyperbaric oxygenation on bone-titanium implant interface strength with and without preceding irradiation, *Int J Oral Maxillofac Implants* 8(4):415-419, 1993.

60. Granstrom G, Tjellstrom A, Branemark PI, Fornander J: Bone-anchored reconstruction of the irradiated head and neck cancer patient, *Otolaryngol Head Neck Surg* 108(4):334-343, 1993.

61. Granstrom G, Bergstrom K, Tjellstrom A, Branemark PI: A detailed analysis of titanium implants lost in irradiated tissues, *Int J Oral Maxillofac Implants* 9:653-662, 1994.

62. Morris HF, Manz MC, Tarolli JH: Success of multiple endosseous dental implant designs to second-stage surgery across study sites, *J Oral Maxillofac Surg* 55(12 suppl 5):76-82, 1997.

63. Lambert PM, Morris HF, Ochi S: Positive effect of surgical experience with implants on second-stage implant survival, *J Oral Maxillofac Surg* 55(12 suppl 5):12-18, 1997.

64. Listgarten MA: Clinical trials of endosseous implants: issues in analysis and interpretation, *Ann Periodontol* 2(1):299-313, 1997.

65. Andersson B, Odman P, Lindvall AM, Branemark PI: Surgical and prosthodontic training of general practitioners for single tooth implants: a study of treatments performed at four general practitioners' offices and at a specialist clinic after 2 years, *J Oral Rehabil* 22(8):543-548, 1995.

66. Iyer S, Weiss C, Mehta A: Effects of drill speed on heat production and the rate and quality of bone formation in dental implant osteotomies. Part II: Relationship between drill speed and healing, *Int J Prosthodont* 10(6):536-540, 1997.

67. Gristina AG: Biomaterial-centered infection: microbial adhesion versus tissue integration, *Science* 237(4822):1588-1595, 1987.

68. Gristina AG, Costerton JW: Bacterial adherence and the glycocalyx and their role in musculoskeletal infection, *Orthop Clin North Am* 15(3):517-535, 1984.

69. Gristina AG, Costerton JW: Bacterial adherence to biomaterials and tissue: the significance of its role in clinical sepsis, *J Bone Joint Surg Am* 67(2):264-273, 1985.

70. Costerton JW, Irvin RT, Cheng KJ: The bacterial glycocalyx in nature and disease, *Annu Rev Microbiol* 35:299-324, 1981.

71. Johnson GM, Lee DA, Regelmann WE, Gray ED, Peters G, Quie PG: Interference with granulocyte function by *Staphylococcus epidermidis* slime, *Infect Immun* 54(1):13-20, 1986.

72. Peters G, Gray ED, Johnson GM: Immunomodulating properties of extracellular slime substance. In: Bisno AL, Waldvogel FA, editors: Infections associated with indwelling medical devices, Washington, DC, 1989, American Society for Microbiology, pp 61-74.

73. Gristina AG, Hobgood CD, Webb LX, Myrvik QN: Adhesive colonization of biomaterials and antibiotic resistance, *Biomaterials* 8(6):423-426, 1987.

74. Gristina AG, Jennings RA, Naylor PT, Myrvik QN, Webb LX: Comparative in vitro antibiotic resistance of surface-colonizing coagulase-negative staphylococci, *Antimicrob Agents Chemother* 33(6):813-816, 1989.

75. Nichols WW, Evans MJ, Slack MP, Walmsley HL: The penetration of antibiotics into aggregates of mucoid and non-mucoid *Pseudomonas aeruginosa*, *J Gen Microbiol* 135(5):1291-1303, 1989.

76. Lazzara RJ: Immediate implant placement into extraction sites: surgical and restorative advantages, *Int J Periodontics Restorative Dent* 9(5):332-343, 1989.

77. Lazzara RJ, Porter SS, Testori T, Galante J, Zetterqvist L: A prospective multicenter study evaluating loading of osseotite implants two months after placement: one-year results, *J Esthet Dent* 10(6):280-289, 1998.

78. Peleg M, Mazor Z, Chaushu G, Garg AK: Sinus floor augmentation with simultaneous implant placement in the severely atrophic maxilla, *J Periodontol* 69(12):1397-1403, 1998.

79. Tatum H Jr: Maxillary and sinus implant reconstructions, *Dent Clin North Am* 30(2):207-229, 1986.

80. Razavi R, Zena RB, Khan Z, Gould AR: Anatomic site evaluation of edentulous maxillae for dental implant placement, *J Prosthodont* 4(2):90-94, 1995.

81. Garg AK, Quinones CR: Augmentation of the maxillary sinus: a surgical technique, *Pract Periodontics Aesthet Dent* 9(2):211-219, 1997.

82. Moy PK, Lundgren S, Holmes RE: Maxillary sinus augmentation: histomorphometric analysis of graft materials for maxillary sinus floor augmentation, *J Oral Maxillofac Surg* 51(8):857-862, 1993.

83. Kent JN, Block MS: Simultaneous maxillary sinus floor bone grafting and placement of hydroxylapatite-coated implants, *J Oral Maxillofac Surg* 47(3):238-242, 1989.

84. Jensen J, Simonsen EK, Sindet-Pedersen S: Reconstruction of the severely resorbed maxilla with bone grafting and osseointegrated implants: a preliminary report, *J Oral Maxillofac Surg* 48(1):27-32, 1990.

85. Raghoebar GM, Brouwer TJ, Reintsema H, Van Oort RP: Augmentation of the maxillary sinus floor with autogenous bone for the placement of endosseous implants: a preliminary report, *J Oral Maxillofac Surg* 51(11):1198-1203, 1993.

86. Adell R, Lekholm U, Grondahl K, Branemark PI, Lindstrom J, Jacobsson M: Reconstruction of severely resorbed edentulous maxillae using osseointegrated fixtures in immediate autogenous bone grafts, *Int J Oral Maxillofac Implants* 5(3):233-246, 1990.

87. Adell R, Eriksson B, Lekholm U, Branemark PI, Jemt T: Long-term follow-up study of osseointegrated implants in the treatment of totally edentulous jaws, *Int J Oral Maxillofac Implants* 5(4):347-359, 1990.

88. Kahnberg KE, Nystrom E, Bartholdsson L: Combined use of bone grafts and Branemark fixtures in the treatment of severely resorbed maxillae, *Int J Oral Maxillofac Implants* 4(4):297-304, 1989.

89. Nystrom E, Kahnberg KE, Gunne J: Bone grafts and Branemark implants in the treatment of the severely resorbed maxilla: a

2-year longitudinal study, *Int J Oral Maxillofac Implants* 8(1):45-53, 1993.

90. Lane JM: Bone graft substitutes, *West J Med* 163(6):565-566, 1995.

91. Rummelhart JM, Mellonig JT, Gray JL, Towle HJ: A comparison of freeze-dried bone allograft and demineralized freeze-dried bone allograft in human periodontal osseous defects, *J Periodontol* 60(12):655-663, 1989.

92. Mellonig JT: Decalcified freeze-dried bone allograft as an implant material in human periodontal defects, *Int J Periodontics Restorative Dent* 4(6):40-55, 1984.

93. Tatum OH Jr, Lebowitz MS, Tatum CA, Borgner RA: Sinus augmentation: rationale, development, long-term results, *N Y State Dent J* 59(5):43-48, 1993.

94. Tatum OH Jr: Osseous grafts in intra-oral sites, *J Oral Implantol* 22(1):51-52, 1996.

95. Schepers E, de Clercq M, Ducheyne P, Kempeneers R: Bioactive glass particulate material as a filler for bone lesions, *J Oral Rehabil* 18(5):439-452, 1991.

96. Schepers EJ, Ducheyne P, Barbier L, Schepers S: Bioactive glass particles of narrow size range: a new material for the repair of bone defects, *Implant Dent* 2(3):151-156, 1993.

97. Koole R, Bosker H, van der Dussen FN: Late secondary autogenous bone grafting in cleft patients comparing mandibular (ectomesenchymal) and iliac crest (mesenchymal) grafts, *J Craniomaxillofac Surg* 17(suppl 1):28-30, 1989.

98. Wood RM, Moore DL: Grafting of the maxillary sinus with intra-orally harvested autogenous bone prior to implant placement, *Int J Oral Maxillofac Implants* 3(3):209-214, 1988.

99. Jensen J, Sindet-Pedersen S: Autogenous mandibular bone grafts and osseointegrated implants for reconstruction of the severely atrophied maxilla: a preliminary report, *J Oral Maxillofac Surg* 49(12):1277-1287, 1991.

100. Second-hand bones? *Lancet* 340(8833):1443, 1992.

101. Meffert RM: Current usage of bone fill as an adjunct in implant dentistry, *Dent Implantol Update* 9(2):9-12, 1998.

102. Furusawa T, Mizunuma K: Osteoconductive properties and efficacy of resorbable bioactive glass as a bone-grafting material, *Implant Dent* 6(2):93-101, 1997.

103. Boyne PJ: Animal studies of application of rhBMP-2 in maxillofacial reconstruction, *Bone* 19(1 suppl):83S-92S, 1996.

104. Betts NJ, Miloro M: Modification of the sinus lift procedure for septa in the maxillary antrum, *J Oral Maxillofac Surg* 52(3):332-333, 1994.

105. Ulm CW, Solar P, Krennmair G, Matejka M, Watzek G: Incidence and suggested surgical management of septa in sinus-lift procedures, *Int J Oral Maxillofac Implants* 10(4):462-465, 1995.

106. Garg AK, Morales MJ, Navarro I, Duarte F: Autogenous mandibular bone grafts in the treatment of the resorbed maxillary anterior alveolar ridge: rationale and approach, *Implant Dent* 7(3):169-176, 1998.

107. Jensen J, Sindet-Pedersen S, Oliver AJ: Varying treatment strategies for reconstruction of maxillary atrophy with implants: results in 98 patients, *J Oral Maxillofac Surg* 52(3):210-216, 1994.

108. Breine U, Branemark PI: Reconstruction of alveolar jaw bone: an experimental and clinical study of immediate and preformed autologous bone grafts in combination with osseointegrated implants, *Scand J Plast Reconstr Surg* 14(1):23-48, 1980.

109. Misch CM, Misch CE: The repair of localized severe ridge defects for implant placement using mandibular bone grafts, *Implant Dent* 4(4):261-267, 1995.

110. Garg AK: Nasal sinus lift: an innovative technique for implant insertions, *Dent Implantol Update* 8(7):49-53, 1997.

111. Garg AK: Subnasal elevation and bone augmentation. In: Jensen O, editor: The sinus bone graft, Chicago, 1998, Quintessence, pp 177-181.

chapter 17

Considerations for Implants in the Geriatric Patient

I T has been predicted that there will be an increase in the proportion of people older than age 80 by the year 2020.[1] Most elderly people are healthy and active, and many are seeking dental care to improve their oral function as they continue to age (Figure 17-1). Over the past decade, the number of patients presenting with more teeth and fewer prostheses has increased. This trend is the result of increased emphasis by dental professionals on prevention and the need for patients to improve their oral hygiene practices.[2] However, the prosthodontic needs of elderly patients are extensive, and these patients will expect to maintain high standards of oral function.[1]

The use of removable dentures does not allow for adequate oral function in many geriatric patients, and these patients may have difficulty adapting to full dentures (Figure 17-2). Firmly retained, functional prostheses should be used in these patients for physiological and psychological reasons, as well as for the role that adequate oral function plays in proper digestion and nutrition.[1] Patients who do not receive adequate oral rehabilitation to improve function and esthetics may withdraw from society and experience a loss of self-esteem.[2]

Dental implants and implant-supported prostheses have been used successfully in geriatric patients (Figure 17-3). In a study of implant placement in elderly patients, Kondell et al found that the success rate was similar to that

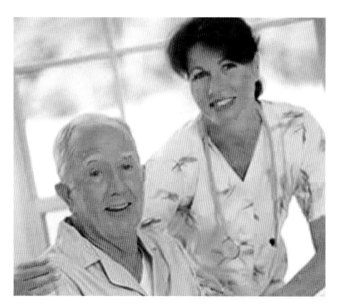

FIGURE 17-1 ■ As more senior citizens live healthier and longer lives, the need for oral care and treatment has increased.

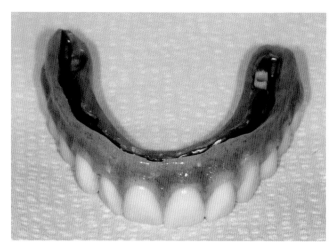

FIGURE 17-3 ■ Implant-supported prosthesis with a bar.

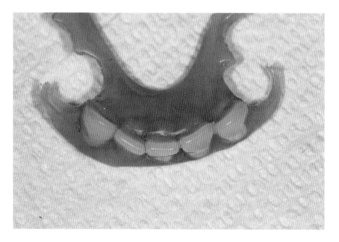

FIGURE 17-2 ■ The use of partial dentures is very common in geriatric patients.

found when implants were placed in younger patients.[1] However, a single type of implant is not appropriate for all patients. The size, shape, quality, and quantity of bone are different in each patient. Clinicians who place dental implants in elderly patients must be aware of the systemic influences that affect alveolar bone and must understand bone physiology, metabolism, and the response of alveolar bone to systemic changes. It is important for clinicians to understand that alveolar bone responds similarly to systemic challenges as bone in other skeletal sites. Factors related to initial integration of the implants, such as maintaining vital osseous peri-implant margins, preserving subperiosteal osteogenic capacity, and stabilizing the implant

firmly within bone, can be affected by the status of the alveolar bone and its associated structures.[3]

Age-related Considerations

As people age, their oral tissue undergoes change. Many physical, endocrine, and metabolic changes are associated with aging, and clinicians must be aware of how these changes can affect implant placement in older patients. Geriatric patients may present with a variety of problems that are not encountered when one is treating younger patients. Severe resorption of the alveolar process usually occurs following tooth loss in the posterior maxilla, resulting in an inadequate amount of bone for implant placement.[4] Common problems encountered in elderly patients include diabetes, which can cause decreased bone density; systemic disease and osteoporosis, both of which can cause alveolar bone loss; compromised oral tissues from irradiation, which can cause impaired wound healing; and xerostomia, which can contribute to plaque formation and an increased incidence of caries.[2]

In addition, many elderly patients present with a variety of nutritional deficiencies. Deficiencies in vitamins A, B, and C can result in decreased cohesiveness and integrity of the epithelial layer, reduction in cell metabolism, and poorly differentiated connective tissue cells and fibers, respectively, leading to friability of the oral mucosa. Vitamin B deficiency can lead to loss of papillae on the tongue. Deficient protein and zinc intake can cause a delay in the renewal of taste buds, resulting in a depressed sense of taste. Degeneration of the olfactory receptors in the roof of the nasal cavity also occurs with aging. Patients may not notice the decrease in their sense of taste and smell until the time of placement of a new prosthesis, when attention is drawn to the mouth. As a result, patients may blame the prosthesis for the decrease noted in these senses. Clinicians should obtain a written dietary history from their patients, including how food is prepared, to determine whether patients have satisfactory mineral intake to undergo implant surgery and the placement of prosthodontics.[5]

Smith et al studied the risks associated with the placement of dental implants to determine whether a medically compromised status, the age or gender of a patient, or the number of implants placed affected implant failure or led to an increased incidence of complications.[6] They found that the patient's medical status and the number of medical problems were not statistically associated with complications related to implant surgery or implant failure. However, patients with surgical risks must be assessed before implants are placed. Local factors, such as the trajectory, quantity, and quality of bone, and surgical and prosthetic techniques probably are more significant indicators of a favorable outcome than are a patient's associated medical conditions. It was shown that the age and gender of the patient were not statistically associated with implant failure. According to the authors, a more accurate risk assessment of elderly patients would include their biological age, rather than their chronological age. The authors also found that patients undergoing implant surgery do not have an increased incidence of anesthetic-related complications.[6]

A statistically significant finding of this study was that implant failure and/or increased risk for a surgical complication was affected by the number of implants placed. This increased complication rate may be the result of increased mucoperiosteal stripping, operating time, and wound contamination that occur with the placement of multiple implants.[6]

Campbell et al studied the incidence of cardiac arrhythmia in geriatric patients undergoing minor oral surgical procedures.[7] Half of the patients in this study were receiving pharmacological treatment for known cardiovascular disease. Results showed that the overall incidence of rhythm disturbances was no different between patients with known cardiovascular disease and those without known disease, with increasing age, or between men and women. None of the arrhythmias that occurred during the study were considered to be life threatening. According to the authors, these findings suggest that patients who are taking medication for cardiovascular disease are not at increased risk for rhythm disturbances during simple, in-office, oral surgical procedures. On the other hand, it cannot be assumed that patients who are not taking medications for cardiovascular disease are disease-free. Special treatment considerations or monitoring techniques may not be necessary, because it has been shown that the risk for adverse medical outcomes is minimal for most patients with cardiovascular disease. In addition, even though rhythm disturbances are common in ambulatory geriatric patients, they usually are benign in nature, and pharmacological treatment for cardiovascular disease is not indicative of their presence.[7]

Discussion

The importance of proper oral hygiene and adequate oral function in elderly patients cannot be underemphasized. With a larger proportion of older people living healthy and active lives, clinicians are going to be expected to provide dental services to maintain satisfactory oral function in these patients. However, extensive treatment may be required. Overall poor dental and prosthodontic status has been seen in cross-sectional studies of institutionalized elderly patients. In a study of geriatric patients, Mojon et al found that only 17% of single crowns and fixed partial dentures were considered to be adequate for proper oral function.[8] Increased plaque accumulation and gingival inflammation have been associated with poorly fitting restorations. The authors found a loss of periodontal attachment in natural teeth adjacent to removable partial dentures, even when the denture was well maintained. An increased incidence of caries was seen in patients with removable partial dentures compared with those without dentures[8].

Implants and implant-supported prostheses are a viable treatment option in geriatric patients. However, successful results depend on careful attention to detail during surgical and prosthodontic procedures. In addition, specific patient selection criteria must be met. Patients should be motivated and cooperative and should not smoke or have parafunctional habits. Patients must understand their specific dental procedure and must not have unrealistic demands and/or expectations. Clinicians must make patients aware of the fact that esthetic compromises often are necessary.[2]

When implants are placed in elderly patients, immediate loading of the implants has been suggested.[9] Immediate loading eliminates the need for a second surgical procedure to uncover the implants, as well as an interim prosthesis, and decreases postoperative discomfort, treatment time, and the cost of the procedure.

Vassos recommended using this procedure in elderly patients with an adequate amount of type I or type II bone. A minimum of four 12-mm or five 10-mm root form, hydroxyapatite-coated implants are used in the mandibular anterior symphysis with a bar-retained overdenture, which is inserted on the third postoperative day.[9]

Immediate extraction and implant placement reduces the healing time between extraction, implant placement, exposure, and function. Because of this reduction in healing time, immediate implant placement has been recommended in patients with a compromised medical status (Figure

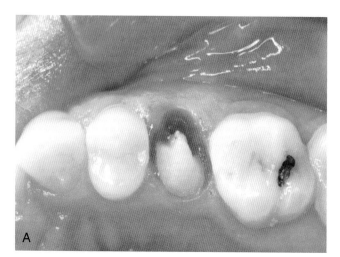

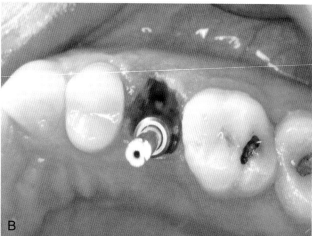

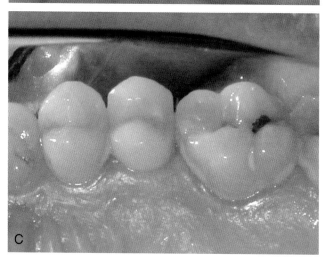

FIGURE 17-4 ■ **A** through **C,** Immediate extraction and implant placement reduces healing time and has been recommended for patients with a compromised medical status.

17-4).[10] In addition, there is usually an ample amount of bone to ensure initial stability of the implant with immediate implant placement. Delaying placement until after extraction may result in an alveolar process that is too thin for implant placement.[10]

The primary disadvantage of immediate implant placement is the need for more complicated soft tissue techniques to achieve an esthetically pleasing result. In addition, surgically related problems, such as premature implant exposure due to problems with the flap design, inadvertent placement of implants too far apically, and damage to the alveolar bone resulting from complications during extraction, may occur. The incidence of premature implant exposure can be reduced by submerging the implant slightly below the osseous crest and using horizontal mattress sutures.[11]

It has been shown that implant failure occurs most frequently in the posterior maxilla. In patients with inadequate bone quantity for implant placement, bone grafting of the floor of the maxillary sinus has been performed, followed by implant placement. A study by Ulm et al showed that the height, not the width, of the alveolar ridge was the limiting factor in the placement of implants in the posterior maxilla.[4] Thin bone walls were found with some alveolar ridges that appeared to be high and wide from the outside, indicating that pneumatization appears to considerably influence bone loss. In the posterior maxilla, a decrease in the density of alveolar bone may be caused by mechanical and inflammatory factors, osteoporotic changes, the type of prosthetic treatment used, and long-term edentulousness. However, these factors do not have a direct influence on bone volume and ridge configuration.

When implant failure occurs, questions are raised regarding the quality and quantity of the recipient bone and the adequacy of the surgical technique, as well as whether disturbance of the healing conditions in general occurred (Figure 17-5). Using osteometry, Blomqvist et al showed that there were significant differences in relative bone mass density between patients with failed implants (mean bone mass density, 89.2%) and age- and sex-matched controls (mean bone mass density, 98.6%).[12] With the use of osteometry, the bone mass density can be assessed quantitatively. Results of this study suggested that osteometry may be useful for future patient selection. The authors evaluated the risk for implant failure in each patient using an equation of multiple response: $y = 131.8 - 1.2 \times BMD\%$, in which y represents the relative total implant loss (%), and $BMD\%$ signifies the mean value for bone mineral density matched for age and sex. They found that the use of this equation produced accurate results; however, additional studies are needed.

SUMMARY

Many factors need to be taken into account when implants are placed in geriatric patients. With proper patient selection and consideration of specific age-related factors, and how they can affect implant placement, a successful and esthetically pleasing outcome can be achieved.

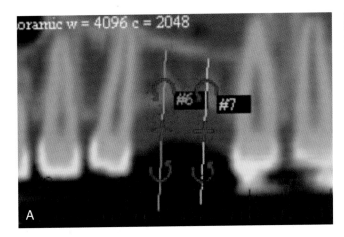

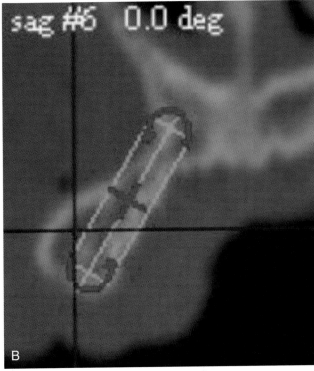

FIGURE 17-5 ■ **A, B,** To minimize implant failures, the clinician should make a treatment plan based on the patient's conditions, such as the height and width of available bone. This generally means cone beam CT scans to determine bone width and angulation, which is especially important in the geriatric patient.

REFERENCES

1. Kondell PA, Nordenram A, Landt H: Titanium implants in the treatment of edentulousness: influence of patient's age on prognosis, *Gerodontics* 4:280-284, 1988.
2. Garg AK, Winkler S, Bakaeen LG, Mekayarajjananonth T: Dental implants and the geriatric patient, *Implant Dent* 6(3):168-173, 1997.
3. Shapiro S: A discussion of alveolar bone physiology relative to implants for the elderly, *J Oklahoma Dent Assoc* 83:34-37, 1992.
4. Ulm CW, Solar P, Gsellmann B, et al: The edentulous maxillary alveolar process in the region of the maxillary sinus—a study of physical dimension, *Int J Oral Maxillofac Surg* 24:279-282, 1995.
5. Winkler S, Mekayarajjananonth T, Garg AK, Tewari DS: Nutrition and the geriatric patient, *Implant Dent* 6(4):291-294, 1997.
6. Smith RA, Berger R, Dodson TB: Risk factors associated with dental implants in healthy and medically compromised patients, *Int J Oral Maxillofac Implants* 7:367-372, 1992.
7. Campbell JH, Huizinga PJ, Das SK, et al: Incidence and significance of cardiac arrhythmia in geriatric oral surgery patients, *Oral Surg Oral Med Oral Pathol* 82:42-46, 1996.
8. Mojon P, Rentsch A, Budtz-Jorgensen E: Relationship between prosthodontic status, caries, and periodontal disease in a geriatric population, *Int J Prosthodont* 8:564-571, 1995.
9. Vassos DM: Immediate loading of implants: an improved treatment for the elderly, *Dental Implantol Update* 7:81-82, 1996.
10. Rosenquist B, Grenthe B: Immediate placement of implants into extraction sockets: implant survival, *Int J Oral Maxillofac Implants* 11:205-209, 1996.
11. Arlin M: Immediate placement of dental implants into extraction sockets: surgically-related difficulties, *Oral Health* 83:23-31, 1993.
12. Blomqvist JE, Alberius P, Isaksson S, et al: Factors in implant integration failure after bone grafting: an osteometric and endocrinologic matched analysis, *Int J Oral Maxillofac Surg* 25:63-68, 1996.

chapter 18

Peri-implantitis: Prevention, Diagnosis, and Treatment

P ERI-IMPLANTITIS has become one of the most significant barriers to the extended use of permanently or temporarily implanted biomaterial components in humans. These components include joint replacements, heart valves, vascular prostheses, sutures, intravascular catheters, and dental implants.[1-3] This chapter describes the soft tissue–dental implant interface, normal flora within the oral cavity, the development of subgingival microflora around dental implants, the prevention of peri-implantitis, its diagnosis, and possible treatments for the ailing and failing implant.

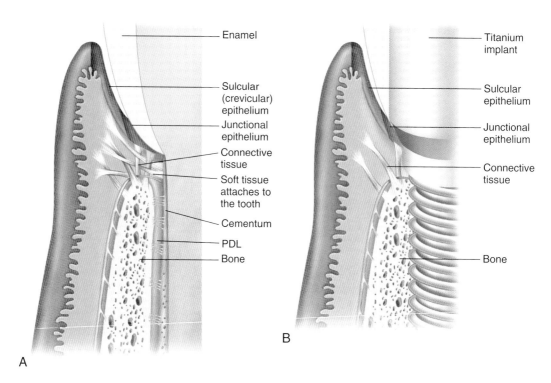

FIGURE 18-1 ■ A comparison of the soft and hard tissues approximating a natural tooth versus a dental implant. (From Rose RJ, Mealey BL: *Periodontics: medicine, surgery, and implants,* St. Louis, 2004, Mosby.)

Soft Tissue–implant Interface

Much research has focused on the soft tissue–implant interface.[4-8] Most implant failures, especially during the first 10 to 15 years of modern oral implantology, were associated with clinical signs of inflammation in the peri-implant soft tissue, such as gingivitis, suppuration, soft tissue edema, bleeding, and increased pocket depth. Inflammation at the soft tissue–implant interface is rarely a major complication. In current practice, this complication is rarely a problem because today's implants are biocompatible, have a highly polished transmucosal surface, and are osseointegrated (stable).

Now, the critical factor for implant success is the site chosen where the implant post penetrates the mucosal covering of the bone. Clinically, the site should be comparable with that of a natural tooth. When inflammation is not present, the keratinized gingiva is tightly apposed to the implant, and a periodontal probe can be inserted only a short distance into the peri-implant gingival sulcus (Figure 18-1). At a healthy site, an adequate functional attachment will exist between the implant and the soft tissue.[9] Some authors though, dispute this description, argue that the sulcular area around the implant more closely resembles an epithelized "crypt" rather than junctional epithelium.[10] According to these authors, if the sulcular area were actually attached in some manner to the titanium–implant surface, removal of

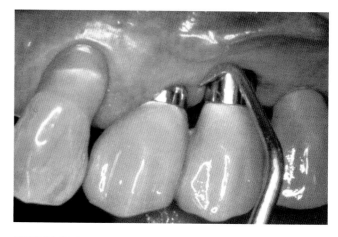

FIGURE 18-2 ■ Due to the lack of soft tissue attachment to the implant abutment, it is important for the dental hygienist to not overinstrument into the sulcus.

the collar of the abutment would result in both resistance and bleeding points. Clinically, though, this result does not occur (Figure 18-2). Thus, even though soft tissue has been shown to bond to the abutment surfaces, the premise of junctional epithelium and hemidesmosomal attachment is widely disputed.

At the implant site, the epithelial junction with peri-implant connective tissue is comparable with the oral junctional epithelium. However, the epithelia differ greatly. Investigations in the mid-1980s showed that the epithelium at the implant site was able to attach via hemidesmosomes

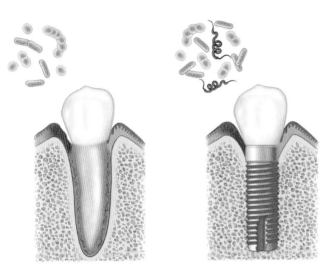

FIGURE 18-3 ■ Marginal health on a natural tooth depicting some redness, loss of attachment, and presence of cocci and rod-like types of bacteria *(left)*, and slight inflammation on an implant indicating some redness but no loss of osseointegration, presence of cocci, rods, and spirochete types of bacteria.

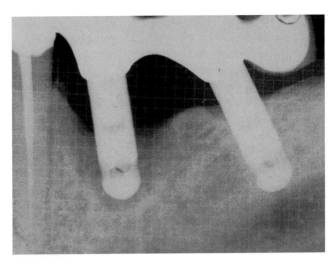

FIGURE 18-4 ■ Implant bone loss shown on a periapical radiograph around a cylindrical hydroxyapatite-coated implant.

to the surface of titanium, ceramic, or aluminum oxide ceramic implants.[11,12] As in the natural tooth, this condition is characterized by a high cell turnover and marked left displacement in the inflammatory infiltrate. According to periodontal investigations, the health of the underlying structures determines the success of the epithelial attachment.[13] A successful attachment requires that the implant be tightly enclosed by inflammation-free supra-alveolar connective tissue.

The tissue around the implant collar consists of a free gingival margin composed of collagenous stroma, covered by squamous epithelium. From the marginal crest down to the bottom of the sulcus, tissue histology gradually changes from keratinized to nonkeratinized epithelium. In addition, the width of the sulcular epithelium narrows as it progresses to the lower recess of the sulcus, with the outermost epithelial cells appearing more flattened than the basal cells.[4,5] All of these morphologic features make the peri-implant sulcus very similar to that seen around natural teeth. Perhaps the most prominent difference between the two is the absence of Sharpey's fibers around the implant, which leaves it without a very important defense mechanism. Thus, the only barrier against bacterial penetration into the sulcus of the implant is the adhesive property of the junctional epithelium.

Subepithelial gingival fibers attached to the cementum are crucial to the gingival/periodontal health of the natural tooth. However, it is unlikely that this healthy attachment can exist around the neck of the implant, although some researchers attest to such a possibility.[14-17] Instead, only a mere cuff of fibrous connective tissue supports the epithelial seal. The lack of a definitive connective tissue–implant attachment with an interposed fibrous tissue interface between the bone and the implant appears to be an area of weakness with implants.[1-3] If this interface gradually widens, peri-implant pocket

formation occurs, and the implant failure process ensues (Figure 18-3).[9,18,19]

The presence of implant mobility is a reliable measure of the likelihood of failure.[20-23] To achieve osseointegration in modern implantology, there should be absolutely no implant mobility, as is the case for ankylosed teeth, which are, in many ways, the biological model for osseointegration in implants (Figure 18-4).

Normal Flora within the Oral Cavity

Bacterial colonization of the oral cavity of a neonate begins within a few days of birth. *Streptococcus salivarius* predominates at this age, probably because of its enhanced ability to attach to mucosal surfaces. Other streptococci, such as *Streptococcus mutans* and *Streptococcus sanguis*, cannot be isolated before tooth eruption, which is consistent with their ability to adhere only to hard surfaces, and it is important to note that they are not found in the oral cavity after the loss of all teeth.

Gram-positive rods, such as *Actinomyces naeslundii* and *Actinomyces viscosus*, also appear very early in life. *A. naeslundii* predominates in saliva samples and can be found in most neonates and in nearly all teenagers and adults. *A. viscosus* usually appears at the time of tooth eruption and is more commonly associated with dental plaque. The initial colonizers usually are gram-positive anaerobic bacteria. Anaerobic bacteria, such as *Bacteroides* species and *Fusobacterium* species, appear later in life and are isolated more frequently after puberty.[9]

It is well established that the oral flora varies from site to site, and it appears that certain bacteria have a specific ecological niche within the oral cavity. The specificity of oral flora apparently results from their ability to selectively attach themselves to various surfaces. At the time of eruption of the complete dentition, gram-positive streptococci make up a large percentage of the normal flora, although the actual percentages differ from site to site. *S mutans* and *S sanguis* generally are found in dental plaque, whereas *S salivarius* is found in dental plaque on the mucosa and in the saliva.

Gram-negative cocci, such as *Veillonella parvula* and *Veillonella alcalescens*, are also present in relatively high numbers. *Neisseria* are among the initial colonizers of cleansed enamel surfaces. Gram-positive rods and filaments common to the normal flora are *Actinomyces* species, *Rothia dentocariosa*, *Corynebacterium*, and *Lactobacillus*. Gram-negative rods and filaments, such as *Fusobacteria*, black-pigmented *Bacteroides* (BPB), and spirochetes, can be isolated from the flora of healthy periodontal sites; however, they represent a very small proportion of the cultivable flora.[9]

(Figure 18-6, 18-7).[9] Dental plaque and calculus on implants is categorized by its relationship to the peri-implant sulcus as supracrevicular or crevicular (Figure 18-8). The pellicle formed on tooth surfaces has been studied extensively, and it is likely that similar films form on titanium oxide surfaces and the natural tooth. Anodic proteins bind selectively to the hydroxyapatite (HA) surface, and we can hypothesize that they bind to a cathodic surface by means of hydrophilic side chains rotated toward the metal. Such absorption apparently occurs without any serious decrease in protein activity. The low surface energy of the titanium surface results in a low binding affinity to the protein, which may explain the clinical observation that plaque adheres less to a titanium surface than to a natural tooth.

Microscopic and cultural studies of supracrevicular plaque taken from teeth and from implants in partially edentulous mouths show that the growth rate of supracrevicular plaque is not significantly influenced by the presence

Development of Subgingival Microflora Around Dental Implants

Research has shown that the subgingival flora around dental implants is derived from the natural flora within the oral cavity.[24-26] A comparison of supragingival plaque on vitallium, titanium, and aluminum oxide implants versus that of control teeth reveals a flora similar in composition to subgingival flora[27] (Figure 18-5).

Only weak evidence suggests that plaque accumulation results in peri-implant mucosal inflammation similar to that seen with gingivitis; however, rapid bone loss can occur with concomitant deepening of the peri-implant sulcus

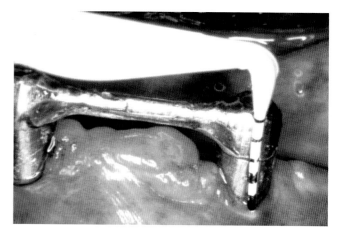

FIGURE 18-6 ■ Verify the health of the gingiva around the implant by measuring the depth of the pocket.

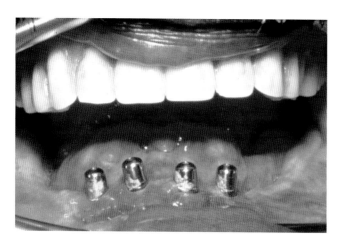

FIGURE 18-5 ■ Dental plaque accumulation around dental implants for many patients begins shortly after stage 2 surgery. Patients generally require good oral hygiene instruction soon after surgery.

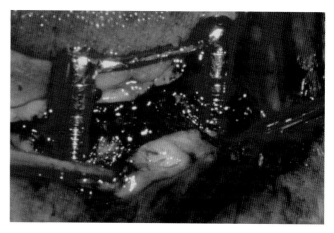

FIGURE 18-7 ■ One of the causative factors of alveolar bone loss is long-lasting marginal inflammation resulting from plaque accumulation.

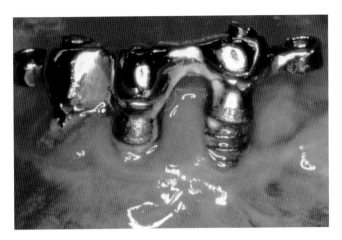

FIGURE 18-8 ■ Bone loss on implants due to excessive plaque and calculus also can occur.

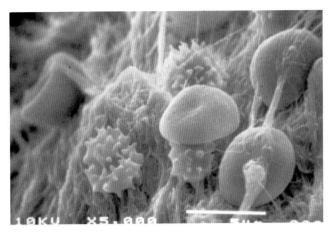

FIGURE 18-9 ■ Clinical inflammation is characterized histologically by increased numbers of plasma cells, lymphocytes, macrophages, and polymorphonuclear leukocytes in the connective tissue.

of a titanium surface.[28-30] Only a few studies have attempted to establish the microflora "profile" of the peri-implant sulcus. Bacterial flora is characterized by the morphology and motility patterns visible in darkfield and phase-contrast microscopy. Culturing techniques further identify and type the microflora in terms of gram staining, anaerobic growth, predominance, and speciation. In periodontal studies, these techniques have been used to establish the differences between microflora at healthy and diseased sites.[28] The microflora found around implants is similar to that found around natural teeth. In both cases, the main species are cocci, motile rods, *Fusiformis*, nonmotile rods, small spirochetes, and large spirochetes.[31-34]

Microbial plaque constitutes the main risk for natural periodontal structures. In one clinical study, when various implant materials were mounted on special vehicles and left in the oral cavity, after 10 days, a distinct, visible plaque could be detected on all material samples.[28] Polished titanium oxide and aluminum oxide samples with microscopically smooth surface profiles were coated with plaque to the same extent as polished or roughened titanium samples. Profile sections demonstrated that the plaque could be removed more easily from aluminum oxide ceramic than from titanium. The physical surface properties of the different materials provided an explanation for the variation in plaque adherence. The surface composition of titanium promotes the binding of organic structures, even in the region of the implant neck, whereas the electrically neutral surface of aluminum oxide ceramic prevents such molecular binding.

However, when a pocket begins to develop, an alteration in the flora on the implant occurs. Even at pocket depths of 3 to 4 mm, the flora is dominated by gram-negative (mainly anaerobic) rods. Bacteria of the *Bacteroides* species and *Fusobacteria* can be differentiated according to their pathogenic properties.[35] The predominance of these bacteria, even in minor gingival pockets, rapidly leads to osteolysis and thus to the endangerment of the implant. Researchers have

theorized that electrochemical influences may be responsible for this pathogenic flora; possible pH shifts, such as those observed in vitro[36-38] and in vivo,[39] can result in an alteration in the ecosystem that is advantageous to anaerobic bacteria.

Although there are obvious differences in the periodontium around teeth and oral perimucosal implants, recent investigations indicate that there are also numerous similarities. Thus, until additional data are obtained, clinicians must continue to rely on traditional periodontal parameters (including use of the periodontal probe, clinical immobility of individual implants, and absence of ongoing marginal bone loss) to objectively assess gingival inflammation or changes in the attachment level (Figure 18-9). In addition, prognostic indicators for the natural tooth still are not available, and very few microbiological reports pertain to different implant surface characteristics. Therefore, the current limited knowledge in this field prevents the drawing of any definitive conclusions.

Available data indicate that, compared with deep pockets around dental implants, deep pockets around natural teeth harbor a greater number of organisms associated with periodontal inflammation. Patients who practice regular oral hygiene usually have fewer periodontal pathogens around perimucosal titanium implants than around natural teeth. However, in partially edentulous mouths (where pockets around natural teeth act as reservoirs for bacteria), implant surfaces are colonized more rapidly. Although studies have documented a greater resistance to periodontitis by some implant systems compared with the area around natural teeth, this resistance cannot be interpreted as absolute because severe gingivitis has been associated with increased marginal bone loss even around implants; thus, clinically, it is essential to carefully monitor plaque control and periodontal tissue reaction around perimucosal oral implants to avoid problems that can result in eventual failure.[19,40,41]

Prevention of Peri-implantitis

Dental implants play a major role in enabling millions of people who are at least partially edentulous to smile, speak, and eat comfortably and confidently.[42-44] The past two decades have been a testament to the predictability and reliability of the most commonly used implant, the endosteal implant. Although the high skill level of the clinician performing dental implants remains a decisive factor in the long-term success of implants (because of the surgical and prosthetic risks that still exist), just as important are ongoing patient maintenance and dental care. In all branches of medicine, often the best treatment is prevention. Implant dentistry and the treatment of peri-implantitis are no exceptions. Patients selected for dental implants must be taught from the very first appointment, if possible, proper home care for their "new" teeth. Additionally, after implantation, regular follow-up will help to ensure the success of the treatment.

Patient Home Care

The success of an implant depends on many factors, including the patient's understanding of the necessity for having the skills for daily care of the prosthesis and surrounding soft tissues. A careful screening is essential for potential implant patients with generally acceptable physical health and a genuine desire to go through the required treatment.[45] Diagnosis and treatment planning based on a risk-benefit analysis follow a detailed medical, dental, and behavioral history, as well as oral and radiographic examinations.[46-49] Contraindications for implant surgery include radiation therapy to the affected part, uncontrolled diabetes mellitus, alcoholism or heavy alcohol intake, substance abuse, an immunosuppressive disease or medication, anticoagulant medication, and psychosis or paranoia.

Plaque control must begin immediately after the uncovering of implants. The dentist, the dental hygienist, and the patient must understand the importance and necessity of good plaque control because it will influence the long-term success of an implant. Hygiene maintenance with dental implants is tedious and requires considerable effort on the part of the patient and dental team. The dental professional's role is to determine the patient's individual and specific home care needs. Recommendation and instruction often are determined by the location and angulation of the implants, the length and position of the transmucosal abutments, and the prosthesis design, as well as by patient habits, motivation, manual dexterity, and oral health.[50-53]

Because the metal abutment is not as hard as a natural tooth, hard-bristled brushes and abrasive powders and pastes are not recommended. A small, soft-bristled toothbrush is effective for cleaning easily accessible areas of the abutment and/or prosthesis. Partially edentulous patients should be instructed in circular brushing according to the Bass technique. Small, soft-textured brushes usually are most efficient for this cleaning technique. Caution must be used with interproximal brushes, which are available with interchangeable brush tips of various shapes. The brushes may have an exposed tip of metal wire that can easily scratch the abutment titanium surface. In addition, if enough pressure is exerted or if the bristles are worn, the wire substructure can scratch the titanium surface. These brushes can be used, but only after their correct use has been properly demonstrated to the patient. Other adjunctive cleaning aids, such as flossing cords and perio-aids, are recommended for cleaning the transmucosal abutment. The lingual side of the abutment and the gingival surface of the prosthesis are areas that are often overlooked by the patient.

For selected patients, several adjunctive treatment regimens that use twice-daily antimicrobial mouth rinses are appropriate. As was noted above, bacterial flora in adult periodontal and peri-implant pockets have been found to be similar. Studies of infected peri-implant pockets have revealed higher levels of spirochetes and gram-negative motile rods, primarily *Peptostreptococcus micros, Fusobacterium,* and enteric rod species.[54,55] Other studies of failing implant sockets revealed increased levels of gram-negative rods, mainly of the *Bacteroides* and *Fusobacterium* species.[2,56] Gram-negative bacteria possess endotoxin, a heat-stable lipopolysaccharide that can produce an acute inflammatory action with associated bone destruction.[57,58]

Chemotherapeutic solutions, such as chlorhexidine, have been recommended for both short-term and long-term use. They can be prescribed for a limited time after abutment connection or to reestablish peri-implant sulcus health. Their long-term use may be indicated when access to abutments is difficult, or when physical impairment prevents proper daily abutment maintenance. Staining of the superstructure can be minimized by applying the antimicrobial with a cotton-tipped applicator or by dipping an interproximal brush in the mouth rinse solution and gently working the brush around the transmucosal abutments.[50-53]

Chlorhexidine gluconate mouth rinse has been prescribed for various periodontal problems and is widely accepted as part of the maintenance therapy in implant dentistry. Patients should be placed on rinse therapy immediately after undergoing the second-stage surgery and should be advised to continue use of the rinse throughout the life of the implants. The mechanism of action of chlorhexidine is related to a decrease in pellicle formation, an alteration of bacterial adsorption to teeth, and a change in the cell wall of the bacteria, resulting in lysis.[59] The agent interacts with negative charges on the bacterial cell wall, bonding to the cell wall and altering its permeability.

By binding to soft and hard tissues in the oral cavity, the action of chlorhexidine is extended. Almost 100% kill of the oral bacteria has been reported up to 5 hours after a

30-second rinse of a 0.12% concentration of the agent.[60] Chlorhexidine has been shown to suppress gram-positive and gram-negative organisms and *Actinomyces* in plaque after 3 to 6 months of use.[61,62]

Follow-up Treatment

Most of today's dental implant systems use titanium because of the metal's superior biocompatibility and the ability of bone to bond to it.[63] The strength, low density, and biocompatibility of titanium make it an ideal implant complement, but it is also a soft metal that is subject to physical wear.[64,65] Conventional periodontal scalers can scratch and irreversibly damage the surface of titanium implants.[66,67] Commercially pure titanium is passive under physiological conditions and forms a layer of titanium oxide when exposed to air.[68,69] This oxide layer separates the metal ions on the implant surface from the tissues and prevents possible cytotoxic reactions. If this oxide layer is damaged by any prophylactic devices, the protective barrier is lost, exposing the metal ions to the tissues. To help prevent this from occurring during implant maintenance, the use of a modified ultrasonic instrument, in which a conventional tip has been adapted to accept a custom-designed plastic tip, has been recommended.[70,71]

Supragingival and subgingival deposits should be removed during each patient visit. Plaque can be removed using floss, gauze, or fine pumice in a rubber cup. Because calculus is not as tenacious on artificial surfaces as it is on natural teeth, it usually can be easily removed with specially designed rigid plastic or titanium instruments. Titanium curettes that break away calculus should be used with caution to avoid scratching the implant surface. Ultrasonic scalers and interdental brushes with exposed metal tend to scratch the implant surface. Interdental brushes with coated wires should be utilized and recommended to patients. A chlorhexidine mouth rinse can be used to decrease the bacterial count on the implant superstructure, as well as within the sulcus.[72] This mouth rinse, along with systemic metronidazole, can help to reduce any gingival hyperplasia seen around the implants.[73]

The sulcular area around the implant is of primary concern. The dental team should check for signs of inflammation or exudate around the implant, implant mobility, and pocket depths. The clinical assessment of peri-implant soft tissues should begin with gentle probing of the peri-implant sulci; probe readings are taken from at least four sites. The average probing depth of the peri-implant sulcus ranges from 1.3 to 3.8 mm.[50-53] The progressive probing depth over time may be a better indicator of disease activity than the absolute probe reading. Zero mobility is expected around stable implants. If abutment movement is found, the abutment screws should be examined for breakage.[50-53]

In addition to clinical assessment of implant mobility, radiographic evaluation of the surrounding bone–implant interface is a traditional mode of evaluating the success of the osseointegrated implant. Radiographs are useful in assessing bone height and density, as well as in showing the functional relationship between the prosthesis, implant, and abutment components.[50-53]

Panoramic baseline radiographs usually are taken 1 week after second-stage surgery is performed. After placement of the prosthesis, individual periapical films of each implant are taken to provide further baseline information. Usually, annual radiographs are taken for the first 3 years. An average marginal bone loss of 1.5 mm usually occurs during the first year of prosthesis connection, and an average of 0.1 mm every year thereafter. Bone loss exceeding these averages should be viewed with concern because progressive bone loss is an indication of implant failure.[50-53]

The peri-implant examination and assessment procedures are performed at each maintenance visit. The patient is often seen for comprehensive oral hygiene instructions and the recording of baseline data within the first week after the prosthesis is seated. A follow-up appointment is scheduled 1 month later to review home care instruction and reevaluate the health of the peri-implant tissues. Soft and hard deposits are carefully removed. A 3-month recall appointment follows this first monthly maintenance visit. If home care is adequate and the patient is symptom-free at the end of the first year, a 4-month to 6-month recall thereafter could be sufficient. During the first 2 years, no more than 6 months should elapse between hygiene visits. However, the patient's individual needs must determine the appointment interval.

Calculus that forms on the transmucosal cylinders is primarily of the supragingival type and is similar to calculus forming on a natural tooth. As was mentioned, using metal instruments to scale or probe around implants is not contraindicated. Although plastic scalers have been developed for use on implants, cavitrons, prophy jets, and sonic units are fine for implants and are definitely not contraindicated for implant prophylaxis. Buffing "shoeshine style" with unwrapped 2-inch by 2-inch gauze strips or with tin oxide on a prophy cup is also recommended.

Diagnosis of Peri-implantitis

Today's implant procedures are performed using a low drill speed and profuse irrigation. These innovations keep the bone temperature below the critical 47°C and allow for the formation of new bone cells around the implant. Thus, "osseointegration,"[63,64] defined as direct bone anchorage to an implant body, occurs, and this can provide a foundation to support the prosthesis and transmit occlusal forces to bone. Progressive changes in traditional periodontal parameters, such as gingival probing depths, clinical attachment levels, bleeding levels, bleeding on probing, and gingival and plaque indices, are important indicators of impending implant failure.[3,50-53]

Radiographs are helpful in diagnosing peri-implantitis. In most cases, a combination of periapical and vertical bitewing radiographs will provide sufficient information regarding the bone–implant interface. However, sometimes right angle radiographs are needed because the thin line that is often visible around failing implants can be easily obscured by small changes in angulation. If the clinician needs a right angle view of the entire implant, it may be necessary to remove the overlying prosthesis or to make a specially designed holder. Generally, implants can be expected to lose about 1.5 mm of bone during the first postoperative year.

There are differences of opinion regarding the probing of implants. Because little evidence supports the existence of a direct connective tissue interface, probing can strip away the epithelial attachment. Despite this potential risk, probing seems to be a reasonable approach to assess gingival health and to monitor pocket depths. As indicated earlier, a plastic probe is less likely to scratch the implant.

It is particularly important that no bleeding occurs during probing because patients with poor oral hygiene tend to experience more rapid breakdown around implants than do patients who practice good dental hygiene. Gingival color should be the same as that around a healthy tooth. The tissue tone should be tight, although some osseointegrated implants do well despite a lack of attached gingiva. At present, however, periodontal literature and clinical experience suggest that a band of keratinized tissue is desirable.[73]

The cause of peri-implantitis has been suggested as bacterial or occlusal in origin. These traditional pathways are primarily related to gingivitis and apical bone loss due to bacterial proliferation, and to the retrograde pathway, which is basically occlusal in origin and results in bone loss at the crest and the absence of a peri-mucosal seal.[3,10] The lack of a peri-mucosal seal allows for increased penetration of bacteria, which results in even greater bone loss, thus creating a vicious cycle that ends with failure of the implant(s) affected by the process.

Although osseointegrated implants can successfully support greater loading than fibro-osseous implants of similar size, excessive occlusal loads should be avoided, because these forces (especially in the form of bruxing) can accelerate breakdown. Some clinicians argue that the quantity and quality of bone around the implant actually increase in patients who have parafunctional habits.[73]

The implant prosthesis should be checked to ensure that there is no movement, and that the screws or cement seals remain tight; otherwise, fractures can occur. Small discrepancies in the prosthetic device can result in very significant detrimental effects on the implants themselves.[73] In a small number of cases, total or partial implant failure can be caused by under-engineering of the prosthesis or faulty techniques during placement, such as overheating the bone or contaminating the implant surface. Such mistakes can lead to a complete or partial lack of osseointegration or bio-integration.

Changes in the biochemical configuration of the crevicular fluid may be an indicator of implant failure; for example, in one study, the concentrations of glycosaminoglycans in the crevicular fluid of healthy implants and failing implants were measured by electrophoretic separation.[74] The process of bone resorption around implants was reported to produce a higher level of glycosaminoglycans, particularly chondroitin-4-sulphate (C4S), similar to the reaction found around teeth with periodontal problems.

Treating the Ailing and Failing Implant

Although dental implants have become a highly successful and widely accepted method for treating edentulous conditions, with hundreds of thousands of implants being placed each year in the United States, it is inevitable that with this large a number of procedures being performed, implant failures will occur (Figure 18-10). When this happens, dentists need to be aware of appropriate management techniques needed to repair and rejuvenate the bone around failed implants.

Osseointegration, the direct apposition between normal remodeled bone and an implant surface without the interposition of nonbone or connective tissue, is the key to successful dental implantation and has to be maintained as such to prolong the life of dental implants and the prostheses they support. The following criteria have long been established as necessary for dental implantation to be considered successful: (1) The individual, unattached implant must be immobile when tested clinically; (2) there must be no radio-

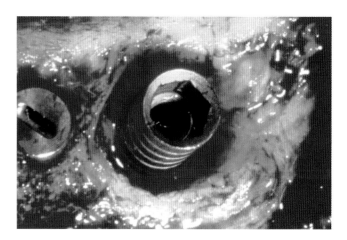

FIGURE 18-10 ■ Implant failure showing bone loss around a titanium structure when it is this extensive, the solution is generally removal of the implant and bone grafting the site after complete debridement of the site.

graphic evidence of peri-implant radiolucency; (3) after the first year of placement, there must be no more than 0.2 mm of vertical bone loss annually; and (4) no pain, infection, neuropathy, or paresthesia can be associated with the individual implants.[75]

The term "ailing" implant suggests that there are means by which to manage or improve the prognosis of fixtures that present with progressive peri-implant bone loss and pocketing as a result of peri-implantitis.[3,76,77] Treatment will depend on the severity of the case. A correct diagnosis must be established, keeping in mind the clinical findings of mobility, pain, swelling, prosthetic fitting, and occlusal force distribution. It is also important to evaluate the implants radiographically and to monitor the patient's hygiene habits and dexterity. Treatment may be nonsurgical or surgical.

Based on traditional periodontal therapy, nonsurgical procedures should be attempted first. Plaque control, oral hygiene instructions, implant cleaning with fine pumice and a rubber cup, and scaling would be the initial steps taken to address the problem. In addition, the condition of the prosthesis should be evaluated, with attention directed toward fitting, mobility, occlusion, and the ability of the patient to properly clean the abutments. As was noted above, most of these same procedures are considered preventative measures for implant failure.

A number of chemotherapeutic agents have been used with varying degrees of success in the treatment of periodontal disease. Chlorhexidine gluconate and stannous fluoride have been used during subgingival irrigation to inhibit local microflora.[72] Treatments with citric acid and sodium hypochlorite have been used to remove bacterial endotoxin (lipopolysaccharides [LPS]). Various chemotherapeutic agents have been shown to detoxify HA-coated implant surfaces infected by endotoxins.[78]

Detoxification of the implant surface can be accomplished by using a citric acid and/or tetracycline slurry. Various chemical and mechanical modalities used to clean and detoxify the surfaces of the implants have been evaluated.[78] It appears that citric acid (pH 1.0) applied for 30 to 60 seconds is effective in removing endotoxins from the surface of HA-coated implants. However, application for longer periods resulted in a significant loss of HA coating because of decalcification, and substantially altered the calcium-to-phosphorus ratio.

Tetracycline is a broad-spectrum antibiotic that prevents bacterial protein synthesis. It has been found to concentrate in the gingival crevicular fluid when used systemically.[79,80] Tetracycline has been shown to promote fibroblastic growth and attachment on root surfaces in vitro.[81,82] However, it does not detoxify the endotoxin-contaminated surfaces of implants. Before the clinician uses bone grafting for a defect, a brief (1 minute) application of citric acid, followed by application of a tetracycline slurry (250 mg mixed with saline in a dappen dish) on the implant surface, is recommended.[61,62] This procedure detoxifies the implant surface

and provides antimicrobial coverage during the healing period.

Surgical procedures for peri-implantitis include mucogingival therapy, open debridement, apical positioning of tissue, grafting, membrane-assisted guided tissue regeneration, and removal of the implant.[83,84] Removal should always be a last resort procedure that may, however, be necessary depending on the severity of the problem.

When the bone is resorbed one-third of the total length of the implant, surgical salvage should be attempted. A flap is reflected, all soft tissue is meticulously curetted and copiously irrigated with a 0.12% solution of chlorhexidine gluconate, citric acid is applied to the implant surface, and freeze-dried bone is placed level with the implant. The area then is covered with a barrier membrane, and primary closure is obtained with a monofilament suture material.

After peri-implant infection or a failing implant has been diagnosed, the following surgical salvage protocol is recommended. Careful periodontal probing to assess pocket depth and bone loss should be performed. Periapical radiographs should be taken to determine horizontal (saucerization) or vertical bone loss. The patient should be treated with the appropriate antibiotics and anti-inflammatory medications for 1 week.

After local anesthesia is applied, a mucoperiosteal flap should be reflected to gain access to the area of the bone defect around the implant. Any granulation tissue present should be removed, and the implant surface should be debrided with plastic-tipped scalers. If the patient has an HA-coated implant, the implant surface should be treated with citric acid (pH 1.0, 40% concentration) for 30 to 60 seconds. If the implant has a plasma-sprayed titanium surface, it should be treated with tetracycline paste slurry.

To freshen the bone surface at the area of bone loss and to keep the host site free of infection by eliminating any endotoxins that may have leached into surrounding bone, a thin layer of bone should be removed with a round bur on a slow-speed handpiece under irrigation. An autogenous or allogenic bone graft, along with some tetracycline powder, should be packed into the defect. Bone grafts for defects around implants can be autografts, allografts, xenografts, or alloplastic grafts.[85] Autogenous grafts, harvested and grafted within the same individual usually at the same time, provide live osteocompetent cells and volume to the grafted sites and are considered to be the best type of graft. Allografts, harvested from one individual, sterilized, and freeze-dried, are grafted into a different individual belonging to the same species. Xenografts are grafts from different species, and alloplastic grafts are synthetic substances that are biocompatible with human tissues and may or may not be resorbable.

A membrane barrier should be placed to promote guided bone regeneration. Guided tissue regeneration (GTR) is based on the principle that different cells in the body have different rates of migration into a healing wound area.[86,87] A membrane is used to act as an occlusive barrier that impedes the entry of rapidly proliferating epithelial (gingival) cells into the osseous defect, while osteocompetent cells, which migrate at a slower rate, gradually fill the defect with bone. The membrane may or may not be resorbable, and may be synthetic or derived from mammalian tissue. The advantage of using a resorbable membrane is the elimination of a subsequent surgery to remove the membrane. Primary closure of tissue over the treated site should be performed. If the prosthesis is found to be impinging on the grafted/treated site, the prosthesis should be adjusted to avoid pressure on the area.

SUMMARY

The prevention of a peri-implant inflammatory reaction is prudent and requires a highly motivated patient who is willing to present for regular follow-up visits. During each visit, the dentist should carefully examine the soft tissues surrounding the implant and record their condition for future comparison and prognostic assessment. The dental implant clinician must thoroughly understand the soft tissue–implant interface, the normal flora of the oral cavity, how subgingival microflora develops around dental implants, and how to prevent, diagnose, and treat peri-implantitis, so that implant patient satisfaction remains high.

REFERENCES

1. Haanaes HR: Implants and infections with special reference to oral bacteria, *J Clin Periodontol* 17(7 Pt 2):516-524, 1990.
2. Lee KH, Maiden MF, Tanner AC, Weber HP: Microbiota of successful osseointegrated dental implants, *J Periodontol* 70(2):131-138, 1999.
3. Ashley ET, Covington LL, Bishop BG, Breault LG: Ailing and failing endosseous dental implants: a literature review, *J Contemp Dent Pract* 4(2):35-50, 2003.
4. Bauman GR, Rapley JW, Hallmon WW, Mills M: The peri-implant sulcus, *Int J Oral Maxillofac Implants* 8(3):273-280, 1993.
5. Weber HP, Cochran DL: The soft tissue response to osseointegrated dental implants, *J Prosthet Dent* 79(1):79-89, 1998.
6. Koka S: The implant-mucosal interface and its role in the long-term success of endosseous oral implants: a review of the literature, *Int J Prosthodont* 11(5):421-432, 1998.
7. Maksoud MA: Manipulation of the peri-implant tissue for better maintenance: a periodontal perspective, *J Oral Implantol* 29(3):120-123, 2003.
8. Karoussis IK, Muller S, Salvi GE, Heitz-Mayfield LJ, Bragger U, Lang NP: Association between periodontal and peri-implant conditions: a 10-year prospective study, *Clin Oral Implants Res* 15(1):1-7, 2004.
9. Krekeler G: Peri-implant problems. In: Schroeder A, Sutter F, Krekeler G, editors: *Oral implantology: basic-ITI hollow cylinder*, New York, 1991, Thieme.
10. Meffert RM: Treatment of failing dental implants, *Curr Opin Dent* 2:109-114, 1992.
11. Gould TR, Westbury L, Brunette DM: Ultrastructural study of the attachment of human gingiva to titanium in vivo, *J Prosthet Dent* 52(3):418-420, 1984.
12. McKinney RV Jr, Steflik DE, Koth DL: Evidence for a junctional epithelial attachment to ceramic dental implants: a transmission electron microscopic study, *J Periodontol* 56(10):579-591, 1985.
13. Ten Cate AR: The gingival junction. In: Branemark PI, Zarb G, Albrektsson T, editors: *Tissue-integrated prostheses*, Chicago, 1986, Quintessence.
14. Donley TG, Gillette WB: Titanium endosseous implant-soft tissue interface: a literature review, *J Periodontol* 62(2):153-160, 1991.
15. Weber HP, Fiorellini JP: The biology and morphology of the implant-tissue interface, *Alpha Omega* 85(4):61-64, 1992.
16. Areva S, Paldan H, Peltola T, Narhi T, Jokinen M, Linden M: Use of sol-gel-derived titania coating for direct soft tissue attachment, *J Biomed Mater Res A* 70(2):169-178, 2004.
17. Atsuta I, Yamaza T, Yoshinari M, Goto T, Kido MA, Kagiya T, Mino S, Shimono M, Tanaka T: Ultrastructural localization of laminin-5 (gamma2 chain) in the rat peri-implant oral mucosa around a titanium-dental implant by immuno-electron microscopy, *Biomaterials* 26(32):6280-6287, 2005.
18. Cornelini R, Artese L, Rubini C, Fioroni M, Ferrero G, Santinelli A, Piattelli A: Vascular endothelial growth factor and microvessel density around healthy and failing dental implants, *Int J Oral Maxillofac Implants* 16(3):389-393, 2001.
19. Quirynen M, De Soete M, van Steenberghe D: Infectious risks for oral implants: a review of the literature, *Clin Oral Implants Res* 13(1):1-19, 2002.
20. Piattelli A, Scarano A, Favero L, Iezzi G, Petrone G, Favero GA: Clinical and histologic aspects of dental implants removed due to mobility, *J Periodontol* 74(3):385-390, 2003.
21. Wijaya SK, Oka H, Saratani K, Sumikawa T, Kawazoe T: Development of implant movement checker for determining dental implant stability, *Med Eng Phys* 26(6):513-522, 2004.
22. Salvi GE, Lang NP: Diagnostic parameters for monitoring peri-implant conditions, *Int J Oral Maxillofac Implants* 19(suppl):116-127, 2004.
23. Shibli JA, Marcantonio E, d'Avila S, Guastaldi AC, Marcantonio E Jr: Analysis of failed commercially pure titanium dental implants: a scanning electron microscopy and energy-dispersive spectrometer x-ray study, *J Periodontol* 76(7):1092-1099, 2005.
24. Heimdahl A, Kondell PA, Nord CE, Nordenram A: Effect of insertion of osseo-integrated prosthesis on the oral microflora, *Swed Dent J* 7(5):199-204, 1983.
25. Bollen CM, Papaioanno W, Van Eldere J, Schepers E, Quirynen M, van Steenberghe D: The influence of abutment surface roughness on plaque accumulation and peri-implant mucositis, *Clin Oral Implants Res* 7(3):201-211, 1996.
26. Baena-Monroy T, Moreno-Maldonado V, Franco-Martinez F, Aldape-Barrios B, Quindos G, Sanchez-Vargas LO: *Candida albicans, Staphylococcus aureus* and *Streptococcus mutans* colonization in patients wearing dental prosthesis, *Med Oral Patol Oral Cir Bucal* 10(suppl 1):E27-E39, 2005.
27. Lekholm A: Microorganisms in peri-implant sites. In: Branemark PI, Zarb G, Albrektsson T, editors: *Tissue-integrated prostheses*, Chicago, 1986, Quintessence.
28. Krekeler G, Kappert H, Pelz K, Graml B: [Affinity of plaque for various materials], *Schweiz Monatsschr Zahnmed* 94(7):647-651, 1984. German.
29. Frolov AG, Triandafillidis S, Novikov SV, Fedorov SIu, Karasev MV, Tsimbalistov A: [An experimental study of the tissue compatibility of titanium implants coated with hydroxyapatite and aluminum oxide by plasma spraying], *Stomatologiia (Mosk)* 74(3):9-11, 1995. Russian.

30. Muster D, Demri B, Moritz M, Hage-Ali M: [What is thought of the various surface treatments of biomaterials used in dental and maxillofacial implantology?], *Rev Stomatol Chir Maxillofac* 99(suppl 1):89-93, 1998. French.

31. Palmisano DA, Mayo JA, Block MS, Lancaster DM: Subgingival bacteria associated with hydroxylapatite-coated dental implants: morphotypes and trypsin-like enzyme activity, *Int J Oral Maxillofac Implants* 6(3):313-318, 1991.

32. Papaioannou W, Quirynen M, Nys M, van Steenberghe D: The effect of periodontal parameters on the subgingival microbiota around implants, *Clin Oral Implants Res* 6(4):197-204, 1995.

33. Danser MM, van Winkelhoff AJ, van der Velden U: Periodontal bacteria colonizing oral mucous membranes in edentulous patients wearing dental implants, *J Periodontol* 68(3):209-216, 1997.

34. Morris HF, Ochi S, Spray JR, Olson JW: Periodontal-type measurements associated with hydroxyapatite-coated and non-HA-coated implants: uncovering to 36 months, *Ann Periodontol* 5(1):56-67, 2000.

35. Gessert R, Krekeler G, Pelz K: [Microbiology of postjuvenile periodontitis], *Dtsch Zahnarztl Z* 40(7):788-790, 1985. German.

36. Zitter H, Plenk H Jr: The electrochemical behavior of metallic implant materials as an indicator of their biocompatibility, *J Biomed Mater Res* 21(7):881-896, 1987.

37. Fathi MH, Salehi M, Saatchi A, Mortazavi V, Moosavi SB: In vitro corrosion behavior of bioceramic, metallic, and bioceramic-metallic coated stainless steel dental implants, *Dent Mater* 19(3):188-198, 2003.

38. Assis SL, Rogero SO, Antunes RA, Padilha AF, Costa I: A comparative study of the in vitro corrosion behavior and cytotoxicity of a superferritic stainless steel, a Ti-13Nb-13Zr alloy, and an austenitic stainless steel in Hank's solution, *J Biomed Mater Res B Appl Biomater* 73(1):109-116, 2005.

39. Hild A: Electromechanical charges in endosteal implants with metal and aluminum ceramic oxide charges, Freiburg Conference, 1985.

40. van Steenberghe D, Quirynen M, Callens A: The reactions of periodontal tissues to implants and teeth. In: Laney WR, editor: *Tissue integration in oral, orthopedic and maxillofacial reconstruction*, Hanover Park, IL, 1992, Quintessence.

41. van Steenberghe D, Naert I, Jacobs R, Quirynen M: Influence of inflammatory reactions vs. occlusal loading on peri-implant marginal bone level, *Adv Dent Res* 13:130-135, 1999.

42. ADA Council on Scientific Affairs: Dental endosseous implants: an update, *J Am Dent Assoc* 135(1):92-97, 2004.

43. Albrektsson T, Wennerberg A: The impact of oral implants—past and future, 1966-2042, *J Can Dent Assoc* 71(5):327, 2005.

44. Eckert SE, Choi YG, Sanchez AR, Koka S: Comparison of dental implant systems: quality of clinical evidence and prediction of 5-year survival, *Int J Oral Maxillofac Implants* 20(3):406-415, 2005.

45. McNutt MD, Chou CH: Current trends in immediate osseous dental implant case selection criteria, *J Dent Educ* 67(8):850-859, 2003.

46. Barbosa F: Patient selection for dental implants, Part 1: data gathering and diagnosis, *J Indiana Dent Assoc* 79(1):8-11, 2000.

47. Barbosa F: Patient selection for dental implants, Part 2: contraindications, *J Indiana Dent Assoc* 80(1):10-12, 2001.

48. Sugerman PB, Barber MT: Patient selection for endosseous dental implants: oral and systemic considerations, *Int J Oral Maxillofac Implants* 17(2):191-201, 2002.

49. Julian JM: Diagnosis and treatment planning for implant placement, *Dent Today* 23(4):104-109, 2004.

50. Orton GS, Steele DL, Wolinsky LE: Dental professional's role in monitoring and maintenance of tissue-integrated prostheses, *Int J Oral Maxillofac Implants* 4(4):305-310, 1989.

51. Lord BJ: Maintenance procedures for the implant patient, *Aust Prosthodont J* 9(suppl):33-38, 1995.

52. Silverstein L, Garg A, Callan D, Shatz P: The key to success: maintaining the long-term health of implants, *Dent Today* 17(2):104, 106, 108-111, 1998.

53. Hancock EB, Newell DH: The role of periodontal maintenance in dental practice, *J Indiana Dent Assoc* 81(2):25-30, 2002.

54. Rosenberg ES, Torosian JP, Slots J: Microbial differences in 2 clinically distinct types of failures of osseointegrated implants, *Clin Oral Implants Res* 2(3):135-144, 1991.

55. Listgarten MA, Lai CH: Comparative microbiological characteristics of failing implants and periodontally diseased teeth, *J Periodontol* 70(4):431-437, 1999.

56. Mombelli A, van Oosten MA, Schurch E Jr, Land NP: The microbiota associated with successful or failing osseointegrated titanium implants, *Oral Microbiol Immunol* 2(4):145-151, 1987.

57. Rizzo AA, Mergenhagen SE: Local Shwartzman reaction in rabbit oral mucosa with endotoxin from oral bacteria, *Proc Soc Exp Biol Med* 104:579-582, 1960.

58. Ramirez-Hernandez C, Hernandez-Vidal G, Wong-Gonzalez A, Gutierrez-Ornelas E, Ackermann MR, Ramirez-Romero R: Mast cell density during initiation and progression of the local Shwartzman reaction, *Inflamm Res* 53(3):107-110, 2004. Epub 2004 Feb 16.

59. Ciancia SG: Pharmacology of oral antibiotics. In: *Perspective on oral antimicrobial therapeutics*, Littleton, MA, 1987, PSG Publishing.

60. Buckner RY, Kayrouz GA, Briner W: Reduction of oral microbes by a single chlorhexidine rinse, *Compendium* 15(4):512, 514, 516, 1994, passim; quiz 520.

61. Meffert RM: Chemotherapeutic mouthrinses as adjuncts in implant dentistry, *Am J Dent* 2(Spec No):317-321, 1989.

62. Lambert PM, Morris HF, Ochi S: The influence of 0.12% chlorhexidine digluconate rinses on the incidence of infectious complications and implant success, *J Oral Maxillofac Surg* 55(12 suppl 5):25-30, 1997.

63. Cochran DL: A comparison of endosseous dental implant surfaces, *J Periodontol* 70(12):1523-1539, 1999.

64. Branemark PI: Tissue integrated prosthesis: osseointegration in clinical dentistry. In: Branemark PI, Zarb GA, Alberktsson T, editors: *Introduction to osseointegration*, Chicago, 1985, Quintessence.

65. Rapley JW, Swan RH, Hallmon WW, Mills MP: The surface characteristics produced by various oral hygiene instruments and materials on titanium implant abutments, *Int J Oral Maxillofac Implants* 5(1):47-52, 1990.

66. Thomson-Neal D, Evans GH, Meffert RM: Effects of various prophylactic treatments on titanium, sapphire, and hydroxyapatite-coated implants: an SEM study, *Int J Periodontics Restorative Dent* 9(4):300-311, 1989.

67. Augthun M, Tinschert J, Huber A: In vitro studies on the effect of cleaning methods on different implant surfaces, *J Periodontol* 69(8):857-864, 1998.

68. Parr GR, Gardner LK, Toth RW: Titanium: the mystery metal of implant dentistry: dental materials aspects, *J Prosthet Dent* 54(3):410-414, 1985.

69. Kim TI, Han JH, Lee IS, Lee KH, Shin MC, Choi BB: New titanium alloys for biomaterials: a study of mechanical and corrosion properties and cytotoxicity, *Biomed Mater Eng* 7(4):253-263, 1997.

70. Kwan JY, Zablotsky MH, Meffert RM: Implant maintenance using a modified ultrasonic instrument, *J Dent Hyg* 64(9):422, 424-425, 430, 1990.

71. Brookshire FV, Nagy WW, Dhuru VB, Ziebert GJ, Chada S: The qualitative effects of various types of hygiene instrumentation on commercially pure titanium and titanium alloy implant abutments: an in vitro and scanning electron microscope study, *J Prosthet Dent* 78(3):286-294, 1997.

72. Heitz F, Heitz-Mayfield LJ, Lang NP: Effects of post-surgical cleansing protocols on early plaque control in periodontal and/or periimplant wound healing, *J Clin Periodontol* 31(11):1012-1018, 2004.

73. Wilson TG, Kornman KS, Newman MG, editors: *Advances in periodontics*, Hanover Park, IL, 1992, Quintessence.

74. Last KS, Cawood JI, Howell RA, Embery G: Monitoring of Tubingen endosseous dental implants by glycosaminoglycans analysis of gingival crevicular fluid, *Int J Oral Maxillofac Implants* 6(1):42-49, 1991.

75. Albrektsson T, Zarb G, Worthington P, Eriksson AR: The long-term efficacy of currently used dental implants: a review and proposed criteria of success, *Int J Oral Maxillofac Implants* 1(1):11-25, 1986.

76. Meffert RM: How to repair the ailing, failing implant, *CDS Rev* 84(3):56-60, 1991.

77. Meffert RM: Maintenance and treatment of the ailing and failing implant, *J Indiana Dent Assoc* 73(3):22-24, 1994; quiz 25.

78. Zablotsky MH, Diedrich DL, Meffert RM: Detoxification of endotoxin-contaminated titanium and hydroxyapatite-coated surfaces utilizing various chemotherapeutic and mechanical modalities, *Implant Dent* 1(2):154-158, 1992.

79. Gordon JM, Walker CB, Murphy JC, Goodson JM, Socransky SS: Concentration of tetracycline in human gingival fluid after single doses, *J Clin Periodontol* 8(2):117-121, 1981.

80. Needleman IG, Grahn MF, Pandya NV: A rapid spectrophotometric assay for tetracycline in gingival crevicular fluid, *J Clin Periodontol* 28(1):52-56, 2001.

81. Terranova VP, Franzetti LC, Hic S, DiFlorio RM, Lyall RM, Wikesjo UM, Baker PJ, Christersson LA, Genco RJ: A biochemical approach to periodontal regeneration: tetracycline treatment of dentin promotes fibroblast adhesion and growth, *J Periodontal Res* 21(4):330-337, 1986.

82. Gamal AY, Mailhot JM, Garnick JJ, Newhouse R, Sharawy MM: Human periodontal ligament fibroblast response to PDGF-BB and IGF-1 application on tetracycline HCl conditioned root surfaces, *J Clin Periodontol* 25(5):404-412, 1998.

83. Kwan JY, Zablotsky MH: Periimplantitis, the ailing implant, *Implant Soc* 2(1):6-9, 1991.

84. Zablotsky MH: A retrospective analysis of the management of ailing and failing endosseous dental implants, *Implant Dent* 7(3):185-191, 1998.

85. Habal MB, Reddi AH: *Bone grafting and bone substitutes*, Philadelphia, 1992, WB Saunders.

86. Meffert RM: What causes peri-implantitis? *J Calif Dent Assoc* 19(4):53-54, 56-57, 1991.

87. Schou S, Berglundh T, Lang NP: Surgical treatment of peri-implantitis, *Int J Oral Maxillofac Implants* 19(suppl):140-149, 2004.

chapter 19

Guidelines for Handling Complications Associated With Implant Surgical Procedures

M OST POSTOPERATIVE COMPLICATIONS associated with dental implant surgery are minor and temporary. As with any surgical procedure, however, prevention is the best cure. This means paying close attention to patient screening and treatment planning, as well as strictly adhering to sound surgical and prosthetic protocols.

Preventing early complications following implant surgery entails using topical ice packs and anti-inflammatories to reduce swelling, prescribing analgesics for pain control, and instructing the patient about the importance of meticulous oral hygiene, including regular use of an antiplaque rinse. Thereafter, the patient should be seen or telephoned for a routine follow-up 1 to 2 days following surgery.

At this point, it is common for some patients to still experience mild discomfort or numbness, which typically subsides within a few days. If no signs of more serious complications are noted at this visit, another appointment is scheduled 1 to 2 weeks following surgery for suture removal and another examination of the healing site. In some cases, however, problems continue for the patient beyond this early postsurgical window. This chapter provides guidelines for addressing some of these.

Postsurgical Complications

Chronic Pain

Pain is rarely mentioned in the literature as a complication of dental implant placement. Immediately following surgery, patients are routinely prescribed Tylenol with codeine to ward off pain symptoms. Although some patients still report minor postoperative discomfort—particularly following first-stage surgery or procedures involving dermal grafts—this should resolve within 1 to 2 days.[1]

Pain that persists, although rare, indicates a greater problem. Most chronic pain problems begin shortly after delivery of the final prosthesis. Initial clinical and radiographic examinations may be negative, and identifying the source may require removing the prosthesis. Although causes of chronic pain may vary, two very common ones are a loose abutment and excessive stress on the implant caused by a poor-fitting prosthesis.[2]

If an abutment does not fit precisely on a fixture, the patient may feel considerable sharp pain as soft tissue is pinched between the implant and the abutment (Figure 19-1). This can be relieved by tightening the fixing screw. Beforehand, the soft tissues should be infiltrated with a local anesthetic and the cuff around the abutment retracted by gently running a probe in the crevice surrounding the abutment. A similar problem can occur if bone that has grown over the cover screw was not completely cleared, resulting in an abutment that is not fully seated.

Excessive stress on the implant can be caused by a poor-fitting superstructure or microscopic discrepancies in the fit of the cast substructure framework. This type of pain is typically a dull ache or a feeling of pressure or clamping, and relief typically occurs when the superstructure is removed. Before reseating, the fit should be checked from all sides of the abutment. Identifying a problem with the substructure may require extraoral analysis of a new master cast. The solution in this case would be a new master impression and a totally new prosthesis framework. Again, an ounce of prevention is worth a pound of cure. Preventing this problem entails assessing the abutment connector–fixture relationship before the master impression is taken. In addition, exceptionally accurate impression methods followed by exact duplication of the clinical relationships on the master cast are essential for making the framework. Meticulous inspection and analysis of the casting fit before the final prosthesis is delivered are also crucial.

Other sources of chronic pain may include failure of the implant to integrate (often noted when the clinician tightens the abutment screw), sinusitis or rhinitis (which may cause pain in the posterior maxilla), nerve injuries, particularly to the inferior alveolar nerve (associated with pain in the mandible), and implant periapical lesions (characterized by

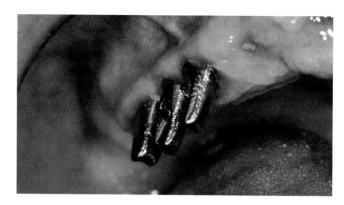

FIGURE 19-1 ■ The abutment should be completely seated into the implant to minimize pain and optimize soft tissue health and prosthetic function. This is best accomplished with a torque wrench.

persistent dull pain).[17] Radiographs typically can identify these pain triggers.

Altered/Lost Sensation

Altered or lost sensation following implant surgery is typically associated with mandibular implant treatment. The cause is usually compression, impingement, or, in some cases, tearing of the inferior alveolar nerve or the mental neurovascular bundle by the implant or instrumentation. Postoperative wound edema can be another cause, and associated disturbances almost always resolve when swelling subsides. In rare cases, temporary sensory disturbances may be attributed to needlestick injuries or the accumulation of metabolites following local anesthesia.[7]

Altered sensation—which typically surfaces following first-stage surgery—can vary from insignificant to debilitating. Sometimes, only the sensation of pain is disturbed (hypersensitivity, hyposensitivity, anesthesia); other cases may involve changes in tactile and temperature sensations. The lower lip and the chin are the most common areas of altered sensation following mandibular implant surgery.[5-7] Occasionally, the gingival tissues or the tongue is affected.

If a patient reports this complication immediately after surgery, a radiograph is warranted to identify any contact between the implant and the nerve.

If the problem involves communication of the implant tip with the mandibular canal, and not overpenetration of the drill, partially withdrawing the implant or replacing it with a shorter implant may alleviate the sensory symptoms. A follow-up radiograph should then be taken to confirm relief to the neurovascular bundle.

Overdrilling is most often the cause of nerve injury, however.[19] When instrumentation has damaged the nerve, it is critical to recognize this immediately and treat and/or refer the patient soon.

An unusual complication that can cause sensory disturbance is displacement of an implant into the inferior alveolar canal. This may be due to the less dense cancellous bone in the posterior mandible and to a large amount of low-density medullary space.[10] If this occurs, the implant must be removed and grafting procedures undertaken before implant treatment can proceed.

Neurosensory disturbances have been the most often reported postoperative complication to date.[18] The literature varies considerably, however, with regard to how frequently sensory disturbances occur, with some authors reporting this complication in less than 1% of cases and others in as many as 43% of cases.[3,4] Although most are transient and resolve on their own, occasionally, sensory alterations can be long term (taking 6 to 12 months to resolve) or, in rare cases, even permanent (with a few patients still reporting neurosensory disturbances at 5 years post surgery).[4,6,7,18] This makes it difficult for the clinician to accurately inform the patient about the potential for this complication, but it is important to warn each patient about the possibility before implant surgery is undertaken. For patients experiencing discomfort postoperatively, a frank discussion and documentation are advisable, as this can be a significant area of legal action, particularly when patients are not informed.[8]

To reduce the risk for this complication, it is crucial for the clinician to preoperatively assess the amount of vertical bone above the nerve using radiographs or, in severely atrophic cases, computed tomography (CT) scans with three-dimensional (3D) reformatted images. Clinicians may not realize how much the bone in the posterior mandible varies from patient to patient and from place to place in the same patient. Bone grafting should be undertaken as needed. In addition, preoperative panoramic radiographs or CT scans are necessary to identify the location of the inferior alveolar nerve and the possible existence of more than one inferior alveolar nerve and canal.[9] Use of a drill guard can also deter overpenetration.

Persistent Edema

Edema is very common following first-stage surgery, although intensity can vary. In most cases, swelling swiftly decreases during the first 2 days postoperatively, and complete dissipation occurs within 1 week.

Most persistent inflammatory conditions are hygiene related and can be resolved with improved patient cleaning and professional prophylaxis. General postoperative edema occasionally can lead to wound dehiscence, but these gaps usually close with granulation tissue formation and re-epithelization, if hygiene is not problematic. Additional sutures at the dehisced site would be necessary only if bone becomes exposed.

In some cases, persistent edema may arise as the result of poor implant positioning, and this may require the clinician to recontour the soft tissues to improve access for cleaning.

Unfortunately, this can lead to poor esthetics, necessitating prosthesis and/or implant replacement in severe cases.

Persistent edema can also signal a loose abutment (with or without concomitant pain), excess cement, or infection at the implant site, which should be treated immediately and thoroughly to prevent integration problems.

Many inflammatory problems can be prevented with an atraumatic surgical technique, incorporating slow drilling speeds and copious irrigation.

A similar problem that can occur is enlargement or proliferation of the soft tissues following placement of the superstructure. In these cases, the tissue usually is firm and is not inflamed. Soft tissue proliferation sometimes is seen beneath the supporting bars of overdentures. This condition may be associated with poor oral hygiene and often can be controlled by using thick floss to clean beneath the bar.[11] If adequate keratinized tissue is present apical to it, a simple excision is all that is typically needed. If the tissues are not inflamed and do not prevent thorough cleaning, the problem may be left alone. Otherwise, an inverse bevel resection is used to thin out the excess tissue while preserving keratinized tissue around the abutment.[12]

Hemorrhage/Hematoma

The submental and sublingual arteries can course closely under the lingual cortical plate in the floor of the mouth. Thus, the risk for hematoma or profuse bleeding is greatest when an implant patient presents with a severely atrophic mandible. This can occur during site preparation when the lingual mandibular cortical bone is severely perforated and a vessel underlying the floor is injured, causing excessive bleeding into the submandibular space that results in massive swelling with acute dyspnea. In many cases, a latency period of several hours may occur.[19]

Although this is a fairly unusual complication, several cases of life-threatening hemorrhage and airway obstruction secondary to hematoma have been reported.[18,20-23]

Damage to the muscles and other soft tissues, without direct arterial damage, can cause profuse bleeding.

Direct exploration of a hematoma or active bleeding in the floor of the mouth is often difficult and is not always effective. In some cases, external carotid artery angiography and endovascular therapy are required.

In many cases, hemorrhage in the floor of the mouth stops spontaneously after a few minutes as the result of pressure from surrounding soft tissue.[22] If a perforation occurs during drilling, the osteotomy should be irrigated with copious amounts of sterile saline. As a safeguard, pressure should be applied to the bleeding area by placing gauze and compressing it with one finger inside and one outside the mouth. In addition, it is prudent to secure and maintain an adequate airway. Because severe bleeding can be delayed, however, it is important to follow closely any case that has involved significant penetrating trauma to the floor of the mouth.

If complication surfaces during surgery, the planned implant should be placed at another site. If this is not possible, the surgery should be halted and the area allowed to heal for 3 to 6 months before surgery is attempted again with redirection or reangulation of the implant.

For a sublingual hematoma that occurs when implants are placed following an undetected perforation, draining aspiration or close monitoring is warranted, depending on the size of the hematoma. If a hollowed basket-type implant has been placed, however, the fixture must be removed immediately.

If bleeding does not resolve, arterial ligation is necessary. In a well-regarded dissection study reviewing the arterial supply to the floor of the mouth, Bavitz et al suggested that it is more effective to ligate first the sublingual artery or its parent facial artery. If this does not control bleeding, then the lingual artery should be ligated.[24] External ligation is done only in severe, uncontrollable cases. Ligation procedures are technically sophisticated and require the skill of an experienced surgeon.

Various preoperative steps can minimize the risk for hematoma or hemorrhage when implants are placed in an atrophic mandible. The lingual surface may be palpated to determine the likelihood of perforation, and continued palpation while the bur is slowly advanced during site preparation can help. CT scans are useful for identifying the locations of structures beneath the mandibular floor.[19]

Peri-implant Complications

Soft Tissue Compromise (Peri-implant Mucositis)

Peri-implant mucositis refers to reversible soft tissue inflammation without radiographic loss of supporting bone. Plaque accumulation is seen around the abutment, and bleeding occurs on probing. This condition usually is caused by bacterial (plaque) contamination (Figure 19-2).

The patient should be reinstructed on proper hygiene and prescribed temporary chlorhexidine as an adjunct if the tissues are severely inflamed or home care is difficult for the patient. If calculus is evident on the abutments, they should be debrided with plastic or other gentle instruments. The prosthesis and involved abutments may be removed and cleaned to remove debris.

The clinician should re-evaluate the marginal fit and design of the prosthesis for accuracy, as well as the quality of soft tissue. Enough keratinized attached tissue should remain to create a peri-implant seal against bacterial invasion. If additional keratinized tissue is needed, a soft tissue mucogingival graft should be performed.

Unchecked plaque accumulation can lead to dehiscence and fistulas. Most dehiscences close on their own, but occa-

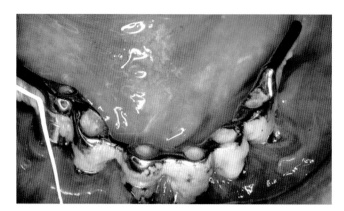

FIGURE 19-2 ■ Peri-implantitis is a complication that may occur post implant surgery.

sionally they lead to exposure of implants before stage 2 surgery. This requires repositioning or resuturing of the flaps for complete coverage to prevent peri-implant bone loss. In highly esthetic areas, this deficit may require a soft tissue graft to achieve an acceptable result.

Fistulas at the abutment–implant connection have been reported to occur in up to 25% of patients and occur most often with single crown replacements.[18] This usually is caused by poor oral hygiene and/or gaps between the components caused by loose abutment screws or misfitting frameworks. A tight seal between the crown and firmly connected abutments will deter this soft tissue complication.[25] Whether deeper subgingival placement of implants prevents these soft tissue problems is still controversial.[18]

More serious inflammatory and infectious peri-implant complications are described in the next section.

Peri-implant Infections (Peri-implantitis)

Peri-implantitis is a rather vague term, but it usually refers to a condition involving soft tissue inflammation (peri-implant mucositis), bleeding, and suppuration, which progress to fairly rapid bone loss. The overall incidence of peri-implantitis appears to be between 5% and 10% of all implant cases.[26]

Some elevated risk may be associated with a history of periodontal disease or the placement of surface-coated or hollow implants with vents versus machined implants.[28,29] Peri-implantitis also appears to occur more rapidly in partially edentulous patients than in totally edentulous ones; this may have something to do with differences in the microflora.[30]

Considerable debate, however, has arisen about whether bacterial contamination, occlusal overload, or some combination of the two is the primary factor responsible for inducing peri-implantitis.[27] Whatever triggers the problem, however, poor oral hygiene clearly accelerates the process.

A peri-implant infection can occur a any time after implant insertion but is most common immediately afterward. Risk for infection falls after sutures are removed and then rises again after the second-stage surgery.[11]

Early attention to this complication is critical to prevent or minimize bone loss around the implant. Once peri-implantitis has progressed, controlling occlusion and inflammation often is not sufficient to promote the healing mechanism.[31] Unchecked, it can lead to implant failure and other serious complications.

To control an early infection, hot salt water mouthwashes and chlorhexidine rinses accompanied by excision, drainage, and systemic antibiotics where appropriate should be used. If the prosthesis has already been placed, treatment calls for removing it and cleaning away any plaque. The prosthesis may require modification to provide easier access for cleaning.

The patient should be reinstructed on hygiene, including meticulous flossing, brushing, and chlorhexidine use. A follow-up visit usually is scheduled 2 weeks later to identify any continued purulence or bleeding on probing. If this persists, an access flap is used to expose the pocket and allow debridement of soft tissues. Success is usually indicated if soft tissue pockets measure no greater than 3 mm, bleeding on probing has subsided, and bone levels are maintained. Guidelines for addressing bone loss—a sign of advanced infection—are outlined in the next section.

Preoperative and perioperative antibiotics may reduce the occurrence of peri-implant infection. Dent et al showed that appropriate dosages of preoperative antibiotics reduced by more than half the number of early implant losses related to infection.[32] A study by Lambert et al suggested that using 0.12% chlorhexidine digluconate rinse perioperatively (at implant placement and uncovering) reduced by half the number of infectious complications.[33] It may be useful to conduct microbiological testing on partially edentulous patients with a history of periodontitis—who are at greater risk for peri-implantitis—to determine what type of antimicrobial therapy should be applied before implant placement.[30]

Other preventative measures include controlling periodontitis prior to implant surgery, avoiding overheating during osteotomy, properly creating emergence profiles and placing the implant–abutment junction, eliminating microgaps and irregular contours, and carefully screening patients for systemic disorders that can impair healing.[27]

Peri-implant Bone Loss

Slight crestal bone loss following implant surgery is common and usually is attributed to remodeling after countersinking, stress distribution to the bone caused by tightening of the implant in place, and excessive loading force.[18] Unfortunately, the literature does not provide consistent information about how much marginal bone loss is acceptable before the risk for implant failure is certain. One recent

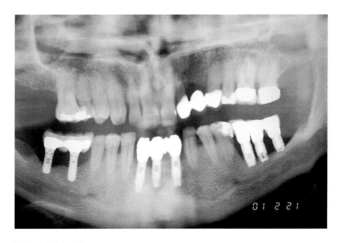

FIGURE 19-3 ■ Severe bone loss can be seen around the dental implants.

literature review reported an average of about 1 mm of marginal bone loss during the first year following implant placement and 0.1 mm per year thereafter. Only a small percentage of successful implant cases exhibited more than 2 mm of total bone loss long term.[18]

Peri-implantitis, as discussed in the preceding section, is a major cause of peri-implant bone loss (Figure 19-3). Late implant failures following successful osseointegration commonly are attributed to this complication, and various studies indicate that complete recovery of osseointegration may be difficult once the peri-implant bone is destroyed.[34] Thus, early attention to this complication is critical.

Occlusal trauma alone may induce peri-implant bone loss, and this often is caused by premature loading of the implant. When this occurs, resulting bone loss occurs uniformly around the implant–bone interface, although it is not limited to the cervical implant bone area. The risk for occlusal trauma and related bone complications can be reduced by inserting enough implants to support the prosthesis.

When occlusal trauma is deemed the cause of bone loss, and not just a contributory factor, correcting the occlusion or parafunctional habit often is sufficient to trigger a reverse of bone loss. It is important to note, however, that occlusion problems can quickly facilitate bacterial invasion and infection. Any micromotion caused by the overload can disrupt the fragile contact area between the implant and soft tissue, creating a pathway for bacteria to reach the apical portion of the implant.

Once any occlusal problems are corrected and infection and inflammation are controlled, the clinician can attempt to improve or reestablish osseointegration. This requires removing the abutment heads from the implant body and elevating a flap. Most clinicians use a nonresorbable expanded polytetrafluoroethylene (e-PTFE) membrane to promote new bone growth; some add allografts or alloplasts.[34,35] Some authors recently reported reosseointegrative success in controlled laboratory studies using rhBMP-2, a bone morphogenic protein.[36] At least 4 months should be allowed for graft consolidation. By then, the implants are reexposed, abutment heads are replaced, and the restoration is replaced or refabricated as needed.

How well this approach minimizes the risk for late implant failure is unclear. Clinical and radiographic evidence supports success of this treatment, but histologic evidence of true osseointegration in humans is still lacking.[26,34]

In cases of severe bone loss, the implant must be removed. Indications for removal include peri-implant bone loss along more than half of the length of the implant or that results in a one-wall defect, bone loss from implant vents and holes, bone destruction that has rapidly advanced (within 1 year of loading), and bone loss that is not amenable to treatment.[54]

Preventing bone loss and implant morbidity is strongly correlated with using proper surgical placement and technique, maintaining physiological distribution of loading forces with sufficient bone quantity and quality, preserving keratinized tissue, and encouraging meticulous patient hygiene.[37]

Damage to Adjacent Teeth

Placing dental implants into severely resorbed, partially edentulous ridges increases the risk for damage to adjacent teeth—particularly in single-tooth restoration cases. This can result from contact with the drilling bur or the implant itself.

During drilling, damage can occur in single-tooth restoration cases when the drilled recesses are reamed. Using burs of inadequate length may cause the contra-angle to contact an adjacent tooth and alter the desired angle or prevent drilling as deeply as planned (Figure 19-4).

Handling this drilling complication depends on how severely the adjacent tooth has been injured. If the bur damages only the cementum, treatment usually is unnecessary because the cementum will regenerate on its own. If the bur enters the dentin, a wait-and-see approach may be followed. If pain or pathology develops at the root apex or the area of bur damage, however, a root canal is probably required. A bur that enters into the canal calls for an immediate root canal and removal of the root portion apical to the damage.[13]

An implant that abuts an adjacent natural tooth can cause many problems. Micromovements of the natural tooth, for instance, can be sufficient to prematurely load or move the implant, thus disrupting its osseointegration. Such implants should be immediately removed and repositioned. In some cases, a narrower implant may be useful, if there is limited space for osseointegration.[14] If the root and/or periodontal membrane are damaged by the implant, treatment may call for apical curettage, root canal therapy, root apex amputation, or even extraction as deemed appropriate. Access for hygiene and esthetic outcome can be affected.

To avoid this complication, a surgical template with the proper position and inclination is helpful, as are radio-

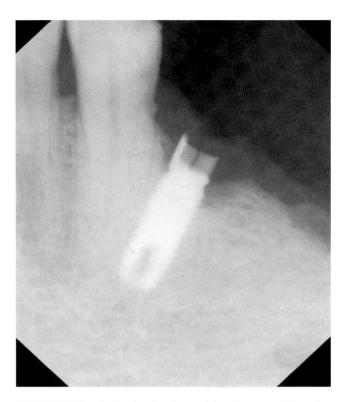

FIGURE 19-4 ■ The implant is touching the root of the adjacent tooth. This problem could have avoided with the use of a surgical template or implant guidance system. In this case, the implant also fractured at the neck during placement.

graphic or study model analyses, appropriately sized implants, and attention to the direction of longitudinal axes of adjacent teeth during reaming.

Retention of Excess Cement

Cemented crowns are a popular alternative that deters the problem of screw loosening that can occur with screw-retained restorations. It can be difficult, however, to visualize and remove excess cement at the abutment–crown interface. This can lead to swollen, sore peri-implant tissues, as well as infection, marginal bone loss, and increased probing depth around the implant. These symptoms often do not surface until months after the prosthesis is placed.

The problem is not always irritation caused by the cement itself. More often, the rough texture enhances plaque accumulation in the gingival sulcus, and the overhanging margins of the restoration increase the presence of pathogenic bacteria consistent with periodontitis.[15]

Identifying this problem typically calls for raising a flap over the site, examining the area for excess cement, then removing it and closing the flaps. It is not unusual for the clinician who placed the crown originally to report having had difficulty with fully seating it.[15] Occasionally, resulting gingival recession may require treatment, lost bone may call for membrane placement or grafting to regenerate bone, and poor-fitting crowns may require replacement.

To prevent problems associated with excess cement, a luting agent that is easy to manipulate and remove without damaging implant parts is useful. A minimal amount of lute should be used, and excess cement should be completely removed with scratch-deterring plastic scalers after the crown is completely seated. Zinc phosphate cement has been deemed easier to remove than resins.[16] Temporary cement is another alternative.

Deep subgingival margin placement is best avoided because this makes it difficult to ensure that all cement is removed.

Important Surgical Complications

With Split-Ridge Techniques

Bone augmentation for the posterior mandible has variable success long-term rates. As an alternative, the split-ridge (or split-crest) technique was developed in the early 1990s to optimize this surgical site in cases with extreme horizontal bone resorption, while maintaining as much as possible the structure of the bone.[38,39] This procedure involves splitting the atrophic crests into two parts with a longitudinal greenstick fracture and then placing an implant (with or without graft material) between them.[40] This is a highly technique-sensitive procedure and should be undertaken only by a well-experienced surgeon.

One complication to guard against is breaking a portion of the bony plate, causing the periosteum to be reflected off the bone. When this occurs, plates or wire should be used to fixate the broken portion. Following a 6-month healing period, the split-ridge technique may be attempted again.

If the resulting horizontal bone fracture extends beyond the intended greenstick fracture, the implant can still be placed if there is adequate bone apical to the planned implant sites. Blood supply would not be disrupted because the tissues and underlying periosteum should still be attached to the bone.

Proper incision and flap design are two key factors in ensuring a successful split-ridge technique. The tissues should be minimally reflected, and this should be followed by the osteotomy and expansion of the ridge with the use of osteotomes.

With Inferior Alveolar Nerve Repositioning

Nerve repositioning surgery sometimes is undertaken to protect the nerve from damage or resection during implant placement in the atrophic posterior mandible or during resection of benign tumors or cysts in the mandible.

Although the goal of this technique is to protect neurosensory function, the principal risk is altered sensation of the inferior alveolar nerve. Some degree of neurosensory dysfunction seems to afflict most patients undergoing nerve repositioning, but this is usually a slight alteration that does not significantly bother the patient.[47] It can vary from a tingling or burning sensation to anesthesia, paresthesia, and so on. This is not a complication to be viewed lightly, however, because some patients may experience more problematic sensory disturbances, and many patients do not experience complete resolution of symptoms for 3 to 6 months.[48,49] Neurosensory alterations seem to occur more often and to last longer with nerve transposition than nerve lateralization.[50]

In most cases, these alterations are caused by overstretching or compression of the nerve, which causes a diffuse axonal injury. It is important to remember that any traction greater than a 5% increase in length can lead to a permanent disturbance.[48]

Nerve severing may occur during the clinician's attempt to uncover it. This should be immediately repaired under magnification for less serious injuries to the nerve during repositioning.

Even when complete sensory function does not return, most patients are satisfied with the procedure and indicate that they would go through with it again.[50] This is particularly true among patients who are informed in detail about this possible complication, as well as the pros and cons of this surgery, before they undergo it.[8]

To prevent complications associated with nerve repositioning, thorough presurgical evaluation and planning are necessary. Three-dimensional visualization of the surgical site is important. Routine radiological evaluation must be performed, and CT scanning may be used. Many variations in the buccolingual or occlusoapical position of the nerve and in nerve direction can be seen easily radiographically.

Nerve retraction should always be done with a blunt, dull instrument, and the neurovascular bundle must not be stretched excessively nor compressed. The anterior loop of the canal near the mental foramen requires the greatest care to avoid damage.

Unexpected anatomical variations, such as more than one mental foramen, may be seen, however. In some cases, two or more smaller foramina are present with narrower nerves extending through them, rather than the normal trunk of the mental nerve. These multiple, small foramina are harder to detect radiographically and are more susceptible to rupture during flap reflection. To prevent this complication once the area has been exposed, the osteotomy should be made at least 5 mm behind the most distal foramen.

A modified nerve repositioning technique involving two osteotomies has been shown to minimize the risk for and duration of any postoperative neurosensory disturbances by preventing inadvertent overstretching or compression of the nerve.[47]

With immediately placed implants, nerve paresthesia may occur when the nerve contacts sharp implant threads, so cylindrical implants are recommended.[47,50,51] The use of a resorbable membrane as a cushion between the implant and the nerve may help to protect the nerve.[52]

Other complications that occur much less commonly with nerve repositioning include infection (typically associated with graft material placed in the region), mandibular fracture, and implant loss (particularly when fracture occurs).[48]

Sinus Membrane Perforations

Sinus membrane perforation is the most common complication of sinus augmentation (Figure 19-5). This membrane, also known as the Schneiderian membrane, lines the sinus cavity and is firmly attached to the bordering bone of the maxillary sinus. When intact, the membrane and its periosteum supply blood to the graft. Although perforations do not necessarily require aborting the surgery, they are a concern because the maxillary sinus communicates with all other sinuses in the respiratory system, and infection can spread quickly. Sinus pneumatization can occur in this area.

The most common cause of sinus membrane perforation is overly vigorous reflection in one area of the osteotomy site without adequate freeing up and elevating of the adjacent membrane area.[42] Perforations can occur during infracture of the lateral wall. Perforations usually occur at the level of the greenstick fracture (when the infracture technique is used), at the level of the superior osteotomy line, and in the inferomedial part of the membrane.

To cover small perforations (1 to 2 mm diameter), a small piece of collagen, a resorbable cellulous membrane, Collatape, Gelfoam, or Surgicel may be used. This should extend over the unaffected membrane by at least 3 mm in all directions. A resorbable collagen wound dressing can be placed below antral lacerations to provide a temporary interface between the antrum and the graft material to be placed.

For larger perforations (greater than 2 mm diameter), the torn membrane can be elevated off the medial wall, folded onto itself to approximate the lacerated membrane of the lateral wall, and then covered with a resorbable collagen wound dressing. This requires the membrane to be of adequate consistency.

If the defect is too large and the margins of the membrane surrounding the perforation have been well elevated, resorbable suture material (5.0 or 6.0) can be used to close the defect. This suturing technique can be unpredictable and very difficult, however, if the membrane cannot be elevated around the margins of the perforation. This may require perforating the bone surrounding the osteotomy to provide a site through which to suture.

Another alternative is to stop the procedure and then suture the outer soft tissues. After 2 to 3 months of healing, the sinus elevation procedure can be performed again. This approach is difficult and is not always practical.

If all else fails, a final—although not always stable—approach to repairing large perforations is to shape and place a large lamellar bone sheet within the osteotomy site, thereby creating a pouch over the perforate region. Graft material is placed along the borders of the bone sheet to stabilize it and then in the middle of the sheet over the perforation.

To prevent sinus membrane perforation, a split-thickness flap design is suggested and a brushstroke type of contact should be used to penetrate the bone when the lateral wall of the sinus membrane is osteotomized. This allows good access while minimizing perforation risk. A No. 8 surgical diamond round bur is recommended for this procedure.

The osteotomy design should consist more of a rounded edge rectangle involving a complete osteotomy on the lateral and inferior walls, as opposed to a hinged-door type of osteotomy window.[42] The osteotomy design should be changed if extensive bony septa are discovered because reflection over these membrane-adhering septa increases the risk for perforation.

Fractured Mandible

Mandibular fracture after implant placement is rare but has been reported in conjunction with severely resorbed edentulous mandibles.[18] The risk is particularly high when numerous implants are placed, and when the bone has been mechanically weakened.[45] The risk for mandibular fracture also increases following nerve repositioning with implant placement.[48]

Patients with fracture tend to present with pain and swelling in the mandible and chin area. Occasionally, they report sensory disturbances of the lower lip and chin.

If a pathologic fracture occurs after implant placement, certain things must be considered in determining how to proceed. The basic goals for all fracture treatment approaches are reduction and immobilization to restore form and function.[43]

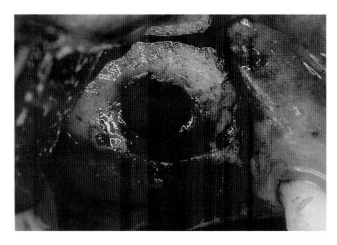

FIGURE 19-5 ■ Sinus membrane perforation can occur from vigorous reflection of the membrane area. A collagen membrane can be used to repair 1- to 20-mm sinus membrane perforations.

In most cases, the implant is in the line of the fracture, and the segments must be evaluated for mobility and displacement of the fracture site. If there is neither clinical evidence of mobility nor radiographic evidence of segment displacement, the fracture should be left untreated and the patient placed on a soft diet. Patients should be instructed to avoid extreme movements, such as yawning, if possible. If these restrictions are followed, uncomplicated healing and implant integration are possible.

If mobility is detected but no radiographic evidence of displacement is noted, the fracture can be reduced in a closed manner. Regular intermaxillary fixation can be used in partially edentulous patients with teeth mesial and distal to the line of fracture. Two options are available for treating partially edentulous patients with a fracture in the free-end area or for completely edentulous patients. If the patient has a transitional prosthesis, circumferential wiring of the mandible and the prosthesis can be accomplished to reduce the fracture. In patients without dentures, open reduction of the fracture should be performed.

Open reduction is the best treatment approach in patients with marked mobility and displacement after a fracture.[43]

For elderly or seriously infirm patients, fracture immobilization is best not attempted, as these patients do not tolerate the usual methods well, and they are prone to failure.[43,46]

To prevent mandibular fracture, the clinician must thoroughly evaluate the height and the labial-lingual width of available bone. Ideally, a few millimeters of cortical bone should remain on both the labial and lingual sites after the osteotomy has been created.[45] If necessary, grafting should be done to strengthen the mandible.

For nerve repositioning cases, a fracture can be prevented by minimizing the amount of buccal cortical plate removed during nerve localization and by maintaining the integrity of the inferior cortex of the mandible.[48]

The osteotomy must be carefully undertaken with copious irrigation, as the thin mandible is vulnerable to thermal injury because of its dense cortical nature.

Multiple implant sites also weaken the mandibular bone. When an atrophic mandible is present, it is prudent to place fewer implants than normal, at least until the mandible has been back in function for 2 years or longer.[44] Use of specially designed transmandibular implants, which distribute masticatory forces along the severely atrophied mandible, may be useful in some cases. Patients should be cautioned about limiting stress to the vulnerable jaw during the healing period.

Tool/Component Aspirations

Accidentally ingested hardware—such as tiny screws, screwdrivers, and other small components—usually passes through the alimentary canal without complication. Often there are no clinical signs or symptoms requiring immediate removal, but radiographs and continued observation

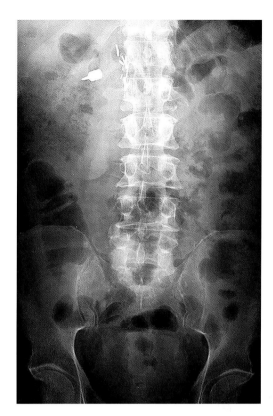

FIGURE 19-6 ■ This chest film shows an implant driver, which was inadvertently swallowed.

are warranted. Aspiration of these tools or components, however, presents a complex problem, and removal should be attempted immediately. Ingestion or aspiration can lead to risks such as airway or intestinal obstruction, bleeding, perforation, and infection, necessitating operative removal (Figure 19-6).

To prevent this error, safety ligatures or tethers made of floss or suture material should be secured to all small tools to allow easy retrieval. A thin gauze screen may be placed across the patient's oropharynx.

Mechanical Complications

Screw Loosening/Fracture

The most common mechanical complication following implant surgery is loosening or fracture of the abutment screw.[18] This occurs most often with single-implant crown replacements in the anterior premolar and molar areas and usually presents as a loose crown. The patient may complain of soreness at the interface between soft tissue and fixture, swelling or fistula formation, and difficulty chewing.

Possible causes of screw loosening or fracture include poor-fitting frameworks, bone remodeling with release of pretension in the screw joint, reduced clamping force and screw joint movement, and heavy occlusal force.[18]

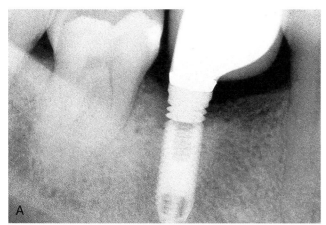

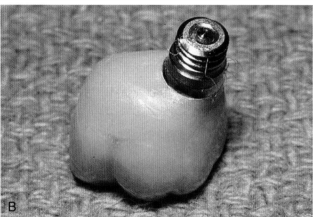

FIGURE 19-7 ■ **A, B** Most fractures occur between the third and fourth implant threads, and this frequently corresponds to the last thread of the abutment screw and the location of a weak spot in many implant systems.

A loose abutment may lead to fistula or sinus formation, loss of integration, or fracturing of abutment or porcelain facings.[14]

Problems with loose or fractured locking or abutment screws commonly occur repeatedly in the same patient (Figure 19-7). This usually indicates that the design concept is inappropriate, the framework does not fit well, mechanical or material components are incompatible, or the occlusal scheme and masticatory function are not harmonious. These factors can be compounded by poor implant distribution within the arch or poor angulation. Neglecting the underlying cause of repeated screw-related problems can result in more serious complications.[57]

Retrieving a mobile crown can be difficult and time consuming. If the screw head can be accessed through the palatal cingulum area, the crown may be perforated to allow retrievability. If the screw head emerges buccally, the crown requires sectioning. The screw then may be tightened or, if fractured, its surface can be engaged with a sharp probe or a special retrieval kit. Abutment screws usually are easy to rotate counterclockwise. The screw is then replaced and attention directed to the cause of loosening or fracture.

To minimize the risk for screw loosening, the clinician should use gold alloy abutment screws, which yield a higher screw preload than titanium screws when properly torqued.[58] Some authors have demonstrated the usefulness of a hexagonal bar that interlocks with the fixation screw to better secure the superstructure on single implants.[59] Screw fracture risk can be minimized by avoiding overtightening.

Taking care to properly place the implant's antirotational device may also help. When placed too shallow, it is difficult to locate during component seating and can lead to vibration and micromovement of the crown from occlusal forces. This can cause the screw joint to fail.[60]

The screw-retained framework must fit passively to eliminate permanent strain on the screws, framework, and veneers. When supragingival abutments are used, the retainer's fit can be assessed using the single-screw test. With subgingival abutments, fit can be evaluated by determining how the screw feels during tightening. If the framework is passive, each screw should become tight immediately after the clinician feels resistance to tightening. On the contrary, if a screw becomes gradually tighter during turning, the implant and the framework are likely being drawn together, indicating a nonpassive fit.[56]

Implant Fracture

Implant fracture is an uncommon but significant complication. In a review of nine different studies following 6,560 implants for up to 15 years, less than 2% of the implants endured fracture.[18] Most fractures occur between the third and the fourth implant thread, which corresponds to the last thread of the abutment screw.[18]

A greater risk for fracture has been reported with fixed partial dentures supported by one or two implants, particularly in the posterior partially edentulous jaw, where occlusal loads are higher and laterally directed jaw forces can be excessive.[18,53]

The primary causes are framework misfit and occlusal overload. Other factors that can contribute to fracture risk include superstructure design, implant diameter (narrow fixtures tend to fracture more easily, especially in the posterior), bone resorption around the implant, implant mobility, and manufacturer design or production flaws (rarely)[41] (Figure 19-8).

Treatment for an implant fracture depends on whether the clinician plans to replace the implant. If so, both implant fragments must be removed. Additional and wider implants may be placed and a new prosthesis made. Ridge augmentation may be necessary in some cases.

If the implant will not be replaced, the clinician may choose to leave the apical fragment in situ, burying it under the mucosa. This approach requires only minimal adjustments at the prosthesis. Its benefit derives from avoiding the often difficult fracture removal procedure and the large bony defect this creates, which requires additional healing time and treatment.

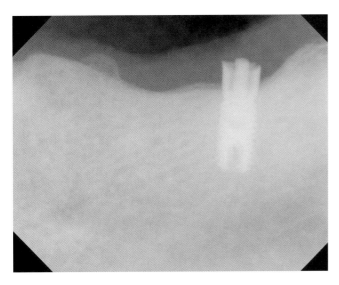

FIGURE 19-8 ■ Fractured implant due to manufacturer design flaw.

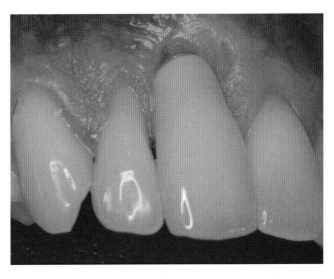

FIGURE 19-9 ■ Buccal gingival recession around an anterior dental implant due to poor placement positioning (implant is placed too far buccally).

For implant-supported fixed partial dentures, which seem to be at greatest risk for implant fracture, at least three implants (in a tripod configuration) should be placed to minimize stress and torque distribution.[53] Placing wider implants, avoiding extensions, staggering placement to avoid a straight line configuration, and putting patients with parafunctional problems on protective splints may prevent implant fractures.[55]

Esthetic/Prosthetic Complications

Gingival Recession

Gingival recession can be a long-term complication that initially causes a long clinical crown and graying at the gingival margin (Figure 19-9). If it progresses, the metal margins or the implant–abutment junction may become exposed. This requires remaking the crown with a modification to the titanium abutment or exchanging it for a ceramic one to improve the esthetic result.

A common cause of gingival recession is positioning the implant too labially, which can leave a deficiency of attached gingivae.

One of the most common soft tissue esthetic problems is loss of the interdental papilla or apical positioning of the labial gingival margin. This occurs during postsurgical healing, causing the appearance of black triangles on either side of the restoration and a gingival margin that does not harmonize with the rest of the dentition. This can be prevented by taking care of the patient's soft tissue needs before or during stage 2 surgery.[56]

Improper Implant Positioning/Alignment

Even with careful planning and use of a surgical template, implant misplacement may occur occasionally. The effect will vary depending on how much flexibility the case presents for modifying the abutment choice and superstructure. An overdenture generally provides somewhat more latitude than a fixed prosthesis. The lower jaw offers greater flexibility than the upper jaw, as does the edentulous patient compared with the partially edentulous patient.[11]

Several manufacturers offer component alternatives, such as angled or bendable abutments, that can be used to address improper implant alignment. These are poor substitutes for properly aligned implants, however, because they may be unesthetic and cause problems due to unfavorable loading. Some implants accommodate a tapered abutment that can be used with a single crown with its margin placed below the mucosa.

Different positioning errors lead to varying problems and warrant different remedies. Implants angled too far labially can require placement of screw-access holes through the labial or buccal surfaces of replacement teeth. Angulated abutments or mesostructure may be necessary in this case to correctly place screw-access holes.

Implants placed too far lingually may irritate the free mucosa of the mouth floor and cause difficulty with hygiene. Implants placed too far buccally may cause the superstructure to be too prominent, while those placed too palatally may have the opposite effect and may interfere with tongue movement and speech (Figure 19-10).

Extreme divergence of the implant long axis from that of remaining teeth or other implants can cause major problems with prosthetic treatment. Widely diverging and crowded implants make impression taking difficult.

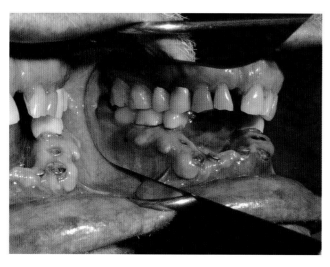

FIGURE 19-10 ■ Poor implant placement and positioning.

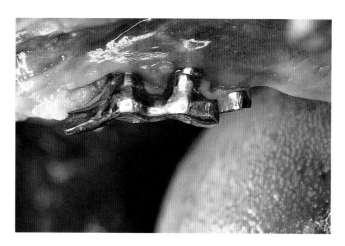

FIGURE 19-11 ■ Overdenture bar is fractured.

Esthetic, hygiene, and biomechanical compromises almost always have to be accepted if implants are placed too far labially or bucally.

Aside from modifying abutment component choice, the clinician may have other options. For instance, if one implant is misplaced, it may be kept as a "sleeper" fixture and the prosthesis design modified accordingly. For more extreme cases, a removable rather than the planned fixed superstructure may be warranted to allow greater freedom in designing it (if space allows such modification.)

Sometimes poor positioning is so extreme that the implants must be excluded from the treatment plan and removed altogether.

Proper treatment planning, team communication, and continual reference to the opposing arch with prosthetic requirements in mind help to prevent angulation problems. The use of a surgical stent during placement is also important. This problem highlights the importance of bone grafting as needed, so the clinician does not simply place the implant wherever any existing bone is found at the site.

Fractured Prostheses

After the various screws involved in an implant-supported restoration, the superstructure is the next most likely component to endure fracture.[11] Failure usually occurs as the result of excessive loads (e.g., long cantilevers, opposing teeth, heavy occlusal loads, bruxism) or poor stress distribution and design leading to overload or fatigue failure.[57]

A fractured fixed superstructure must be refabricated after the cause of fracture has been identified and addressed. If the fracture affects a distal cantilever, the rest of the superstructure can continue to be used in the interim. If the fracture occurs in the middle of a fixed superstructure, a

temporary repair with wire and cured resin can be done. A temporary denture could be made for use until the new final prosthesis is received.

Overdenture fractures present a different scenario. Because these are stabilized by both the underlying mucosa and the implants, care must be taken to control load distributions—which usually involve linear vertical movement and rotation—between the two. It is important that attachments allow for both types of movement. Spacers may facilitate this.

Without adequate interocclusal space, excessive forces on the attachment can cause fracture of the denture base, the superstructure, or the attachments (Figure 19-11). This can result from bone resorption, which causes the denture to sink in relation to the implants. Rebasing of overdentures may be required to correct effects of bone resorption or design/construction errors.

If a bar-type attachment is used, distal cantilevers may be incorporated to reduce rotation of the denture away from the mucosa.

These bars can be subject to heavy occlusal loads if bone resorbs or a spacer is not used when the clips are located. This can cause the bar or gold cylinder to fracture. Thus cantilevers normally should be no longer than 8 mm.[11]

Patients who clench or brux can rapidly wear down or fracture acrylic teeth; using teeth with a hard, wear-resistant surface can reduce this problem.[14] Malpositioned implants can increase the incidence of overdenture fracture; this can be avoided by using a surgical stent.

SUMMARY

Complications can be minimized by following sound surgical and prosthetic principles as well as appropriate treatment planning. Of course, it is also important to use well-researched implant systems and components.

REFERENCES

1. Muller E, del Pilar Rios Calvo M: Pain and dental implantology: sensory quantifications and affective aspects, Part I: at the private dental office, *Implant Dent* 10:14-22, 2001.
2. Balshi TJ: Preventing and resolving complications with implants, *Dent Clin North Am* 33:821-868, 1989.
3. Adell R, Lekholm H, Rockler B, Branemark P-I: A 15-year study of osseointegrated dental implants in the treatment of the edentulous jaw, *Int J Oral Surg* 10:387-416, 1981.
4. Kiyak HA, Beach BH, Worthington P, et al: The psychological impact of osseointegrated dental implants, *Int J Oral Maxillofac Implants* 5:61-91, 1990.
5. Wismeijer D, van Waas MAJ, Vermeeren JIJF, Kalk W: Patients' perception of sensory disturbances of the mental nerve before and after implant surgery: a prospective study of 110 patients, *Br J Oral Maxillofac Surg* 35:254-259, 1997.
6. van Steenberghe D, Lekholm U, Bolender C, et al: The rehabilitation of partial edentulism: a prospective multicenter study on 558 fixtures, *Int J Oral Maxillofac Implants* 5:272-281, 1990.
7. Ellies LG, Hawker PB: The prevalence of altered sensation associated with implant surgery, *Int J Oral Maxillofac Implants* 8:674-679, 1993.
8. Worthington P: Medicolegal aspects of oral implant surgery, *Austral Prosthodont J* 9:13-17, 1995.
9. Delcanho RE: Neuropathic implications of prosthodontic treatment, *J Prosthet Dent* 73:146-152, 1995.
10. Theisen FC, Shultz RE, Elledge DA: Displacement of a root form implant into the mandibular canal, *Oral Surg Oral Med Oral Pathol* 70:24-28, 1990.
11. Surgical problems. In: Hobkirk JA, Watson RM, editors: *Color atlas and text of dental and maxillo-facial implantology*, London, 1995, Mosby-Wolfe.
12. Palmer R, Palmer P, Howe L: Complications and maintenance, *Br Dent J* 187:653-658, 1999.
13. Mehlman S: A review of implant-related damage to adjacent tooth: a case report. Observations and remarks, *Implant Dent* 9:279, 2000.
14. Watson CJ, Tinsley D, Sharma S: Implant complications and failures: the single-tooth restoration, *Dent Update* 27:35-42, 2000.
15. Pauletto N, Lahiffe BJ, Walton JN: Complications associated with excess cement around crowns on osseointegrated implants: a clinical report, *Int J Oral Maxillofac Implants* 14:865-868, 1999.
16. Agar JR, Cameron SM, Hughbanks JC, Parker MH: Cement removal from restorations luted to titanium abutments with simulated subgingival margins, *J Prosthet Dent* 78:43-47, 1997.
17. Scarano A, Di Dmoisio P, Petrone G, et al: Implant periapical lesion: a clinical and histologic case report, *J Oral Implantol* 26:109-113, 2000.
18. Goodacre CJ, Kan JYK, Rungcharassaeng K: Clinical complications of osseointegrated implants, *J Prosthet Dent* 81:537-552, 1999.
19. Tepper G, Hofschnader UB, Gahleither A, Ulm C: Computed tomography diagnosis and localization of bone canals in the mandibular interforaminal region for prevention of bleeding complications during implant surgery, *Int J Oral Maxillofac Implants* 16:68-72, 2001.
20. Niamtu J: Near-fatal airway obstruction after routine implant placement, *Oral Surg Oral Med Oral Pathol* 92:597-600, 2001.
21. Givol N, Chaushu G, Halamish-Shani T, Taicher S: Emergency tracheostomy following life-threatening hemorrhage in the floor of the mouth during immediate implant placement in the mandibular canine region, *J Periodontol* 71:1893-1895, 2000.
22. Mordenfeld A, Andersson L, Bergstrom B: Hemorrhage in the floor of the mouth during implant placement in the edentulous mandible: a case report, *Int J Oral Maxillofac Implants* 12:558-561, 1997.
23. ten Buggenkate CM, Krekeler G, Kraaijenhagen HA, et al: Hemorrhage of the floor of the mouth resulting from lingual perforation during implant placement: a clinical report, *Int J Oral Maxillofac Implants* 8:329-334, 1993.
24. Bavitz JB, Harn SD, Homze EJ: Arterial supply to the floor of the mouth and lingual gingivae, *Oral Surg Oral Med Oral Pathol* 77:232-235, 1994.
25. Andersson B, Odman P, Lindvall AM, Lithner B: Single-tooth restorations supported by osseointegrated implants: results and experiences from a prospective study after 2 to 3 years, *Int J Oral Maxillofac Implants* 10:702-711, 1995.
26. Mombelli A: Prevention and therapy of peri-implant infections. In: Lang NP, Karring T, Lindhe J, editors: Proceedings of the 3rd European Workshop on Periodontology, Berlin, 1999, Quintessence, pp 281-303.
27. Callan DP, Hahn J, Hogan B, et al: Perspectives: (A follow-up to a report on implant failure), *Implant Dent* 11:109-117, 2002.
28. Weyant RJ: Characteristics associated with the loss and peri-implant tissue health of endosseous dental implants, *Int J Oral Maxillofac Implants* 9:95-102, 1994.
29. Esposito M, Hirsch J-M, Lekholm U, Thomsen P: Biological factors contributing to failures of osseointegrated oral implants: (II) etiopathogenesis, *Eur J Oral Sci* 106:721-764, 1998.
30. van Winkelhoff AJ, Goene RJ, Benschop C, Folmer T: Early colonization of dental implants by putative periodontal pathogens in partially edentulous patients, *Clin Oral Implants Res* 11:511-520, 2000.
31. Miyata T, Koabyashi Y, Araki H, et al: The influence of controlled occlusal overload on peri-implant tissue, Part 4, a histologic study in monkeys, *Int J Oral Maxillofac Implants* 17:384-390, 2002.
32. Dent CD, Olson JW, Farish SE, et al: The influence of preoperative antibiotics on success of endosseous implants up to and including stage II surgery: a study of 2641 implants, *J Oral Maxillofac Surg* 55:19-24, 1997.
33. Lambert PM, Morris HF, Ochi S: The influence of 0.12% chlorhexidine digluconate rinses on the incidence of infectious complications and implant success, *J Oral Maxillofac Surg* 55:25-30, 1997.
34. Persson LG, Berglundh T, Lindhe J, Senneby L: Reosseointegration after treatment of peri-implantitis at different implant surfaces, *Clin Oral Implants Res* 12:595-603, 2001.
35. Hurzeler MB, Quinones CR, Schupbach P, et al: Treatment of peri-implantitis using guided bone regeneration and bone grafts, alone or in combination, in beagle dogs, Part 2, histologic findings, *Int J Oral Maxillofac Implants* 12:168-175, 1997.
36. Hanish O, Tatakis DN, Osmotic MM, et al: Bone formation and re-osseointegration in peri-implantitis defects following surgical implantation of rhBMP-2, *Int J Oral Maxillofac Implants* 12:604-610, 1997.
37. Block MS, Kent JN: Factors associated with soft-and hard-tissue compromise of endosseous implants, *J Oral Maxillofac Surg* 48:1153-1160, 1990.

38. Simion M, Baldoni M, Zaffe D: Jawbone enlargement using immediate implant placement associated with a split-crest technique and guided tissue regeneration, *Int J Periodontics Restorative Dent* 12:463-473, 1992.

39. Bruschi GB, Sciopioni A: Alveolar augmentation: new approaches for implants. In: Heimke G, editor: *Osseointegrated implants, vol II, implants in oral and ENT surgery*, Boca Raton, FL, 1990, CRC Press.

40. Garg AK: Complications associated with dental implants, *Dent Implantol Update* 8:1-4, 2002.

41. Tagger Green N, Machtei EE, Horwitz J, Peled M: Fracture of dental implants: literature review and report of a case, *Implant Dent* 11:137-143, 2002.

42. Vlassis JM, Fugazzotto PA: A classification system for sinus membrane perforations during augmentation procedures with options for repair, *J Periodontol* 70:692-699, 1999.

43. Buchbinder D: Treatment of fractures of the edentulous mandible, 1943 to 1993, *J Oral Maxillofac Surg* 51:1174-1180, 1993.

44. Worthington P: Clinical aspects of severe mandibular atrophy. In: Worthington P, Branemark P-I, editors: *Advanced osseointegration surgery: applications in the maxillofacial region*, Chicago, 1992, Quintessence.

45. Raghoebar GM, Stellingsma K, Batenburg RHK, Vissink A: Etiology and management of mandibular fractures associated with endosteal implants in the atrophic mandible, *Oral Surg Oral Med Oral Pathol Oral Radiol Endod* 89:553-559, 2000.

46. Alpert B: Discussion of Eyrich G, Gratz KW, Sailer HF: Surgical treatment of fractures of the mandible, *J Oral Maxillofac Surg* 55:1081-1087, 1997.

47. Peleg M, Mazor Z, Chaushu G, Garg AK: Lateralization of the inferior alveolar nerve with simultaneous implant placement: a modified technique, *Int J Oral Maxillofac Implants* 17:101-106, 2002.

48. Louis PJ: Inferior alveolar nerve transposition for endosseous implant placement: a preliminary report, *J Oral Maxillofac Surg Clin North Am* 13:265-281, 2001.

49. Sethi A: Inferior alveolar nerve repositioning: a preliminary report, *Int J Periodont Rest Dent* 15:475-481, 1995.

50. Kan JYK, Lozada JL, Goodacre CJ, et al: Endosseous implant placement in conjunction with inferior alveolar nerve transposition: an evaluation of neurosensory disturbance, *Int J Oral Maxillofac Implants* 12:463-471, 1997.

51. Babbush CA: Transpositioning and repositioning the inferior alveolar and mental nerves in conjunction with endosteal implant reconstruction, *Periodontology* 17:183-190, 2000.

52. Kahnberg K-E, Henry PJ, Tan AES, et al: Tissue regeneration adjacent to titanium implants placed with simultaneous transposition of the inferior dental nerve: a study in dogs, *Int J Oral Maxillofac Implants* 15:119-124, 2000.

53. Rangert B, Krogh PH, Langer B, Van Roekel N: Bending overload and implant fracture: a retrospective clinical analysis, *Int J Oral Maxillofac Implants* 10:326-334, 1995.

54. Jovanovic SA: Recognition and treatment of peri-implantitis. In: Block MS, Kent JN, editors: pp 591-601.

55. Purton, DG, Hunter KM: Success and failure in partially edentulous bridge with implant supported bridges, *New York Dent J* 90:98-102, 1994.

56. Baumgarten HS, Chiche GJ: Diagnosis and evaluation of complications and failures associated with osseointegrated implants, *Compend Contin Educ Dent* 16:814-823, 1995.

57. Tolman DE. Laney WR: Tissue-integrated prosthesis complications, *Int J Oral Maxillofac Implants* 7:477-484, 1992.

58. Jorneus L, Jemt T, Carlsson L: Loads and designs of screw joints for single crowns supported by osseointegrated implants, *Int J Oral Maxillofac Implants* 7:353-359, 1992.

59. Artzi Z, Dreinangel A: A screw lock for single-tooth implant superstructures, *J Am Dent Assoc* 130:677-682, 1999.

60. Binon P: The role of screws in implant systems, *Int J Oral Maxillofac Implants* 9:48-63, 1994.

Glossary

A

Aberrant deviating from the norm or the usual.

Abrade to grind, rub, scrape, or wear away the surface of a part by friction.

Abrasion a surface or a part worn away by natural or artificial means.

Abscess an abscess is an enclosed collection of pus on the body as a result of the body's defensive reaction to an infection. Most abscesses can occur anywhere in the body.

Absorbable See: BIOABSORBABLE.

Absorption the reception of substances through, by, or into biological tissue.

Abutment the portion of an implant or implant component(s) above the neck of the implant that serves to support and/or retain a fixed, fixed-detachable, or removable dental prosthesis.

Abutment attachment a mechanical device for the fixation, retention, or stabilization of an implant-borne dental prosthesis.

Abutment clamp 1. any device used for positioning a dental implant abutment upon a dental implant body. 2. forceps used to assist in the positioning of an abutment on the implant platform.

Abutment connection a procedure for securing an abutment to an implant.

Abutment level impression the impression of an abutment either directly (using conventional impression techniques) or indirectly (using an abutment impression coping). See: IMPLANT LEVEL IMPRESSION.

Abutment screw a screw used to secure the abutment to the implant, usually torqued to a final seating position.

Abutment selection the decision during prosthodontic treatment concerning the type of abutment used for the restoration, based on implant angulation, interarch space, soft tissue (mucosal) height, planned prosthesis, occlusal factors (e.g., opposing dentition, parafunction), and esthetic and phonetic considerations.

Abutment swapping See: PLATFORM SWITCHING.

Abutment transfer device See: ORIENTATION JIG.

Access hole the channel in a screw-retained implant prosthesis that receives the abutment or prosthetic screw, usually through the occlusal or lingual surface of the prosthesis.

Accessory ostium occasional opening of the maxillary sinus either into the infundibulum or directly in the wall of the middle meatus. See: OSTIUM (MAXILLARY SINUS).

Acellular having no cells.

Acellular dermal allograft a substitute for autogenous soft tissue grafts in root coverage procedure that replaces lost dermis and is used as a synthetic or biosynthetic material. Also referred to as skin grafts.

Acid-etched implant external surface of an implant body modified by the chemical action of an acidic medium intended to enhance osseointegration.

Acid-etched surface an implant surface treated with acid to increase the surface area by subtraction. See: SUBTRACTED SURFACE.

Acrylic resin a self-cured or heat-cured plastic consisting of monomers (usually liquid) and polymers (usually powders).

Actinobacillus actinomycetem comitans a species of gram-negative, facultatively anaerobic spherical or rod-shaped bacteria; frequently associated with some forms of human periodontal disease as well as subacute and chronic endocarditis; occurs with actinomycetes in actinomycotic lesions.

Actonel an oral bisphosphonate; brand name for active ingredient risedronate sodium; used to treat Paget's disease of the bone, and to prevent and treat postmenopausal osteoporosis and ucocorticoid-induced osteoporosis in men and women. Several cases of bisphosphonate-related osteomyelitis (BON, also referred to as osteonecrosis of the jaw) have been associated with the use of the oral bisphosphonates (Fosamax [alendronate], Actonel [risedronate] and Boniva [ibandronate]) for the treatment of osteoporosis; these patients may have had other conditions that could put them at risk for developing BON.

Added surface syn: Additive surface treatment; alteration of an implant surface by addition of material. See: SUBTRACTED SURFACE, TEXTURED SURFACE.

Additive surface treatment See: ADDED SURFACE.

Adduct to pull or draw medially.

Adhesion the sticking together of dissimilar materials.

Adjustment a modification of a restoration of a tooth or of a prosthetic after insertion in the mouth.

Adsorption   adhesion of molecules to solid or liquid surfaces.

Ailing implant   general term for an implant affected by implant mucositis, without bone loss; an implant with a history of bone loss. See: PERI-IMPLANT MUCOSITIS, PERI-IMPLANTITIS.

Ala nasi   the wings of the nose.

Ala-tragus line   a line extending from the midpoint of the tragus to the nasal wings.

Algipore   a biological HA derived from calcifying maritime algae.

Alkaline phosphatase   a hydrolase enzyme used to remove phosphate groups from many types of molecules, including nucleotides, proteins, and alkaloids.

Allogenic   transplantation tissues of the same species but antigenically different.

Allogenic graft   tissue transplanted between members of the same species; a homograft. See: ALLOGRAFT.

Allograft   syn: Allogenic graft; graft tissue from genetically dissimilar members of the same species. Three types exist: frozen, freeze-dried bone allograft (FDBA), and demineralized freeze-dried bone allograft (DFDBA). Allograft bone is processed and prepared from tissue banks. See: HOMOGRAFT, ALLOPLAST.

Alloplast   syn: Alloplastic graft; synthetic, inorganic material used as a bone substitute or as an implant; a relatively inert synthetic material, generally metal, ceramic, or polymeric, used to construct, reconstruct, or augment tissue. See: IMPLANT.

Alloplastic graft   See: ALLOPLAST; graft of a relatively inert synthetic material.

Alloplastic material   relatively inert synthetic material, usually metal, ceramic, or polymeric.

Aluminum oxide   a metallic oxide. 1. Alpha Single Crystal: an inert, highly biocompatible, strong ceramic material from which some endosseous implants are fabricated. 2. Polycrystal: constituent of dental porcelain used to increase viscosity and strength.

Aluminum oxide (alpha single crystal)   an inert, strong, highly biocompatible ceramic material from which endosseous implants are fabricated through crystal culture techniques.

Aluminum oxide (polycrystal)   a fused A1203 biocompatible material.

Alveolar   pertaining to an alveolus. See: ALVEOLUS.

Alveolar augmentation   A surgical procedure designed to enlarge the morphology of a ridge. See: AUGMENTATION.

Alveolar bone   See: BONE; the portion of the jaw bone that retained or retains teeth.

Alveolar crest   the most coronal portion of the alveolar process.

Alveolar defect   a deficiency in the contour of the alveolar ridge. The deficiency can be in the vertical (apicocoronal) and/or horizontal (buccolingual, mesiodistal) direction.

Alveolar distraction osteogenesis   See: DISTRACTION OSTEOGENESIS.

Alveolar mucosa   syn: Lining mucosa; mucosa covering the alveolar process apical to the cogingival junction, consisting of a nonkeratinized epithelium lining, a connective tissue that is loosely attached to the periosteum and movable; the mucous membrane covering the basal part of the alveolar process, continuing without demarcation into the vestibular fornix and the mouth's floor. See: ORAL MUCOSA.

Alveolar nerve   a terminal of the mandibular nerve that passes through the lower teeth, periosteum, and gingiva of the mandible and finally to the skin of the chin and the mucous membrane of the lower lip. See: INFERIOR ALVEOLAR, INFERIOR DENTAL NERVE.

Alveolar process   the portion of the maxillae or mandible forming the dental arch and serving as a bony investment for the teeth; the compact and cancellous portion of bone surrounding and supporting the teeth. See: ALVEOLAR RIDGE, RESIDUAL RIDGE, RIDGE.

Alveolar recess   a cavity formed in the maxillary sinus floor formed by a septum. See: SEPTUM (MAXILLARY SINUS).

Alveolar reconstruction   surgical procedure designed to reshape or restore the alveolar ridge; alveoloplasty.

Alveolar ridge   the bony ridge of the maxillae or mandible containing the alveoli (teeth sockets); the remainder of the alveolar process after the teeth are removed. See: RESIDUAL RIDGE, RIDGE.

Alveolar ridge augmentation   See: AUGMENTATION.

Alveolar ridge resorption   See: RIDGE RESORPTION.

Alveolectomy   removal of a portion of the alveolar process, usually performed to achieve acceptable bone contour. See: OSTECTOMY.

Alveoloplasty   conservative contouring of the alveolar process to achieve acceptable ridge morphology. See: OSTEOPLASTY.

Alveolus   the socket in the bone in which a tooth is attached via the periodontal ligament; tooth socket.

Amorphous   free of crystalline structure.

Amoxicillin   an antibiotic effective against different bacteria found in and around the oral cavity including but not limited to *Haemophilus influenzae*, *Neisseria gonorrhoea*, *Escherichia coli*, Pneumococci, Streptococci, and certain strains of Staphylococci, particularly infections of the middle ear, tonsillitis, throat infections, laryngitis, bronchitis, and pneumonia. Amoxicillin is also used in treating urinary tract infections and some skin infections.

Analgesic   a chemical that generally relieves pain without causing the patient to lose consciousness.

Analog (Analogue)   syn: replica. A replica of an implant, abutment, or attachment mechanism, usually incorporated within a cast for a prosthetic reconstruction; an implant replica on the laboratory bench used for purposes of prosthetic reconstruction.

Anatomy branch of science that describes the morphology of organs; the art associated with separating the parts of an organism to determine the position, relations, structure, and function of those parts.

Anesthesia absence of sensation to stimuli.

Angiogenesis formation and differentiation of new blood vessels.

Angle, E.H. occlusal conditions classified by anteroposterior relationships (Class 1, normal; Class 2, bilateral or partial protrusion of the maxilla; Class 3, protrusion of the mandible).

Angled abutment a prosthetic coupling component of an implant (available in a variety of angles, up to 35 degrees), which is specially designed to be fitted with a crown or other anchorage attachment. See: ANGULATED ABUTMENT.

Angled implant allows for implant placement within available bone while the restorative platform is located at an optimal esthetic angle.

Angular cheilitis inflammation of the corners of the mouth, frequently caused by bite overclosure and sometimes by riboflavin deficiency.

Angulated abutment syn: angled abutment; abutment with a body that is not parallel to the long axis of the implant. It is used when the implant is at a different inclination in relation to the proposed prosthesis; the portion of an endosteal implant that deviates from its long axis as it passes permucosally to serve as an anchorage device for a crown. See: NONANGULATED ABUTMENT.

Animal model a laboratory animal used for medical research because it has specific characteristics, based on its breed and species, that can be affected similar to a human afflicted by a specific disease or disorder. It can be created by transferring genes into them.

Anisotropic surface surface with a directional pattern. See: ISOTROPIC SURFACE.

Ankylosis bony consolidation in a joint between a tooth or implant and the jaw (see osseointegration); stiffness of a joint that is caused by disease or by surgery; the joining or union of distinct bones or separate hard parts to form one bone or part.

Anneal to heat and then cool (metals or glass) by a slow process to prevent brittleness, add toughness, and maintain pliability.

Anodization is an electrolytic passivation process used to increase the thickness of the natural oxide layer on the surface of metal to deter tarnish or corrosion. Anodization changes the microscopic texture of the surface and can change the crystal structure of the metal near the surface.

Anterior the forward part or front part in anatomy.

Anterior loop an extension of the inferior alveolar nerve, anterior to the mental foramen, and before exiting the mandibular canal.

Anterior nasal spine See: NASAL SPINE.

Anteroposterior spread (AP spread) the distance from the center of the most anterior implant to a line joining the distal aspects of the most distal implants; a measurement that provides a guideline for the amount of acceptable cantilever within the bilateral distal extensions of an implant-supported prosthesis.

Antibiotic substance produced by fungi that is able to inhibit bacterial growth used to treat infections caused by bacteria and other microorganisms.

Antirotation a feature or characteristic that prevents the rotation of two joint components.

Antirotation component a component of the implant body—hexagonal, tapered (Morse), or with some other internal design—placed to prevent unwanted abutment rotation.

Antral floor bony floor of the maxillary sinus cavity, typically lower than the nasal floor and tending to be wider.

Antral mucosa See: SCHNEIDERIAN MEMBRANE.

Antrum based on Greek antron, meaning "cave"; a cavity or chamber within the bone. See: SINUS.

Antrum of Highmore See: MAXILLARY SINUS.

Apatite calcium phosphate; the mineral component of teeth and bones.

Aperture an opening or hole.

Apex the highest point or tip.

Apex region (or apical region) the area surrounding the root tips of teeth.

Aphagia the inability to swallow.

Aphasia the inability to speak.

Apical referring to the apex.

Apical (retrograde) peri-implantitis See: IMPLANT PERIAPICAL lesion.

AP spread the acronym for anteroposterior spread.

Appliance a general reference to a prosthesis, splint, stent, template, guide, or denture.

Apposition a description of the relationship of two parts when the parts are placed together or co-adapted.

Approximation near or adjacent; the process of drawing parts together.

Arch form the shape of the arch when viewed from above or below; the shape may be square, oval, round, or tapering, or a combination of these.

Arch length discrepancy a reference to the differences between maxillary and mandibular arch forms, widths, lengths, and other dimensions.

Artery A vessel that carries blood high in oxygen content away from the heart to the farthest reaches of the body.

Articulation the natural relationship between upper and lower teeth in both static and dynamic function. Artificial articulation is the use of a mechanical device that simulates the movements of the temporomandibular joint, permitting the orientation of casts so as to duplicate or simulate various positions or movements of the patient.

Articulator a complex or simple mechanical device used to simulate the jaws and their movements in order to fabricate a prosthesis.

Artifact a foreign object revealed in the tissues through the use of diagnostic imaging, during palpation, or during surgery.

Asepsis prevention of contact with microorganisms; the state of the surgical field desirable for implant surgery.

Asleep term used to describe a non-pathologic implant left submerged.

Asymmetry a lack of balance or sameness.

Atrophic characterized by atrophy, in other words, by a decrease in the size of the ridge because of resorption of the bone.

Atrophy decrease in size of a cell, organ, tissue, or part. See: DISUSE ATROPHY, RIDGE ATROPHY.

Attached gingiva part of the gingiva extending from the base of the sulcus to the mucogingival junction around teeth. The gingival is "attached" to bone by the periosteum; to cementum by the gingival fibers; and to cementum, enamel, or dentin by the epithelial attachment. Alternately, the portion of the gingiva extending from the dental cervical margin to the alveolar mucosa; it is fairly dense, tightly bound to the underlying periosteum, tooth, and bone.

Attachment a mechanical device for the fixation, retention, and stabilization of a dental prosthesis; the attachment may consist of one part or several parts; it is made of metal, plastic, or other materials.

Attachment device See: ATTACHMENT.

Attachment screw a threaded device used to fasten prostheses to implants, driven in or removed by using a specially designed driver, which is inserted in a geometric pattern in its widened head.

Attrition the grinding or wearing down or away of hard tissues as a result of functional friction.

Augmentation placing autogenous or alloplastic materials in an attempt to correct deficiencies in the bone; alternately, the placement of a graft or any procedure that attempts to correct a soft tissue or hard tissue deficiency. See: BONE AUGMENTATION.

Auricular prosthesis a device that artificially replaces all or part of an ear.

Autocrine secretion of a chemical substance, such as hormones and growth factors that stimulate the secretion within the cell itself.

Autogenous self-generated.

Autogenous bone graft bone harvested from one site and transplanted to another site in the same individual.

Autogenous graft syn: autograft, autologous graft; tissue taken from one site and transplanted to another site in the same individual.

Autograft a graft taken from one part of the patient's body and transplanted to another part. See: AUTOGENOUS GRAFT.

Autologous See: AUTOGENOUS.

Autologous graft See: AUTOGENOUS GRAFT.

Available bone a reference to that portion of an edentulous ridge that is available for the predictably stable insertion of an endosseous implant.

Avascular lacking blood vessels.

Avascular necrosis cell death that has occurred due to loss of blood supply.

Avulsion a traumatic or surgical separation of a body part from its anatomic site.

Axial inclination a reference to the alignment of the long axis of a tooth to a horizontal plane.

Axial loading natural forces of function that are directed on the long axis of a tooth or implant; a reference, most often, to any force applied in the direction of the long axis of an implant. See: NONAXIAL LOADING.

B

Balanced occlusion the simultaneous contact of the upper and lower teeth on the right and left and in the anterior and posterior areas in centric and eccentric positions within the functioning range; used primarily to ensure alignment of dentures or prosthetics.

Bar syn: connecting bar; a type of connector between two or more implants or teeth, used to provide retention, stability, and/or support for a prosthesis.

Barium sulfate (BaSO4) finely ground radiopaque powder used in the construction of a radiographic template.

Bar overdenture (implant) a removable partial or complete denture, which may be either implant-supported or implant-tissue-supported. Implants in this type of reconstruction are connected with a bar incorporating attachment mechanisms for retention and support of the prosthesis.

Barrier membrane syn: occlusive membrane; a device that helps to confine a grafted area, thus preventing movement or loss of grafting material and controls the growth of undesirable cells into a site with or without a graft material.

Basal bone refers to the portion of the jaw bone not including the alveolar processes. See: BONE.

Base metal any metal that fails to resist a corrosive or oxidizing agent.

Basic multicellular unit (BMU) refers to a functional unit consisting of cellular elements responsible for bone formation and resorption (i.e., remodeling).

Basket endosteal dental implant generally, a perforated or fenestrated cylindrical endosteal implant that has been designed to permit bone growth within its basket.

Beading the placement of small balls or other devices for the adhesion of acrylic, cement, or other materials to a prosthesis.

Bending stress refers to stress forces caused by a load that tends to bend an object. See: STRESS.

Bevel a slanted edge.

BIC acronym: bone-to-implant contact.

Bicortical stabilization   the substantive engagement of an implant with the crestal cortical bone of the edentulous ridge and the cortical bone of the base of the mandible or the floor of the maxillary sinus or floor of the nasal cavity. This term may also apply to the engagement of the facial and lingual cortices or any two cortices by an implant.

Bifid   split or double-headed.

Bifurcation   splitting into two parts (for example, a split at the point of mandibulomental separation).

Bilateral   referring to two sides.

Bilateral stabilization   See: CROSS-ARCH STABILIZATION.

Bimaxillary protrusion   a reference to the pronation of both jaws.

Bioabsorbable   syn: absorbable; the property of a material that degrades and dissolves in vivo. Breakdown products from such material are incorporated into normal physiologic and biochemical processes (for example, bioabsorbable membranes or sutures).

Bioacceptability   See: BIOCOMPATIBLE.

Bioactive   having the quality of interfacial metabolism after implantation; having an effect on, or eliciting a response from, living tissue. See: BIOINERT.

Bioactive fixation   fixation or stabilization that involves the direct physical or chemical attachment mechanisms between biological materials and an implant surface at the ultra-structural level.

Bioactive glass   absorbable alloplastic material composed of the metal oxides Si02, Na20, and P205. It has the ability to form a chemical bond with living tissues and thereby to help stabilize a filled defect site and maintain a rigid scaffold upon which cells can migrate and grow.

Biocompatible   ability of a material to function without a negative host response (immune response or inflammation) in a specific application. In general, biocompatibility can be measured on the basis of allergenicity, carcinogenicity, localized cytotoxicity, and systemic responses; also used to refer to a material that has qualities that permit it to remain in a biologic environment successfully.

Biodegradable   a reference to the property of a material that causes it to break down when placed in a biologic environment. See: BIOABSORBABLE.

Bioinert   the property of a material that elicits no host response. See: BIOACTIVE.

Biointegration   the process by which living tissue bonds to the surface of a biomaterial or implant, which is independent of any mechanical interlocking mechanism. The term is often used to describe the bond of living tissue to hydroxyl apatite-coated implants. See: OSSEOINTEGRATION. Such bonding implies that contact is established without interposition of nonbony tissue between implant surface coating and host-remodeled bone; thus, a bond between the materials is formed biochemically, at the light microscopic level.

Biologic width   a reference to the combined width of the epithelial tissues and connective tissues above the bone level; alternately, the combined apicocoronal height of connective tissue and epithelial attachment. Such width exists around teeth as well as around dental implants once the implants are exposed to the oral cavity.

Biomaterial   non-viable material used to replace part of a living system or to function in contact with a living system; additionally, the term used to describe a relatively inert, naturally occurring, or manmade material that can be used to implant in or interface with living tissues or biologic fluids without resulting in untoward reactions with those tissues or fluids; such material can be used to fabricate devices designed to replace body parts or functions.

Biomechanical test   a test that measures the physical properties of any biomechanical device, device-tissue interface (e.g., bone-implant), or the properties of tissues themselves.

Biomechanics   the science of applying mechanical laws to living structures; the field of science dealing with the mechanical properties of biologic structures as well as the interaction between mechanical devices and living tissues, organs, and organisms.

Bioengineering   the application of engineering methods and techniques to solve issues in medicine and biology, including structure and movement, or the design of prosthetics.

Biofilm   a layer of extracellular matrix containing quiescent, non-proliferating microorganisms.

Biomimetic   able to replicate or imitate a body structure (anatomy) and/or function (physiology).

Biopsy   an evaluation and diagnosis of tissues removed from a living body.

Bioresorbable   See: RESORBABLE.

Bisphosphonate   an oral antiresorptive medicine that stops or slows the natural process that dissolves bone tissue, resulting in maintained bone density and strength. Note: Use of these medications has recently been linked to cases of jawbone decay or osteonecrosis of the jaw (ONJ). ONJ or "dead jaw" is a rare bone disease in which the jaw bone deteriorates and dies. The discovery of this link was published in the Journal of Oral and Maxillofacial Surgeons.

Bite raising   a term used to refer to increasing the occlusal all-vertical dimension.

Blackspace   See: BLACK TRIANGLE.

Black triangle   syn: black space; a condition resulting from papilla missing or not totally filling the embrasure space.

Blade endosteal dental implant   See: BLADE IMPLANT.

Blade implant   an endosteal implant consisting of an abutment, cervix, and body (or infrastructure) that is buccolingually thin and has fenestrations to permit the ingrowth of bone/connective tissue for purposes of anchorage. Laminar endosseous implant designed to be placed within the bone in a surgically prepared thin groove.

Blanching   making white or pale; usually in reference to pen-implant or periodontal soft tissue (for example, during prosthetictry-in/insertion).

Bleeding on probing   bleeding that is induced by gentle manipulation of the tissue at the depth of the gingival sulcus, or interface between the gingiva and a tooth with a periodontal probe. The dentist records this in order to determine the periodontal health of a patient.

Block graft   graft consisting of a monocortical piece of autogenous bone (for example, chin or ramus) or a piece of bone replacement graft, usually stabilized in the recipient site with screws.

Block out   eliminating harmful undercuts from human bone or study casts using surgery or putty-like materials.

Blood cell   any of the cell types, red, white, or platelet normally found in blood. In mammals, they are anucleate as they mature in order to provide more space for hemoglobin.

Blood clot   a semisolid mass in the bloodstream resulting from coagulation of the blood, primarily from platelets and fibrin.

BMP   acronym: bone morphogenetic protein.

BMU   acronym: basic multicellular unit.

Boil out   the elimination of wax using elevated temperatures.

Bond   a force that hold units of matter together.

Bone   the material of the skeleton of most vertebrate animals; the tissue constituting bones; the hard portion of the connective tissue constituting the majority of the skeleton. Bone consists of an inorganic component (67%, minerals such as calcium phosphate) and an organic component (33%, (collagenous matrix and cells). 1. Alveolar bone: bony portion of the mandible or maxilla in which the roots of the teeth are held by periodontal ligament fibers. Alveolar bone is formed during tooth development and eruption. 2. Basal bone: bone of the mandible or maxilla, excluding the alveolar bone. 3. Bundle bone: type of alveolar bone, so called because of the continuation into it of the principal (Sharpey's) fibers of the periodontal ligament. 4. Cancellous bone: syn: medullary bone, Spongy bone, Trabecular bone. Bone in which the trabeculae form a three-dimensional latticework with the interstices filled with bone marrow. 5. Cortical bone: syn: compact bone. The noncancellous hard and dense portion of bone that consists largely of concentric lamellar osteons and interstitial lamellae. 6. Lamellar bone: the normal type of mature bone, organized in layers (lamellae) that may be concentrically arranged (compact bone) or parallel (cancellous bone). 7. Woven bone: syn: nonlamellar bone, Primary bone, Primitive bone, Reactive bone. Immature bone encountered where bone is healing or being regenerated.

Bone atrophy   bone resorption manifested externally by morphologic change and internally by changes in density; decrease in the dimensions of bone due to its resorption.

Bone augmentation   the application of one of a variety of surgical procedures to enhance the dimensions of a potential operative site; placement of an autogenous graft and/or a bone replacement graft, or any procedure that corrects a hard tissue deficiency.

Bone, basal   the part of the mandible and maxillae from which the alveolar process develops.

Bone biopsy   a portion of bone under pathological examination for diagnosis.

Bone, bundle   the bone that forms the immediate attachment of the numerous bundles of collagen fibers incorporated into bone.

Bone, cancellous   the bone that forms a trabecular network and surrounds marrow spaces that may contain either fatty or hematopoietic tissue; this bone lies subjacent to the cortical bone and makes up the main portion (bulk) of a bone; also referred to as spongiosa, spongy bone, supporting bone, medullary bone, trabecular bone.

Bone cell   bone-forming osteoblasts, mature osteocytes, and degenerative osteoclasts that resorb. See: BONE.

Bone, compact   hard, dense bone constituting the outer, cortical layer and consisting of an infinite variety of penosteal bone, endosteal bone, and Haversian system.

Bone condenser   See: OSTEOTOME.

Bone, curettage   gentle moving of medullary bone by use of hand instruments to create an implant receptor site or to remove diseased intraosseous tissue; surgical shaving or smoothing of the bone surface.

Bone density   1. Clinical: Tactile assessment of bone quality reflecting the percentage of calcified bone to marrow, determined during osteotomy preparation. Usually classified from Dl (dense) to D4 (porous). Other classifications exist. 2. Histological: The "density" is calculated from the percentage of all bone tissue constituted by mineralized bone. 3. Radiographic: An estimate of the total amount of bone tissue (as bone mineral) in the path of one or more x-ray beams, as measured by Hounsfield units. When in quotes, "density" is as defined in absorptiometry. The term does not mean density as used in physics.

Bone derivative   one of the substances extracted from bone (for example, such as bone morphogenetic proteins).

Bone expander   See: OSTEOTOME.

Bone expansion   immediate or longer-term increases of bone width via surgery. See: RIDGE EXPANSION.

Bone factor   the relationship between osteogenesis and osteolysis.

Bone graft   syn: osseous graft; autogenous bone used for grafting.

Bone grafting   a surgical procedure performed to establish additional bone volume, using autogenous bone and/or a bone replacement graft, before or simultaneously with implant placement. See: BONE GRAFT, BONE REPLACEMENT GRAFT, BONE SUBSTITUTE.

Bone growth factors histochemicals, proteins, and enzymes that have been shown to be responsible for assisting or enhancing bone growth (for example, bone morphogenic protein [BMP]).

Bone implant interface See: IMPLANT INTERFACE.

Bone loss (implant) Physiologic or pathologic bone resorption around an implant. See: CRESTAL BONE LOSS, EARLY CRESTAL BONE LOSS, IMPLANT PERIAPICAL LESION, PERI-IMPLANTITIS.

Bone marrow Soft spongy tissue found in the center of bone that contains fat and/or hematopoietic tissues; the soft, highly vascularized tissue within the intermedullary space responsible for hematopoiesis and osteogenetic cells.

Bone mass a term used to reference the amount of bone tissue, frequently estimated by absorptiometry, and viewed as volume minus the marrow cavity. Quotations around the definition are used to distinguish it from the term "mass" in physics.

Bone matrix the intercellular element of bone; the matrix consists of osteocollagenous fibers, which are embedded in anamorphous substances as well as in organic salts.

Bone milling process by which particulate harvested bone is progressively transformed into smaller particles.

Bone morphogenetic protein (BMP) osteogenic protein produced by osteoblast sand stored in bone, capable of causing growth in nonosseous tissues. See: OSTEOINDUCTION.

Bone morphogenetic protein 2 (BMP-2) apoly-peptide protein known to stimulate secretion of alpha 1, a core-binding factor. It is an important factor in the development of bone and cartilage.

Bone morphogenetic protein 7 (BMP-7) member of the family of super proteins TGF-ß that plays a key role in the transformation of mesenchymal cells into bone and cartilage. Its inhibitors are noggin and a similar protein, chordin.

Bone necrosis See: Osteonecrosis.

Bone quality an assessment of bone based on its density.

Bone regeneration the renewal and/or repair of bone tissue.

Bone remodeling See: REMODELING (BONE).

Bone replacement graft a hard tissue graft (though not autogenous bone) used to stimulate new bone formation in an area where bone formerly existed.

Bone resorption Bone loss as a result of osteoclastic activity.

Bone sounding See: RIDGE SOUNDING.

Bone spreader See: OSTEOTOME.

Bone substitute a bone graft consisting of alloplastic material.

Bone tap See: TAP.

Bone-to-implant contact (BIC) direct contact between surfaces of bone and implant at the light microscope level. See: PERCENTAGE BONE-TO-IMPLANT CONTACT.

Bone trap refers to a device employed to harvest bone chips, osseous coagulum.

Bone trephine See: TREPHINE.

Bony ankylosis osseous joining; concerning teeth, a reference to periodontal tissue loss, and cementum bonding to alveolus.

Brittle fragile, non-elastic, and fracture-prone.

Buccal index a recorded impression of the facial aspect of teeth, with reference to a cast.

Bundle bone See: BONE.

Button implant See: MUCOSAL INSERT, INTRAMUCOSAL INSERT.

C

CAD/CAM acronym: computer-aided design/computer-aided manufacturing. Computer-assisted design; manufacturing accomplished through computer-assistance; a milling accomplished through computer control or stereolithography.

Calcium carbonate(CaCO3) See: CORALLINE.

Calcium phosphate 1. Types of minerals (usually from surrounding bone or blood supply) required for mineralization of new bone within a graft site. 2. Class of ceramics (with varying calcium-to-phosphorous ratios) used as a grafting material due to their ability to directly bond with bone. See: ALLOPLAST.

Calcium sulfate (CaSO4) See: DENTAL STONE, PLASTER; PLASTER OF PARIS.

Caldwell-Luc a surgical procedure that attempts to relieve chronic sinusitis by an incision into the maxillary canine fossa to improve the drainage of the maxillary sinus; sinus through the bone in the Named after American physician, George Caldwell, and French laryngologist, Henry Luc.

Callus tissue forming around fractured bone segments for maintaining structural integrity and facilitating the generation of bone.

Calvarial graft bone harvested for a graft from the superior portion of the cranium. Most often, this graft is taken from the parietal region, usually the right side (non-dominant hemisphere) behind the coronal suture, approximately 3 cm lateral to the sagittal suture.

Calvarium refers to the bones of the skull, specifically consisting of three layers, including outer (cortex), middle diploe (medullary), and inner (cortex).

Cancellous bone See: BONE, CANCELLOUS.

Canine protected articulation separation of the buccal segments during eccentric movements of the mandible caused by overlap of the canines.

Cantilever a beam segment or bridge segment supported at only one end.

Cantilever fixed partial denture a fixed bridge most often at the distal end with unsupported pontics.

Cartilage   mesenchyme-derived tissue from a protective medium that is both compliant and flexible.

Case report   diagnostic and treatment documentation describing patient progress and outcomes.

Case sequencing   for a patient undergoing dental implant therapy, this term refers to the order of treatment (for example, time of treatment related to healing and prosthodontic restoration).

Castable abutment   syn: UCLA abutment; cast component fabricated by waxing a plastic burn out pattern with or without a prefabricated cylinder; used to fabricate a custom abutment for either a cement-retained or screw-retained prosthesis.

CAT   computerized axial tomography.

CAT scan   acronym: computed axial tomography scan.

CBCT Scanners   See: CONE BEAM COMPUTED TOMOGRAPHY.

Cellulitis   inflammation (purulent) of loose connective tissue.

Cement   a substance designed to bond (temporarily or permanently) prostheses to implants or natural teeth.

Cement-retained   refers to the use of cement for retention of a prosthesis to an abutment. See: SCREW-RETAINED.

Center of the ridge   the site of the linea alba.

Centric   pertaining to or situated at the center.

Centric occlusion   maximum intercuspation of teeth.

Centric relationship   when the condyles are in their most posterior positions in the glenoid fossa, this relationship is the most posterior one of the mandible to the maxillae.

Ceramic   afloplastic material used for bone grafting and to fabricate abutments and prostheses. See: ALLOPLAST.

Ceramics   strong, hard, brittle, and inert nonconductors of thermal and electrical energy; metal and oxygen compounds formed of chemically and biochemically stable substances; characterized by ionic bonding.

Cervix   See: IMPLANT NECK; the connection between the infrastructure of the implant with the abutment; the neck of the implant.

Chamfer   a beveled edge that connects two surfaces.

Chemotaxis   directed movement of a cell or organism along chemical concentration gradient either toward or away from a chemical stimulus source. Also called chemotropism.

Chin graft   a mostly cortical bone graft that is harvested from the facial aspect of the symphyseal area of the mandible; this area is located between the mental foramina, apical to the roots of the teeth; it is usually above the mandible's lower border.

Chisel   An instrument with a beveled cutting edge used for cutting or cleaving hard tissue.

Chlohexidine   C22H30Cl2N10, syn: Chlorhexidine.

Chronic   a reference to a patient's condition that is long-standing and non-acute.

Chronic abscess   a long-standing collection of pus surrounded by fibrous tissue without signs of inflammation. Usually develops slowly.

Chronic infection   Chronic infections can last for days to months to a lifetime and typically develop from acute infections.

Circumferential subperiosteal implant   See: SUBPERIOSTEAL IMPLANT.

Clamping force   When torque is used to screw two components together, elastic deformation of the screen can result: this result is known as clamping force. See: PRELOAD.

Clean technique   the use of sterile instruments, implants, grafts, and irrigation solution during a surgical procedure in a clinical setting, and although operating room level sterility is not achieved, the surgeons wear sterile gloves, and the surgeons and assistants wear non-sterile attire. Under such conditions, the patient may or may not be covered by sterile drapes. See: STERILE TECHNIQUE.

Clip   an overdenture element used for fixation to a bar; the element usually grasps by spring action and is composed of plastic or metal. See: BAR OVERDENTURE.

Closed tray impression   Syn: indirect impression. This technique uses an impression coping with positioning features; a rigid, elastic impression material is injected around these features. Once the impression is removed, the coping is unthreaded from the mouth and then connected to a laboratory analog; subsequently, it is repositioned into the impression before pouring. See: OPEN TRAY IMPRESSION.

Closure screw   See: COVER SCREW.

Coating   1. Abutment: surface treatment used to alter optical transmission characteristics. 2. Implant: a substance applied to all or a portion of the dental implant's surface.

Coatings   a technique for making implant substrates more biocompatible by covering them with layers of materials designed for this purpose.

Cohesion   molecular bonding; the joining or attraction of similar materials.

Cohort study   a longitudinal study conducted by choosing a cohort group exhibiting a specific characteristic and following this group over a specified time to discover related characteristics (presumably).

Col   an interdental gingival depression between the facial and ingual papillae that conforms to the shape of the interproximal area.

Collagen   the proteinaceous white fibers, often used in grafting procedures, which occupy over half of bone, muscle, and connective tissue. A molecule whose characteristics include a triple helical structure and a high content of certain substances, namely glycine, proline, and hydroxyproline. Collagen represents a major constituent of a number of anatomical elements, including connective tissue fibers, the organic matrix of bone, dentin, cementum, and basal laminas. Fibroblasts, chondroblasts, osteoblasts, and odontoblasts are used to synthesize collagen. The human body consists of several types of collagen, including Type I, which is one of the first products the body synthesizes during bone formation.

Collagen membrane   a bioabsorbable membrane composed of collagen (mainly Type I); membrane properties: semi-permeable, hemostatic, and chemotactic, and tolerated well by surrounding tissues.

Collar   See: IMPLANT COLLAR.

Combination syndrome   a condition of significant maxillary anterior alveolar resorption when lower anterior teeth are present and the posteriors are absent.

Comfort cap   See: HYGIENE CAP.

Commercially pure titanium (CP-Ti)   a metal alloy (99 wt. % titanium) commonly used for dental implants because of its biocompatibility. Oxygen amounts (from 0.18 to 0.40 wt. %) within the alloy determine its grade. Trace elements include less than 0.25 wt. % of iron, carbon, hydrogen, and nitrogen. See: TITANIUM, TITANIUM ALLOY.

Compact bone   dense bone of the outer layer or cortex. See: BONE.

Compatible   a reference to a high degree of interchangeability of prosthetic components between one implant system and another.

Complete arch subperiosteal implant   a subperiosteal implant that is designed for an arch that is completely edentulous.

Complete subperiosteal implant   See: SUBPERIOSTEAL IMPLANT.

Complication   a reversible or irreversible unfavorable condition.

Composite graft   a graft consisting of a combination of different materials.

Composite resin   a tooth-colored plastic mixture filled with a bisphenol A-glycidylmethacrylate BISMA or urethane dimethacrylate (UDMA), and an inorganic filler such as silicon dioxidesilica. Primarily used to restore decayed areas, but also for cosmetic dental improvements of the color or shaping of the teeth.

Compression   refers to a force that is delivered to the surface of an object at right angles.

Compressive stress   an induced force that usually leads to the shortening or compression of a body or object when two forces are applied toward one another in the same straight line. See: STRESS.

Computed axial tomography (CAT scan)   See: COMPUTED TOMOGRAPHY.

Computed tomography (CT)   the use of x-rays to produce a digital description of an image for display on a computer monitor or on a film for diagnostic studies of internal body structures; the x-rays produce a series of scans along a single axis of a bodily structure to con-struct a three-dimensional, panoramic, or cross-sectional image of that structure.

Computer-aided design / computer-aided manufacturing (CAD/CAM)   the use of computer-acquired or computer-generated data to prepare a physical object.

Computer-aided navigation   the use of high-resolution computed tomography for surgical placement of implants.

Cone beam computed tomography (CBCT)   a scanner that uses a cone-shaped x-ray beam instead of a conventional linear fan beam to produce images of the bony structures of the skull; such scanners have been available for craniofacial imaging in Europe (since 1999) and the United States (since 2001).

Configuration   refers to the specific size and shape of an implant or an implant component.

Congenital   a condition that exists at or dates from the birth of an individual, of nongenetic etiology.

Connecting bar   a fixed bar connecting two or more permucosal extensions (for example, an integral part of the substructure of the ramus frame or subperiosteal implant). See: BAR.

Connective tissue   binding and supportive tissue composed of fibroblasts, primitive mesenchymal cells, collagen fibers, and elastic fibers; connective tissue is also composed of associated blood and lymphatic vessels, nerve fibers, and so on. Connective tissue is considered primary tissue, but it has many forms and functions, including support, storage, and protection. Its larger proportion of extracellular matrix makes it distinct from other types of tissue.

Connective tissue attachment   the mechanism by which connective tissue attaches to the tooth or the implant. Connective tissue fibers run parallel to the implant surface and compose the apical part of biologic width.

Connective tissue graft   also known as a subepithelial connective tissue graft, it is a thin piece of tissue grafted from the roof of the mouth, or harvested from an adjacent area, to augment attached gingival around the tooth. The gingival graft is placed to cover an exposed portion of the root, to create a stable band of attached tissue around the root.

Consolidation period   See: DISTRACTION OSTEOGENESIS.

Contact osteogenesis   this term refers to the direct migration of bone-building cells; the migration takes place through the clot matrix to form new bone first on the implant surface. See: DISTANCE OSTEOGENESIS.

Contour   an object's outline, shape, or silhouette.

Contralateral   refers to the side opposite another side.

Contraindication   when a treatment would involve a greater-than-normal risk to the patient, based on a certain condition or factor, and is therefore not recommended. When the patient is at higher risk of complications and there is no circumstance important enough to undertake the risky treatment, the contraindication is called "absolute." If the patient is at higher risk of complications, but these risks may be outweighed by other considerations or mitigated by other measures, the contraindications are called relative.

Coolant   an irrigating fluid used to reduce the heat generated during drilling in the alveolar bone.

Coping   a prefabricated (or custom) component that fits on an implant or on an abutment; a thimble made of metal, ceramic, or plastic to fit an abutment.

Coping screw   See: PROSTHETIC SCREW.

Coralline   ceramic used as a grafting material and made from the calcium carbonate skeleton of coral.

Coral-derived hydroxyapatite   a non-biodegradable structure derived from natural coral through a hydrothermic process used to promote bone in growth (osseointegration) into prosthetic implants. The high temperature used to create it also burns off proteins, preventing graft-versus-host disease (GVHD).

Corrode   a term used to refer to the chemical deterioration of a metal placed in a biologic or saline environment.

Cortical bone   the peripheral layer of compact osseous tissue; the average thickness of which is 2mm. See: BONE, COMPACT.

Corticocancellous bone   a piece of bone that contains both cortical bone full of morphogenetic proteins, and cancellous bone, that functions as graft.

Corticotomy   a surgical procedure during which only the bony cortex is cut.

Countersink   to enlarge an osteotomy in the coronal part using a specific drill to accommodate the implant platform.

Countersink drill   drill for enlarging the coronal part of an osteotomy.

Cover screw   syn: closure screw, healing screw; a cap-type screw for sealing the platform of an implant during osseointegration.

Cover screw mill   device to remove excess bone growth over a cover screw.

CP-Ti   acronym: commercially pure titanium.

Crestal   pertaining to the most coronal portion of the ridge.

Crestal bone loss   resorption of the most coronal aspect of the ridge surrounding the implant neck.

Crestal implant placement   placing an implant with the edge of the platform at the crest of bone. 1. Subcrestal: placement with the edge of the platform apical to the crest of bone. 2. Supracrestal: placement with the edge of the platform coronal to the crest of bone.

Crestal incision   incision made at the crest of the edentulous ridge. See: MIDCRESTAL INCISION, MUCOBUCCAL FOLD INCISION.

Crest of the ridge   See: ALVEOLAR CREST.

Crevicular   a reference to the gingival crevice.

Crevicular epithelium   the nonkeratinized epithelium of the gingival crevice. See: SULCULAR EPITHELIUM.

Critical-sized defect   osseous defects of a size that will not heal during the lifetime of the organism may be termed critical size defects (CSDs).

Cross-arch stabilization   syn: bilateral stabilization; a form of stabilization resulting from resistance to dislodging or rotational forces when a prosthetic design uses implants and/or natural teeth on opposite sides of the dental arch and are splinted together.

Crossbite   a form of malocclusion resulting from the mandibular teeth being buccal to the maxillary teeth.

Crossbite occlusion   an occlusion in which the mandibular teeth overlap the maxillary teeth.

Cross-sectional study   A type of study that involves the observation of a defined population at a single point in time or time interval.

Crown   the tooth portion protruding into the mouth for chewing; also a reference to a prosthetic replacement for such a structure.

Crown-implant ratio   ratio of crown height to the length of the implant when surrounded by bone; "crown height" is the extension from the most coronal bone-to-implant contact to the most coronal aspect of the prosthetic reconstruction that is connected to that implant.

Crown-root ratio   the mathematical ratio of crown length to root length.

CT   computerized tomography; connective tissue.

Cumulative success rate   percentage of implant success over time. See: SUCCESS RATE.

Cumulative survival rate   the percentage of implant survival overtime. See: SURVIVAL RATE.

Curettage   Scraping or scooping infected or inflamed tissue, or cavity in teeth.

Curve of Spee   an anatomic curvature of the occlusal alignment of teeth, beginning at the tip of the lower canine, following the buccal cusps of the natural premolars and molars, and continuing to the anterior border of the ramus.

Custom abutment   a component machined or cast for a unique circumstance.

Cylinder (Cylindrical) implant   endosseous root-form, press-fit implant with parallel-sided walls; a threaded or press-fit round endosteal implant.

Cylinder root form   See: CYLINDER IMPLANT.

Cylinder wrench   device used to place an implant into its osteotomy and to tighten the implant after placement.

Cytokine   a category of signal ling proteins and glycol proteins that, like hormones and neurotransmitters, are used extensively in cellular communication.

D

DBM   acronym: demineralized bone matrix.

Debridement   exposing healthy tissue by removing foreign material and contaminated or devitalized tissue from or adjacent to a traumatic or infected lesion.

Decortication   removal, in whole or in part, of the bony cortex to induce bleeding and release of bone-forming cells from the marrow.

Definitive prosthesis   a dental prosthesis to be used over a prescribed period of time, or long term.

Deglutition   swallowing.

Dehiscence   1. Incomplete coverage or cleft-like absence of bone at localized areas of teeth or implants, extending for a variable distance from the crest. See: FENESTRATION. 2. Premature opening of primary soft tissue closures.

Dehiscence, implant   a break in the covering epithelium, resulting in an isolated area of an implant or bone exposed to the oral cavity.

Dehiscence, mandibular   extreme resorption of the mandible resulting in exposure of the inferior alveolar nerve so that bone no longer covers the roof of the mandibular, leaving soft tissue alone to separate the contents of the canal from the oral cavity.

Delayed loading   time of applying force on an implant after initial placement when prosthesis is attached or secured after a conventional healing period. See: EARLY LOADING.

Demineralization   mineral loss.

Demineralized bone matrix (DBM)   a chemical process of mineral extraction resulting in a composite of collagenous proteins, noncollagenous proteins, and bone growth factors remaining.

Demineralized freeze-dried bone allograft (DFDBA)   Collagen (mainly Type I) that remains after demineralization of freeze-dried bone allograft (FDBA).

Dense cortical bone   See: CORTICAL BONE.

Dental implant   a permucosal, biocompatible, and biofunctional device placed on or within the bone of the oral cavity to support fixed or removable prostheses; Iso definition: "A device designed to be placed surgically within or on the mandibular or maxillary bone to provide resistance to displacement of a dental prosthesis" (ISO 1942-5).

Dental implant body   portion of an endosteal blade or root form implant that is attached by the cervix to the abutment and designed to achieve intraosseous retention.

Dental plaster   See: DENTAL STONE.

Dental stone   alpha-form of calcium sulfate hemihydrate, not used as a grafting material. See: PLASTER.

Denture   artificial substitute for missing natural teeth and adjacent tissues, not necessarily a removable prosthesis, or a device to completely cover an arch. See: FIXED PROSTHESIS, REMOVABLE PROSTHESIS.

Denture adhesive   substance used to adhere a prosthesis to the mucosa.

Denture flange   that portion of the denture base that extends from the teeth to the vestibules; the denture margins.

Denture flask   metal container for fabricating acrylic prostheses.

De-osseointegration   loss of achieved osseointegration from peri-implantitis and/or occlusal overload.

Depassivation   loss or removal of a metal's surface oxide layer caused by local conditions that produce an acidic environment. See: PASSIVATION.

Depth gauge   graduated instrument whose markings measure the vertical extent of an osteotomy.

Dermal graft   de-epithelialization and de-cellularized immunologically inert avascular connective tissue obtained from a cadaver.

Design (implant)   form, shape, configuration, surface macrostructure, and micro-irregularities of the three-dimensional structure of an implant or component.

Device orientation   distraction device position, usually relative to the anatomical axis of bone segments for distracting.

DFDBA   acronym: demineralized freeze-dried bone allograft.

Diagnostic wax-up   lab procedure creating teeth in wax according to the planned restoration; used to evaluate the feasibility of a plan and to fabricate a radiographic template, a surgical guide, or laboratory guides.

Diarthrodial joint   an articulation that is freely moving.

Direct bone impression   a negative recording of jawbone that is surgically exposed, usually used to fabricate a subperiosteal implant.

Direct impression   See: OPEN TRAY IMPRESSION.

Direction indicator   a device that is inserted into an osteotomy to assess its orientation or position relative to adjacent teeth and anatomic structures. This term is also used to verify and assist in achieving parallelism when the clinician is preparing multiple osteotomies.

Disc implant   an implant whose endosteal design consists of a thin, plate-like component that is placed into a horizontal osteotomy and attached to a post-like vertical component that protrudes permucosally.

Disclusion (disocclusion)   a reference to the separation of the teeth in opposing jaws.

Disk implant   a reference to a kind of endosseous implant that consists of a plate, a neck, and an abutment that is inserted into the edentulous ridge laterally.

Distance osteogenesis   a gradual process of bone healing that occurs from the edge of the osteotomy and towards the implant. In this process, bone does not grow directly on the implant surface. See: CONTACT OSTEOGENESIS.

Distraction   See: DISTRACTION OSTEOGENESIS

Distraction axis   the direction that the distal bone segment is distracted.

Distraction device   an appliance allowing gradual movement of bone segments away from each other incrementally.

Distraction osteogenesis   syn: osteodistraction; an invasive surgical technique that employs specialized instruments allowing bones to become lengthened as much as 500 mu per day. Formation of new soft tissue and bone between vascular bone surfaces that is created by an osteotomy and separated by gradual, controlled distraction. The process begins with the development of a reparative callus. Placing the callus under tension by stretching generates new bone. Distraction osteogenesis takes place in three sequential periods: 1. Latency: from bone division (i.e., surgical separation of bone into two segments) to the onset of traction, representing the time allowed for callus formation. 2. Distraction: from the application of gradual traction to the formation of bone segments and new tissue (regenerate tissue). 3. Consolidation: syn: fixation period; corticalization of the distraction regenerate, after the discontinuation of traction forces and segment movement.

Distraction parameters the biological and biomechanical variables affecting the quality and quantity of bone formed during distraction osteogenesis.

Distraction period See: DISTRACTION OSTEOGENESIS.

Distraction protocol the sequence and duration of events during the process of distraction osteogenesis.

Distraction rate daily total of distraction achieved.

Distraction regenerate See: REGENERATE.

Distraction rhythm the division rate of distraction osteogenesis based on the number of increments per day.

Distraction vector a reference to the final direction and magnitude of traction forces that occur during distraction osteogenesis.

Distraction zone See: REGENERATE.

Distractor See: DISTRACTION DEVICE.

Disuse atrophy inactivity resulting in diminution in dimension and/or density.

DO acronym: distraction osteogenesis.

Dolder bar a device used as a connector for multiple prosthetic elements, lending strength and retaining an overdenture or superstructure; often accompanied by special clips for grasping.

Donor site an anatomic location used for contributions of tissues for a graft, including skin, mucosa, connective tissue, and bone.

Doxycycline Doxycycline is a semi-synthetic tetracycline antibiotic developed in the early 1960s by Pfizer Inc. It works by slowing the growth of bacteria in the body. It is linked to both inhibiting tooth growth and tooth discoloration.

Drill extender See: EXTENDER.

Drilling sequence using specific drills in a specific step-by-step manner to prepare and increase the diameter of an osteotomy gradually before implant placement.

Ductility the characteristic of a material ability to be strained plastically but suffering no permanent deformation from tension.

Dysfunction an organ's or body part's inability to perform satisfactorily.

Dysthesia a spontaneous or evoked condition in which the sense of touch is distorted and interpreted by the body as an unpleasant sensation. Sometimes perceived as painful such as burning, itching, or prickling.

E

Early crestal bone loss an event involving crestal bone loss around an implant during the first year after exposure to the oral environment; the loss is usually attributed at least in part to the formation of the biologic width.

Early implant failure syn: primary implant failure; a root-form implant's failure due to the inability to establish osseointegration, resulting in mobility. See: LATE IMPLANT FAILURE.

Early implant placement a treatment option in post-extraction sites of teeth in the anterior maxilla that involves the placement of an implant into a prepared socket immediately or soon after tooth extraction. Recent clinical studies show that dental implants placed directly into prepared sockets immediately after tooth extraction achieved successful results compared with late implantation.

Early loading a reference to when force is applied to an implant soon after initial placement; a prosthesis is attached to the implant(s), earlier than after the conventional healing period. Loading time should be stated in days/weeks. See: DELAYED LOADING.

ECM acronym: extracellular matrix.

Eccentric a reference to a deviation from a central path.

Ectopic generally, a reference to an object being out of place.

Edema swelling that is secondary to the retention of fluid (e.g., lymph).

Edentulism the absence or complete loss of all natural dentition.

Edentulous refers to a patient who is experiencing a complete loss of all natural dentition.

Edentulous space the space caused by a missing tooth that is located between teeth.

Elasticity the characteristic allowing a structure or material to return to its original form after an external force is removed.

Elastic modulus refers to the level of stiffness of a material within an elasticity range.

Elastomer a material consisting of a base and catalyst that, after being mixed, sets into a supple but firm substance.

Electric discharge method (EDM) syn: spark erosion; a process involving the removal of precision metal via a series of electrical sparks that erode material from a work piece in a liquid medium under carefully controlled conditions.

Electron microscopy the projection of images via electron beams thousands of times shorter than visible light, creating much greater magnification.

Elements   the fundamental aspects of an object or subject.

Elevator   multipurpose dental surgical tool used to elevate, prop up, strip, or scrape soft tissue and bones.

Elevator muscle   one of a group of muscles whose contraction closes the mandible.

Embrasure   a space between teeth (lesser = above the contact point; greater = below the contact point) that resembles a triangle in shape.

EMD   acronym: enamel matrix derivative.

Emergence angle   refers to the angle created by an imaginary extension of the long axis of an implant vs the corrected axis of the abutment.

Emergence profile   a reference to the contour of tooth (restored) or implant relative to surrounding tissues.

Emergence profile   a reference to the part of the axial contour of a tooth or prosthetic crown extending from the sulcus base beyond the margin of free soft tissue. This profile extends to the contour's height and produces a straight or convex profile in the apical third of the axial surface.

Enamel matrix derivative (EMD)   a derivative of sterile protein aggregate from the enamel matrix, amelogenin, the precursor of developing teeth's enamel; these proteins are specially harvested from developing pig embryo teeth.

Endochondral ossification   is one of the two processes in which long bone tissue is formed, lengthened, and healed. It requires a pre-existing cartilage model.

Endocrine   a function by which the body's chemical compounds, such as hormones, are secreted and get transported throughout the body to exact cell recipients through the bloodstream.

Endodontic endosteal implant   a (smooth or threaded) pin implant extending through the root into periapical bone and stabilizing a mobile tooth.

Endodontic implant   syn: endodontic pin, endodontic stabilizer; a pin placed into a root canal, extending beyond the apex into the bone.

Endodontic pin   See: ENDODONTIC ENDOSTEAL IMPLANT, ENDODONTIC IMPLANT.

Endodontic stabilizer   See: ENDODONTIC IMPLANT.

Endodontic stabilizer implant   See: ENDODONTIC ENDOSTEAL IMPLANT.

Endosseous blade implant   See: BLADE IMPLANT.

Endosseous distractor   syn: intraosseous distractor; distraction device placed into the edentulous ridge and/or basal bone (maxilla or mandible) and used in distraction osteogenesis.

Endosseous implant   syn: endosteal implant; a device placed into the alveolar and/or basal bone of the maxilla or mandible to support a prosthesis.

Endosseous ramus implant   a type of implant that is used if the lower jawbone is too thin for a root form or subperiosteal implant. A ramus implant is embedded in the jawbone in the back corners of the mouth (near the mandibular third molars) and near the chin. A thin metal bar around the top of the gum will then be fitted for prosthesis. Ramus implants can stabilize weak jaws and help prevent them from fracturing.

Endosteal dental implant abutment   See: ABUTMENT.

Endosteal dental implant body   See: DENTAL IMPLANT BODY.

Endosteal implant   a device placed within alveolar or basal bone to serve as a prosthetic abutment. See: ENDOSSEOUS IMPLANT.

Endosteal root form implant   that portion of an endosteal implant (blade or root form) attached by the cervix to the abutment and designed to achieve intraosseous retention.

Endosteum   tissue lining the medullary cavity of bone, composed of a single layer of osteoprogenitor cells and a small amount of connective tissue.

Endothelial progenitor cell   bone marrow-derived cells that circulate in the blood, have the ability to adhere or bind, and contain LDL and differentiate into endothelial cells, the cells that make up the lining of blood vessels. There is evidence that circulating endothelial progenitor cells play a role in the repair of damaged blood vessels after a myocardial infarction. In fact, higher levels of circulating endothelial progenitor cells detected in the bloodstream predict for better outcomes and fewer repeat heart attacks.

Endotoxin   potentially toxic, natural compound found inside part of the outer membrane of the cell wall of gram-negative bacteria.

Envelope flap   a flap elevated from a horizontal linear incision, parallel to the free gingival margin, with no vertical incision, either sulcular or submarginal.

Epidermal growth factor   a small mitogenic protein that is involved in the regulation of normal cell growth, oncogenesis, and wound healing and plays an important role in proliferation and differentiation.

Epithelial attachment   the attachment mechanism of the junctional epithelium to the tooth or implant (i.e., hemidesmosomes). See: JUNCTIONAL EPITHELIUM; the continuation of the sulcular epithelium, joined to the tooth or adherent to implant structure, located at the base of the sulcus or pocket.

Epithelial cuff, implant   the band of tissue constricted around an implant cervix.

Epithelial implant   See: MUCOSAL INSERT.

Epithelialization   a reference to the kind of healing that takes place when epithelium grows over connective tissue.

Epithelium   the outer layer that covers the underlying connective tissue stroma; the issue lining the intraoral surfaces and extending into the sulcus while adhering to the implant/tooth.

Epithelization   a reference to the secondary healing of epithelium.

Eposteal implant a device that receives primary bone support by resting upon bone. See: SUBPERIOSTEAL IMPLANT.

ePTFE acronym: expanded polytetrafluoroethylene.

Epulis an oral pathologic condition that appears in the mouth as a tumor in the gingival; is a mucosal hyperplasia that results from chronic low-grade trauma induced by a lesion caused by denture.

Erosion the loss of hard or soft tissue resulting in a saucer-shaped configuration and caused by pathologic tooth wear; alternatively caused by trauma to the integument (an ulcer).

Erythrocyte A mature red blood cell that contains hemoglobin and can carry oxygen to the body.

Esthetic pertaining to beauty.

Esthetic zone any dentoalveolar region that is visible during a patient's full smile. The relationship between gingiva, lips, and teeth determines a particular smile's description as high or low.

Etching the use of acids or other agents (etchants) for increasing the surface area of an implant or other materials.

Etiology contribution to the cause of a disease or condition.

Exclusion criteria the characteristics preventing a participant entering a clinical trial. See: INCLUSION CRITERIA.

Exfoliation loss of implanted materials or of implant-associated devices.

Expanded polytetrafluoroethylene (ePTFE) a polymer of tetrafluoroethylene that is stretched to allow fluid but not cells to pass; the polymer is used as a nonresorbable membrane in guided bone regeneration (GBR) and guided tissue regeneration (GTR). Titanium reinforcement may or may not be used in conjunction with this polymer to maintain its shape. This polymer can also be used as a non-absorbable suture material.

Expanded polytetrafluoroethylene (ePTFE) membrane surgical membrane for grafting believed to be an inert material for vascular prosthesis, made up of tetrafluoroethylene; it can be varied in porosity to fill clinical and biological requirements of its applications. Typically used to guide bone regenerative substances.

Expert witness a person who has the training, education, or experience on a particular subject and who is formally found to be qualified as an expert by a judge.

Exposure 1. Implant: the dehiscence of soft tissue that leads to the exposure of the implant covers crew, neck, body, or threads. This is a colloquial term for stage- two surgery. 2. Barrier membrane: the dehiscence of soft tissue that leads to the exposure of an occlusive membrane during the healing period.

Extender a surgical component used as an intermediary between the handpiece or wrench and another component (e.g., drill, implant mount) to increase the reach of the latter part; a device for lengthening a bur, drill, or instrument.

External connection a prosthetic interface external to the implant platform (e.g., an external hexagon) See: INTERNAL CONNECTION.

External hexagon a connection interface of the platform of an implant that extends coronally and prevents rotation of attached components. See: INTERNAL HEXAGON.

External irrigation method used during the drilling of osteotomies for the implants whereby a cooling solution is directed at the drilling bur, delivering the cooling solution at the entrance of the osteotomy; this cooling solution may be delivered through tubing connected to the handpiece and drilling unit; alternatively, it maybe from a handheld system. See: INTERNAL IRRIGATION.

External oblique ridge a smooth area on the buccal surface of the body of the mandible extending with diminishing prominence from the anterior border of the ramus both downward and forward to the region of the mental foramen; the ridge changes only a small degree in size and direction over time and is an important landmark in the design of a subperiosteal implant.

Extirpate to remove an organ, body part, or neoplasm.

Extracellular matrix (ECM) a reference to any material produced by cells and excreted into the tissue's extracellular space. The matrix takes the form of both ground substance and fibrous elements, proteins involved in cell adhesion, and glycosaminoglycans, as well as other space-filling molecules. The matrix can serve as a scaffolding to hold tissues together; additionally, its form and composition help determine tissue characteristics.

Extraction socket the alveolus resulting from tooth removal.

Extraction socket graft See: RIDGE PRESERVATION.

Extraoral (external) distraction device device located outside the oral cavity and used in distraction osteogenesis; the bone segments are usually attached to percutaneous pins connected externally to device fixation clamps.

Extraosseous distractor a device placed outside the edentulous ridge or basal bone of the maxilla or mandible and used in distraction osteogenesis.

Exudate a reference to the fluids, cells, and cellular debris that have escaped from blood vessels and deposited in tissues or on tissue surfaces (frequently as a result of inflammation); fluid with a high content of protein that has escaped from blood vessels and deposited in tissues as a result of infection; pus; purulence.

F

Fabrication structure or prosthesis construction.

Facebow a device used to record the relationship of the maxillae to the opening axis of the mandible and to orient the casts in this same relationship to the opening axis of an articulator.

Facial augmentation implant prosthesis a polymeric device that is shaped to restore a depressed or inadequate portion of the facial skeleton; it is implanted subperiosteally.

Facial moulage impression of facial structures from elastomeric materials.

Failed implant a mobile implant (failed to achieve or has lost osseointegration) or symptomatic in spite of osseointegration.

Failing implant a general term for an implant that is progressively mobile; the implant may exhibit increased probing depth and purulence but remains clinically stable. See: PERI-IMPLANTITIS.

Failure rate percentage of failure in a study or clinical trial of a procedure or device (e.g., implant) not meeting the success criteria, or falling into the failure criteria, defined in the study protocol.

Fatigue progressive weakening of a structure; steady embrittlement and crack formation/propagation; breaking or fracturing of a material caused by repeated cyclic or applied loads below the yield limit.

Fatigue failure fracture of a material from loading, resulting from stresses beyond tolerance; a structural failure caused by multiple loading when all loads lie below the structure's ultimate strength. Typically, such failures occur only after thousands or millions of loading episodes.

Fatigue fracture structural failure caused by repetitive stresses, resulting in a slowly propagating crack to cross the material.

FDBA acronym: freeze-dried bone allograft.

FEA acronym: finite element analysis.

Fenestration a single, isolated area where the root or implant surface is denuded of bone but not involving the crestal bone. See: DEHISCENCE.

Fibrinolysis the process wherein a fibrin clot, the product of coagulation, is broken down. Its main enzyme plasmin cuts the fibrin mesh at various places, producing circulating fragments cleared by other proteases or by the kidney and liver.

Fibroblast the cell type found within the connective tissue responsible for synthesis of collagen fibers and the ground substance of connective tissue.

Fibroblast growth factor (FGF) from the family of cytokines, FGFs promote the growth of new blood vessels from the pre-existing vasculature and give rise to granulation tissue, which fills up a wound space/cavity in the early wound-healing process. FGFs also have important roles in angiogenesis, neurogenesis, and tumor growth. Human have about 23 FGFs, with FGF-2 being the one used for regenerative treatments.

Fibro-integration See: FIBRO-OSSEOUS INTEGRATION.

Fibronectin a high-molecular-weight extracellular matrix glycoprotein that binds to receptor proteins, acting as binding sites for cell surface receptors. Fibronectin helps create a cross-linked network within the ECM by having binding sites for other ECM components. Fibronectin also serves as a plasma opsonin.

Fibro-osseous integration incorporation of a blade implant into an osseous host site that is lined with fibrous tissue.

Fibro-osteal integration See: FIBRO-OSSEOUS INTEGRATION.

Fibrosis a reference to the process leading to formation of fibrous tissue (often degenerative).

Fibrous composed of or containing fibers.

Fibrous encapsulation layer of connective tissue in between implant and surrounding bone.

Fibrous integration refers to soft tissue-to-implant contact; often refers to the interposition of healthy, dense, collagenous ligament tissue existing between a blade implant and bone transmitting load from the implant to the bone. See: FIBROUS ENCAPSULATION.

Finite element analysis (FEA) software technique used for the study of stresses and strains on mechanical parts. CAD software automatically generates the simulated mechanical loads for FEA measurements.

First-stage dental implant surgery surgery during which the body of a two-piece implant is inserted.

Fissure a cleft or groove.

Fistula refers to the abnormal passage or communication (an abnormal epithelial-lined tract) between two internal organs or the passage leading from an internal organ to body surface. 1. Oroantral: an opening between oral cavity and maxillary sinus. 2. Orofacial: opening between the cutaneous surface of the face and oral cavity. 3. Oronasal: opening between the nasal cavity and oral cavity.

Fixation period See: DISTRACTION OSTEOGENESIS.

Fixation screw screw used to stabilize a block graft or a barrier membrane.

Fixation tack See: TACK.

Fixed nonremovable.

Fixed bridge a prosthetic dental appliance replacing lost teeth and supported and held in position by attachments to natural teeth or implants nonremovably.

Fixed-detachable prosthesis fixed to an implant or implants, but removable by the dentist. See: FIXED PROSTHESIS, CEMENT-RETAINED, HYBRID PROSTHESIS, IMPLANT-SUPPORTED PROSTHESIS, REMOVABLE PROSTHESIS, SCREW-RETAINED.

Fixed partial denture See: FIXED BRIDGE.

Fixed prosthesis restoration not removable by the patient; may be partial arch (FPD: fixed partial denture), or complete arch (FCD: fixed complete denture). See: DENTURE, REMOVABLE PROSTHESIS.

Fixed-removable prosthesis fixed to an implant or implants, but removable by the dentist. See: FIXED PROSTHESIS, CEMENT-RETAINED, HYBRID PROSTHESIS, IMPLANT-SUPPORTED PROSTHESIS, REMOVABLE PROSTHESIS, SCREW-RETAINED.

Fixed/removable   a prosthesis affixed with screws but removable by the patient; fixed-detachable.

Fixture   See: ROOT-FORM IMPLANT.

Fixture cover   healing screw.

Flapless implant surgery   implant placement technique whereby neither soft tissue flaps are raised nor a circular piece of tissue is removed.

Flipper   claspless interim all-acrylic denture.

Food and Drug Administration (FDA)   a U.S. Department of Health and Human Services agency responsible for ensuring the safety, efficacy, and security of human and veterinary drugs, biological products, medical devices, U.S. food supply, cosmetics, and products that emit radiation, through testing and regulation.

Force   influence acting on a body and tending to produce or alter motion, and tending to deform the surface of a stable body.

Fossa   anatomic pit or depression.

Fracture   break, rupture, or tear; failure caused by crack growth.

Framework   a reference to the structure of a prosthetic reconstruction; alternatively, the armature or skeleton of a prosthesis.

Free gingiva   keratinized gum surrounding but not attached to the teeth.

Free gingival margin   refers to that distance that is the most coronal portion of the gum tissues surrounding the dental cervix.

Free soft tissue autograft   See: GINGIVAL GRAFT.

Free-standing implant   an implant not splinted to adjacent teeth or implants.

Freeze-dried bone allograft (FDBA)   refers to bone harvested from donor cadavers, and then washed, immersed in ethanol, frozen in nitrogen, freeze-dried, and ground into particles. Particles range in size from 250 to 750 microns. This substance acts primarily osteoconductively as inductive proteins, often found in only minute quantities; the substance's arc is only released after the resorption of the mineral.

Freeze-drying   a dehydration process used to preserve tissue that allows the frozen water in the material to sublime directly from the solid phase to gas.

Frenulum   small fold of integument or mucous membrane checking, limiting, or curbing movements of an organ or part.

Friction-fit   refers to the retention state of an implant at the time of insertion, resulting from slight compression of the implant body walls in the osteotomy. This term also applies to components retained to an implant by friction. See: PRESS-FIT.

Fulcrum   a prop or support upon which a lever turns.

Full-thickness graft   a graft section of epithelium removed for distant or adjacent repair.

Functional loading   See: OCCLUSAL LOADING.

Functional occlusion   contact of teeth providing the highest efficiency in the centric position and during all excursive movements of the jaw essential to mastication without producing trauma.

G

Galvanism   refers to the electropotential difference of dissimilar metals occurring in dental metallurgy in the presence of an electrolyte (such as saliva).

GBR   acronym: guided bone regeneration.

Genial tubercles   refers to mental spines, small round elevations (usually two pairs) that are clustered around the midline on the lingual surface of the lower portion of the mandibular symphysis; tubercles serve as attachments for the genioglossus and geniohyoid muscles; these tubercles serve as critical landmarks for the subperiosteal implant.

Genioplasty   the use of surgery to alter the chin.

Gingiva   part of the masticatory mucosa covering the alveolar process, surrounding the cervical portion of teeth, and consisting of an epithelial layer and an underlying connective tissue layer (lamina propria).

Gingivae   gum tissues.

Gingival crevice   the space located between the marginal gingivae and a tooth or implant.

Gingival crevicular fluid   Fluid originating in the gingival connective tissue that seeps through the sulcular and junctional epithelium, containing sticky plasma proteins that improve adhesions of the epithelial attachment and have antimicrobial and antibody properties. Flow increases in the presence of inflammation.

Gingival graft   syn: free soft tissue autograft; surgical procedure to establish adequate keratinized soft tissue around a tooth or an implant or to increase the quantity of soft tissue of an edentulous ridge.

Gingival recession   The apical migration of the marginal gingiva, resulting in exposure of the root surface of the tooth, causing hypersensitivity. One of the main causes of gingival recession is abnormal tooth positioning or trauma.

Glossoplasty   surgical alteration of the tongue.

Glucocorticoid   hormone that affects the metabolism of carbohydrates, fats, and proteins made in the adrenal gland and chemically classified as steroids. They act as immunosuppressants to prevent acute transplant rejection and the graft-versus-host disease. Effective in treating oral lesions.

Glycoprotein   a protein containing one or more covalently linked carbohydrates, plus a protein. Glycoproteins play essential roles in the body such as acting as key molecules in the immune system.

Glycosaminoglycan   (mucopolysaccharide) a binding membrane protein, an important component of connective tissues.

Gnathic   pertaining to the jaw.

Gold cylinder   See: PREFABRICATED CYLINDER.

Graft   material used to replace a body's defect; a substance inserted into another substance and intended to become an integral part of the latter. In the case of bone grafts, either artificial or synthetic bone, this graft is usually for the purpose of increasing its strength and/or dimension.

Grafting material   a substance (natural or synthetic) used to repair a tissue defect or deficiency.

Grinding in   a reference to the correction of occlusion.

Grit blasting   delivery of a high-velocity stream of abrasive particles propelled by compressed air to an implant surface, to increase its surface area.

Groove   a long, thin depression.

Growth factor   any highly specific protein that is used to stimulate the division and differentiation of cells.

Guide   See: RADIOGRAPHIC TEMPLATE, STEREO-LITHOGRAPHIC GUIDE, SURGICAL GUIDE.

Guided bone regeneration (GBR)   bone regenerative technique using physical means (e.g., membranes) to seal an anatomic site for bone regeneration. The goal of GBR is to direct bone formation and to prevent other tissues (e.g., connective tissue) from interfering with osteogenesis.

Guided tissue regeneration   a procedure designed to direct epithelial and supporting soft tissue restoration and to inhibit epithelial invagination by the use of synthetic membranes.

Guide drill   a round drill used to mark an osteotomy site by making an initial entry into cortical bone.

Guide pin   1. device placed within an osteotomy to determine the location and angulation of the site relative to adjacent teeth, implants, or other landmarks. 2. extended occlusal or abutment screws used during prosthesis fabrication in the laboratory.

Gustation   the sense of taste.

H

HA   acronym: hydroxyapatite.

Hadar bar   See: DOLDER BAR.

Harvest   gathering or collecting hard or soft tissue for grafting.

Haversian canal   freely anastomosing channels within cortical bone; the channels contain blood and lymph vessels and are surrounded by concentric lamellae of bone.

Healing   regeneration or repair of injured, lost, or surgically treated tissue, occurring by first (primary) intention or by second (secondary) intention.

Healing abutment   syn: healing collar, permucosal extension, second-stage permucosal abutment, temporary healing cuff; an abutment connecting to the implant and protruding through the soft tissue. Temporary cuff used after uncovering to facilitate soft tissue healing in the permucosal areas.

Healing by first (primary) intention   syn: primary closure; wound healing involving the close reapproximation of edges; minimal granulation tissue and scar formation after union.

Healing by second (secondary) intention   syn: secondary closure; wound healing in which a gap is left between edges; granulation tissue formation from the base and the sides remains after union. A large amount of epithelial migration, collagen deposition, contraction, and remodeling during healing is required.

Healing cap   See: HYGIENE CAP.

Healing collar   See: HEALING ABUTMENT.

Healing period   syn: healing phase; time allocated for healing following a surgery, after which the next procedure is performed at the same site.

Healing phase   See: HEALING PERIOD.

Healing screw   refers to the final intra-implant screw placed after first-stage surgery. See: COVER SCREW.

Hematopoietic stem cell   progenitor cells from which every lineage, including red blood cells, platelets, and a variety of lymphoid and myeloid cells, in the body are generated. HSCs are able to generate some of the most important lymphoid cells and myeloid cells including natural killer (NK) cells, T cells, and B cells, granulocytes, monocytes, macrophages, microglial cells, and dendritic cells. HSCs can generate these for many years.

Hemidesmosome   microscope structures that serve as cementing media at the surfaces of epithelial cells; their combinations are called desmosomes when they serve two such adjacent cells.

Hemi-maxillectomy   surgical removal of one portion of the upper jaw, including the premaxilla, maxilla, or hard palate.

Hemisection   process of dividing or cutting a tooth or structure into two parts.

Hemocytoblasts   See: STEM CELLS.

Hemorrhage   internal or external excessive bleeding.

Hemostasis   the physiologic process of halting bleeding involving three basic mechanisms: vasoconstriction serotonin, ADP, and Thromboxane A_2, and finally, coagulation. Also may refer to the process of manually clamping a blood vessel with hemostatic clamps during surgery.

Heterogeneous graft   See: XENOGRAFT.

Heterograft   tissue taken from one species and placed into another. See: XENOGRAFT.

Hex   a hexagonally shaped interface connection.

Hex-lock   a six-sided screwdriver or matching screw.

Hexed   component or implant with a hexagonal connection interface.

High lip line   condition in which gingival tissue and crown margins are revealed during smiling.

High-water prosthesis   See: HYBRID PROSTHESIS.

Histomorphometry   the study of microstructures; quantitative study of the microscopic tissue organization and structure, especially the computer-assisted analysis of images acquired from a microscope.

Hollow basket implant   a root-form implant with an internal channel that penetrates the implant body at or from its apical aspect.

Homogenous graft   See: HOMOGRAFT.

Homograft   syn: homogenous graft, homologous graft; a graft transplanted between genetically non-identical individuals of the same species (e.g., a graft taken from one human subject and transplanted into another). See: ALLOGRAFT.

Homologous graft   See: HOMOGRAFT.

Horseshoe denture   palateless, U-shaped prosthesis.

Host response   local or systemic response of the host organism to the implanted material or device.

Host site   See: RECIPIENT SITE.

Hounsfield Unit (HU)   x-ray unit attenuation for CT scans to measure bone density; each pixel is assigned a value on a scale (air is—1000, water 0, and compact bone + 1000).

HU   acronym: Hounsfield unit.

Hybrid denture   partial or full denture prosthesis affixed with screws to a mesostructure bar.

Hybrid implant   endosseous, root-form implant consisting of different surface textures at different levels.

Hybrid prosthesis   syn: high-water prosthesis (using long standard abutments with several millimeters of space between the prosthesis and the mucosa of the edentulous ridge); screw-retained, metal-resin, implant-supported, fixed complete denture; implies a combination of a metal framework with a complete denture (i.e., prefabricated resin teeth and heat polymerized resin). See: HYBRID DENTURE.

Hydroxyapatite (HA), $Ca_{10}(PO_4)_6(OH)_2$ general term for calcium hydroxyapatite; the primary inorganic and natural component of bone; used as an alloplast and to coat some implant surfaces. See: ALLOPLAST.

Hydroxyapatite ceramic   dense, relatively nonresorbable ceramic that displays a highly attractive generic profile featuring a lack of local or systemic reactivity when implanted into bone (pentahydroxyapatite).

Hydroxylapatite   See: HYDROXYAPATITE.

Hygiene cap   syn: comfort cap, healing cap, sealing screw; component that is inserted over a prosthetic abutment. The cap's function is to prevent debris and calculus from invading the internal portion of the abutment (between prosthetic appointments).

Hyperbaric oxygenation   administering oxygen under greater than normal pressures, used for therapeutic purposes in the treatment of aerobic infections (or in areas of ischemia, postradiation.

Hyperbaric oxygen therapy   treatment modality in which a patient is placed in a pressurized chamber (hyperbaric chamber), allowing for delivery of oxygen in high concentrations, sometimes used before implant therapy for patients who have undergone radiation therapy in the head and neck areas, thus reducing the risks of osteoradionecrosis.

Hyperesthesia   a reference to abnormally increased sensitivity of skin, mucosa, or an organ of special sense.

Hyperocclusion   Premature tooth contact during mouth closure, such as grinding and clenching teeth, which causes a great deal of dental trauma.

Hyperparathyroidism   a chronic disorder of the parathyroid glands involving oversecretion of parathyroid hormone that results in increased bone resorption and increased calcium absorption in the intestines. The main cause of renal failure.

Hyperplasia   abnormal multiplication or increase in the number of normal tissue cells; excessive enlargement of a tissue or structure due to cell number increase.

Hyperplastic tissue   a reference to the enlargement of tissue secondary to a proliferation of normal cells.

Hyperpneumatized sinus   sinus within creased air space. See: PNEUMATIZED MAXILLARY SINUS.

Hypertension   commonly known as high blood pressure, a chronic condition in which the blood pressure is excessively high.

Hypertrophy   a reference to the increase in tissue bulk beyond normal limits, caused by an increase in size, but not number, of cellular elements.

Hypogeusia   diminished tasting ability.

Hypoplasia   development that is defective or incomplete.

I

Iatrogenic   a result caused by the activity of the doctor.

Idiopathic   of unknown origin.

IGF   acronym: insulin-like growth factors.

Iliac crest   superior part of the ilium used as a grafting source of autogenous bone. See: ILIAC GRAFT.

Iliac graft   a bone graft that is harvested from the iliac bone's crest; such bone can be removed from the anterior iliac crest posteriorly to the anterosuperior iliac spine or to the posterior ilium. Additionally, this graft may be cancellous, cortical, or cortico-cancellous.

Ilium   The uppermost of the three bones that make up the innominate bone, (or hip bone), the crest of which is a source of bone for mandibular and chin reconstruction and enhancement in dentistry.

Immediate denture   a prosthesis designed for insertion directly after teeth removal.

Immediate functional loading   See: IMMEDIATE OCCLUSAL LOADING.

Immediate implant placement   placement of an implant into the extraction socket at the time of tooth extraction.

Immediate loading   See: IMMEDIATE OCCLUSAL LOADING, IMMEDIATE NONOCCLUSAL LOADING; the placement into function of newly inserted implants.

Immediate nonfunctional loading   See: IMMEDIATE NONOCCLUSAL LOADING.

Immediate nonocclusal loading   a clinical protocol for placing an implant in a partially edentulous arch (at the same clinical visit) with a fixed or removable restoration not in occlusal contact with the opposing dentition. See: NONOCCLUSAL LOADING.

Immediate occlusal loading   a clinical protocol for the placement and application of force on implants (at the same clinical visit) with a fixed or removable restoration in occlusal contact with the opposing dentition. See: OCCLUSAL LOADING.

Immediate placement   See: Immediate implant placement.

Immediate provisionalization   clinical protocol for placing an interim prosthesis with or without occlusal contact with the opposing dentition, at the same clinical visit of implant placement. See: IMMEDIATE NON-OCCLUSAL LOADING, IMMEDIATE OCCLUSAL LOADING.

Immediate restoration   See: IMMEDIATE PROVISION-ALIZATION.

Immediate temporization   See: IMMEDIATE PROVI-SIONALIZATION.

Immunologic response   a bodily defense in the form of a reaction that recognizes an invading substance (an antigen: such as a virus, fungus, bacterium, or transplanted organ) and produces antibodies specific against that antigen.

Implant (noun)   device designed for surgical insertion into the body, including an alloplastic material or device that is surgically placed into the oral tissue, for anchorage, functional, therapeutic, and/or esthetic purposes.

Implant (verb)   the surgical act of placing a device into the body.

Implant abutment   See: ABUTMENT.

Implant-abutment junction   syn: microgap; margin of connection between the implant's coronal aspect and the prosthetic abutment or restoration.

Implant anchorage   support for orthodontic tooth movement or arch expansion provided by an implant.

Implant-assisted prosthesis   any prosthesis completely or partly supported by an implant or implants. See: IMPLANT-SUPPORTED PROSTHESIS, IMPLANT-TISSUE-SUPPORTED PROSTHESIS; CEMENT-RETAINED, FIXED PROSTHESIS, HYBRID PROSTHESIS, REMOVABLE PROSTHESIS, SCREW-RETAINED.

Implant attachment   See: ATTACHMENT.

Implant body   syn: implant shaft; the portion of a root-form implant available for bone-to-implant contact; the infrastructure.

Implant collar   the smooth part that can be found just apical to the edge of the platform or the implant-abutment junction, the root-form implant has a collar.

Implant connecting bar   a cast or welded bar that connects one implant to another.

Implant crown   a casting placed over an implant abutment, which is designed to assume the role of a natural crown.

Implant dentistry   type of dentistry concerned with the diagnosis, design, and insertion of implant devices and implant restorations to provide increased function, comfort, and esthetics for the edentulous or partially edentulous patient. syn: oral implantology.

Implant denture   a denture receiving stability and retention from a dental implant.

Implant exposure   a postoperative condition whereby an implant is not completely covered by soft tissue due to a bursting open or splitting along sutured lines.

Implant fixture   See: IMPLANT.

Implant head   the segment of the subperiosteal or blade implant above the neck, used to connect to the prosthetic reconstruction. Syn: Abutment.

Implant infrastructure   that segment of an implant of any type designed to achieve retention. See: IMPLANT BODY.

Implant integration   a reference to tissue-to-implant contact.

Implant interface   a reference to that site created by an implant and its adjacent supporting tissues; area of contact between tissues (for example, bone, connective tissue) and the implant surface.

Implant length   data for implants involving the straight-line measurement from the implant crown surface to the end tip of the implant screw.

Implant level impression   the impression of the implant platform that uses an implant impression coping. See: ABUTMENT LEVEL IMPRESSION.

Implant loading   placement of prosthetic devices so that an implant can be brought into function.

Implant micromovement   microscopic movement of a dental implant amidst soft tissue. Primary stability of dental implants is critical for their osseointegration.

Implant mount   device used to transfer an implant to the prepared surgical site.

Implant neck   syn: cervix. 1. Root-form implant: the most coronal aspect of an implant. 2. Subperiosteal or blade implant: the transmucosal segment that connects the implant to the head or abutment.

Implantology   the art and science of diagnosis, treatment, maintenance, and problem management of implant dentistry.

Implant periapical lesion   radiolucency localized at the apex of a root-form implant, either asymptomatic or symptomatic (acute), which may include fistula with purulent exudates and/or pain on palpation.

Implant prosthesis   a denture that is supported wholly or partly by implants. Any (fixed, removable, or maxillofacial) prosthesis using dental implants for retention, support, and stability.

Implant prosthodontics   implant dentistry concerned with the diagnosis, presurgical planning, construction, and placement of fixed or removable prostheses on any dental implant device; concerns the construction and placement of fixed or removable prostheses on any implant device.

Implant-retained prosthesis   any prosthesis completely or partly supported by an implant or implants. See: IMPLANT-CEMENT-RETAINED, FIXED PROSTHESIS, HYBRID PROSTHESIS, REMOVABLE PROSTHESIS, SCREW-RETAINED.

Implant shaft   See: IMPLANT BODY.

Implant site   the area in the alveolar ridge where the implant is to be inserted in restorative surgery.

Implant soft tissue management   use of special techniques during the pre-implant phase and during implant integration to maintain the periodontal health and restorative aspects of soft tissue in and after implant surgery.

Implant splinting   connection of restorative components with a bar or an overdenture typically between implant abutments and natural teeth to enhance strength.

Implant stability   the variables in movement of an implant within the surrounding bone after testing. Implant stability is dependent to local bone density and subject to changes due to bone remodeling.

Implant stability quotient (ISQ)   the measure of implant stability (from 1 to 100, 100 being the highest degree of stability) obtained from resonance frequency analysis.

Implant substructure   See: INFRASTRUCTURE.

Implant success   implant status based on predetermined success criteria. See: IMPLANT SURVIVAL.

Implant superstructure   prosthesis permitted to rest on implants, on a mesostructure bar, or on natural tissue and implants.

Implant-supported prosthesis   a restoration whose entire support is from dental implants. This type of restoration may be fixed or removable, partial, or a complete arch. See: FIXED PROSTHESIS, REMOVABLE PROSTHESIS.

Implant surface   See: SURFACE CHARACTERISTICS (IMPLANT).

Implant surgery   portion of implant dentistry that concerns the placement and exposure of implant devices; the area of implant dentistry concerning the placement, surgical repair, and removal of implant devices.

Implant survival   implant longevity within the oral cavity. See: IMPLANT SUCCESS.

Implant system   a set of instruments and supplies designed to perform the various steps of implant insertion and prosthetic reconstruction.

Implant thread   See: THREAD.

Implant-tissue-supported prosthesis   restoration deriving its support from a combination of intraoral tissues and dental implants, always removable and either partial or complete arch. See: FIXED PROSTHESIS, REMOVABLE PROSTHESIS.

Implant try-in   See: TRIAL FIT GAUGE.

Impression   a negative likeness (reverse copy) of the surface of an object or anatomic part.

Impression coping   device for registering the position of a dental implant or dental implant abutment in an impression. The coping may be retained in the impression (direct) or may require a transfer from intraoral usage to the impression after the attachment of the corresponding analog (indirect).

Impression tray   special trays made from acrylic or shellac consisting of a body with a handle used to contain a material (e.g., rubber, hydrocolloid, or alginate) to place against the palatal tissues for making a mold of teeth.

Incisive foramen   a critical landmark for implant dentistry, and one of many openings of incisive canals into the incisive fossa, located in the midline on the anterior extreme of the hard palate; it transmits the left (more anterior) and right (more posterior) nasopalatine (Scarpa's; long sphenopalatine) nerves and vessels.

Incisive papilla   soft tissue mound that overlies the incisive foramen and neurovascular bundle, found immediately palatal to the central incisors.

Inclusion criteria   specific characteristics that all participants must have to enter a clinical trial. See: EXCLUSION CRITERIA.

Index   mold for recording the relative position of an implant or tooth to its surroundings. See: Buccal index.

Indirect impression   See: CLOSED TRAY IMPRESSION.

Indirect transfer coping   prosthetic device permitting the laboratory technician to restore the case on a cast.

Indurated   hard.

Inferior alveolar artery   (arteria alveolaris inferior) the artery that runs through the mandibular canal to supply the lower teeth.

Inferior alveolar canal   See: MANDIBULAR CANAL.

Inferior alveolar nerve   one of the terminal branches of the mandibular nerve, a division of the trigeminal nerve, entering the mandibular canal and branching to the lower teeth, periosteum, and gingival of the mandible. One branch, the mental nerve, passes through the mental foramen, supplying the skin and mucosa of the lower lip and chin.

Inflammation   a process by which the body's white blood cells and chemicals protect it from infection and foreign substances, such as bacteria and viruses, by forming a protective wall, accompanied by heat, redness, soreness, pain, itching, and/or swelling.

Informed consent   a process of communication between a patient and oral surgeon that results in the patient's full awareness of risks and benefits of, and subsequent authorization to undergo a specific medical procedure.

Infracture   controlled fracture of: 1. The lateral wall of the maxillary sinus for a window. 2. The floor of the maxillary sinus through an osteotomy prepared in the ridge.

Infraocclusion   below the biting plane.

Infrastructure   framework upon which a denture is processed; implants supporting a prosthetic reconstruction.

Initial stability   syn: primary stability; degree implant tightness immediately after placement in the prepared osteotomy. Implant initial stability is measured by clinical immobility at placement.

Insertion torque torque value used to insert an implant into an osteotomy, expressed in Newton's centimeter.

Insulin-like growth factors (IGF) peptides that behave similarly to insulin and stimulate cell proliferation. See: PLATELET-RICH PLASMA.

Integration melding of an implant surface with its supporting tissues.

Interdental bone height vertical distance from the crest of bone to the height of the interproximal papilla between two teeth or adjacent implants.

Interdental papilla portion of the free gingiva that occupies the interproximal space confined by adjacent teeth in contact; triangular projections of gingival tissue extending between the teeth. See: PAPILLA.

Interdigitation interlocking of protruding processes (fingers, teeth).

Interface See: IMPLANT INTERFACE.

Interfacial zone between an implant and adjacent supporting tissue.

Interim endosteal dental implant abutment temporary abutment to retain an interim prosthesis.

Interimplant distance horizontal distance between the platforms of two adjacent implants.

Interimplant papilla soft tissue that occupies the interproximal space confined by adjacent implant-supported fixed partial dentures in contact. See: PAPILLA.

Interim prosthesis/restoration syn: provisional prosthesis/restoration; denture used during healing or while a final prosthesis is being fabricated. A fixed or removable prosthesis, designed to restore and enhance esthetics, stabilization, or function for a limited time; used as a diagnostic tool to mimic the planned definitive prosthesis; may be tissue-borne, tooth-supported, implant-supported, or any combination of these.

Interlock male-female device used to create a relationship between two prostheses, one of which must be fixed.

Interleukins a class of proteins that are secreted mostly by macrophages and T lymphocytes and induce growth and differentiation of lymphocytes and hematopoietic stem cells. Linked to periodontal and peri-implanter disease.

Intermediate abutment tooth or implant located between natural or tooth abutments; a pier abutment.

Internal connection prosthetic connection interface internal to the implant platform (e.g., hexagon and Morse taper). See: EXTERNAL CONNECTION.

Internal hexagon hexagonal connection interface of the platform of an implant within coronal aspect; prevents rotation of attached components. See: EXTERNAL HEXAGON.

Internal irrigation irrigation during drilling of osteotomies for placement of root form implants so that cooling solution passes inside the shaft of the drilling bur and is delivered through an exit at the working end.

The cooling solution is delivered inside the osteotomy. See: EXTERNAL IRRIGATION.

Internally-threaded thread pattern within the implant body.

Interocclusal distance the distance between the occlusal surfaces of opposing teeth of the mandibular and maxillary arches.

Interproximal space (embrasure) area between two adjacent teeth, which may be gingival to (greater embrasure) or incisal to (lesser embrasure) the contact point.

Interpupillary line imaginary line that connects the centers of the pupils and is helpful for frontal facial symmetry when arranging prosthetics and implants.

Intramembranous ossification sheet-like connective tissue membranes (not cartilage) with bony tissue. Bones formed in this manner include flat bones of the skull and some of the irregular bones.

Intramucosal insert alloplastic devices placed into tissue-borne surface of a removable prosthesis to mechanically maintain the mucostatic seal; the insert is generally made of titanium or surgical stainless steel and shaped with a narrow permucosal neck, a wider retentive head, and a broad, flat, denture-attaching base; general utilization: maxillary complete denture or mandibular and maxillary removable partial dentures; also called mucosal insert or subdermal implant. See: MUCOSAL INSERT.

Intraoral distraction procedure in which a device is located completely within the oral cavity for distraction osteogenesis.

Intraoral (internal) distraction device device located within the oral cavity and used in distraction osteogenesis. The device can be attached to the bone (bone-borne), to the teeth (tooth-borne), or simultaneously to the teeth and bone (hybrid).

Intraosseous within the bone.

Intraosseous distractor See: ENDOSSEOUS DISTRACTOR.

In vitro outside the organism or natural system; refers to artificial experimental systems such as cultures or cell-free extracts.

In vivo within the living organism or natural system.

Irrigation 1. Technique of using a solution, usually saline, to cool the surgical bur and wash the debris off the flutes. 2. Act of flushing an area with a solution. See: EXTERNAL IRRIGATION, INTERNAL IRRIGATION.

Ischemia loss of tissue blood supply due to pathologic or mechanical obstruction, which may result in cell death and necrosis. Blood deficiency due to functional constriction or actual obstruction of a blood vessel(s).

Isogeneic graft See: Isograft.

Isograft syn: isogeneic graft, isologous graft, syngeneic graft; tissue graft transplanted from one genetically identical individual to another, as in monozygotic twins.

Isologous graft See: ISOGRAFT.

Isometric contraction muscle tightening with no change in muscle length.

Isotonic contraction   muscle tightening with change in muscle length and constant tension.

Isotropic surface   Surface textures that are randomly distributed so that the surface is identical in all directions. See: ANISOTROPIC SURFACE.

J

Jacob-Creuzfeldt disease   transmissible degenerative brain disorder technically termed spongiform encephalopathy; symptoms may include forgetfulness, nervousness, trembling hand, unsteady gait, muscle spasms, chronic dementia, balance disorder, and loss of facial expression; can be caused by consumption of "mad cow" meat or squirrel brains.

Jaw   one of two bony structures where teeth are found.

Jig   a dental restoration device in which dowels are employed to locate and register teeth. See: ORIENTATION JIG, VERIFICATION JIG.

Joint-separating force   force attempting to disengage screw-joined parts.

Junctional epithelium   epithelium adhering to the surface of an implant or tooth at the base of the sulcus; constitutes the coronal part of the biologic width and formed by single or multiple layers of nonkeratinizing cells. The junctional epithelial cells have a basal membrane and hemidesmosomal attachments to the surface of implant or tooth. See: EPITHELIAL ATTACHMENT.

K

Kaplan-Meier analysis   statistical method to estimate a population (e.g., implants) survival curve from a sample. Survival over time can be estimated even if patients drop out or are studied for different lengths of time.

Keratin   a protein found in all comified body structures (e.g., hair, nails, teeth, and fixed gingiva).

Keratinized gingiva   portion of the mucosa covered by keratinized epithelium; part of the oral mucosa covering the gingiva and hard palate, extending from the free gingival margin to the mucogingival junction. It consists of the free gingiva and the attached gingiva.

Knife-edge   (knife-edge ridge) a term used to describe a residual ridge's extremely sharp, narrow morphology.

Knoop hardness testing   method of using varying pressures with a diamond stylus to test a material's surface hardness.

L

Labial   pertaining to the lip; in the direction of the lip.

Laboratory analog   See: ANALOG.

Lamellar bone   See: BONE.

Lamina dura   thin cortical bone plate bone that functions as tooth socket lining.

Lapping tool   instrument used for precise finishing of surfaces; instrument used to remove the uneven surface produced during a lab's casting process of an abutment.

Laser   (Light Amplification by the Stimulated Emission of Radiation) a device that emits a very narrow, highly concentrated beam of light that can be focused on tight areas. Lasers have a variety of uses. They function by pumping photons out of a chamber with mirrors at both ends. Output can be continuous or pulsed.

Laser etching   the use of a laser beam selectively to ablate a material from a surface (e.g., implant).

Laser welding   connecting titanium implants, bars, and so on by using the noninvasive electrons of a machine developed by Arturo Hruska.

Late implant failure   syn: secondary implant failure; failure of a root-form implant after osseointegration due to or accompanied by peri-implantitis or overload. See: EARLY IMPLANT FAILURE.

Latency period   See: DISTRACTION OSTEOGENESIS.

Lateral   sideways; to the side.

Lateral window technique   creation of an access to the maxillary sinus through the lateral wall to elevate the Schneiderian membrane for graft placement in the sinus through the prepared opening.

Le Fort osteotomy   a surgery separating the maxilla and the palate from the skull above the roots of the upper teeth. The maxilla is repositioned in its new position with titanium screws and plates. There are three types: Le Fort I, II, and III.

Leukocyte   A white blood cell. A blood cell that does not contain hemoglobin. Cells are made by bone marrow that help the body fight infection and other diseases.

Life table analysis   Statistical method for describing the survival in a sample (e.g., implants). Survival time is divided into a certain number of intervals, and for each interval, computation can determine the number and proportion of cases that entered the respective interval "alive," the number and proportion of cases that failed in the respective interval (i.e., number of cases that "died"), and the number of cases that were lost or censored in said interval.

Light microscopy   method for viewing specimens via a device offering conventional enlargement.

Linea alba   white line; a reference to the midcrestal scar caused by extractions and secondary healing.

Lingual   pertaining to the tongue; on the side of the tongue.

Lining mucosa   See: ALVEOLAR MUCOSA, ORAL MUCOSA.

Lip line   the point or level during smiling where the lip can be found.

Load   a reference to any external mechanical force that is applied to a prosthesis, implant, abutment, tooth, skeletal organ, or tissue.

Loading   a reference to the placing of an implant or tooth into functional occlusion; application of a force directly or indirectly to an implant.

Localization film(s)   a method used to determine the site of a foreign body by using one or several multi-angle radiographs.

Longitudinal study   observations of the same subjects at two or more different times.

Lute   to attach, cement, affix, join, spot-weld, or solder.

Lyophilization   preferred method of preservation in the medical industry, regularly used to preserve vaccines, pharmaceuticals, blood, plasma, and other fragile substances. Commonly known as "freeze-drying."

M

Machined surface   syn: turned surface; an implant surface that has undergone the milling process of a cylindrical titanium rod. Tooled etches on the implant form a machined implant surface. See: SURFACE CHARACTERISTICS (IMPLANT), TEXTURED SURFACE.

Macroglossia   enlargement of the tongue.

Macrointerlock   mechanical interlocking between bone and implant macro-irregularities such as threads, holes, pores, grooves, and so on, which have dimensions in the range of l00 µm or greater.

Macromotion   excess movement that prevents bone healing and osseointegration, resulting in fibrous tissue encapsulation. See: MICROMOTION.

Macrophage   a mononuclear, actively phagocytic cell originating from specific monocytic stem cells in bone marrow, widely distributed throughout the body that vary in morphology and digest cellular debris and pathogens and stimulate lymphocytes and other immune cells to respond to the pathogen. Large, long-lived cells with nearly round nuclei and abundant endocytic vacuoles, endosomes, lysosomes, and phagolysosomes.

Magnet   device used for retention of overdentures.

Magnetic resonance imaging (MRI)   a diagnostic radiologic modality, using nuclear magnetic resonance technology in which the magnetic nuclei (especially protons) of a patient absorb energy from radiofrequency pulses, and emit radiofrequency signals then converted into sets of high-quality, three-dimensional images of their point sources, without use of x-rays or radioactive tracers.

Maintenance   procedures at selected time intervals to maintain prosthetic reconstruction and periodontal and peri-implant health.

Malleable   material capable of enlargement or shaping by pressure rollers or a mallet.

Malpositioned implant   dental implants that are ill-fitting or faulty, inserted incorrectly in the alveolar ridge, and unusable.

Malpractice litigation   a part of tort law, in which negligence is the predominant theory of liability. Medical malpractice is improper, illegal, or negligent professional activity or treatment by a medical practitioner. A person who alleges medical malpractice must prove four elements: (1) a duty of care was owed by the physician; (2) the physician violated the applicable standard of care; (3) the person suffered a compensable injury; and (4) the injury was caused in fact and proximately caused by the substandard conduct. The plaintiff has the burden of proof and the critical element is "standard of care."

Mandible   the bone of the lower jaw consisting of a "body," which is a curved, horizontal portion and the "rami," which are two perpendicular portions uniting the ends of the body nearly at right angles. It is the largest and strongest bone of the face.

Mandibular block graft   Intraoral source of autogenous block graft taken from the ramus buccal shelf or the mandibular symphysis, and surgically attached to a prepared site to enhance bone volume and density, allowing for placement of implants to facilitate stress distribution.

Mandibular canal   syn: inferior alveolar canal; canal within the mandible holding the inferior alveolar nerve and vessels. The posterior opening is the mandibular foramen, and anterior opening is the mental foramen.

Mandibular flexure   deformation in the body of the mandible caused by contraction of the pterygoid muscles during opening and protrusion.

Mandibular foramen   opening into the mandibular canal on the medial surface of the ramus giving passage to the inferior alveolar nerve, artery, and vein.

Mandibular nerve   the third division of the trigeminal nerve, leaving the skull through the foramen ovale and providing motor innervation to the muscles of mastication and to the tensor tympani, the anterior belly of the digastric, and the mylohyoid muscles; this nerve also provides general sensory innervation to the teeth, gingivae, the mucosa of the cheek, floor of the mouth, the epithelium of the anterior two thirds of the tongue, the meninges, and the skin of the lower portion of the face.

Mandibular staple implant   syn: transmandibular implant; also called a bone plate; a form of a transosseous implant; a plate is placed at the inferior border and a series of retentive pins is placed partially into the inferior border, with two continuous screws placed transcortically and penetrating the mouth in the canine areas for abutments.

Mandrel   device used in a handpiece, permitting the mounting of a stone or disc for grinding or finishing a restoration.

Marginal peri-implant area   The mucosal peri-implant tissues and marginal bone.

Master cast   the final model representing the exact positioning of the abutments for fabrication of a prosthesis.

Masticate   chew.

Masticatory mucosa   keratinized and attached oral mucosa of gingival and hard palate. See: ORAL MUCOSA.

Matrix   intricate network of natural or synthetic fibers aiding the reinforcement and development of tissues by supplying a scaffold for cells to grow, migrate, and proliferate.

Maxillary antroplasty See: SINUS GRAFT.

Maxillary antrum See: MAXILLARY SINUS.

Maxillary artery The maxillary artery, the larger of the two terminal branches of the external carotid artery that starts behind the neck of the mandible and supplies the face with blood.

Maxillary sinus syn: antrum of Highmore, maxillary antrum; bilateral cavities in the maxillary bone located above the dentition, lateral to the nose, inferior to the orbits, and lined with respiratory epithelium. Air cavity within the maxilla, lined by the Schneiderian membrane, consisting of a pseudostratified ciliated columnar epithelium. The maxillary sinus lies superior to the roots of premolars and molars, generally extending from the canine or premolar region posterior to the molar or tuberosity region. The cavity is pyramidal, with thin, bony walls corresponding to the orbital, alveolar (floor), facial, and infratemporal aspects of the maxilla. The apex extends into the zygomatic process, and its base is medial, forming the lateral wall of the nasal cavity. The sinus communicates with the nasal cavity through an opening (ostium) in the middle meatus. The floor of the maxillary sinus is formed by the maxillary alveolar process and by the hard palate. The floor of the maxillary sinus has recesses and depressions in the premolar and molar regions. Each of the sinuses usually has a volume of about 15 ml. See: ALVEOLAR RECESS, SEPTUM (MAXILLARY SINUS).

Maxillary sinusitis inflammation of the maxillary sinuses that produces pain over the cheeks just below the eyes, a toothache, and headache. It may or may not be as a result of infection, from bacterial, fungal, viral, allergic, or autoimmune issues.

Maxillary sinus membrane thin mucous membrane lining the sinus cavity.

Maxillary sinus pneumatization air cells or cavities in tissue, which are usually fluid-filled at birth. The growth of these sinuses is biphasic with growth during years 0-3 and 7-12. During the later phase, pneumatization spreads more inferiorly as permanent teeth take their place.

Maxillary tuberosity most distal structure of the maxillary alveolar ridge; bulbous in configuration, the tuberosity is usually located behind the third molars.

Maxillofacial prosthesis an artificial replacement of the jawbone.

Maxillofacial prosthetics a branch of dentistry that deals with congenital and acquired defects of the head and neck. Maxillofacial prosthetics integrates parts of multiple disciplines, including head and neck oncology, congenital malformation, plastic surgery, speech, and other related disciplines.

Mean (arithmetic) measure of central tendency, calculated by adding all the individual values in the group and dividing by the number of group values.

Mechanical failure implant (or abutment or restorative component or material) fracture or deformation.

Mechanicoreceptor nerve endings that respond to mechanical stimuli.

Median measure of central tendency; the middle score in a distribution or set of ranked scores. The median is computed as the average of the two middle values when the number of values in the sample is even.

Medical-grade calcium sulfate a ceramic filling material in bone cavities that is resorbable and has been used to fill cavities for more than 100 years. The main sources of calcium sulfate are naturally occurring gypsum.

Medullary pertaining to the bone marrow.

Medullary bone See: BONE.

Membrane thin layer of tissue or material (usually a lining). See: BARRIER MEMBRANE, SCHNEIDERIAN MEMBRANE.

Mental foramen anterior opening of the mandibular canal on the lateral aspect of the body of the mandible; the foramen gives passage to the mental artery and nerve.

Mental nerve a branch of the inferior alveolar nerve, arising in the mandibular canal and passing through the mental foramen; the mental nerve provides sensation to the chin and lower lip.

Mensenchymal cell also known as the mesenchymal stem cell or MSC that contributes to regeneration of mesenchymal tissues such as bone, cartilage, muscle, ligament, and tendons. The best source for MSC is bone marrow. Known to stimulate growth of hemopoietic cells within bone marrow.

Mesostructure that part of a construction that joins the implant complex (infrastructure) to the superstructure.

Meta-analysis quantitative method for combining the results of independent studies that meet specified protocol criteria (usually drawn from the published literature) and synthesize summaries and conclusions that may be used to evaluate therapeutic effectiveness and to plan new studies.

Metal strong, relatively ductile substance providing electropositive ions to a corrosive environment; can be highly polished.

Metal encapsulator See: METAL HOUSING.

Metal housing syn: metal encapsulator; part of an attachment mechanism incorporated in a removable prosthesis; the interchangeable plastic retentive component that is inserted in the metal housing and replaced when necessary.

Metal tap See: TAP.

Methylmethacrylate an organic compound with the formula $CH_2–C(CH_3)CO_2CH_3$ that is used in the production of the transparent plastic polymethyl methacrylate (PMMA); also known as resin.

Metronidazole (Flagyl) an antibiotic that fights bacteria in the body, mainly in the treatment of infections caused by susceptible organisms; used to treat periodontitis and peri-implantitis.

Microfracture minuscule crack in solid material caused either by stress or (manufacturing) flaw that could lead to structural failure.

Microgap space (usually measured in microns) between two structures or devices. See: IMPLANT-ABUTMENT JUNCTION.

Microglossia small tongue.

Micrognathia small jaw.

Microinterlock fixation from mechanical interlocking of bone to micro-irregularities at the implant surface (e.g., machined surfaces, texture from grit blasting, coating, ion bombardment, or irregularities from plasma spraying, and so on); the interlocking has dimensions in the range of microns.

Microlock very small device designed to securely and reliably affix a prosthesis.

Micromotion movement that does not stop bone ingrowth of an implant, resulting in direct bone anchorage of the implant (osseointegration). See: MACROMOTION.

Microstomia small oral orifice.

Microtia small ear.

Midcrestal incision incision in the middle of the alveolar crest. See: CRESTAL INCISION, MUCOBUCCAL FOLD INCISION.

Millipore filter a trade name for filters made of a meshwork of cellulose acetate or nitrate with a defined pore size. They can be autoclaved and are used for filtering out microorganisms. They are about 150 μm thick.

Mini-implant implant that is smaller than standard dental root form implant, cheaper, and allows for immediate loading. They are 1.8 mm in diameter and come in four lengths, depending on the amount of bone available to retain the implant, as well as an assessment of the density of the bone. Mini-implants are used for supporting crowns in situations in which there is not enough room for a standard implant.

Mobile loose or movable.

Mode score or value occurring most frequently in a distribution.

Modeling (bone) independent sites of formation and resorption resulting in shape or size change of bone. Modeling occurs during growth and healing.

Modulus of elasticity stress-over-strain ratio when deformation is elastic. A measure of material stiffness or flexibility. Stiff material has a high modulus of elasticity, while flexible material has a low modulus (also called Young's modulus). See: ELASTICITY.

Monocortical a specimen or bone with a single external dense covering.

Monocyte a large white blood cell formed in bone marrow and the spleen that removes dead or damaged tissues, destroys cancer cells, and regulates immunity against foreign substances.

Monomer chemical (usually liquid) that can undergo polymerization, either by itself or with a compatible powder.

Morse taper connection an internal connection interface that consists of a converging circular surface forming a mechanical locking friction-fit. syn: cold weld.

Moulage a facial moulage; a procedure used to record the contours of the face by making a molding (moulage) and model of the face.

Mucobuccal fold cul-de-sac formed by the mucous membrane when turning from the upper or lower gingivae to the cheek.

Mucobuccal fold incision syn: vestibular incision; an incision made in the mucobuccal fold. See: CRESTAL INCISION, MIDCRESTAL INCISION.

Mucocele an oral mucous retention cyst, from a ruptured salivary gland duct usually caused by local trauma, commonly found in children and young adults.

Mucogingival junction demarcation that occurs between the masticatory mucosa and the alveolar mucosa. Border that exists between fixed and areolar gingivae.

Mucogingival surgery surgical procedures to augment the band of soft-tissue defects around the teeth used in periodontics, one of which is to create a flap of gingival tissue repositioned apically to maintain a functionally adequate zone of attached gingiva.

Mucoperiosteal flap a full-thickness flap of mucosal tissue, including the periosteum, gingival, and alveolar mucosa, reflected from a bone.

Mucoperiosteum layer of mucosa, connective tissue, and periosteum covering bone in the oral cavity, sometimes giving rise to muscle attachments.

Mucosa a membrane composed of epithelium and lamina propria lining the oral cavity and other organs and cavities of the body; also called mucous membrane. The epithelial lining of body cavities, consisting of a mucous membrane and opening to the outside. See: ORAL MUCOSA.

Mucosal implant See: MUCOSAL INSERT.

Mucosal insert syn: button implant, epithelial implant, intramucosal insert, mucosal implant; a mushroom-shaped device that is fastened to the tissue surface of a removable denture and that fits within a prepared gingival receptor site and, in conjunction with other, multiple inserts, enhances denture retention and stability.

Mucosal peri-implant tissues soft tissues (epithelium and connective) around an implant.

Mucositis inflammation of the mucosa. See: PERI-IMPLANT MUCOSITIS.

Multicenter study clinical trial conducted on a single protocol but at more than one research center and by more than one investigator.

Muscle mold the shaping of material by manipulation or action of the tissues adjacent to the impression's borders; also called border mold.

Mylohyoid ridge   oblique ridge on the lingual surface of the mandible, extending from the level of the roots of the last molar as a bony attachment for the mylohyoid muscles that form the floor of the mouth; the ridge determines the lingual boundary of the mandibular subperiosteal implant.

Myositis   muscle inflammation.

Nasal spine   median, sharp process that is formed by the forward prolongation of two maxillae at the lower margin of the anterior aperture of the nose; used to support a maxillary subperiosteal implant.

Nasopalatine nerve   branch of the pterygopalatine ganglion passing through the sphenopalatine foramen, crossing to and then down the nasal septum and through the incisive foramen; this nerve supplies the mucous membrane of the anterior hard palate.

Navigation   See: COMPUTER-AIDED NAVIGATION.

Ncm   acronym: Newton's centimeter.

Nd:YAG laser   a crystal that is used as a medium for solid-state lasers. Nd: YAG lasers are used for soft tissue surgeries in the oral cavity, such as gingivectomy, periodontal sulcular debridement, frenectomy, and coagulation of graft donor sites.

Necrosis   death of cells or tissue, caused by loss of blood supply, by bacterial toxins, or by physical and chemical agents.

Nerve lateralization   See: NERVE REPOSITIONING.

Nerve repositioning   syn: nerve lateralization, nerve transpositioning; surgical procedure during which the course of the inferior alveolar nerve is redirected so as to increase the clinician's ability to place longer implants in a mandible that has experienced extensive resorption of the posterior ridge.

Nerve transpositioning   See: NERVE REPOSITIONING.

Neuralgia   pain experienced along a sensory nerve pathway.

Neuritis   inflammation of a nerve.

Neurovascular bundle   a term applied to the body's nerves, arteries, veins, and lymphatics lying between the innermost and the inner intercostal muscles. Neuropathy: any functional disturbance or change to a nerve.

Newton's centimeter   (Ncm) Unit of rotational torque.

Nidus   a place or central point from which organisms emanate.

Nightguard   See: OCCLUSAL GUARD.

Noble metals   elements resistant to oxidation, corrosion, and tarnishing during heating operations in a saline environment.

Nonabsorbable   description of a material that does not degrade in vivo overtime. See: NONRESORBABLE.

Nonangled abutment   See: NONANGULATED ABUTMENT.

Nonangulated abutment   seen: NONANGLED ABUTMENT, STRAIGHT ABUTMENT; abutment with a body parallel to the long axis of the implant. See: ANGULATED ABUTMENT.

Nonaxial loading   the application of forces off the implant long-axis. See: AXIAL LOADING.

Nonfunctional loading   See: NONOCCLUSAL LOADING.

Nonhexed   implant component or an implant without a hexagonal connection interface.

Nonlamellar bone   See: Bone.

Nonocclusal loading   restoration not in occlusal contact with the opposing dentition in maximal intercuspal position or in excursions, although there may be restoration contact with the cheeks, tongue, lips, and food. See: OCCLUSAL LOADING.

Nonresorbable   description of material that does not degrade over time or that shows relatively limited in vivo degradation. See: NONABSORBABLE.

Nonsubmergible   not buried.

Nonsubmergible implant   See: ONE-STAGE IMPLANT.

Nonthreaded implant   endosseous, root-form implant with no threads, maybe parallel-sided (i.e., cylindrical) or tapered.

O

Obtundent   material used to obdurate or seal.

Obturator   prosthesis designed to seal an acquired or congenital defect.

Occlude   to close.

Occlusal dysesthesia   refers to unusual perceptions of the bite.

Occlusal equilibration   balance between opposing elements of the masticatory apparatus.

Occlusal guard   removable appliance designed to minimize effects of bruxism and other occlusal habits that may damage dental implants, dentition, and prosthetic reconstruction.

Occlusal loading   refers to the restoration's occlusal contact with the opposing dentition in maximal intercuspal position and/or excursions. See: NONOCCLUSAL LOADING.

Occlusal overload   See: OVERLOAD.

Occlusal table   the masticating surfaces of the bicuspid and molar teeth, and other posterior teeth.

Occlusion   the manner in which the maxillary (upper) and mandibular (lower) teeth come together when they approach each other, as occurs during chewing, or when the mouth is closed.

Occlusive membrane   See: BARRIER MEMBRANE.

Odontalgia   toothache.

Oligodontia   fewer than the normal complement of teeth.

One-part implant   syn: one-piece implant; implant without a surface joint exposed to tissues since the endosseous and transmucosal portions consist of a single unit. See: TWO-PART IMPLANT.

One-piece abutment   abutment connecting to the implant without an additional screw, retained by cement, friction (press-fit), or screw threads. See: TWO-PIECE ABUT-MENT.

One-piece implant   See: ONE-PART IMPLANT.

One-screw test   a method for checking the fit of a mul-tiple-unit screw-retained restoration. A single screw is placed in the terminal abutment, and evaluation is made on the opposite side. Fit is inaccurate when a clinical or radiological examination determines that the framework rises or has a ledge.

One-stage implant   syn: nonsubmergible implant, single-stage implant; endosseous implant designed with a transmucosal coronal portion (one-piece implant with no microgap) and placed in a one-stage surgery proto-col. See: TWO-STAGE IMPLANT.

One-stage implant placement   single surgical procedure where the site is prepared, implant placed, and there is no need for a second surgical procedure.

One-stage surgery   placing an endosseous root-form implant in the bone and leaving it in contact with the oral environment during the healing process, eliminating a second surgical procedure. See: TWO-STAGE SURGERY.

Onlay graft   an autogenous bone or bone replacement graft or both placed on or over bone to increase length or width, or both.

Open-ended wrench   instrument for applying torque during removal of an implant mount.

Open tray impression   syn: direct impression; technique using an impression coping with retentive features around which a rigid elastic impression material is injected. The impression coping is first unthreaded through an opening on the occlusal surface of the tray before removal. See: CLOSED TRAY IMPRESSION.

Oral flora   organisms in the mouth.

Oral implant   biomaterial or device made of one or more biomaterials, biologic or alloplastic, surgically inserted into soft or hard tissues for functional or cosmetic pur-poses or both. See: DENTAL IMPLANT.

Oral implantology   See: IMPLANT DENTISTRY.

Oral mucosa   Epithelial lining of the oral cavity continu-ous with the skin of the lips and mucosa of the soft palate and pharynx, consisting of 1. Masticatory mucosa of the gingiva and hard palate, 2. Specialized mucosa of the dorsum of the tongue, and 3. Lining mucosa of the remainder of the oral cavity. Syn: Alveolar mucosa.

Orientation jig   syn: abutment transfer device; laboratory fabricated device for maintaining the correct position of a component transferred from the cast to the mouth.

O-ring   the doughnut-shaped, resilient overdenture attach-ment with the ability to bend with resistance and return to its approximate original shape; the O-ring attaches to a post with a groove or undercut area.

Oro-antral fistula   abnormal communication between the maxillary sinus and oral cavity, most often a complica-tion after tooth extraction, but may also occur after api-cectomy or due to severe periodontal disease. The teeth most frequently involved are the upper second molar, followed by the first molar. Small fistulae may close independently, but larger fistulae may require surgical closure.

Oronasal fistula   abnormal opening between the mouth and nose.

Orthodontic implant   any implant used as anchorage for tooth movement.

Orthodontics   a specialty of dentistry that deals with the study and treatment of malocclusions, tooth irregularity, disproportionate jaw relationships, or all of these. Also known as dentofacial orthopedics.

Osse(o)   syn: osteo; pertaining to bone or containing a bony element.

Osseointegration   direct contact between living bone and a functionally loaded implant surface without interposed soft tissue at the light microscope level, with, clinically, the absence of mobility and including a sustained trans-fer and distribution of load from the implant to and within the bone tissue.

Osseoperception   special feeling or special sensory perception result from a changed impact force through implant-bone interface, in contrast to the cushioning effect of the skin under the socket prosthesis perhaps with intraosseous or periosteal neural endings involved.

Osseous   of the nature or quality of bone.

Osseous coagulum   mixture consisting of small bone particles and blood.

Osseous graft   See: BONE GRAFT.

Ossification   calcification or mineralization of bone.

Osteal   Bony, osseous.

Ostectomy   excision of bone. See: OSTEOPLASTY.

Osteo   See: OSSE(O).

Osteoblast   fully differentiated cell originating in the embryonic mesenchyme and functioning in bone tissue formation during the skeleton's early development. Osteoblasts produce inorganic salts and synthesize the collagen and glycoproteins that form the bone matrix; they develop into osteocytes.

Osteocalcin   bone-specific protein produced by the osteoblast; plays a possible role in osteoclast recruit-ment. Osteocalcin is an indicator of bone remodeling or mineralization.

Osteoclast   large, multinucleated cell arising from mono-nuclear precursors of the hematopoietic lineage; the osteoclast plays a role in the breakdown and resorption of osseous tissue.

Osteoconduction   bone growth by apposition from sur-rounding bone; during the process, an inorganic material provides scaffolding for bone growth. See: OSTEOIN-DUCTION.

Osteoconductive graft   allografts, autografts, and bone substitutes that act as a conductive means for formation of osteoids, the bone matrix, especially before calcifica-tion.

Osteocyte   osteoblast embedded within the bone matrix and occupying a flat oval cavity (bone lacuna). Cells found in bone lacunae send slender cytoplasmic processes through canaliculi that make contact with processes of other osteocytes.

Osteodistraction   See: DISTRACTION OSTEOGENESIS.

Osteogenesis   formation and development of bone; the development of bony tissue; ossification; the histogenesis of bone.

Osteogenetic   1. Forming bone. 2. Concerned in bone formation.

Osteogenic   syn: osteogenous; promoting the development and formation of bone exclusively from the action of osteoblasts.

Osteogenous   See: OSTEOGENIC.

Osteoid   1. Resembling bone. 2. The nonmineralized bone matrix laid down by the osteoblasts and later calcified into bone with inclusion of osteoblasts as osteocytes within lacunae.

Osteoinduction   bone formation in the absence of a bony host site; new bone formation occurs as a result of osteoprogenitor cells from primitive mesenchymal cells that have come under the influence of one or more agents that emanate from the bone matrix; a process involving cellular change or cellular interaction when cells are coerced to differentiate; osteoinduction is used during autogenous bone grafting. See: BONE MORPHOGENETIC PROTEIN, OSTEOCONDUCTION.

Osteointegration   See: OSSEOINTEGRATION.

Osteomyelitis   bone inflammation from infection, which may remain localized or spread through the bone to the marrow, cortex, cancellous tissue, and periosteum.

Osteon   basic structural unit of compact bone, comprising a Haversian canal and its concentrically arranged lamellae, which may be 4 to 20, each 3µ to 7µ thick, in a single (Haversian) system, mainly directed in the long axis of the bone.

Osteonecrosis   syn: bone necrosis; the death of bone.

Osteonecrosis of the jaw (ONJ)   Literally, the death of bone in the jaws; several cases of bisphosphonate-related osteomyelitis (BON, also referred to as osteonecrosis of the jaw) have been associated with the use of the oral bisphosphonates (Fosamax [alendronate], Actonel [risedronate] and Boniva [ibandronate]) for the treatment of osteoporosis; these patients may have had other conditions that could put them at risk for developing BON.

Osteonectin   phosphoprotein in bone and blood platelets, binding both collagen and calcium and regulating mineralization.

Osteoplasty   surgical modification of bone by removal. See: OSTECTOMY.

Osteopontin   acidic calcium-binding phosphoprotein involved in bone mineralization with a high affinity for hydroxyapatite.

Osteoporosis   medical problem often seen in postmenopausal females and characterized by demineralization and diminution of bone mass, decreased density, and enlarged intrabony spaces.

Osteoprogenitor cell   undifferentiated cell able to transform into a bone-forming cell.

Osteopromotion   sealing off an anatomical site physically (e.g., barrier membrane) to direct bone formation and prevent soft tissue proliferation (i.e., connective tissue) from interfering with osteogenesis.

Osteoradionecrosis   bone necrosis caused by excessive exposure to radiation.

Osteotome   instrument (circular in cross-section) to expand an osteotomy apically or laterally, with or without grafting.

Osteotome lift   See: OSTEOTOME TECHNIQUE.

Osteotome technique   1. Sinus grafting technique involving the careful infracturing of the maxillary sinus floor and elevation of the Schneiderian membrane via an osteotomy prepared and extended in the ridge with an osteotome. 2. The surgical expansion of an osteotomy laterally with or without grafting. See: RIDGE EXPANSION.

Osteotomy   1. Site prepared in bone for the placement of an implant or graft. 2. Any surgical procedure when bone is transected or cut.

Ostium (maxillary sinus)   opening connecting the maxillary sinus to the middle meatus of the nasal cavity.

Overdenture   removable partial or complete denture whose built-in secondary copings overlay (or telescope over) the primary copings, fitting over the prepared natural crowns, posts, or studs. Syn: Overlay denture.

Overdenture (implant)   removable partial or complete denture, which may be implant-supported or implant-tissue-supported. The prosthesis is retained by attachments.

Overlay denture   See: OVERDENTURE.

Overload (occlusal)   a reference to masticatory forces exceeding the withstanding capacity of a bone-implant interface, implant, or componentry.

Oxidized surface treatment   modification of the surface oxide properties of titanium implants by alteration of the titanium oxide layer thickness.

P

Paget disease   a malfunction in the normal process of bone growth. Normal bone growth includes a breaking down and regeneration. Paget's disease causes a malfunction in regrowth. The bone grows back weak, soft, and porous, which bends easily and leads to shortening of the affected part of the body.

Palatal implant   See: ORTHODONTIC IMPLANT.

Palatal vault   the deepest portion of the roof of the mouth, usually found in the midline.

Palliative   offering relief of pain, symptoms, and stress, but not a cure.

Palpate to examine by touching (bimanual palpation: using two hands, usually with the examined part compressed between the hands; bi-digital palpation; using two fingers, each of a different hand).

Palsy See: PARALYSIS.

Panoramic radiograph radiographic view of the maxilla and mandible extending from the left to the right glenoid fossae.

Panoramic radiography dental tomogram that reveals the jaws, teeth, and surrounding osseous components.

Papilla small, V-shaped gingival extensions between healthy teeth; soft tissue in the interproximal space confined by adjacent crowns in contact. See: INTERDENTAL PAPILLA, INTERIMPLANT PAPILLA.

Papilla-sprang incision parasulcular incision excluding the papilla in the flap elevation.

Paracrine of or relating to hormones or secretion released by endocrine cells into adjacent cells or surrounding tissue instead of directly into the bloodstream.

Parallel(ing) pin See: DIRECTION INDICATOR.

Parallel-sided implant syn: parallel-walled implant, straight implant; an endosseous root-form implant with the body of the implant the same diameter at the coronal and apical ends. The platform of such an implant may have a larger diameter.

Parallel-walled implant See: PARALLEL-SIDED IMPLANT.

Paralysis syn: palsy, paresis; loss of motor function from disease.

Paresthesia partial loss of sensation; spontaneous or evoked abnormal sensations, not painful, often unpleasant (e.g., tingling, burning, prickling, or numbness), usually caused by nerve injury and sometimes resulting from surgical procedures.

Partially edentulous absence of one of more teeth in one portion or either the mandible or maxilla or both. To have some, but not all teeth missing.

Partial-thickness flap a surgical flap consisting of the mucosa and submucosa but not including the periosteum. Also known as the split-thickness flap.

Particulate graft graft consisting of particles.

Passivate literally, to make passive; to create an oxide layer on a metal implant.

Passivation process by which metals and alloys are made more resistant to corrosion by the creation of a thin and stable oxide layer on the external surfaces. See: DEPASSIVATION.

Passive without resistance, inert.

Passive fit a fit not inducing strain between two or more implants.

Patent open, unobstructed; not closed.

Path of placement corridor of passivity permitting the seating or removal of a prosthesis or other intraoral device.

PDGF acronym: platelet-derived growth factors.

Pedical flap a skin flap that during surgery is elevated through connective tissue only and used to increase the width of attached gingiva.

Peer-reviewed journal academic periodical that requires approval by a panel of peers on each article submitted before publication.

Penicillin one of the oldest and most widely used antibiotics derived from the mold, *penicillium notatum*, which is toxic to a number of pathogens by blocking the peptidoglycan synthesis, destroying the cell wall.

Percentage bone-to-implant contact a measure expressed as a percentage of the total implant surface of the linear surface of an *implant* in direct contact with the bone. See: BONE-TO-IMPLANT CONTACT.

Perforate to pierce or make a hole; to fenestrate.

Perforation 1. Cortical: hole created in the cortical bone by a drill or implant. See: DECORTICATION. 2. Schneiderian membrane: Tearing or creation of an opening in the maxillary sinus membrane during sinus graft surgery or following tooth extraction.

Periabutment round the abutment.

Periapical around or about the apex of the tooth.

Pericervical saucerization Pathologic crestal bone loss from peri-implantitis. The bone loss is cup-shaped or saucer-like around the coronal aspect of the implant when viewed in a radiograph. See: PERI-IMPLANTITIS.

Peri-implant around the implant.

Peri-implant crevicular epithelium nonkeratinized epithelium that lines the mucosal crevice.

Peri-implant disease inflammatory reactions in soft or hard tissues surrounding implants.

Peri-implantitis inflammatory reactions in the hard or soft tissues, with loss of supporting bone, surrounding an implant or other implanted materials; the condition can be traumatic, ulcerative, resorptive, or exfoliative (e.g., periodontitis).

Peri-implant mucositis reversible inflammatory reactions in the soft tissues surrounding an implant.

Periodontal biotype two types of periodontal tissue that not only affect natural dentition, but may also affect the esthetic result in an implant-supported prosthesis. In most cases when the patient has a thick-flat periodontium, the papillae can be preserved. When the patient has the thin-scalloped periodontium, there will be papillary recession.

Periodontal dressing a bandage and controller of hemorrhage, placed over the areas where a gingivectomy has been performed, after periodontal surgery.

Periodontal ligament a thin, connective tissue that surrounds the root of a tooth and attaches it to the alveolar bone.

Periodontal plastic surgery involves regenerative and reconstructive procedures designed to restore form and function in the oral cavity by eliminating gingival deficits and deformities and to also enhance esthetics. Also known as mucogingival surgery.

Periodontal pocket   abnormally deepened gum tissues surrounding a tooth that have become inflamed and infected. Periodontal pockets make it hard to remove plaque and lead to periodontitis and bone destruction.

Periosteum   membrane of fibrous connective tissue covering all bone except at the articular surfaces (cartilaginous extremities).

Periotome   Instrument used to sever the periodontal ligament fibers before tooth extraction.

Permucosal   passing through or across the mucosa or epithelium.

Permucosal extension   portion of an implant extending through and beyond the epithelium. See: HEALING ABUTMENT.

Permucosal seal   junctional epithelium separating connective tissues from the environment outside an implant. See: JUNCTIONAL EPITHELIUM.

PGA   acronym: polyglycolic Acid.

Phase-1 bone regeneration   the first step toward total bone regrowth in a healing bone, involving formation of the woven bone in conjunction with a graft.

Physiologic rest position   the natural postural position of the mandible when at rest in the upright position and the condyles are in a neutral unstrained position in the mandibular fossae. Also known as the postural position.

Pick-up impression   an impression made with the super-structure frame in place on the abutments in the mouth after the implant has been surgically inserted and the mouth has healed. The superstructure frame is included in the impression material, and an accurate impression of the oral mucosal tissue over the implant is obtained.

Pier abutment   See: INTERMEDIATE ABUTMENT.

Pilot drill   drill used to enlarge the coronal aspect of an osteotomy, so that the path of the subsequent drill can be directed.

PLA   acronym: polylactic Acid.

Placement   insertion of an implant or other device or prosthesis.

Plasma-containing growth factor   (IGF-1) the main naturally-occurring, growth factor in plasma, found in the bone matrix, which acts like insulin.

Plasma spray   implant surface treatment during which a dense or porous coating is formed after high temperature deposition of metal or ceramic powders that have been totally or partially melted and then rapidly resolidified.

Plasma spray-coated with titanium   a reliable technique for coating the surface of a titanium implant with small, irregular particles of titanium.

Plasmid   an extra-chromosomal DNA molecule capable of replicating independently of the chromosomal DNA. They occur naturally in bacteria.

Plaster   syn: dental plaster; the beta-form of calcium sulfate hemihydrate powder; it is produced by heating gypsum to eliminate water and is used as modeling material in dentistry when mixed with water to reform

gypsum. In guided bone regeneration, plaster can also be used as a bone graft or membrane. See: DENTAL STONE.

Plaster of Paris $CaSO_4 \cdot \frac{1}{2}H_2O$ See: PLASTER.

Plastic   a description of the degree to which a material can be formed, shaped, or molded.

Plateau   an elevated flat plane or area of tissue.

Platelet   an irregular, disc-shaped, nonnucleated, disklike cytoplasmic element in the blood that assists in blood clotting. Also called blood platelet or thrombocyte. Actually fragments of large bone marrow cells called megakaryocytes.

Platelet-derived growth factors (PDGF)   growth factors released by platelets that initiate connective tissue healing (e.g., bone regeneration and repair). These factors also increase mitogenesis, angiogenesis, and macrophage activation.

Platelet gel   referring to an autogenous hematopoetic tissue graft a surgeon creates from harvesting an individual's own natural healing factors (stem cells, growth factors, platelets, and white cells) from that person's blood.

Platelet-poor plasma (PPP)   lesser concentration of active platelets that remain after the separation process to derive platelet-rich plasma.

Platelet-rich plasma (PRP)   autologous product derived from whole blood through the process of gradient density centrifugation, the purpose of which is to derive a substance able to incorporate high concentrations of growth factors PDGF, TGF-El, TGF-L2, IGF, VEGF, FGF-1, and fibrin into a graft mixture.

Platform   syn: prosthetic table, restorative platform, seating surface; the coronal aspect of an implant to which abutments, components, and prostheses may be connected.

Platform switching   syn: abutment swapping; using an abutment with a diameter narrower than that of the implant platform and, in so doing, moving the implant-abutment junction away from the edge of the platform.

Pneumatization   a process by which air-filled cavities become an increasing part of a body. See: PNEUMATIZED MAXILLARY SINUS.

Pneumatized maxillary sinus   maxillary sinus enlargement; gradual thinning of the sinus walls as a result of the increase in size of the maxillary sinus. Usually the result of aging and loss of maxillary teeth (and masticatory forces).

Polish   to treat with abrasives of graduated fineness (machined finish).

Polished surface   machined (smoother) surface.

Polishing cap   component connected to the abutment's apical part to protect the base and allow the lab to polish the prosthesis and abutment without excessive reduction of the base diameter or rounding of edges.

Polyglactin   multifilament braided purified lactides and glycolides used as absorbable sutures or membranes.

Polyglycolic acid (PGA)   polymer of glycolic acid used for absorbable sutures or membranes.

Polylactic acid (PLA)   polymer of lactic acid used for absorbable sutures or membranes.

Polymer   natural or synthetic substance composed of giant molecules formed from smaller molecules of the same substance.

Polymorphonuclear leukocyte   a type of white blood cell with a nucleus that is divided so that the cell looks to have multiple nuclei.

Polysulfide rubber   an elastomeric impression material; Thiokol.

Polytetrafluoroethylene   a synthetic fluoropolymer commonly known as Teflon. Used in a variety of surgical material such as guided tissue regeneration.

Polyvinylsiloxane   elastomeric impression material.

Pontic   a false tooth in a dental bridge.

Porosity   having minute openings or pores.

Porous   characterized by pores or voids within a structure (e.g., grafting material, implant surface).

Porous coralline hydroxyapatite   a bone substitute from Porite coral shown to facilitate growth of bone into the desired shape, which is nonresorbable but osteoconductive.

Porous surface   See: PLASMA SPRAYED, SINTERED (POROUS) SURFACE.

Posterior palatal seal, postdam   postpalatal seal; the seal at the posterior border of a denture.

Posterior superior alveolar artery   One of three arteries (along with infraorbital and posterior lateral nasal arteries) supplying them axillary sinus, all of which are ultimate branches of the maxillary artery. During lateral approach sinus elevation surgery, any of these arteries may be encountered.

Postpalatal seal   See: POSTERIOR PALATAL SEAL.

PPP   acronym: platelet-poor plasma.

Prefabricated abutment   machine-manufactured abutment.

Prefabricated coping   thimble prepared to fit an abutment.

Prefabricated cylinder   component made of a noble alloy and connecting to an implant or abutment; to form a custom abutment for a cement-retained or screw-retained prosthesis, a compatible alloy is cast to the cylinder.

Preload   energy transferred to a screw after torque is applied during tightening. The result of such stretching is that the screw threads are tightly secured to the screw's mating counterpart, holding them together by producing a clamping force between the screw head and seat.

Prepable abutment   abutment prepared and modified from its original manufactured design.

Preprosthetic surgery   surgery performed to improve the prognosis of planned prostheses.

Press-fit   retention of a root-form implant from close proximity of the bone; alternatively, a reference to the retention of certain components into the implant. See: FRICTION-FIT.

Primary bone   See: BONE.

Primary closure   bringing the flaps of a wound together to prevent tension and to enable a traumatic suturing. See: HEALING BY FIRST (PRIMARY) INTENTION.

Primary implant failure   See: EARLY IMPLANT FAILURE.

Primary stability   See: INITIAL STABILITY.

Primitive bone   See: BONE.

Prions   proteinaceous infectious particles that show marked resistance to conventional inactivation procedures, including irradiation, boiling, dry heat, and chemical treatment; these particles cause and transmit bovine spongiform encephalopathy and similar encephalopathies. However, other deactivating agents can be successfully used against prions, including denaturing organic solvents, chaotropic agents, and alkali.

Probing depth   as measured by a periodontal probe, the distance from the free mucosal or gingival margin to the base of the pen-implant or periodontal sulcus.

Probing depths   pocket depths adjacent to implants or teeth.

Profiler (bone)   burs (with different profiler diameters to accommodate a desired component diameter) for removing bone around the platform of a root-form implant, thus allowing the connection of components to the implant.

Profilometer   device used to trace and record the roughness of a surface at high magnification.

Progenitor cell   undifferentiated cell able to transform into one or more types of cells.

Prognathism   a protruding mandible.

Prognosis   a prediction of the outcome of therapy.

Progressive loading   placing a series of increasingly hard prostheses into function, usually beginning with acrylic and ending with porcelain; gradually increasing the application of load on a prosthesis and implant.

Proprioception   ability of sensory nerves to determine the position of body parts.

Prospective study   study planned to observe events that have not yet occurred.

Prosthesis   syn: restoration; artificial replacement of a missing part of the body; artificial device used to substitute for a lost or underfunctioning body part.

Prosthetic   artificial.

Prosthetic screw   syn: retaining screw; screw used in a prosthetic reconstruction to connect a prosthesis to an implant or an abutment.

Prosthetic table   See: PLATFORM.

Prosthodontic abutment   See: ABUTMENT.

Prosthodontics   the art and science of diagnosis, treatment, maintenance, and follow-up care of patients requiring artificial dentures or oromaxillofacial parts.

Protocol   details for a proposed activity, such as surgical protocol, prosthetic protocol, and research protocol.

Provisional implant   See: TRANSITIONAL IMPLANT.

Provisionalization   the process of creating a temporary and alterable prosthesis.

Provisional prosthesis/restoration   See: INTERIM PROSTHESIS/RESTORATION.

Provisional restoration   prostheses made for temporary purposes.

Proximal   toward the center of a body.

PRP   acronym: platelet-rich plasma.

Pterygoid implant   root-form implant originating near the former second maxillary molar; its end point encroaches in the scaphoid fossa of the sphenoid bone. The implant follows an intrasinusal trajectory in a dorsal and mesio-cranial direction, perforating the posterior sinus wall and the pterygoid plates.

Pterygoid notch   groove at the pyramidal process of the palatine bone between the pterygoid plates and the maxillary tuberosity.

Pterygomaxillary notch   bony groove between the maxillary tuberosity and the pterygoid bone (lesser sphenoidal wing).

Punch technique   exposure of the implant by the removal of a circular piece of soft tissue over a submerged implant; the incision is approximately the diameter of the implant platform.

P-value   probability that a test statistic will assume a value as extreme as or more extreme than that seen under the assumption that the null hypothesis is true.

Q

Quadrant   any one of four parts created by dividing an object with two right-angled intersecting lines.

R

RAD   radiation absorbed dose.

Radicular   referring to root.

Radiograph   an x-ray.

Radiographic guide   See: RADIOGRAPHIC TEMPLATE.

Radiographic marker   radiopaque structure of known dimension, or a material incorporated in or applied to a radiographic template to yield positional or dimensional information.

Radiographic template   guide used for diagnosis and planning phases for dental implants; the template is derived from a diagnostic wax-up and worn during the radiographic exposure to show the tooth position to nearby anatomical structures.

Radiolucent   the quality of appearing dense or black on exposed x-ray film; allowing the passage of x-rays or other radiation.

Radiopaque   the quality of appearing light or white on exposed x-ray film; capable of blocking x-rays.

Ramus endosteal implant   blade implant designed for placement in the anterior ramus of the mandible.

Ramus frame endosteal implant   three-component blade complex composed of an anterior foot and bilateral ramus extensions.

Ramus frame implant   full-arch mandibular implant with a tripodal design consisting of a horizontal supragingival connecting bar with endosseous units placed into the two rami and symphyseal area.

Ramus graft   bone graft harvested from the lateral aspect of the ascending ramus of the mandible, consisting of mostly cortical bone.

Radionecrosis   osteonecrosis due to excessive exposure to radiation. Typically seen to occur in patients who have undergone chemotherapy for tumors that were located anywhere from the neck up.

Radiopaque marker   a marker used to interpret an object's length, angulation, or localization within an x-ray image. It is made of metal or any other radio-opaque material, meaning that it does not let x-rays or other types of radiation penetrate.

Ramus   the posterior vertical part of the mandible on each side that extends from the corpus to the condyle, and makes a joint at the temple.

Random controlled trial   prospective study detailing the effects of a particular procedure or material; in such a study, subjects are randomly assigned to either test or control groups. The former receives the procedure or material, while the latter receives a standard procedure, or material, a different test procedure, or a placebo.

RAP   acronym: regional acceleratory phenomenon.

Ratchet   wrench for threaded implants to facilitate final implant seating.

RBM   acronym: resorbable blast media.

Reactive bone   See: BONE.

Reamer   tool for finishing the mating surface of a metal cylinder/coping, specifically the screw seat interface.

Receptor sites   areas in the maxillary mucosa into which are nestled the heads of intramucosal inserts.

Recipient site   See: HOST SITE; site that receives a soft or hard tissue graft.

Recombinant human bone morphogenetic protein (rhBMP)   osteoinductive protein produced by recombinant DNA technology.

Record base   a temporary form representing the base of a denture and used to help establish maxillomandibular relation records for facilitating trial placement in the oral cavity. Also known as a base plate.

Re-entry   surgical reopening of a site to improve or observe results from the initial procedure.

Reflection   elevation or folding back of the mucoperiosteum to expose the underlying bone.

Refractory   resistant to treatment.

Regenerate   syn: distraction zone; tissue forming between gradually separated bone segments in distraction osteogenesis.

Regenerate maturation   completion of mineralization and remodeling of the regenerate tissue.

Regeneration   reproduction or reconstitution of a lost or injured part to its original state; restoration of body parts after trauma. See: REPAIR.

Regional acceleratory phenomenon (RAP)   local response to a stimulus in which tissues form 2 to 10 times more rapidly than the normal regeneration process. The duration and intensity are directly proportional to the kind and amount of stimulus as well as to the site where it was produced.

Reimplantation   act of reinserting a tooth into the alveolar socket from which it has been removed.

Rejection   immunological response of incompatibility in a transplanted organ or implanted device.

Releasing incision   an incision made to allow for periodontal flap repositioning and/or mobility for suture closure.

Remodel   morphologic change in bone as it adapts to environmental stimuli.

Remodeling (bone)   turnover of bone in small packets by basic multicellular units (BMUs) of bone remodeling.

Removable prosthesis   restoration that the patient can remove partially (RPD: removable partial denture) or completely (RCD: removable complete denture). See: DENTURE, FIXED PROSTHESIS.

Removal torque   rotational force applied to remove the implant from its placement within the bone.

Removal torque value (RTV)   syn: reverse torque value; measure of rotational force to rupture the bone-implant interface of a root-form implant.

Repair   healing of a wound by tissue that does not fully restore the architecture or function of the lost part. See: REGENERATION.

Replica   See: ANALOG.

Replicate   to reproduce.

Residual ridge   remnant of the alveolar process and soft tissue covering after tooth removal.

Resilient   springing back into shape or position.

Resin   a compound made by condensation or polymerization of low-molecular-weight organic compounds, clear to translucent yellow or brown, which begins in a highly viscous state and hardens with treatment. Typically, resin is soluble in alcohol, but not in water.

Resonance frequency analysis (RFA)   technique for clinical measurement of implant stability/mobility, registering by means of a transducer attached to the abutment or implant, which records the resonance frequency arising from the implant-bone interface (change in amplitude over induced frequency band).

Resorbable   ability of an autogenous graft to dissolve physiologically. See: BIOABSORBABLE.

Resorbable blast media (RBM)   surface treatment obtained by blasting the implant surface with a biocompatible material (e.g., tricalcium phosphate).

Resorpable membrane   a natural or synthetic absorbable membrane that goes over the bone grafting before dental implantation, which does not need to have a second surgery to remove it.

Resorption   loss of substance or bone by physiologic (natural) or pathologic means. See: BONE RESORPTION.

Restoration   See: PROSTHESIS.

Restorative platform   See: PLATFORM.

Retainer   any type of clasp, attachment, or device used for the fixation or stabilization of a prosthesis.

Retaining screw   See: PROSTHETIC SCREW.

Rethreading   repair of the damaged internal threads of a root-form implant using a tap instrument.

Retractor   all the instruments used to keep a patient's mouth open wide and steady during procedures.

Retrievability   a reference to the likelihood of removing a prosthesis undamaged.

Retromolar pad   mass of tissue (frequently pear-shaped) located at the distal termination of the mandibular residual ridge and composed of the retromolar papilla and the retromolar glandular prominence.

Retrospective study   study designed to observe events that have already occurred.

Retrusion   a posterior position.

Reverse articulation   full arch crossbite; class III malocclusion.

Reverse torque test (RTT)   an assessment of the extent of osseointegration, specifically the shear strength at the bone-implant interface; the test includes the application of rotational force in a direction opposite that used to place the implant.

Reverse torque value   See: REMOVAL TORQUE VALUE.

Revolutions per minute (rpm)   unit of rotational speed at which a bur or drill turns.

RFA   acronym: resonance frequency analysis.

rhBMP   acronym: recombinant human bone morphogenetic protein.

Ridge   remainder of the alveolar process after teeth extraction. See: ALVEOLAR PROCESS, RESIDUAL RIDGE.

Ridge, alveolar   alveolar process and its soft-tissue covering that remain after teeth are removed.

Ridge atrophy   decrease in volume of the ridge caused by bone resorption.

Ridge augmentation   increasing the dimension of the existing alveolar ridge morphology.

Ridge crest   highest continuous surface of the alveolar ridge.

Ridge defect   deficiency in the contour of the edentulous ridge, both vertical (apicocoronal) and/or horizontal (buccolingual, mesiodistal) direction.

Ridge expansion   surgical widening of the residual ridge with osteotomes and/or chisels in the lateral direction (buccolingually), in order to accommodate the insertion of an implant and/or bone graft.

Ridge lap   portion of a pontic that opposes the edentulous crest (sanitary ridge lap; bullet-shaped ridge lap).

Ridge mapping   creating a diagnostic cast by transposing information obtained after penetrating anesthetized soft tissue with a graduated probe or caliper at several sites; shape of the residual ridge is reproduced by trimming back the stone of the cast to the corresponding depth of soft tissue. See: RIDGE SOUNDING.

Ridge preservation   syn: extraction socket graft, socket graft, socket preservation; immediate placement of a grafting material or any procedure (e.g., guided bone regeneration) performed on the extraction socket following tooth extraction to conserve the bone and soft tissue contours by avoiding bone resorption with a resultant ridge defect.

Ridge resorption   the loss of bone in an edentulous area. See: RESIDUAL RIDGE.

Ridge sounding   syn: bone sounding, sounding; penetration of anesthetized soft tissue to determine the topography of the underlying bone. See: RIDGE MAPPING.

Ridge splitting   See: RIDGE EXPANSION.

Rigid fixation   absence of observed mobility.

Risk factor   condition shown to negatively affect the success of a treatment modality.

Residual ridge resorption   the resorption of alveolar bone after tooth removal.

Root form   similar in shape to a dental root.

Root form endosteal dental implant   endosseous implant, circular in cross-section, and root-shaped; it is supported from a vertical expanse of bone; implants can be in the form of spirals, cones, rhomboids, and cylinders. Additionally, such implants can be smooth, fluted, finned, threaded, perforated, solid, hollow, or vented. Finally, these implants can be coated or textured; they are generally available in submergible and non-submergible forms in a variety of biocompatible materials.

Root-form implant   See: ROOT FORM ENDOSTEAL DENTAL IMPLANT.

Root-form implants shear loading   forces delivered in the plane of the long axis of an implant.

Rotation   the action of turning on an axis.

Rough surface   See: TEXTURED SURFACE.

Round bur   circular bur for marking site for an osteotomy or to decorticate bone. It may also be used in the outline of a lateral window access for sinus grafting.

Rpm   acronym: revolutions per minute.

Rugae   ridges and folds running horizontally in the anterior palatal mucosa.

R-value   two-dimensional roughness parameter calculated from the experimental profiles after filtering. Ra: arithmetic average of the absolute value of all points of the profile, also called central line average height. Rt: maximum peak-to-valley height of the entire measurement trace.

S

Saddle   part of a complete or partial denture to which the teeth are attached and that rests on the ridge.

Sagittal plane   any vertical section parallel to the median plane of the body, dividing it into right and left parts.

Sandblasting   grit blasting of an implant surface with sand.

Saucerization   See: PERICERVICAL SAUCERIZATION.

Saucerization   pericervical implant bone loss adjacent to all implants.

Scaffold   framework or armature; three-dimensional biocompatible construct (may be seeded with cells) acting as a framework and providing a structure on which tissue grows. It may be replaced by natural tissue.

Scalloped implant   A root-form implant with the level of the implant-abutment junction more coronal interproximally than facially or lingually.

Scanning microscopy   an image recorded point-by-point by means of a beam of electrons and projected to a television monitor.

Scanographic template   radiographic template used for CT-scanning. See: RADIOGRAPHIC TEMPLATE.

Scar   fibrous tissue that replaces normal tissues after healing.

Schneiderian membrane   syn: sinus membrane (maxillary); layer of pseudostratified ciliated columnar epithelium cells lining the maxillary sinus. See: PERFORATION.

Screw endosteal dental implant   Threaded root-form implant, parallel-sided or tapered. See: ROOT-FORM IMPLANT, THREADED IMPLANT, ENDOSTEAL ROOT FORM IMPLANT.

Screw implant   See: ROOT-FORM IMPLANT.

Screw joint   junction of two parts held together by a screw (e.g., implant-abutment screw joint).

Screw loosening   prosthetic complication occurring when a screw loses its preload, causing the restoration or abutment to loosen.

Screw-retained   description of an abutment or a prosthesis whose retention is accomplished by a screw. See: CEMENT-RETAINED.

Screw tap   See: TAP.

SD   acronym: standard deviation.

Sealing screw   See: HYGIENE CAP.

Seating surface   See: PLATFORM.

Secondary closure   See: HEALING BY SECOND (SECONDARY) INTENTION.

Secondary Implant failure   See: LATE IMPLANT FAILURE.

Second-stage implant surgery   subperiosteal implant: reopening of the tissue and placement of the infrastructure that was constructed after the first-stage surgery; endosteal submerged implants: re-exposure of the portion of the implant that receives the attachment or abutment.

Second-stage permucosal abutment   See: HEALING ABUTMENT.

Second-stage surgery   See: STAGE-TWO SURGERY.

Self-tapping   feature of the apical aspect of a threaded implant or screw to create its thread path in the bone.

Semiadjustable articulator   adjustable device simulating jaw movements so that it conforms to actual mandibular functions.

Semiprecious metal alloy   mixture of base metal(s) with gold, platinum, or both.

Senile atrophy   a condition of tissue or organ losing morphology or function because of the age of the patient.

Septum   a compartment or wall between two cavities.

Septum (maxillary sinus)   syn: Underwood cleft; spine-like bony structure or web formation in some maxillary sinuses that may divide the inferior portion of the sinus into sections. See: ALVEOLAR RECESS.

Sequestration   to separate a portion of necrotic from the whole surrounding bone.

Serum CTX   a marker of bone resorption (serum C-terminal cross-linking telopeptide of type I collagen); serum CTX testing may be used to help determine the stage of biosphosphonate-induced osteonecrosis of the jaws.

Set screw   prosthetic or retention screw, lab-prepared in the prescribed location on the prosthesis (usually lingual); the set screw joins the crown to the abutment or the superstructure to the mesostructure and may also complement a cement-retained restoration.

Sharpey connective tissue fibers   periosteal connective tissue collagen becomes incorporated into the matrix that is being laid down by the surface osteoblasts and serves to anchor the periosteum to the cementum.

Shear stress   stress caused by a load that tends to slide one portion of object over another. The forces applied in such stress are toward one another but not in the same straight line. See: STRESS, ROOT-FORM IMPLANTS SHEAR LOADING.

Shoulder finish line   the casting endpoint on a tooth after its preparation.

Simultaneous placement   insertion of a root-form implant in conjunction with another surgical procedure performed at the same site (e.g., grafting).

Single crystal sapphire   material for implantation composed of a single crystalline alpha aluminum oxide identical in crystalline structure to a gem sapphire.

Single-stage implant   See: ONE-STAGE IMPLANT.

Single-stage surgery   single-stage (implant) surgery is to graft or insert into the body in one single step.

Sinter   to fuse together; in biomaterials, with hydraulic pressure.

Sintered   treated by sintering. See: SINTERING.

Sintered (porous) surface   implant surface produced when spherical powders of metallic or ceramic materials become a coherent mass with the metallic core of the implant body; porous surfaces are characterized by pore size, pore shape, pore volume, and pore depth, which are affected by the size of the spherical particles and the temperature and pressure conditions of the sintering chamber.

Sintering   heating a powder below the melting point of any component to permit agglomeration and welding of particles by diffusion alone, with or without applied pressure.

Sinus   air space within bone.

Sinus augmentation   the use of open or osteotome techniques for placement of bone grafting materials in the antral floor. See: SINUS GRAFT.

Sinus elevation   See: SINUS GRAFT.

Sinus floor elevation   antroplasty; sinus floor augmentation; bone grafting via a modified Caldwell-Luc approach to improve the posterior maxilla for placement of an endosteal implant; often preferable to subantral augmentation.

Sinus graft   syn: maxillary antroplasty, Sinus augmentation, sinus elevation, sinus lift, subantral augmentation; augmentation of the antral floor with autogenous bone and/or bone to improve conditions for placement of a dental implant.

Sinus perforation   when a direct connection between the sinus and mouth is created by a perforation of the maxillary sinus membrane following a tooth extraction or a sinus grafting procedure.

Sinusitis (maxillary)   inflammation of the sinus; signs include sensitivity of teeth to percussion, fever, and facial swelling. Symptoms: nasal congestion, postnasal discharge, facial pain/headache, rhinorrhea, halitosis, popping of ears, and muffled hearing.

Sinus lift   See: SINUS GRAFT.

Sinus membrane (maxillary)   See: SCHNEIDERIAN MEMBRANE.

Sinus pneumatization (maxillary)   maxillary sinus enlargement; gradual thinning of the sinus walls as a result of the increase in size of the maxillary sinus, usually the result of aging and loss of maxillary teeth (and masticatory forces).

Site development   augmenting the quantity and quality of soft and/or hard tissues before implant placement.

Sleeper implant   an implant that is nonfunctioning, nonprotruding through the mucoperiosteum into the oral cavity that serves in to fix a fracture or to conserve a bone.

Sluiceway   a slot or passage permitting the passage of fluids.

Smile line   the imaginary gingival line that follows the contour of the lower lip when the patient is smiling.

Socket   an alveolus; depression such as those placed in special wrenches.

Socket graft   See: RIDGE PRESERVATION.

Socket preservation   See: RIDGE.

Soft tissue cast   cast with the implant laboratory analog platform surrounded by an elastic mucosal simulating material.

Solid   dense mass.

Solid screw   root-form threaded implant of circular cross-section with no vents or holes penetrating the body.

Sounding   See: RIDGE SOUNDING.

Spark erosion   See: ELECTRIC DISCHARGE METHOD.

Specialized mucosa   See: ORAL MUCOSA.

Sphincter   round band of muscle designed to permit the closing of a passageway.

Spirochete   a microscopic bacterial organism of the order Spirochaetales, many of which are pathogenic, causing syphilis, relapsing fever, yaws, and periodontitis.

Splint (noun)   device designed to hold or stabilize weakened or injured hard tissues; a series of connected crowns.

Splint (verb)   to apply a supporting device to aid weakened or injured hard tissues.

Splinting   joining of two or more abutments into a unit; joining two or more teeth or implants into a rigid or nonrigid unit via fixed or removable restorations or devices.

Split crest technique   See: RIDGE EXPANSION.

Split ridge technique   See: RIDGE EXPANSION.

Split thickness graft   slice of epithelium taken for transplantation.

Spongy bone   See: BONE.

Staged protocol   treatment sequence involving the completion of one procedure followed by another at a later date.

Stage-one surgery   syn: first-stage dental implant surgery; surgical procedure consisting of placing an endosseous implant in the bone and suturing the soft tissue over the implant to submerge the implant for healing.

Stage-two surgery   syn: second-stage surgery; surgical procedure consisting of exposing a submerged implant to the oral environment by connecting an abutment extruding through the soft tissue.

Standard abutment   machined titanium, cylindrical abutment to support a screw-retained prosthesis. See: HYBRID PROSTHESIS.

Standard deviation (SD)   statistical term indicating the variability or dispersion of a distribution of scores; the more scores clustering around the mean, the smaller the standard deviation.

Staple implant   implant inserted via a submental skin incision through the inferior border of the mandible and exiting through the alveolar ridge as one or multiple abutments. The implant's retention is established by a screw-fastened foot plate. See: MANDIBULAR STAPLE IMPLANT.

Static   body at rest.

Stem cell   undifferentiated cell of embryogenic or adult origin that can undergo unlimited division and give rise to one or several different cell types.

Stem cells   cells potentially developing into a significant series ending with red blood cells.

Stent   a prosthetic device used to influence and guide the healing of soft tissues; surgical device used to keep a graft in place or protect a surgical site during initial healing; incorrect term for guide, splint, or template. syn: radiographic template, surgical guide.

Stepping implant   endosseous, root-form implant with parallel walls of different diameter joined to form a step.

Stereolithographic guide   guide generated from a CAM according to a software-planned implant placement.

Stereolithography   syn: three-dimensional imaging, three-dimensional modeling; method for creating a three-dimensional model using lasers driven by CAD software from CT-scan information. The model is used for surgical planning and the generation of a guide.

Sterile technique   surgical procedure performed under sterile conditions, under operating room conditions, and following operating room protocol for setup, instrument transfer and handling, and personnel movement. Clinicians wear surgical scrubs, head covers, shoe covers, and sterile gowns; a standard technique in which an aseptic area is established and maintained to a specific conclusion (e.g., the proper sterilization of instruments, drapes, gowns, gloves, and surgical area); the systematic maintenance of asepsis throughout an implant insertion procedure. See: CLEAN TECHNIQUE.

Sterilization   complete elimination of microbial life; caution must be used during sterilization to preserve the integrity and properties of the implant.

Stomatognathic   relating to the jaws and mouth.

Straight abutment   See: NONANGULATED ABUTMENT.

Straight/angled abutments   See: ABUTMENT.

Straight implant   See: PARALLEL-SIDED IMPLANT.

Strain   an object's dimensional change after being subjected to stress; change in an object's length after application of stress.

Stress   mechanical tensile force: the form divided by perpendicular cross-sectional area over which force is applied; force or load applied to an object. Types of stress include bending, compressive, shear, tensile, and torsion. See: BENDING STRESS, COMPRESSIVE STRESS, SHEAR STRESS, TENSILE STRESS, TORSION STRESS.

Stress breaker   device designed to ameliorate abutment stresses via soft, compliant materials, springs, or hinges.

Stress broken   a description of the after effects of having used devices to relieve the abutment teeth of all or part of the occlusal forces.

Stress concentration   the point at which stress is substantially higher because of the geometry of the stressed object or the point of force application.

Stripped threads   a description of jammed threads of a screw or the internal threads of a root-form implant that have been bent, broken, or otherwise damaged.

Stripping   a reference to damage (i.e., distortion or obliteration) done to the internal threads of an implant or abutment.

Subantral augmentation   See: SINUS GRAFT.

Subcrestal implant placement   See: CRESTAL IMPLANT PLACEMENT.

Sublingual artery   an artery with origin in the anterior margin of the hyglossus that runs from the forward between the genioglossus and mylohyoideus to the sublingual gland.

Submerged implant   implant covered by soft tissue and (so) isolated from the oral cavity.

Submergible   able to be buried.

Submergible implant   See: TWO-STAGE IMPLANT.

Submersible endosteal implant   See: ENDOSTEAL (ENDOSSEOUS) IMPLANT.

Submersible implant   buried or partially buried implant.

Submucosal inserts   See: INTRAMUCOSAL INSERT.

Submucous cleft palate   bony cleft not readily detected by clinical examination.

Subnasal elevation   a surgical technique to enhance anterior bone height in the anterior maxilla.

Subperiosteal dental implant   framework specifically constructed (complete-arch, unilateral, or universal) to fit supporting areas of the mandible or maxillae with permucosal extensions for a prosthesis; the framework consists of permucosal extensions with or without connecting bars and struts (peripheral, primary, and secondary).

Subperiosteal dental implant abutment   See: ABUTMENT.

Subperiosteal dental implant substructure   See INFRASTRUCTURE.

Subperiosteal dental implant superstructure   See: OVERDENTURE.

Subperiosteal implant   implant consisting of a customized casting, made of a surgical grade metal, which rests on the surface of bone and under the periosteum. Prosthetic retention is accomplished by permucosal abutments, posts, and intraoral bars. 1. Complete: for a completely edentulous arch. 2. Unilateral: located on one side of the posterior mandible or maxilla. 3. Circumferential: bypasses remaining teeth or implants.

Subtracted surface   syn: subtractive surface treatment; alteration of an implant surface by material removal. See: ADDED SURFACE, TEXTURED SURFACE.

Subtraction radiography   technique for detecting radiographic density change at two points in time to determine bone formation or loss.

Subtractive surface treatment   See: SUBTRACTED SURFACE.

Success criteria   conditions established by a study protocol for evaluating a procedure's effectiveness.

Success rate   percentage of success of a procedure or device (e.g., implant) in a study or clinical trial based on success criteria as defined by the study protocol. See: SURVIVAL RATE.

Sulcular epithelium   syn: crevicular epithelium; nonkeratinized epithelium of the mucosal sulcus surrounding implants and teeth.

Superstructure   prosthesis that attaches to an implant's abutments or an intermediary casting, called a mesostructure; prosthesis supported by implants with or without a mesostructure.

Suppuration   pus formation.

Supracrestal implant placement   See: CRESTAL IMPLANT PLACEMENT.

Surface alteration   modification of an implant surface by treatment. See: ADDED SURFACE, SUBTRACTED SURFACE.

Surface characteristics (implant)   implant topography, defined by form (the largest structure or profile), waviness, and roughness (the smallest irregularities in the surface). Waviness and roughness are often referred to collectively as texture. Implant surfaces are usually designated as machined or textured. See: MACHINED SURFACE, TEXTURED SURFACE.

Surface roughness   Qualitative and quantitative features of an implant surface determined two-dimensionally by contact stylus profilometry (See: R VALUE) or three-dimensionally by confocal laser scanner (See: S VALUE). See: SURFACE.

Surgical bed   site prepared to receive a graft.

Surgical guide   guide derived from the diagnostic wax-up to assist in the preparation for placement and the placement of implants; the surgical guide determines drilling position and angulation; template fabricated to reveal implant osteotomies to the surgeon.

Surgical indexing   record for registering the position of an implant at stage-one or stage-two surgery.

Surgical jaw relationship, subperiosteal   registration of the vertical dimension in centric relationship of the exposed superior surface of the mandibular or maxillary bone with the opposing arch, providing intermaxillary registration for determination of abutment height of a subperiosteal implant framework.

Surgical navigation   real time computer technology used to aid in the intraoperative navigation of surgical instruments and operation site, allowing for precise operation site localization before and during surgery.

Surgical occlusal rim, subperiosteal   conventional occlusion rim with a base adapted for accurate recording of the surgical vertical-centric relations.

Surgical template   See: SURGICAL GUIDE.

Survival rate   percentage of implant success in a study or clinical trial; success is most often defined as an implant functioning according to predetermined criteria. See: SUCCESS RATE.

Suture   verb: to join together by sewing.

Suturing   wound closure with thread.

S value   three-dimensional roughness parameter calculated from topographical images. Sa: arithmetic average of the absolute value of all points of the profile, a height-descriptive parameter. Scx: space-descriptive parameter. Sdr: developed surface area ratio.

Swage   to press or hammer malleable material to adapt it to an underlying model or form.

Symphysis   immovable dense midline articulation of the right and left halves of the adult mandible.

Syngeneic graft   See: ISOGRAFT.

System (implant)   1. product line of implants (often representing a specific concept, inventor, or patent) with specific surgical protocol and matching prosthetic components. See: CONFIGURATION. 2. ISO definition: "Dental implant components that are designed to mate together. It consists of the necessary parts and instruments to complete the implant body placement and abutment components" (ISO 10451).

T

Tack   syn: fixation tack. Metal or bioabsorbable pin with a flat head to secure the barrier membrane position during guided bone regeneration.

Tap   syn: threader, threadformer. 1. Bone tap: device to create a threaded channel in bone for a fixation screw or before the insertion of an implant. 2. Metal tap: instrument (harder than titanium) used for rethreading the damaged internal threads of an implant.

Tapered implant   endosseous, root-form implant (threaded or nonthreaded) with a wider diameter coronally than apically; the sides converge apically.

Tapping   creating a threaded channel in bone with a bone tap for placing a fixation screw or before the insertion of an implant (also known as pretapping).

TCP   acronym: tricalcium phosphate.

Team approach   The use of a multidisciplinary approach that combines the collaboration of various healthcare providers in the postoperative management of a patient with dental implants.

Teeth in an hour   Nobel Biocare trademark that reflects the general advancements in technology (e.g., CT scans, CAD/CAM software) and procedure (e.g., timely prosthesis fabrication, computer-guided surgery via templates) for using dental implants to provide edentulous patients (upper, lower, or complete) with functionally esthetic tooth function in minimal time. The technique employs pre-made (temporary or final) prosthetics ready for use at the time of surgery, eliminating multiple surgeries and visits.

Telescopic coping   thin metal covering or cap fitted over the prepared tooth or implant abutment to accept a secondary or overlay crown or prosthesis.

Telescopic denture   denture fitting over retentive extensions (tooth or implant borne). See: OVERDENTURE.

Template   guide. See: RADIOGRAPHIC TEMPLATE, STEREOLITHOGRAPHIC GUIDE, SURGICAL GUIDE.

Temporary abutment   syn: temporary cylinder; abutment for the fabrication of an interim restoration, which may be cemented on the temporary abutment. The temporary abutment may be incorporated in the interim restoration as screw-retained.

Temporary cylinder   See: TEMPORARY ABUTMENT.

Temporary healing cuff   See: HEALING ABUTMENT.

Temporary prosthesis/restoration   See: INTERIM PROSTHESIS/RESTORATION.

Tensile stress   stress caused by a load (two forces applied away from one another in the same straight line) tending to stretch or elongate an object; pulling force. See: STRESS.

Tension   pulling or drawing away.

Tension-free wound closure   closure for a postoperative wound that can be performed without flap tension.

Tenting screw   metal screw used to support a barrier membrane to maintain a space under the membrane for guiding bone regeneration.

Tent pole procedure   a surgical procedure whereby the periosteum and soft tissue matrix are elevated through the use of dental implants, creating a tenting effect, which prevent graft resorption. This procedure also offers predictable long-term reconstruction of the severely resorbed mandible without complications.

Tetracycline   antibiotic used to treat bacterial infections, typically used to treat rhinogenic infections.

Textured surface   machined implant surface that has been altered or modified by addition or reduction. See: ADDED SURFACE, MACHINED SURFACE, SUBTRACTED SURFACE, SURFACE CHARACTERISTICS (IMPLANT).

Texturing   process by which the surface area of an implant is increased. See: TEXTURED SURFACE.

TGF-b   abbreviation for the transforming growth factor beta, one of two classes of transforming growth factors that are found in hematopoietic tissue and stimulate bone healing and regeneration.

Thick flat periodontium   Also known as the periodontal biotype; the thick, flat, short, and wide tooth and its supporting structure, including the cementum, the periodontal membrane, the bone of the alveolar process, and the gums.

Thermal expansion   enlargement of a material by heat.

Thermoplastic   heat labile.

Thin scalloped periodontium   a thin, filed-down ends of a tooth, the supporting structures of the teeth including the cementum, the periodontal membrane, the bone of the alveolar process, and the gums.

Thread   extruding feature of the body of certain implants. Geometric characteristics include thread depth, thickness, pitch, face angle, and helix angle. Basic thread geometries include V-thread, buttress thread, and power (square) thread.

Threaded implant endosseous, root-form implant with threads similar to a screw, also known as a screw-shaped implant; sides may be parallel-sided or tapered.

Threader See: TAP.

Threadformer See: TAP.

Thread pitch number of threads per unit length in the same axial plane.

Three-dimensional imaging See: STEREOLITHOGRAPHY.

Three-dimensional implant endosseous implant inserted laterally, from the facial aspect of the edentulous ridge.

Three-dimensional modeling See: STEREOLITHOGRAPHY.

Ti acronym: titanium.

Ti-6A1-4V See: TITANIUM ALLOY.

Tibial bone harvest harvesting of bone from the lateral proximal tibia as a source of autogenous cancellous bone for grafting.

Tinnitus ringing or roaring in the ears.

Tissue bank laboratory specializing in harvesting, processing, and sterilization of tissues from humans or animals.

Tissue-borne See: TISSUE-SUPPORTED.

Tissue conditioner widely used, concentrated polymer solutions based on poly (ethyl methacrylate) (PEMA) in prosthetic dentistry.

Tissue engineering application of the principles of life sciences and engineering to develop biological substitutes for the restoration or replacement of tissue.

Tissue integration intimate implant-to-tissue contact.

Tissue punch technique a surgical technique done with a cutter or laser, to gain access to the underlying bone or implant without raising a full thickness flap or disrupting the integrity of the interdental papilla. There is also no discontinuation of the alveolar blood supply of the surrounding osseous tissue.

Tissue-supported syn: tissue-borne; supported by soft tissue of the edentulous alveolar ridge.

Titanium (Ti) elementary substance, isolated as an iron-gray powder with a metalliccluster. See: COMMERCIALLY PURE TITANIUM, TITANIUM ALLOY.

Titanium alloy biocompatible medical alloy containing approximately 90% titanium, 6% aluminum, and 4% vanadium (e.g., Ti-6Al-4V) and used for the fabrication of dental implants and components; physical properties are superior to most commercially pure titanium. See: TITANIUM, COMMERCIALLY PURE TITANIUM.

Titanium mesh flexible titanium grid used during bone augmentation to maintain a predetermined volume for bone regeneration during healing.

Titanium mesh crib Titanium mesh used for autogenous bone grafting to stimulate bone resorption, promote wound healing, and restoration of normal physiologic function of the maxillary sinus.

Titanium oxide 1. Surface layer of varying surface composition (e.g., Ti02, Ti04) immediately formed when pure metallic titanium and titanium alloy are exposed to air; a corrosion-resistant layer protects the implant against chemical attack in biological fluids. 2. Metal oxide blasted on implant surfaces to increase the surface area.

Titanium plasma sprayed (TPS) description of an implant surface altered by high temperature deposition of titanium powders, totally or partially melted and then rapidly resolidified, forming a dense or porous coating. See: PLASMA SPRAYED.

Titanium reinforced description of a nonabsorbable membrane containing a thin titanium ribbon to increase stiffness and maintain shape during healing.

Tomograph detailed image produced from multiple x-ray measurements of a particular body plane.

Torque 1. Force creating rotation or torsion. 2. Measurement capacity to do work or to continue to rotate under resistance to rotation expressed in Newton's centimeter (Ncm).

Torque controller See: TORQUE DRIVER.

Torque driver syn: torque controller, torque indicator, torque wrench; manual or electronic device used to apply torque.

Torque indicator See: TORQUE DRIVER.

Torque wrench See: TORQUE DRIVER.

Torsion stress stress caused by a load that tends to twist an object. See: STRESS.

Torus exophytic bony prominence at the midline of the hard palate (palatal) or on the lingual aspect of the mandible in the canine premolar area (mandibular). The torus can be used as a source of autogenous bone for grafting.

Toxicity adverse reaction of tissues to a drug, chemical, material, or environment.

TPS acronym: titanium plasma sprayed.

Trabecular bone also known as cancellous bone, in which the spicules form a latticework, with interstices filled with embryonic connective tissue or bone marrow. See: BONE.

Transepithelial through or across the epithelium. See: PERMUCOSAL.

Transfer coping device placed on a tooth or implant that permits the technician to reproduce the oral conditions on a cast after the coping is lifted out in an impression. See: IMPRESSION COPING.

Transforming growth factor (TGF) Any of a group of proteins produced by cells, one of the three growth factors, released by platelets that stimulate the growth of normal cells.

Transforming growth factor beta (TGF-B) growth factor produced by platelets and bone cells that increase the chemotaxis and mitogenesis of osteoblast precursors and also stimulate osteoblast deposition of the collagen matrix for wound healing and bone regeneration.

Transitional implant syn: provisional implant; implant used during implant therapy to support a transitional fixed or removable denture; such an implant is usually an immediately loaded narrow diameter implant and removed at a later stage of treatment.

Transitional prosthesis   See: INTERIM PROSTHESIS.

Transitional prosthesis/restoration   prosthesis replacing a missing tooth or teeth over treatment.

Transmandibular implant   See: MANDIBULAR STAPLE IMPLANT.

Transmission microscopy   See: LIGHT MICROSCOPY.

Transmucosal   passing through or across the oral mucosa.

Transmucosal abutment   a device connecting an implant to the oral cavity through the soft tissue.

Transmucosal healing cap   device designed to prevent loosening of the healing cap when attached by screw to an implant fixture placed in phase one of a two-stage implant surgery. A retaining screw, separate from the cap body, and locking washer help to prevent damage to the cap body and other parts of the implant.

Transmucosal loading   pressure exerted through the soft tissue on a submerged implant (often by a removable denture).

Transosseous implant   syn: transosteal implant. 1. Implant completely penetrating the edentulous ridge buccolingually. 2. Implant completely penetrating the parasymphyseal region of the mandible, from the inferior border through the alveolar crest. See: MANDIBULAR STAPLE IMPLANT.

Transosteal   penetration of both the internal and external cortical plate by a dental implant.

Transosteal dental implant   See: STAPLE IMPLANT.

Transosteal implant   See: TRANSOSSEOUS IMPLANT.

Transport segment   sectioned segment of bone moving coronally in distraction osteogenesis.

Trauma   a physical or emotional wound.

Trephine   a circular opening created during surgery.

Trephine drill   hollow drill to remove a disk or cylinder of bone or other tissue.

Trial fit gauge   syn: implant try-in; replica of an implant body used to test the size of the osteotomy.

Trial placement   temporary or experimental placement of a prosthesis.

Tricalcium phosphate (TCP)   inorganic particulate or solid form of relatively biodegradable ceramic used as a scaffold for bone regeneration and a matrix for new bone growth.

Tripodization   placement of three or more implants with a nonlinear alignment.

Trismus   motor disturbance of the trigeminal nerve, especially a spasm of the masticatory muscles, limiting the opening of the mouth.

T-test   commonly used statistical method to evaluate the differences in means between two groups.

Tuberosity (maxillary)   most distal aspect of the maxillary ridge, bilaterally, often used as a source of autogenous bone.

Tunnel (verb)   to make a passage through and under the soft tissue.

Tunnel dissection   to separate the overlying tissues to reach a surgical goal without performing an open procedure.

Turned surface   See: MACHINED SURFACE.

Turnover   amount of older bone replaced by new bone often expressed as percent per year.

Twist drill   drill used to widen or create a preliminary osteotomy.

Two-part implant   implant combining the endosseous and transmucosal portions to present a joint surface to the tissues (i.e., implant-abutment junction). See: ONE-PART IMPLANT.

Two-piece abutment   abutment connecting to the implant by an abutment screw. See: ONE-PIECE ABUTMENT.

Two-stage grafting procedures   when the bone defect is too large for single-stage, simultaneous placement of the implant, a second surgery is required to place the implant.

Two-stage implant   syn: submergible implant; endosseous implant designed for a two-stage surgery protocol, undergoing osseointegration while covered with soft tissue. See: ONE-STAGE IMPLANT.

Two-stage surgery   protocol consisting of placing an endosseous root-form implant in the bone and leaving it covered with a flap; second surgery exposes the implant to install the prosthesis. See: ONE-STAGE SURGERY, STAGE-ONE SURGERY, STAGE-TWO SURGERY.

U

UCLA abutment   UCLA: University of California at Los Angeles. See: CASTABLE ABUTMENT; custom-made abutment designed for single implants that lack antirotational elements.

Uncover   popular term for the act of surgically exposing a submerged implant following healing from stage-one surgery. See: STAGE-TWO SURGERY.

Undercut   portion of an object that is less than and beneath its widest diameter.

Underwood cleft   See: SEPTUM (MAXILLARY SINUS).

Unilateral   pertaining to one side.

Unilateral subperiosteal implant   partial subperiosteal implant usually located in the posterior area of the mandible or maxillae. See: SUBPERIOSTEAL IMPLANT.

Universal implant   complete subperiosteal implant designed to function with remaining teeth.

V

Van der Waals bond   a bond with weak, inter-atomic attractions.

Vascular endothelial growth factors (VEGF)   factors with potent angiogenic, mitogenic, and vascular permeability, enhancing activities specific for endothelial cells.

Vascularization   infiltration of blood vessels, a critical support for the health and maintenance of living tissue or the healing of a graft.

Velum   curtain or drape; the soft palate.

Vent   opening in the implant body allowing tissue ingrowth for increased retention, stability, and antirotation.

Vented   fenestrated.

Verification cast   cast made from a verification jig. See: VERIFICATION JIG.

Verification index   the accurate positioning of the fixtures or abutment replicas on a working master cast before definitive fabrication of an implant-supported prosthesis.

Verification jig   index of multiple implants fabricated on the master cast and checked in the mouth for accuracy for possible cutting and reconnecting; new cast or an alteration of the master cast is made from the reconnected jig (verification cast). A verification jig can be fabricated in the mouth, from which a cast is poured.

Vertical bone height   the height from the inferior border of the edentulous mandible to the top of the crest of the alveolar ridge.

Vertical dimension   the superinferior dimension of facial height, often altered by depressing or elevating the occlusal plane.

Vertical dimension of occlusion   the vertical dimension of the face when the teeth or occlusion rims are in contact in centric occlusion.

Vestibular incision   See: MUCOBUCCAL FOLD INCISION.

Vestibule   the area or fold found between the lips and the alveolar ridges.

Vestibuloplasty   surgical modification of the gingival mucous membrane relationships in the vestibule of the mouth (may include deepening of the vestibular trough).

Vitreous carbon   biomaterial with a glassy amorphous structure (formerly used for fabrication of endosseous implants or as an implant coating).

Volkmann canal   a channel that runs transversely that transmits blood vessels and nutrients from the periosteum into the bone.

W

Waxing sleeve   castable plastic pattern used to form the framework of a restoration; polymeric, open-ended coping designed for direct wax-ups.

White blood cell   also known as leukocyte; a colorless blood cell that has a nucleus and cytoplasm and forms the foundation of the body's immune system.

Wolff's Law   bone will develop the structure most suited to resist forces acting on it; change in static relationships of a bone leads both to a change in its internal structure and architecture and in its external form and function.

Working occlusion   the occluding contacts of teeth on the side toward which the mandible is moved.

Wound closure   suturing and securing flaps after surgery.

Wound dehiscence   a splitting open of surgical suture lines or poor wound healing due to poor blood supply.

Wound healing   the body's natural process of regenerating dermal and epidermal tissue through a series of steps: inflammatory, proliferative, and maturation.

Woven bone   See: BONE.

Wrench   See: CYLINDER WRENCH, OPEN-ENDED WRENCH, TORQUE DRIVER.

Wrought   worked into shape by swaging, hammering, or pressuring.

X

Xenograft   syn: heterogeneous graft; harvested from a species different from that of the recipient. See: HETEROGRAFT.

Xerostomia   dry mouth.

Y

Yield strength   strength through which a small amount of permanent strain occurs, usually measured in pounds per square inch (psi).

Young's modulus   See: MODULUS OF ELASTICITY.

Z

Zirconia   the oxide of zirconium, a biocompatible ceramic.

Zirconium oxide   zirconium dioxide, ZrO_2, a white, infusible powder used in dental restoration when esthetics are a problem.

Zirconium implants   white ceramic (non-metal) implants for which long-term studies are not available: possible benefits include good esthetics in the anterior region, soft-tissue compatibility, and single-stage structure (lack of microgap); detriments may include inferior osseointegration when compared to titanium and susceptibility to damage.

Zone   anatomic area or segment.

Zygoma   area formed by the union of the zygomatic bone and the zygomatic process of the temporal and maxillary bones, used for support of the subperiosteal implant.

Zygomatic implant   root-form implant originating in the region of the former first maxillary molar and ending in the zygomatic bone, directed laterally and upwardly with an angulation of approximately 45 degrees from a vertical axis, following an intrasinusal trajectory.

appendix *A*

Useful Dental Codes for Dental Implant Surgery and Related Procedures

4265 biologic materials to aid in soft and osseous tissue regeneration

Biologic materials may be used alone or with other regenerative substrates such as bone and barrier membranes, depending upon their formulation and the presentation of the periodontal defect. This procedure does not include surgical entry and closure, wound debridement, osseous contouring, or the placement of graft materials and/or barrier membranes, including, but not limited to, D4240, D4241, D4260, D4261, D4263, D4264, D4266, and D4267.

4266 guided tissue regeneration— resorbable barrier, per site

A membrane is placed over the root surfaces or defect area following surgical exposure and debridement. The mucoperiosteal flaps are then adapted over the membrane and sutured. The membrane is placed to exclude epithelium and gingival connective tissue from the healing wound. This procedure may require subsequent surgical procedures to correct the gingival contours. Guided tissue regeneration may also be carried out in conjunction with bone replacement grafts or to correct deformities resulting from inadequate faciolingual bone width in an edentulous area.

When guided tissue regeneration is used in association with a tooth, each site on a specific tooth should be reported separately with this code. When no tooth is present, each site should be reported separately.

4273 subepithelial connective tissue graft procedures, per tooth

This procedure is performed to create or augment gingiva, to obtain root coverage to eliminate sensitivity and to prevent root caries, to eliminate frenum pull, to extend the vestibular fornix, to augment collapsed ridges, to provide an adequate gingival interface with a restoration, or to cover bone or ridge regeneration sites when adequate gingival tissues are not available for effective closure. There are two surgical sites. The recipient site utilizes a split thickness incision, retaining the overlying flap of gingiva and/or mucosa. The connective tissue is dissected from the donor site, leaving an epithelialized flap for closure. After the graft is placed on the recipient site, it is covered with the retained overlying flap.

6010 surgical placement of implant body: endosteal implant

Includes second-stage surgery and placement of healing cap.

6040 surgical placement: eposteal implant

An eposteal (subperiosteal) framework of a biocompatible material designed and fabricated to fit on the surface of the bone of the mandible or maxilla with permucosal extensions, which provide support and attachment of a prosthesis. This may be a complete arch or unilateral appliance. Eposteal implants rest upon the bone and under the periosteum.

6050 surgical placement: transosteal implant

A transosteal (transosseous) biocompatible device with threaded posts penetrating both the superior and inferior cortical bone plates of the mandibular symphysis and exiting through the permucosa, providing support and attachment for a dental prosthesis. Transosteal implants are placed completely through the bone and into the oral cavity from extraoral or intraoral.

6080 implant maintenance procedures, including removal of prosthesis, cleansing of prosthesis and abutments, and reinsertion of prosthesis

This procedure includes a prophylaxis to provide active debriding of the implant and examination of all aspects of the implant system, including the occlusion and stability of the superstructure. The patient is also instructed in thorough daily cleansing of the implant.

6090 repair implant supported prosthesis, by report

This procedure involves the repair or replacement of any part of the implant-supported prosthesis.

6095 repair implant abutment, by report

This procedure involves the repair or replacement of any part of the implant abutment.

6100 implant removal, by report

This procedure involves the surgical removal of an implant. Describe procedure.

6190 radiographic/surgical implant index, by report

An appliance, designed to relate osteotomy or fixture position to existing anatomic structures, to be utilized during radiographic exposure for treatment planning and/or during osteotomy creation for fixture installation.

6199 unspecified implant procedure, by report

Use for procedure that is not adequately described by a code. Describe procedure.

7941 osteotomy—mandibular rami

7943 osteotomy—mandibular rami with bone graft; includes obtaining the graft

7944 osteotomy—segmented or subapical—per sextant or quadrant

7945 osteotomy—body of mandible

Surgical section of lower jaw. This includes the surgical exposure, bone cut, fixation, routine wound closure, and normal postoperative follow-up care.

7250 surgical removal of residual tooth roots (cutting procedure)

Includes cutting of soft tissue and bone, removal of tooth structure, and closure.

7950 osseous, osteoperiosteal, or cartilage graft of the mandible or facial bones—autogenous or nonautogenous, by report

This code may be used for sinus lift procedure and/or ridge augmentation. It includes obtaining autograft and/or allograft material. Placement of a barrier membrane, if used, should be reported separately.

7953 bone replacement graft for ridge preservation—per site

Osseous autograft, allograft, or non-osseous graft is placed in an extraction site to preserve ridge integrity (e.g., clinically indicated in preparation for implant reconstruction or where alveolar contour is critical to planned prosthetic reconstruction). Membrane, if used, should be reported separately.

7995 synthetic graft—mandible or facial bones, by report

Includes allogenic graft material.

7996 implant-mandible for augmentation purposes (excluding alveolar ridge), by report

7999 unspecified oral surgery procedure, by report

Used for procedure that is not adequately described by a code. Describe procedure.

9230 analgesia, anxiolysis, inhalation of nitrous oxide

9241 intravenous conscious sedation/analgesia—first 30 minutes

Anesthesia time begins when the doctor administering the anesthetic agent initiates the appropriate anesthesia and non-invasive monitoring protocol and remains in continuous attendance of the patient. Anesthesia services are considered completed when the patient may be safely left under the observation of trained personnel, and the doctor may safely leave the room to attend to other patients or duties.

9242 intravenous conscious sedation/analgesia—each additional 15 minutes

Anesthesia time begins when the doctor administering the anesthetic agent initiates the appropriate anesthesia and non-invasive monitoring protocol and remains in continuous attendance of the patient. Anesthesia services are considered completed when the patient may be safely left under the observation of trained personnel and the doctor may safely leave the room to attend to other patients or duties.

9248 non-intravenous conscious sedation

A medically controlled state of depressed consciousness while maintaining the patient's airway, protective reflexes, and the ability to respond to stimulation or verbal commands. It includes non-intravenous administration of sedative and/or analgesic agent(s) and appropriate monitoring.

Useful Codes for Dental Implant Prosthetics and Related Procedures

6053 implant/abutment-supported removable denture for completely edentulous arch

6054 implant/abutment-supported removable denture for partially edentulous arch

6055 dental implant supported connecting bar

A device attached to transmucosal abutments to stabilize and anchor a removable overdenture prosthesis.

6056 prefabricated abutment—includes placement

A connection to an implant that is a manufactured component usually made of machined high noble metal, titanium, titanium alloy, or ceramic. Modification of a prefabricated abutment may be necessary and is accomplished by altering its shape using dental burrs/diamonds.

6057 custom abutment—includes placement

A connection to an implant that is a fabricated component, usually by a laboratory, specific for an individual application. A custom abutment is typically fabricated using a casting process and usually is made of noble or high noble metal. A "UCLA abutment" is an example of this type of abutment.

6058 abutment-supported porcelain/ceramic crown

A single crown restoration that is retained, supported, and stabilized by an abutment on an implant; may be screw retained or cemented.

6059 abutment-supported porcelain fused to metal crown (high noble metal)

A single metal-ceramic crown restoration that is retained, supported, and stabilized by an abutment on an implant; may be screw retained or cemented.

6060 abutment-supported porcelain fused to metal crown (predominantly base metal)

A single metal-ceramic crown restoration that is retained, supported, and stabilized by an abutment on an implant; may be screw retained or cemented.

6061 abutment-supported porcelain fused to metal crown (noble metal)

A single metal-ceramic crown restoration that is retained, supported, and stabilized by an abutment on an implant; may be screw retained or cemented.

6062 abutment-supported cast metal crown (high noble metal)

A single cast metal crown restoration that is retained, supported, and stabilized by an abutment on an implant; may be screw retained or cemented.

6063 abutment-supported cast metal crown (predominantly base metal)

A single cast metal crown restoration that is retained, supported, and stabilized by an abutment on an implant; may be screw retained or cemented.

6064 abutment-supported cast metal crown (noble metal)

A single cast metal crown restoration that is retained, supported, and stabilized by an abutment on an implant; may be screw retained or cemented.

6094 abutment-supported crown— (titanium)

A single crown restoration that is retained, supported, and stabilized by an abutment on an implant; may be cast or milled and is screw retained or cemented.

6065 implant-supported porcelain/ceramic crown

A single crown restoration that is retained, supported, and stabilized by an implant; may be screw retained or cemented.

6066 implant-supported porcelain fused to metal crown (titanium, titanium alloy, high noble metal)

A single metal-ceramic crown restoration that is retained, supported, and stabilized by an implant; may be screw retained or cemented.

6067 implant-supported metal crown (titanium, titanium alloy, high noble metal)

A single cast metal crown restoration that is retained, supported, and stabilized by an abutment on an implant; may be screw retained or cemented.

6068 abutment-supported retainer for porcelain/ceramic FPD

A ceramic retainer for a fixed partial denture that is retained, supported, and stabilized by an abutment on an implant; may be screw retained or cemented.

6069 abutment-supported retainer for porcelain fused to metal FPD (high noble metal)

A metal-ceramic retainer for a fixed partial denture that is retained, supported, and stabilized by an abutment on an implant; may be screw retained or cemented.

6070 abutment-supported retainer for porcelain fused to metal FPD (predominantly base metal)

A metal-ceramic retainer for a fixed partial denture that is retained, supported, and stabilized by an abutment on an implant; may be screw retained or cemented.

6071 abutment-supported retainer for porcelain fused to metal FPD (noble metal)

A metal-ceramic retainer for a fixed partial denture that is retained, supported, and stabilized by an abutment on an implant; may be screw retained or cemented.

6072 abutment-supported retainer for cast metal FPD (high noble metal)

A cast metal retainer for a fixed partial denture that is retained, supported, and stabilized by an abutment on an implant; may be screw retained or cemented.

6073 abutment-supported retainer for cast metal FPD (predominantly base metal)

A cast metal retainer for a fixed partial denture that is retained, supported, and stabilized by an abutment on an implant; may be screw retained or cemented.

6074 abutment-supported retainer for cast metal FPD (noble metal)

A cast metal retainer for a fixed partial denture that is retained, supported, and stabilized by an abutment on an implant; may be screw retained or cemented.

6194 abutment-supported retainer crown for FPD—(titanium)

A retainer for a fixed partial denture that is retained, supported, and stabilized by an abutment on an implant. May be cast or milled and is screw retained or cemented.

6075 implant-supported retainer for ceramic FPD

A ceramic retainer for a fixed partial denture that is retained, supported, and stabilized from an implant; may be screw retained or cemented.

6076 implant-supported retainer for porcelain fused to metal FPD (titanium, titanium alloy, or high noble metal)

A metal-ceramic retainer for a fixed partial denture that is retained, supported, and stabilized from an implant; may be screw retained or cemented.

6077 implant-supported retainer for cast metal FPD (titanium, titanium alloy, or high noble metal)

A cast metal retainer for a fixed partial denture that is retained, supported, and stabilized from an implant; may be screw retained or cemented.

6078 implant/abutment-supported fixed denture for completely edentulous arch

A prosthesis that is retained, supported, and stabilized by implants or abutments placed on implants but does not have specific relationships between implant positions and replacement teeth; may be screw retained or cemented; commonly referred to as a "hybrid prosthesis."

6079 implant/abutment-supported fixed denture for partially edentulous arch

A prosthesis that is retained, supported, and stabilized by implants or abutments placed on implants but does not have a specific relationship between implant positions and replacement teeth; may be screw retained or cemented; commonly referred to as a "hybrid prosthesis."

appendix *B*

Consent Form: Dental Implant(s)

Part 1—Patient and Doctor Information

Patient Name: _____

Doctor Name: _____

    In order for me to make an informed decision about undergoing a procedure, I should have certain information about the proposed procedure, the associated risks, the alternatives, and the consequences of not having it. The doctor has provided me with this information to my satisfaction. The following is a summary of this information. This form is meant to provide me with the information I need to make a good decision; it is not meant to alarm me.

Part 2—Details of Consent

Condition

My doctor has explained the nature of my condition to me: Missing tooth or teeth.

Procedure—Dental Implant

My physician has proposed the following procedure to treat or diagnose my condition: Dental implant This means: Surgically place an implant into the supporting jawbone.

    We believe that patients have a right to be informed about any treatment, but the law requires extensive disclosure of the risks of surgery and anesthesia, many of which are extremely unlikely to occur. These can be alarming for the patient. Please feel free to ask the doctor about the frequency of any risks or complications disclosed herein that might apply to you (based on our clinical experience and that of other oral surgeons and implantologists).

1. After a careful oral examination and study of my dental condition, the doctor has advised me that my missing tooth or teeth may be replaced with artificial teeth supported by an implant. I hereby authorize and direct the doctor and his authorized associates and assistants to treat my condition.

2. The procedure I choose to treat this condition is understood by me to be the placement of root form implant(s). Additional treatment procedures may include a bone graft including materials of human, animal, or plant origin. I understand that the purpose of this procedure is to allow me to have more functional artificial teeth by the implants providing support, anchorage, and retention for these teeth.

3. I understand that this is nonetheless an elective procedure, that such procedures are performed to improve function, and that an alternative option, although less desirable, is to not undergo surgery and do nothing. I have also

293

been advised that other alternative treatments performed for patients in my condition include, but are not limited to, a bridge, a partial denture, full denture, or other options. I understand and choose to undergo the placement of root form implant(s).

4. I understand that my gum tissue will surgically be opened to expose the bone and that implants will be placed immediately by tapping or threading them into holes that have been drilled into my jawbone. I understand that the gum tissue will then be stitched closed over or around the implant to permit healing for a period of 3 to 6 months. I understand that dentures usually cannot be worn during the first few weeks of the healing phase. I understand that the implants placed will be integrated within 3 to 9 months, depending on my personal healing ability.

5. I also understand that during the course of the procedure, unforeseen conditions may arise that necessitate an extension or alteration of the planned procedure contained herein. I therefore authorize and request that the doctor and his associates or assistants under his direction perform such procedure as found necessary and administer such drugs and treatments as required in their professional judgment.

6. I have had the opportunity to discuss with the doctor the planned surgical procedure, implant placement, and my postoperative responsibilities. I understand that following the procedure during the healing process I should not smoke, drink heavily, use any drugs not prescribed by my doctor, should not blow my nose for at least 2 weeks, and thereafter not heavily blow my nose for an additional 2 weeks. I should take any antibiotics prescribed and use pain medication as needed. If I experience an unusual amount of pain, I should contact the doctor or his associates immediately, because it may signify a problem.

7. I understand that anesthesia given during surgery and certain prescription medications used after surgery cause drowsiness and impaired physical performance, and that such effect is increased by the use of alcohol, and that I must not operate a motor vehicle or any other hazardous equipment while taking these drugs. I also agree not to operate a motor vehicle or any other hazardous equipment for at least 48 hours after my release from surgery.

8. I understand no guarantee has been given to me that the proposed treatment will be curative and/or successful to my complete satisfaction. I also understand that due to individual patient differences and the imperfections of the art and science of surgery, there is a risk of failure or necessity of additional treatment despite appropriate care. I have been advised that the placement of root form implants has shown long-term success rates. However, I understand that such disclosure is not to imply that I personally can expect such a favorable long-term result and that there will be no refund of fees from the surgeon or restorative dentist in the event of complications requiring additional surgery to salvage the implant or failure requiring removal of part or all of the implant. I further understand that should removal be required, the doctor will remove the implant at no additional cost. However, If I elect to have another doctor remove the implant, I am solely responsible for all costs and fees incurred in doing so and hereby release the doctor from any such costs and fees imposed by the other doctor.

Alternatives

My physician has explained the following medically acceptable alternatives: A bridge, a partial denture, full denture, or other options.

Also, I can seek specialized care somewhere else, or I can have nothing done.

Consequences of not Having Procedure Performed

If I don't have the procedure, my condition may stay the same or even improve. However, it is the doctor's opinion that the proposed procedure is a better option for me. If I don't have the procedure, the following may also happen: Further loss of supporting tissues or bone. A gap in the teeth.

Other Procedures

During the course of the procedure, the doctor may discover other conditions that require an extension of the planned procedure, or a different procedure altogether. I authorize the doctor to perform the procedures at this sitting rather than later on.

Risks

The doctor will give his or her best professional care toward accomplishment of the desired results. The substantial and frequent risks and hazards of the proposed procedure are restricted mouth opening, gum shrinkage, clicking or pain of the temporomandibular joints (jaw joints), tooth sensitivity to hot or cold for days up to months, loose teeth, food lodging between the teeth requiring flossing for removal, and unesthetic exposure of crown margins of teeth in the surgery area. These are usually temporary. Uncommonly, these effects may persist. Uncommon risks also include interference with speech sounds and permanent nerve injury, which could require nerve graft surgery.

There will be no refund of fees from the surgeon or restorative dentist in the event of complications requiring additional surgery to salvage the implant or failure requiring removal of part or all of the implant. If removal is required, the doctor will remove the implant at no additional cost. If I have someone else remove the implant, I am responsible for all costs and fees and will not ask the doctor to pay for it.

Drugs, Medications, and Anesthesia

Antibiotics, pain medication, and other medications may cause adverse reactions such as redness and swelling of tissues, pain; itching; drowsiness; nausea; vomiting; dizziness; lack of coordination; miscarriage; cardiac arrest (which can be increased by the effect of alcohol or other drugs); blood clots in the legs, heart, lungs, or brain; low blood pressure; heart attack; stroke; paralysis; or brain damage. After injection of a local anesthetic, I may sometimes have prolonged numbness and/or irritation in the area of injection. If I use nitrous oxide, Atarax, chloral hydrate, Xanax, or other sedatives, possible risks include, but are not limited to, loss of consciousness, severe shock, and stoppage of breathing or heartbeat. I will arrange for someone to drive me home from the office after I have received sedation, and I will have someone watch me closely for 10 hours after my dental appointment to observe for side effects such as difficulty breathing or loss of consciousness.

Implant Database

If a device is placed in my body, the doctor may give my name, dental information, social security number, and other personal information to the device manufacturer for quality control purposes.

No guarantee

The practice of dentistry and surgery is not an exact science. Although good results are expected, the doctor has not given me any guarantee that the proposed treatment will be successful, will be to my complete satisfaction, or that it will last for any specific length of time. Due to individual patient differences, there is always a risk of failure, relapse, need for more treatment, or worsening of my present condition despite careful treatment. Occasionally, treated teeth may require extraction.

Part 3—My Responsibility

I agree to cooperate completely with the doctor's recommendations while under his or her care. If I don't fulfill my responsibility, my results could be affected.

Success requires my long-term personal oral hygiene, mechanical plaque removal (daily brushing and flossing), completion of recommended dental therapy, periodic periodontal visits (dental clinic care), regular follow-up appointments, and overall general health.

There may be several follow-up clinical visits for the first year following surgery. It is my responsibility to see the doctor at least once a year for evaluation of implant performance and oral hygiene maintenance.

I have provided an accurate and complete medical and personal history to the best of my ability, including those antibiotics, drugs, medications, and foods to which I am allergic. I will follow all instructions as explained and directed to me and will permit all required diagnostic procedures. I have had an opportunity to discuss my past medical and health history, including any serious problems and/or injuries, with the doctor.

Necessary Follow-up Care and Self-Care. Natural teeth and appliances should be maintained daily in a clean, hygienic manner. I should follow postoperative instructions given after surgery to ensure proper healing. I will need to come for appointments following the procedure so that my healing may be monitored and so that my doctor can evaluate and report on the outcome of the surgery upon completion of healing.

I will not drink alcohol or take non-prescribed drugs during the treatment period. If sedation or general anesthesia is used, I will not operate a motor vehicle or hazardous device for at least 24 hours or more until I have fully recovered from the effects of the anesthesia or drugs.

I will let the doctor's office know if I change my contact information so I can be contacted for any recalls.

Part 4—Miscellaneous

Photography

I give permission for persons other than the doctors involved in my care and treatment to observe this operation (such as company representatives and dentists who are learning the procedure), and I consent to photography, filming, recording, and x-rays of my oral and facial structures and the procedure. Their publication for educational and scientific purposes is authorized, as long as my identity is not revealed. I give up all rights for compensation for publication of these records.

If teeth are removed during treatment, they may be retained for training purposes and then disposed of sensitively.

Fees

I know the fee that I am to be charged. I am satisfied with it and know that it does not include additional postoperative x-rays, injections, or anesthetics that may later be necessary to correct any complications. As a courtesy to me, the office staff will help prepare and file insurance claims should I be insured. However, the agreement of the insurance company to pay for medical expenses is a contract between myself and the insurance company and does not relieve my responsibility to pay for services provided. Some, and perhaps all, of the services provided may not be covered or not considered reasonable and customary by my insurance company. I am responsible for paying all co-pays and deductibles at the time services are rendered and all costs that have not been paid for by my insurance company within 45 days. Otherwise, all payments are due at the time services are rendered. All accounts not paid in full within 90 days shall accrue interest at the rate of 18% per year. I will be liable for all collection costs, including court costs and attorney fees.

Part 5—Signature

Understanding

I read and write English. I have read and understand this form. All blanks or statements requiring insertion or completion were filled in and inapplicable paragraphs, if any, were stricken before I signed.

I have been encouraged to ask questions and am satisfied with the answers. I have read this entire form. I give my informed consent for surgery and anesthesia.

Someone at the doctor's office has explained this form, my condition, the procedure, how the procedure may help me, things that can go wrong, and my other options, including not having anything done. I want to have the procedure done.

I authorize Dr. _____ or his designee (referred to in the rest of this form as the doctor) to perform the procedure listed in the title above.

I know that I am free to withdraw from treatment at any time.

_____   _____

Patient or Representative Signature   Date

If not the patient, what is your relationship to the patient?

_____

I have explained the condition, procedure, benefits, alternatives, and risks described on this form to the patient or representative.

_____   _____

Dentist Signature   Date

Surgical Trays

It is very important that all the appropriate instruments are on the correct trays in the correct order so you can anticipate the doctor's actions. The following is a list of the instruments contained on all six kinds of surgical trays:

1. Implant placement
2. Stage II implant uncovering
3. Implant prosthetics
4. Ridge preservation
5. Maxillary sinus grafting
6. Ridge augmentation and/or osteotomes

When the doctor enters the room, proceed in this order:

1. Post all x-rays, FMX, panorex, and bitewings on CDR.
2. Have the appropriate instrumentation ready for the procedure.
3. Review the health history, noting any changes.
4. Pre-medicate the patient if necessary.
5. Place the napkin around the patient's neck.
6. Position the chair.
7. Hand the doctor topical on a 2 x 2 gauze pad.
8. Hand the doctor the syringe with warm anesthetic.
9. Have additional carpules or anesthetic ready if needed.
10. Comfort the patient. Hold the patient's hand if you think it will help. Reassure the patient that everything will be fine.
11. Divert the patient's attention away from procedure with an interesting conversation.
12. Ask the patient, "Are you okay?"
13. After the injection, allow the patient to rinse.

Extraction Setup Kits and Instruments

Below is a list of the instruments needed for basic extractions:

1. Exam kit
2. Topical and syringe with anesthetic
3. Straight elevator #301
4. Appropriate forceps
5. Surgical suction tips
6. Sterile gauze
7. Consent for Extraction of Teeth for patient to read and sign before the procedure
8. Postoperative instructions
9. CDR
10. Surgical bur
11. Surgical high-speed handpiece

The following information will help you pick the right forceps for each part of the mouth:

MOLARS				
FORCEPS			**ELEVATORS**	
Max	*Pedo*	*Mand*	*Max*	*Mand*
210	150	16 Cowhorns	E/W Crossbars	301 on 77E
10s	151			11 arrowhead

Additional Instruments

- #9 Molt periosteal elevator
- Curette—double sided spoon
- Root Pick—EHB 1
- EHB—13/14
  *East/West—one for left side, one for right side

PREMOLARS	ANTERIOR		
FORCEPS		**FORCEPS**	
Max	*Mand*	*Max*	*Mand*
99c	MD3	150	151

Ridge Preservation Setup

1. Patient drape
2. Topical and syringe with anesthetic
3. One Bard Parker blade handle
4. Suture scissors
5. 4.0 gut or 3.0 silk sutures—check with doctor
6. Large and small periosteal
7. Hemostats
8. Surgical suction tips
9. Sterile gauze
10. Bone graft material—check with doctor

Implant Surgical Setup

Below is a list of the instruments needed for implant surgical setups

1. Patient drape
2. Topical and syringe with anesthetic
3. One #15 blade
4. One Bard Parker blade handle
5. Suture scissors
6. 4.0 gut or 3.0 silk sutures—check with the doctor
7. Large and small periosteal
8. Round and fissure surgical burs
9. Hemostats
10. Surgical suction tips
11. 301 elevator
12. Appropriate forceps
13. Consent for Removal of Teeth for patient to read and sign before the procedure
14. Postoperative instructions to review with patient after extraction
15. Sterile gauze
16. #9 Molt periosteal elevator
17. Impact Air surgical high-speed handpiece
18. Root tip pick elevators

Soft Tissue Grafting Setup

1. Patient drape
2. Topical and syringe with anesthetic
3. One #15 blade
4. Mirror
5. Tissue holder
6. Needle holder
7. One Bard Parker blade handle
8. Suture scissors
9. 4.0 gut or 3.0 silk sutures—check with doctor

10. Large and small periosteal
11. Round and fissure surgical burs
12. Hemostats
13. Surgical suction tips
14. Consent for Gingival Grafting for patient to read and sign before the procedure
15. Postoperative instructions to review with patient after procedure
16. Sterile gauze
17 #9 Molt (periosteal elevator)
18. Soft tissue graft material—check with doctor

Sinus Grafting Setup

1. Patient drape
2. Topical and syringe with anesthetic
3. One #15 blade
4. One Bard Parker blade handle
5. Suture scissors
6. Mirror
7. Tissue holder
8. 4.0 gut or 3.0 silk sutures—check with doctor
9. Large and small periosteal
10. Bone scraper if needed
11. Hemostats
12. Surgical suction tips
13. Consent for Sinus Grafting for patient to read and sign before the procedure
14. Postoperative instructions to review with patient after the sinus graft
15. Sterile gauze
16. Needle holder
17. #9 Molt (periosteal elevator)
18. Sinus graft curettes
19. Bone packer
20. Bone plugger
21. Bowl to mix the bone

Ridge Splitting Setup

1. Patient drape
2. Topical and syringe with anesthetic
3. One #15 blade
4. One Bard Parker blade handle
5. Suture scissors
6. Mirror
7. Tissue holder
8. 4.0 gut or 3.0 silk sutures—check with doctor
9. Large and small periosteal
10. Hemostats
11. Surgical suction tips
12. Consent for Ridge Split for patient to read and sign before the procedure

13. Postoperative instructions to review with patient after the ridge split
14. Sterile gauze
15. Needle holder
16. #9 Molt (periosteal elevator)
17. Curettes
18. Bone packer
19. Bone plugger
20. Bowl to mix the bone
21. Ridge split kit

Possible Infection or Dry Socket Setup

1. Exam kit
2. Topical and syringe with anesthetic
3. Curettes
4. Saline water
5. Dry socket medicate paste (Alvogyl or similate)

Postoperative Setup

Below is a list of the instruments included in the postoperative setup.

1. Exam kit
2. Suture scissors
3. Peroxyl rinse

appendix D

Postoperative Instructions and Menus for Patients of Implant Surgery

Section 1. Easy Postoperative Care

Following surgery, the last thing you want to worry about is a complication due to poor postoperative care.

Bleeding, Pain, and Swelling

Immediately After Surgery

First and foremost, after placement of dental implants, do not disturb the wound. That means avoid any rinsing, spitting, or touching of the wound on the day of surgery. Your doctor may even advise you to avoid nose-blowing in some cases.

A small amount of bleeding, pain, and swelling is perfectly normal. But there are certain tricks you can use to keep these postop nuisances to a minimum.

Bleeding

Keep steady pressure over the surgical site following the procedure. Pressure helps reduce bleeding and permits the formation of a clot. Gently remove the compress after 1 hour. If bleeding persists, place another compress, and again keep steady pressure on the area for 1 hour. Blood or redness in the saliva is normal. However, excessive bleeding, such as your mouth filling up rapidly with blood, can be controlled by biting on a gauze pad, placed directly on the wound for 30 minutes.

If bleeding continues, call your physician for further instructions. A moistened tea bag applied to the site for 30 minutes also may help to stop bleeding. After bleeding has stopped, the patient can cautiously resume oral hygiene.

It's a good idea to limit or reduce your activity as much as possible for several hours after surgery. Avoid any unnecessary eating, drinking, and talking. These oral activities may hinder proper healing, especially in the first few hours.

Swelling

Any swelling can be minimized by applying an icepack on the cheek or on the jaw directly in the area of surgery. If an icepack is unavailable, simply fill a heavy plastic bag with crushed ice. Secure the end and cover with a soft cloth to avoid skin irritation. Frozen bags of peas make wonderful icepacks and can be refrozen and used repeatedly.

Immediately following the procedure, it's advisable to apply the icepack over the affected area—20 minutes on, and 20 minutes off—for 2 to 4 hours, to help prevent the development of excessive swelling and discomfort. Apply the ice as much as necessary for the first 36 hours.

You may expect swelling for up to 10 days and possibly a fever of 99°F to 100°F.

Pain

To minimize any discomfort from the pain, before the anesthesia wears off and feeling has returned to normal, begin taking medication as directed by your doctor.

For moderate pain, over-the-counter Tylenol or ibuprofen comes in 200-mg tablets. Take two (2) to three (3) tablets every 3 to 4 hours as needed to relieve the ache.

For severe pain, the prescribed medication should be taken as directed. Take the prescribed narcotic medication only if you experience significant pain.

If anti-inflammatory medication was prescribed, begin taking the medication with food immediately after the procedure and continue as directed.

If you were not prescribed any anti-inflammatory medication and you don't have a known allergy to aspirin or ibuprofen (Motrin), you can take 600 mg of ibuprofen (Motrin) every 6 hours to control mild to moderate pain. *Note: Do not take any of the above medications if you are allergic, or have been instructed by your doctor not to take it.*

Prescribed antibiotics, to help prevent infection, usually are started an hour or 2 before implant surgery and are continued for several days afterward.

Cold Then Warm

Remember, in terms of compresses and foods, administer cold items for the first 24 hours and then warm afterward.

Ongoing Oral Hygiene

Good oral hygiene is essential to good healing. This includes warm salt water rinses (a teaspoon of salt in a cup of warm water) at least four to five times a day. Repeat after every meal or snack for 7 days. Rinsing is important because it removes food particles and debris and thus helps to promote healing.

You also can brush your tongue with a dry toothbrush to keep bacteria growth down, but be careful not to touch the surgical site. Resume your regular tooth brushing after 2 days, but continue to avoid disturbing the surgical area.

Diet

Eating might seem like the last thing on your mind after dental surgery, but it's important to nourish your body. Drink plenty of fluids. Avoid hot liquids or food. Soft, cool foods and liquids should be consumed on the day of surgery, with return to a normal diet as soon as possible, unless otherwise directed.

Maintain Proper Diet

Have your meals at the usual time. Eat soft, nutritious foods and hydrate your mouth regularly with liquids, during meals and in between. However, always be careful not to disturb the blood clot. Add solid foods to your diet as per the schedule in the upcoming Menu section.

Warning: For 2 weeks after surgery do *not* eat or drink the following:
- Spicy foods
- Acidic juices (orange, grapefruit, etc.)
- Chips
- Popcorn
- Carbonated drinks

Wearing Your Prosthesis

Partial or full dentures should not be used immediately after surgery and for at least 10 days, unless allowed by your doctor.

Activity

It's wise to keep physical activities to a minimum immediately following surgery. Rest up and heal, otherwise you could be setting yourself back by a few days. If you engage in vigorous exercise, throbbing or bleeding may occur. If this does occur, you should discontinue exercising. Keep in mind that you are probably not taking in the normal quantities of calories for normal exercise. This may weaken you and further limit your mobility.

If you should have any problems such as excessive bleeding, pain, or difficulty in opening your mouth, call the dental office immediately for further instructions, assistance, or additional treatment.

Remember your follow-up visit: You will be scheduled to return for a postoperative visit to make certain healing is progressing satisfactorily. While you wait for that appointment, maintain a healthful diet, observe the basic rules for proper oral hygiene, and call the office if you have any questions or concerns.

Postop Care Recap

Here are the Top 10 Tips for Care After Surgery:
1. **Don't Touch!** Keep fingers and tongue away from surgical area.
2. **Cool It!** Use icepacks on surgical area (side of face) for the first 12 hours; apply ice 20 minutes on, 20 minutes off. Bags of frozen peas work quite well for this.
3. **Still Hurts?** For mild discomfort, take Tylenol or ibuprofen every 3 to 4 hours.

4. **In Pain!** For severe pain, please use the prescription medication for pain given to you.

5. **Hydrate Yourself.** Drink plenty of fluids. Do not use a straw.

6. **Chew Gum.** If the muscles of the jaw become stiff, chewing gum at intervals will help relax the muscles. The use of warm, moist heat to the outside of your face beginning on the second day after surgery will help further with relaxation of the muscle.

7. **Eat Soft Foods!** Diet may consist of soft foods, which can be chewed easily and swallowed. Recommended foods and recipes are provided in the Menu section. No seeds, nuts, rice, or popcorn!

8. **Blood?** A certain amount of bleeding can be expected following surgery. Bleeding is controlled by applying pressure to the surgical area for 90 minutes. Then you may eat or drink. If bleeding persists, a moist tea bag should be placed in the area of bleeding firmly for 1 hour straight.

9. **No Smoking, Please!** Do not smoke for at least 5 days after surgery.

10. **Drugs?** If you are on other medications, be sure to discuss this with your doctor or pharmacist to minimize adverse drug interactions. Do start taking a multivitamin daily, however, if you are not already doing so.

Section 2. The First 24 Hours

After dental surgery, some people find it difficult to eat or enjoy their food. This reluctance to sit down at meal times, plus an inability to consume normal, solid food, is especially likely to occur after dental surgery.

It's not difficult to see why—too much chewing, slurping, or sucking can aggravate the treated area, resulting in discomfort and even pain. It also can potentially reopen the area, causing bleeding or infection that will delay healing or cause problems with the surgery if the area is disturbed too much. However, despite any fears or lack of appetite, it's vital that you continue to eat, as nutrients provide energy and facilitate your healing process on the road to recovery.

On the day of your surgery, and for the first 24 hours following, it's a good idea to give your teeth a bit of a break. For this reason, cold soups, smoothies, Jell-o/puddings, and cold drinks should be your main dietary intake. And remember, refrain from using a straw, because the sucking action can cause excess strain and can delay your ultimate recovery.

Suggestions for Day 1

BEVERAGES

Blackberry-Orange Cooler

Throughout the world and throughout history, the citrus fruit has been a symbol of health and beauty. The very wealthy presented citrus to each other as precious gifts, and citrus is still a primary ingredient in perfume and aromatherapy. Blackberries help combat nausea and are also high in Vitamin E, which promotes healing. Here is a recipe that incorporates both, for your enjoyment.

INGREDIENTS
- 4 blackberries
- ½ cup plain yogurt
- ½ cup orange juice
- Sugar or sweetener to taste (Splenda does not raise the glycemic index)
- 1 scoop vanilla whey protein powder (optional)

DIRECTIONS
Place all ingredients in the blender, and blend at high speed for 1 minute, or until blackberries are liquefied. Strain to eliminate all seeds. Pour into a large glass, and drink!

Chocolate Banana Smoothie

This recipe is for your inner child and your outer body. Flax seed oil is full of omega-3, a natural antioxidant. It also helps prevent constipation, a common postop complaint due to antibiotics and pain medication. Pamper yourself with the flavors you craved when you were a kid, with the ingredients you need as an adult.

INGREDIENTS

- 1 tsp cocoa powder
- ½ ripe banana
- ½ cup plain yogurt
- 1 tsp sugar, or 1 packet sweetener
- ½ cup water
- 1 to 2 large ice cubes
- 1 tsp flax seed oil (if available)
- 1 scoop whey protein powder (optional)

DIRECTIONS

Combine all ingredients in a blender, and blend at high speed for 30 seconds. Add 1 or 2 large ice cubes, and blend for another 30 seconds, or until smooth. Enjoy.

MAIN COURSES

French Ratatouille Soup

If cooking is not your strength, then this recipe might intrigue you for many reasons. First, you can create something from nothing (or leftovers). Second, with such a variety of vegetables in this soup, the wide range of vitamins and nutrients available help promote and regulate various chemical processes within your body. And third, this classic Provençal dish is good hot, cold, or pureed.

INGREDIENTS
- 2 tbsp olive oil
- 1 large onion, chopped
- 1 tsp garlic, chopped
- 1 medium zucchini, chopped
- 1 small eggplant, chopped
- 1 bell pepper, chopped (any color)
- 2 lb fresh or canned tomatoes, peeled and chopped
- 1 tsp fresh thyme minced (or $\frac{1}{4}$ teaspoon dried)
- 2 cups vegetable or chicken stock
- Pinch of cayenne pepper
- 1 tsp salt (ideally, sea salt, that great sel de mer from France)
- $\frac{1}{8}$ tsp freshly ground black pepper
- 2 tbsp fresh basil, sliced fine, for garnish
- Balsamic vinegar, for garnish

DIRECTIONS
Heat the olive oil in a large saucepan or Dutch Oven. Sauté the onion and garlic until soft—3 to 4 minutes—over medium heat. Add the chopped eggplant, zucchini, and pepper, sautéing for color and to soften the vegetables, approximately 5 minutes, stirring occasionally. Gradually stir in the tomatoes and their juices, followed by the spices and vegetable stock. Bring the liquid to a boil. Then reduce the heat and simmer for 15 to 20 minutes.

Chill in the refrigerator for 1 hour, then garnish with a little balsamic vinegar over each bowl, and sprinkle with fresh basil.

Gazpacho Soup

Gazpacho soup is the original "V-8." All good comfort food is usually derived from "poor people food," and gazpacho soup is no different, being the food that farm workers enjoyed in Andalusia, Spain. Gazpacho is a sultry mix of everyday garden vegetables, and if you've never had a cold soup before, this rich burst of flavors will make you a convert. Although there are many regional and modern versions of this soup, it's traditionally made with ripe tomatoes, bell peppers, cucumbers, and garlic. But the main reason I've included it here is because all the ingredients reduce inflammation and tissue damage, prevent disease and cell damage, and relieve stress!

INGREDIENTS

- 4 cups tomato juice
- 1 onion, minced
- 1 green bell pepper, minced
- 1 cucumber, chopped
- 2 cups chopped tomatoes
- 2 green onions, chopped
- 1 clove garlic, minced
- 3 tbsp fresh lemon juice
- 2 tbsp red wine vinegar
- 1 tsp dried tarragon
- 1 tsp dried basil
- ¼ cup chopped fresh parsley
- 1 tsp white sugar
- Salt and pepper, to taste

DIRECTIONS

Tomatoes, onion, bell pepper, cucumber, and garlic are pureed with lemon juice, red wine vinegar, and tarragon, then chilled for a refreshing cold soup. In a blender, combine all ingredients, except salt and pepper. Pulse until well combined but still slightly chunky. Taste the soup, adding seasoning (salt and pepper) as needed. Chill at least 2 hours before serving.

Mexican Avocado Soup

For many years, it's been thought that avocados were unhealthy because they contained lots of fat. Now we know those reports were only partially true; avocados are high in fat—"good fat"—the monounsaturated kind. Avocados actually will lower your cholesterol. In fact, they are extremely nutritious and contribute nearly 20 vitamins, minerals, and beneficial plant compounds to your diet. Always with your health in mind, try this delicious all-season treat with a South-of-the-border twist. Serve cold.

INGREDIENTS

- 4 cups vegetable or chicken stock
- 1 cup heavy cream, or half-and-half
- 1 chili pepper, as hot as you dare (from banana to habanero)
- 1 garlic clove
- 2 avocados
- Salt and white pepper
- 2 tbsp cilantro, finely chopped, for garnish
- ¼ cup crisp, fried tortillas, for garnish

DIRECTIONS

In a saucepan, heat the stock and cream, and keep the temperature steady at a simmer. Puree the chili pepper and garlic in a blender, then add the avocado. When ready to serve, gradually add the hot stock mixture and blend until smooth. Season to taste, and serve immediately with cilantro and chips on the side, or refrigerate to make a cold soup. Note that avocados turn bitter when heated, so be careful not to add liquid that is too hot.

DESSERTS

Lush Chocolate Mousse

By now you should know that dark, unsweetened chocolate is great for lowering blood pressure. But did you also know that chocolate helps improve your mood? Indulge in this sumptuous dessert while you recover. You don't need to feel guilty anymore.

INGREDIENTS
- 1½ cups whipping cream
- 8 oz unsweetened dark chocolate, melted
- 2 tbsp sugar
- ½ tsp vanilla

DIRECTIONS
In a saucepan, warm ½ of the whipping cream, and remove from heat. Add sugar and vanilla to the melted chocolate; then combine chocolate mixture with the heated cream. In a separate bowl, whip remaining cream until it has soft peaks. At that point, slowly fold it into the chocolate mixture. Divide into small bowls or glasses, and chill until set, before serving.

Section 3.
Days 2-5

BEVERAGES

Apple Cider

Long touted by ancient Egyptians to be an elixir of eternal youth, apple cider is indeed a natural multivitamin and mineral treasure trove. Even Hippocrates—the father of medicine—acknowledged the vast healing properties of apple cider.

INGREDIENTS
- 2 cups apple juice
- 1 cinnamon stick, 2 inches
- 3 cloves, whole
- 2 tbsp orange peel
- Sugar, if desired

DIRECTIONS
Place all ingredients in a saucepan and bring to a simmer. Continue to simmer with the lid on for 15 to 20 minutes. Taste, and add sugar if desired. Strain and serve warm.

Peach Iced Tea

Tea is known for its antioxidants and healing properties, and peaches, a source of natural sugars, also contain Vitamins A and C. You can even add a bit of peach puree to create a mock Bellini. This beverage is a great twist on an old favorite.

INGREDIENTS
- 3 cups water
- 3 tea bags
- 3 tbsp sugar
- 1 cinnamon stick, 2 inches
- 1 cup peach nectar
- 1 peach, sliced in thin wedges

DIRECTIONS
Boil the water, and make tea. Once steeped to your preference—3 to 5 minutes—remove tea bags. Add sugar and cinnamon while liquid is still warm, and stir to dissolve. Mix in peach juice and peach slices. Chill in the fridge before serving over ice.

BREAKFAST

Hot Oatmeal

In 1997, oatmeal became the first whole food to bear a "claim" label approved by the FDA. This is one of those little labels that claim the food has a property that does something good for your body. Your grandmother was right: Oatmeal may reduce the risk of heart disease. Try it mixed with raisins and brown sugar, so you can also remember how good her cookies were.

INGREDIENTS
- ½ cup small, quick-cooking oats
- 1 cup water
- ¼ cup raisins
- 2 tbsp brown sugar
- 2 tbsp milk

DIRECTIONS
Place oats and water into a large microwaveable bowl. Cook on high for 1½ to 2½ minutes, until oats are soft and cooked. Stir in raisins and top with brown sugar. Once the sugar has "melted," finish with milk and serve.

Pancakes

INGREDIENTS
- 2 cups flour
- ½ tsp salt
- 3 tbsp sugar
- 1 tbsp baking powder
- ½ cup blueberries
- 2 eggs
- 1¼ cups milk
- 1 tbsp melted butter

DIRECTIONS
Combine the dry ingredients and stir together. Add in and coat the blueberries. In a separate bowl, mix the wet ingredients, beating the eggs slightly. Combine dry and wet ingredients together, just until mixed. (They don't need to be smooth.) Spoon the batter in small portions (¼ cup of the mixture) onto a hot, oiled frying pan, on low-medium heat. When the pancakes have "bubbles" on the top, they are ready to flip. The other side will need only 2 to 3 minutes. Should your pancake be overcooked on the underside, before the bubbles appear, turn down the heat for the next batch. Serve with maple syrup, fresh fruit, or simply butter.

SOUPS

Borlotti Bean Soup

Italian Borlotti beans, also known as "tongues of fire," are not like Great Northern White beans. They are creamier and heavier. It's really worth buying them at an Italian goods store, for the real deal. Borlotti is an excellent source of fiber for a healthy digestive system and a source of protein that is low in fat.

INGREDIENTS

- 1 lb Borlotti beans
- 8 cups water
- 15 cloves garlic, peeled and trimmed
- 2 large shallots (or 1 white onion), sliced into thin crescents

- 2 to 3 dried smoked chilis (serrano pepper, if available)
- 2 tsp fine sea salt, plus additional for seasoning
- A drizzle of extra virgin olive oil
- A small handful of cilantro, chopped
- ½ cup Parmesan, grated (optional)

DIRECTIONS

Give the beans a thorough rise, then soak them overnight in a large pot of water, covered with a few extra inches of liquid. When you are ready to use the beans, drain and rinse them again, before using. Preheat oven to 350°, with the racks near the bottom. Put the beans, water, garlic, shallots, and peppers in an oven-proof pot, preferably one with an oven-proof lid. Place the pot on a rimmed baking sheet (in case of accidental overflow), and cook in the oven for 2 hours, or until beans are nice and tender. After the first hour, check every 20 minutes. When the beans are done, remove from the oven and season generously with salt. Stir, taste, and season to your liking. Let the soup rest on the stovetop, covered for 10 minutes, allowing the beans time to absorb the seasoned broth. Taste and adjust seasoning once again, finally drizzling with the olive oil. To serve, first ladle a generous scoop of beans into each bowl, followed by the broth, covering the beans. Sprinkle with fresh cilantro and grated cheese.

Chicken Tortilla Soup

Tortillas, a Mexican flatbread made with ground maize, have experienced a meteoric rise in popularity that has everyone craving wraps. The fresher you can get them, the better they are for your health. When you find a nice Mexican restaurant you can trust, ask if you can buy them in bulk, and then freeze them, so you can use whenever you need. On another note, cumin is a fantastic source of iron and calcium.

INGREDIENTS

- 2 skinless, boneless chicken breasts
- ½ tsp olive oil
- ½ tsp garlic, minced
- ¼ tsp ground cumin
- 4 cups chicken broth
- 1 cup frozen corn kernels
- 1 cup onion, chopped
- ½ tsp chili powder
- 1 tbsp lemon juice
- 1 cup chunky salsa
- 1 cup corn tortilla chips
- ½ cup Monterey Jack cheese, shredded (optional)

DIRECTIONS

First, in a large pot over medium heat, sauté the chicken in the oil for 5 minutes. Add the garlic and cumin, and mix well. Then add the broth, corn, onion, chili powder, lemon juice, and salsa. Reduce heat to low, and simmer for about 20 to 30 minutes. Before serving, break up some tortilla chips in the individual bowls. Then pour soup over the chips; top with the shredded cheese and a dollop of sour cream. Lemon juice brightens the flavors in this gorgeous chicken, corn, and salsa soup. Garnish with tortilla chips, grated cheese, and a dollop of sour cream.

Ham and Potato Soup

INGREDIENTS

- 3½ cups potatoes, peeled and diced
- ⅓ cup celery, diced
- ⅓ cup onion, finely chopped
- ¾ cup cooked ham, chopped
- 3¼ cups water
- 2 tbsp chicken bouillon granules
- ½ tsp salt
- 1 tbsp ground black pepper
- 5 tbsp butter
- 5 tbsp all-purpose flour
- 2 cups milk

DIRECTIONS

Combine the potatoes, celery, onion, ham, and water in a stockpot. Bring to a boil, then reduce the heat to medium and cook until potatoes are tender, about 10 to 15 minutes. Stir in the chicken bouillon, salt, and pepper. In a separate saucepan, melt butter over low heat. Whisk in flour with a fork, and cook, stirring continually until thick—about 1 minute. Slowly stir in milk, a little at a time, as not to allow lumps to form. Continue stirring until thick, 4 to 5 minutes. Add the thickened milk mixture to the stockpot, and cook soup until heated thoroughly.

Vegetable Soup

INGREDIENTS

- 2 tsp butter
- ½ cup onion, chopped
- 2 medium carrots, peeled, sliced, and halved
- 2 medium potatoes, peeled and chopped
- 1 cup green beans, cut
- 4 cups chicken broth
- 1 tbsp chopped fresh parsley
- 1 tsp dried tarragon leaves
- ¼ tsp ground black pepper

DIRECTIONS

Add butter to a large saucepan and stir in onion and carrots, cooking on medium-high heat for 5 minutes or until tender. Add potatoes, green beans, broth, and spices; mix well. Cook 10 minutes or until potatoes are tender, stirring frequently. You can serve this chunky, as is, or puree in a blender, to serve it cold.

LUNCH AND DINNER

Chicken Pesto Pasta

Eating this delicious dish can also prevent infection! Basil, the main ingredient of pesto, is actually a natural, gentle sedative that helps to relieve high blood pressure and the symptoms of peptic ulcers. The unique array of volatile oils, which contain estragole, linalool, cineole, eugenol, sabinene, myrcene, and limonene, found in basil provide protection against unwanted bacterial growth. Some bacteria that basil works best against are strains of bacteria from the genera *Staphylococcus, Enterococcus,* and Pseudomonas, all of which not only are widespread but have now developed a high level of resistance to antibiotics.

INGREDIENTS

- 2 tbsp vegetable oil
- 2 boneless, skinless chicken breasts, chopped
- 1 tbsp salt
- 8 oz fettucini
- 2½ cups basil
- 5 cloves garlic
- ½ cup pine nuts
- ⅔ cup olive oil
- ½ cup Parmesan cheese, grated

DIRECTIONS

In a frying pan, heat the vegetable oil and add the chopped chicken. Sauté the meat and fully cook the chicken before setting it aside. To make the sauce, combine the basil, garlic, and pine nuts in a food processor (or blender) until it reaches a paste-like texture. Slowly pour in the olive oil while still blending together. Then, stir in the cheese. Taste and season with salt and pepper, as needed. At the same time, boil a large pot of salted water. When it reaches a rolling boil, add the fettucini and cook until al dente. Toss the cooked pasta with the pesto sauce, topping the dish off with the cooked chicken pieces.

DESSERTS

Bread and Butter Pudding

This is essentially a baked form of French toast. Best when made with Brioche and served warm with custard and cream. Perfect for tender gums.

INGREDIENTS
- 4 cups white bread, diced
- ½ cup raisins
- ½ cup dried cranberries
- 2 eggs, slightly beaten
- 1¾ cups milk
- 2 tsp vanilla
- 1 tsp cinnamon
- ¾ cup sugar

DIRECTIONS
Preheat oven to 350°. Fill a 9″ × 9″ pan or one of similar size with the bread pieces; scatter the bread with raisins and cranberries. In a mixing bowl, combine eggs, milk, vanilla, cinnamon, and sugar. Pour wet ingredients over the bread, and let sit for 5 to 10 minutes, so the bread can absorb some of the liquid. Bake for 40 to 50 minutes, or until firm and colored on top. Let sit 10 more minutes before serving.

Very Berry Pie

Eat, drink, and be berry! This pie will have any precancerous cells running for cover! Raspberries contain significant quantities of polyphenol antioxidants such as anthocyanin pigments. Buy the frozen organic berries, they work just as well. Raspberries are also a rich source of Vitamin C (about 50% of our daily recommended value). Drench in delicious vanilla ice cream or custard. Enjoy!

INGREDIENTS
- 2 unbaked pie crusts, 9 inch
- 2 cups raspberries, fresh or frozen
- 1 cup strawberries, sliced, fresh, or frozen
- 1 cup blueberries, fresh or frozen
- 1 tsp lemon juice
- ¾ cup sugar
- ¼ cup flour
- 1 tbsp butter

DIRECTIONS
Preheat the oven to 400°. Mix together the berries and lemon juice in a large bowl. In another bowl, stir together the sugar and flour. Combine the dry ingredients with the fruit mixture, coating the berries evenly. Place berries in one of the pie shells, and dot with small pieces of butter. Invert the second pie shell on top of the filled shell, and pinch around the edges to seal. Cut several slits on the top of the pie, allowing steam to escape. Bake at 400° for 15 minutes, then at 375° for 45 minutes, until golden on top. Let rest 15 minutes before serving.

Section 4.
Days 6 to 14

In addition to many of the fine dishes from our previous menus, your mouth will now be ready to enjoy the nourishing and comforting meals below.

- **Main Courses**
  - Almond-Crusted Halibut Crystal Symphony*
- Broiled Tilapia Parmesan*
- Chicken Fettucini Alfredo
- Fish in Ginger-Tamarind Sauce
- Grilled Salmon Kyoto*
- Lasagna
- Orange Roughy
- Salmon Patties*
- Sesame Seared Tuna*

MAIN COURSES

All of the fish in these dishes are a good source of protein and, of course, contain omega-3 fatty acids, which are known to benefit your cardiovascular system and your nervous system. Fatty fish, in particular, is recommended to be eaten at least twice a week.

Broiled Tilapia Parmesan

INGREDIENTS

- ½ cup Parmesan cheese
- ¼ cup butter, softened
- 3 tbsp mayonnaise
- 2 tbsp lemon juice
- ¼ tsp dried basil
- ¼ tsp black pepper
- ⅛ tsp onion powder
- ⅛ tsp celery salt
- 2 lb tilapia fillets

DIRECTIONS

Preheat oven to broiler setting. Grease a broiling pan or line it with aluminum foil. In a small bowl, mix together cheese, butter, mayonnaise, and lemon juice. Then stir in basil, pepper, onion powder, and celery salt, and set aside. Arrange fillets in a single layer on the prepared pan. Broil 3 minutes a side, a few inches from the heat. Remove the fish from the oven, and cover the top side with the cheese mixture. Broil until the topping is brown and fish flakes easily with a fork, about 2 minutes. Be careful not to overcook the fish!

Grilled Salmon Kyoto

INGREDIENTS

- ⅓ cup soy sauce
- ¼ cup orange juice concentrate
- 2 tbsp vegetable oil
- 2 tbsp tomato sauce
- 1 tsp lemon juice
- ½ tsp prepared mustard
- 1 tbsp green onion, minced
- 1 clove garlic, minced
- ½ tsp fresh ginger, minced
- 4 salmon steaks, 1-inch thick
- 1 tbsp olive oil

DIRECTIONS

In a shallow glass baking dish, combine all ingredients, except salmon and olive oil. Then, place salmon in marinade, and turn to coat. Cover and refrigerate for 30 minutes to 1 hour. Once the fish is almost ready, preheat an outdoor grill to high heat. Remove salmon from marinade, reserving the liquid in a small saucepan. Bring the liquid to a boil, and cook for 1 to 2 minutes. Next, lightly oil the grill grate, and brush or spray salmon with olive oil. Place fish on the grill, and cook for 10 minutes or until fish flakes easily with a fork. Turn salmon once, and brush with boiled marinade halfway through cooking time. Delicious fish, Japanese-style!

Salmon Patties

To benefit from antioxidants and omega-3 fatty acids, salmon is an ideal source.

INGREDIENTS

- ½ lb salmon
- 1 red potato, peeled and chopped
- 1 shallot, minced
- 1 egg, beaten
- ¼ cup Italian seasoned bread crumbs
- 1 tsp Italian seasoning
- Salt and pepper, to taste
- ½ cup cornflake crumbs
- 2 tbsp olive oil

DIRECTIONS

Preheat your oven to 350°, and lightly grease a small baking dish. Place the salmon in the prepared baking dish; cover and bake 20 minutes, or until easily flaked with a fork. While the fish is cooking, boil the potato in a small saucepan and cook until tender, 10 to 15 minutes. Once cooked, drain and mash the potato. Next, combine the salmon, potato, shallot, egg, and bread crumbs in a bowl, and add the Italian seasoning, salt, and pepper. In a separate bowl nearby, place the cornflake crumbs. Then, using the salmon mixture, create 1-inch balls of salmon. Roll the balls in the cornflakes, to coat, and press into patties. Heat the olive oil in a medium saucepan, and fry the patties over medium heat, 3 to 5 minutes a side, or until golden brown. Delicious!

Sesame Seared Tuna

INGREDIENTS

- ¼ cup soy sauce
- 1 tbsp mirin (Japanese sweet wine)
- 1 tbsp honey
- 2 tbsp sesame oil
- 1 tbsp rice wine vinegar
- 4 (6-oz) tuna steaks
- ½ cup sesame seeds
- Wasabi paste
- 1 tbsp olive oil

DIRECTIONS

In a small bowl, stir together soy sauce, mirin, honey, and sesame oil. Divide the liquid into two equal parts. Stir the rice vinegar into one part, and set this aside as a dipping sauce. Coat the tuna steaks with the remaining soy sauce mixture. Next, spread the sesame seeds out on a plate, and press the tuna into them, to coat. Heat the olive oil until very hot, in a cast iron skillet on high heat. Place steaks in the pan, and sear for about 30 seconds on each side. Serve with the dipping sauce and wasabi paste.

Day 14 and Beyond

Congratulations! You made it. With a fantastic foundation built within the past 2-week period, during which your mouth has had ample time to heal by eating softer, gum-sensitive nutritional food, you have now reached the 14-day marker, where you can resume a normal diet.

After Day 14, you can eat whatever you wish, but be careful not to disturb any residual swelling that might be present in the surgical site. Add solid foods to your diet as soon as they are comfortable to chew.

But now that you have conscientiously integrated this healthier eating regimen into your life, I believe you will want to continue.

Oral health is a critical part of your overall health. Don't wait until the next oral surgery to focus on taking good care of your teeth and gums.

Fitness 101

Your overall health and well-being are keys to a speedy recovery process from any type of surgery, including oral surgery.

Along with healthy eating, as guided by the menus within the preceding section of this book, you should be conscious of the value of nutrition in your diet and the level of fitness in your daily activities. This ideal combination of a balanced quantity of vitamins and nutrients, along with regular exercise, is critical for postoperative recovery. Not to mention, by being aware of both these factors, you can aim to stay at an optimum health level in the weeks, months, and years to come.

You don't need to enlist a fitness trainer and nutritionist. All you need to do is follow a suitable plan that includes exercises, proper nutrition, vitamins, and minerals and embrace a healthier lifestyle plan.

In the days following surgery, it will be natural to feel tired and achy, so common sense prevails that you shouldn't overexert yourself. This especially means taking care not to exacerbate sensitive or delicate areas, in this case, in your head and mouth area.

It's not recommended that you attempt any vigorous physical exercise that involves head-turning, nodding, neck strain, or inverting your body—for example, strenuous yoga positions, sit-ups, push-ups, or running might be too stressful in these early days of recovery.

However, a moderate amount of fitness and exercise will be a productive way to build your body into a stronger, fitter, and healthier machine.

Exercise has multiple benefits, in addition to controlling weight; it can reduce risk for cardiac disease, lower blood pressure, improve mental function, improve blood glucose levels, reduce the risk of some cancers, and improve the immune system. When it becomes apparent that it is safe to do so, try to get at least 30 minutes of physical activity each day.

Physical activity is defined as activities performed in addition to your normal daily routines such as going to work, shopping, or housekeeping.

Running might be too hard on your body at this time, but fast walking or even a short walk around the block will be worthwhile and rewarding. In fact, you will be amazed at how good it will make you feel!

Five Pillars of Fitness

Supporting your entire fitness plan, the five pillars of fitness are essential elements of healthier, stronger, and longer living.

Strength, Agility, Flexibility, Cardiovascular, and Endurance exercises should be included as part of every well-rounded and balanced fitness regimen. Of course, many different exercises can benefit each pillar from this group; however, all of the exercises that are specially recommended within these five pillars are intended as safe for postoperative patients who are 14 days into their recovery, and onward.

If in doubt, or if you do not feel 100% ready for this type of movement, please do not attempt it.

Strength Building and toning muscles is what strength training is all about. This can involve using weights and repetitions of movement—essentially, fewer reps can be performed with heavier weights to achieve similar results as more reps with lighter weights.

Ultimately though, strength training is not about completing the action once or twice, but repeating it 6 to 12 times (called a "set"). This helps to develop strength and endurance.

Types of weight equipment can include barbells and dumbbells; you can even use your own body weight by performing chin-ups and push-ups.

Push-Ups A classic push-up—lie flat, face down on the floor, with your stomach to the ground; bring your hands up to your shoulders and raise your toes, so the bottom of your toes touch the ground.

With your legs out straight behind you, push up, keeping your back straight and your stomach tight. Then, lower yourself in this horizontal position until your elbows make a right angle and/or your chest almost reaches the floor.

Are you improving? Once a month, do as many push-ups as possible to find out your maximum repetition level. This number should increase over time, with more practice and training.

Target area: Chest and arms (pectoral, triceps, biceps).

Variation: If this is a challenge, try with your knees bent to begin, gradually working up to a full-body push-up.

Crunches Lie on the floor, face up, with your back flat and knees bent, so the soles of your feet are flat on the floor.

Place your arms gently behind your head. Curl your neck and shoulders up off the floor, and feel your abdominal muscles "crunch." Then, release and lower your shoulders back down. You should be using your abdominals to curl you up, and not your arms, which would pull your neck.

Are you improving? Once a month, do as many crunches as possible to find out your maximum repetition level. This number should increase over time, with more practice and training.

Target area: Abdominal muscles.

Variation: Try raising your legs in the air, with bended knees; keep your legs in this position throughout the crunch. Alternatively, try lifting only one shoulder and twisting to target the oblique abdominal muscles; be sure to crunch both sides.

Squats A squat basically involves bending your knees and rising again. To begin, start with your feet shoulder-width apart; bend your knees, and squat as low as possible.

During your bend, bring your arms out in front of you, parallel with the floor. Then straighten back up to a standing position again, and repeat.

Are you improving? Once a month, do as many squats as possible to find out your maximum repetition level. This number should increase over time, with more practice and training. Also, you may notice a difference in the level of squat that you can achieve; with time, you may be able to bend lower, into a deeper squat.

Target area: Lower body—quadriceps, hamstrings, calves, and glutes.

Variation: For more of a challenge, try it on one leg. Support yourself on one leg and lift the other in front of you while bending. Be sure to repeat on the other leg.

Lunges To try this lunge, stand with one foot in front of the next, 2 to 3 feet apart. The goal is to have both knees at a 90° angle when you're bending your knees, so you may need to bring your feet closer or farther apart.

To begin, bend your knees—your front heel stays down on the floor, with the knee directly over the foot, while the back leg/knee is lowered toward the floor. Your upper body should remain straight throughout the movement. Then, push up through your front foot and return to the starting position, keeping your knees bent slightly in the top position. Try doing 2 to 3 sets of 10 to 15 repetitions.

Are you improving? Once a month, do as many lunges as possible to find out your maximum repetition level. This number should increase over time, with more practice and training.

Target area: Glutes, hamstrings.

Variation: As you increase your level of strength and comfort with this exercise, add extra weight. For instance, hold hand-weights in each hand as you perform this exercise. If you don't have barbells, try a can of soup or a bottle of water in each hand instead.

Leg Lift Lie on the floor, face up, on your back, placing your hands under your hips; your legs should be straight in front of you. Slowly lift one leg off the floor, about 6 inches high, and hold it in the air. Then lower and repeat with the other leg.

Once this movement is comfortable, try raising both legs off the ground together. When they're in the air, spread your legs out wide and then bring them back together; lower them to the ground.

Are you improving? Continue until your strength improves to desired level.

Target area: Lower body—Legs, hips, abs.

Variation: Instead of spreading your legs apart, simply keep them hovering 6 inches off the ground, and hold this position for 30 to 45 seconds, before lowering.

Lifestyle Activities That Encourage Strength: Weightlifting, Swimming, Rowing

Agility Agility is all about being able to change the direction your body is headed, quickly. This requires a combo of balance, coordination, reflexes, and speed—particularly useful when playing racquet sports, for instance.

Shuttle Run This exercise has you run from one direction to another and then back again. Mark two parallel lines on the floor, about 10 feet apart (try using a piece of tape on the floor to mark the lines). Starting in the middle of them, run toward the left line and touch it; then run toward the opposite line and touch it, before finally running back to the first line.

You can do this back-and-forth shuttle for a set amount of time, or instead time yourself for three or five re-directions, and try to beat your time.

Are you improving? Either count how many re-directions you can do in a set period (for example, 1 minute), or see how fast you can complete a series of re-directions, continually trying to beat your previous time.

Variation: Change the footwork. Try doing this drill running forward and backward between lines, doing a side-step, side to side between lines, or even running sideways, crossing your feet in front and behind with each step.

Ski Hops Draw two lines, 10 meters long and 1 meter apart. Looking up the length of both lines, and starting on the far side of one line, jump horizontally across to the outside of the other line (so you're jumping over both lines). Jump back and forth, from one side to the next as you move down the length of the lines. When you reach the end, turn around and repeat the exercise.

Are you improving? Depending on your agility, having the lines at 1 meter apart may be too challenging; if so, consider bringing the lines in slightly. To assess improvement, look at your level of ease in jumping this distance repeatedly—is it challenging, can you always do it? etc.

Variation: Face the lines so that you're looking horizontally across both of them. Starting on the far side and at one end, jump forward, across both lines, and then jump backward, trying to jump across both lines. Repeat up, all the way up the lines.

Broad Jump With your feet shoulder-width apart, swing your arms and jump forward with both feet. Continue jumping in succession, for 3 to 5 jumps. The timing of your arm swing can dramatically help with the distance of your jump.

Are you improving? Consider measuring how far your longest jump is, and try to break your record. Also, try jumping three times in a row, and measure the total distance. Compare your results after a month to see if you're jumping farther.

One-Foot Balance Good balance is often associated with agility. Try improving your balance by simply standing on one foot. See how long you can balance. Try your luck on both legs.

Figure 8 Pattern At a brisk walk or jog, follow a large Figure 8 pattern for 3 to 5 minutes. Then, change directions and complete the Figure 8 in the other direction. With practice, decrease the size of the Figure 8, and increase your time completing the exercise.

Lifestyle Activities That Encourage Agility: Soccer, Football, Tennis, Badminton, Basketball

Flexibility A key component in overall fitness, yet many lose their flexibility as they get older, so when you're young, it's great to maintain and/or improve what you have, to help set the stage for later in life. If you're only considering this, or noticing a decline in flexibility later in life, there are still many ways to improve your level of flexibility now.

Repetition and consistency are crucial—being flexible isn't something you achieve after 2 weeks; it takes time and regular effort. Also, this term can apply to a range of different areas of your body. It isn't as easy as a simple, "Can I touch my toes?"

Key points: Always start slow and always *hold* your stretch. Don't bounce. It's easier on your muscles if you're "warmed up" before stretching; so increase your heart rate slightly by lightly running on the spot, or fast walking on the spot before beginning.

Additionally, pain is not a good sign. When stretching, lean into a stretch until you can feel it; then hold it, ideally for 10 to 20 seconds. Release your stretch and relax for 30 seconds, and stretch again and hold.

As a result, you should gain suppleness and the ability to achieve a full range of movements—turning, twisting, and bending—with no stiffness or aching.

Toe Touch

Standing from the waist, bend over slowly, letting your body hang naturally. Then, with straight legs, reach toward the floor. When you've reached as low as you can go, gently hold that part of your legs with your dangling hands. If you can reach the floor, touch it instead, and hold. Release and return to where you body hung over naturally. Repeat. When you straighten back up, be sure to bend your knees initially, and slowly curl your back to the upright position.

Are you improving? With repetition, over time, you should gradually be able to reach farther and farther down, or if you can touch the floor with only the tips of your fingers, then aim to touch the floor with the palm of your hand.

Target area: Lower back and the back of your legs.

Variation: If standing isn't working for you, try doing this stretch while seated on the floor. Place your back against

a wall, legs outstretched flat in front of you, and lean forward to feel the stretch, reaching for your toes.

Chest Lift

Lie flat on your stomach, with your arms behind your back. Slowly and gently lift your chin, shoulders, and chest off the floor, while keeping your hips and legs lying flat. Hold 10 seconds, if possible, and lower your chest, shoulders, and head back down. Then repeat the stretch three to five times. Be careful not to strain your neck with any twisting or rotation.

Are you improving? Over time, you should notice that you can stretch farther up, raising more and more of your torso off the floor. Or, if at the moment, you can lift only your chin and part of your shoulders, then in the future, you may be able to raise the top of your chest off the floor.

Target area: Back, chest.

Variation: If it's more comfortable, try the exercise with your hands by your side.

Shoulder Roll

This is a simple exercise and stretch. Often flexibility is about restoring movement and loosening those muscles that were once supple and had a full range of motion.

While standing or seated at a firm chair, bring your shoulders up to your ears and slowly roll them backward in a circular motion, stopping momentarily in quarters around the circle (that is, at positions 12, 3, 6, and 9 on a clock). Push your shoulders as low as they can go at the bottom of the circle, then bring them to the front and back up. Repeat this slow circle 5 to 10 times, and then rest. Repeat in the opposite direction 5 to 10 times.

Are you improving? With practice, you should find this exercise easier to do. Your shoulders and upper body will be able to move in a larger "circle," and with less internal resistance.

Target area: Shoulders, back.

Extension: Once limber, try swinging your arms, fully extended, one at a time, in the same circular motion. It's important to be in control of your rotating arm, instead of letting it swing freely, as this could result in injury.

Knee Hug

Lie on your back, with your legs outstretched and arms at your side. Slowly, bring up one leg, bent at the knee, toward your chest. Wrap your arms around this bent leg, with your hands meeting below the knee. The goal is to keep the other leg still on the floor, touching the floor, straight, and in line with your hip. However, to begin with, your straight leg may want to come off the floor, and/or it may be difficult to "hug" your knee. Do this stretch three to five times, and repeat with the other leg.

Are you improving? Over time, you should notice the bent knee pull in farther toward your chest, with greater ease, and less internal resistance. Also, the straight leg eventually should feel comfortable at rest on the floor, instead of wanting to pull up.

Target area: Hips and buttocks.

Variation: If this exercise is difficult for you, try isolating the "hug" element. Lying flat on the floor, slowly bring *both* bent knees toward your chest, grasping both legs with your hands; you should resemble a ball. Hold this stretch, breathing deeply, and release. Then repeat.

Side Stretch

Stand upright, feet shoulder-width apart. Reach your right arm slowly over your head, and bend to the left slightly in the waist; your raised arm should be reaching overhead to the left as well. Your left arm stays at rest. You should feel a stretch under your arm and down the exposed side of your body. Hold this stretch, and then straighten up. Repeat three to five times, and then try the stretch on the other side.

Are you improving? You should notice with time that your body can bend farther and more deeply to the side.

Target area: Abdominals, arms.

Variation: Try reaching upward with your raised arm instead of letting it follow your abdominal bend—you should feel a lengthening stretch as well. Or, spread your feet apart, greater than shoulder-width, and try the stretch from this position.

Lifestyle Activities That Encourage Flexibility: Yoga, Tai Chi, Dance/Ballet, Stretching

Cardiovascular Cardiovascular refers to both heart and lung components of fitness. It is the cornerstone of overall health and well-being. A well-tuned cardio system usually results in improvements across your whole body. The basic idea is to get involved in an activity that raises your heart rate and breathing to an elevated level for an extended period of time, ideally for 20 to 40 minutes, depending on your fitness level.

However, you do need to monitor your heart rate, to ensure that it stays within a healthy range, and that you're not overworking yourself.

With regard to your breathing, here's the rule of thumb: You should always be able to carry on a conversation with a friend; if you're too winded to do this, you're working too hard.

When beginning a new cardio program, the key is to build up to the 20 to 40 minutes. If you haven't done any activity for a while, don't start for too long, or you'll never want to do it again. For example, try 10 minutes for the first week, then 5 additional minutes every week, until you build up to your target of 20 to 40 minutes. Also, be sure to warm up, to get your heart rate going, before every session.

Jumping Rope

Get a skipping rope and find a wide area in which to start jumping rope. Skipping is a very difficult exercise to do for prolonged periods. So, start slow; don't jump as fast as you can right away, but instead jump at a rate that you can hopefully sustain for several minutes.

Are you improving? Measure your success by the length of time skipping and the intensity/speed of your jumping.

Both have their advantages and signal your ongoing improvement.

Variation: Try alternating your jumping style: Try on one foot, alternating feet; try jumping with your feet apart, or even try bringing your knees up high when you jump. Also, try varying the intensity: Jump as fast as you can for 1 minute, and then at your regular speed for 5, repeating this pattern throughout your workout.

Swimming

Head to the local swimming pool, or perhaps just outside if you have your own pool, and swim a couple laps. With swimming, you're trying to maintain your increased heart rate, so swimming laps is an ideal activity.

Are you improving? Look for an increase in distance or an ability to swim for a longer period of time. If time is limited, then try to swim harder than you did before (that is, swimming a longer distance in the same amount of time).

Variation: You can use any stroke you like or any combination, or variation, but keep at it, and you can swim like you're Michael Phelps. Note: If you're not swimming in a life-guarded area, never swim alone.

Fast Walking

Grab a sturdy pair of walking shoes or gym shoes, and head outside. You don't need any more equipment, other than healthy determination, to start walking. But to help improve your cardio, you need to walk fast enough to get your heart rate up, so pick up the pace—this isn't a leisurely stroll. In bad weather, try the mall for a dry, covered area in which to walk.

Are you improving? Over time, you should be able to walk faster and for a longer period of time, without adding an uncomfortable amount of stress to your body. You can measure your improvement in terms of distance walked, steps taken, or distances that you walked in a certain amount of time. A pedometer will definitely help keep track of some of these figures.

Variation: Try alternating fast walking with light jogging. For example, try a combination such as the following: Walk 4 minutes, jog 1 minute, for the duration of your workout. Or consider varying your route to include a hill or an incline. Also, terrain makes a difference—walking on sand provides more resistance, while walking in the woods demands more thought and attention.

Squash/Tennis

Racquet sports can be a great way to improve your cardio in a social setting. Get a fitness buddy, and join a squash club. Squash is a great racquet sport that involves both coordination and cardio. Alternatively, if you've previously enjoyed tennis, try picking the sport up again.

Are you improving? With improved skill, you should notice, in squash or tennis, longer rallies of play. It is in these longer rallies that you will notice your improvement—you should be able to keep the play going and not have to stop because of fatigue. Provided you're not playing one of the Williams sisters…

Variation: You can also practice a sport like squash on your own; so try to challenge yourself and see how hard you can work yourself.

Walking Stairs

This is the idea behind the trusty Stair Master, but the authentic version. Head up the stairs in your house, the local sporting arena, or any nearby flight of steps. Then, it's as easy as climbing up and down for your set amount of time. Although climbing up definitely uses more energy and is more of a cardio workout, climbing down also requires effort from your system.

Are you improving? Look for signs such as climbing faster, breathing easier, and being able to climb for longer.

Variation: Once you've mastered this, try adding weight such as wrist weights, or even carrying two bottles of water, to increase the amount of weight your body has to carry up the stairs.

Lifestyle Activities That Encourage Cardio Development: Cycling, Running/Jogging, Boxing, Soccer, Dancing Vigorously, Trampoline Jumping, Gym Activities—Treadmill and Elliptical, As Well As Tennis and Squash, of Course

Endurance Endurance training involves low- to medium-intensity exercise for longer periods, such as jogging several miles instead of sprinting once around the block.

Tips for Building Endurance

- **Aim for longer, slower-paced workouts.**

    When striving to build endurance, slow and steady wins the race. Once you've decided on the time goal, set an appropriate pace, so that you're able to sustain your activity throughout the time period. Pace yourself; this is playing the long game.

- **Dedication goes a long way.**

    Ideally, try to work out several times a week, and build up to daily workouts. Because endurance training doesn't have the same intensity as strength training, daily workouts are fine. However, don't try to do too much at once. Start at 5 or 10 minutes, and work your way up to 30 to 40 minutes of activity.

- **Have a positive mental attitude.**

    A large part of endurance is your mental attitude. Making a commitment to follow a fitness routine requires a certain mental attitude; it is this same perseverance that is required when you're almost at the end of your energy. This means that toward the end of your cycle, jog, or swim, dig deep and keep going. Take it one step at a time, and you can do it.

- **Have a balanced workout.**

    Incorporate all the other elements of fitness—Strength, Flexibility, Agility, and Cardio—because each of these will help you achieve your Endurance goals.

Lifestyle Activities That Encourage Endurance: Swimming, Bicycling, Walking Briskly, Tennis, Volleyball, Rowing, Dancing, Climbing Stairs or Hills, Skiing, Hiking, Jogging

ABCs of Vitamins and Nutrition

When having surgery, you're in the care of a capable health care team, but once you leave, you have to do everything you can for yourself. Thus, this chapter will provide the general nutritional support and advice that are vital for consuming the nutrients that any body requires to function at its peak level of performance.

Naturally, we don't all necessarily stick to a strict dietary regimen of carrots and celery; a hamburger or a tempting bowl of chicken wings is bound to creep into the picture. Yet, especially after surgery, it's important to give your body an added boost, so it can get back on track and repair itself.

Read on to learn some of the ways you can build a good nutritional base to help pave your road to recovery.

A total of 13 vitamins are essentially organic compounds that are necessary for your body's normal metabolic functions. They constantly have to be replenished because we lose them every time we urinate. So, it's important to ensure a daily intake of the nutrients you need.

Nutrition falls into six major nutrition groups: carbohydrates, proteins, fats, vitamins, minerals, and water.

Here's a cheat sheet of vitamins and what they do.

Vitamin A

Why you need it: This vitamin helps you see in the dark and promotes a healthy immune system. This includes aiding the growth and development of cells, keeping your skin healthy, and promoting the formation and maintenance of healthy teeth.

Where you find it: Vitamin A can be found in milk, eggs, liver, fortified cereals, carrots, sweet potatoes, pumpkin, cantaloupe, apricots, peaches, papayas, and mangos—the majority of your orange fruits and vegetables.

Vitamin B_1

Why you need it: All B vitamins help to create energy by breaking down and metabolizing fats and carbohydrates. In addition, Vitamin B_1, also known as thiamine, helps to maintain functions of the heart, as well as the nervous, cardiovascular, and digestive systems.

Where you find it: Oatmeal, brown rice, whole grain flour, asparagus, potatoes, oranges, pork, liver, and eggs.

Vitamin B_2

Why you need it: Vitamin B_2 (or riboflavin) aids the body's antioxidants, to protect against free radicals.

Where you find it: Milk, cheese, green leafy vegetables, liver, kidneys, and legumes.

Vitamin B_3

Why you need it: Vitamin B_3 aids antioxidants and plays a role in our digestive system. Be aware that deficiency of "B_3" (or niacin) can cause the disease, pellagra (a vitamin deficiency); in mild cases, lack of B₃ may slow the body's metabolism, causing intolerance to cold.

Where you find it: Often in pill form.

Vitamin B₄

Why you need it: Vitamin B₄ (or adenine) produces energy, along with the other B vitamins.

Where you find it: Found in whole grains (breads and cereals), raw honey, bee pollen, royal jelly, and most fresh vegetables and fruits.

Vitamin B₅

Why you need it: Vitamin B₅ (or pantothenic acid) is also known as the antistress vitamin because of its support of the release of cortisol from the adrenal gland. It also stimulates the immune system to produce antibodies.

Where you find it: Beef, eggs, fresh vegetables, kidney, legumes, liver, mushrooms, nuts, pork, saltwater fish, whole rye flour, and whole wheat.

Vitamin B₆

Why you need it: Vitamin B₆ (or pyridoxine) is crucial for normal brain function.

Where you find it: Found in a variety of foods, including potatoes, bananas, beans, seeds, nuts, red meat, poultry, fish, eggs, and spinach, as well as being added to some breakfast cereals.

Vitamin B₉

Why you need it: Otherwise known as folate, this vitamin is important in DNA production, producing new cell bodies and preventing changes that may lead to cancer. Particularly important for expecting moms.

Where you find it: Spinach, turnip greens, lettuces, fortified cereal, and sunflower seeds.

Vitamin B₁₂

Why you need it: Vitamin B₁₂ (or cobalamin) helps make red blood cells and gives you energy, of course.

Where you find it: Fish, red meat, poultry, milk, cheese, eggs, and fortified cereals.

Vitamin C

Why you need it: Vitamin C is essential for healthy bones, teeth, and gums. It also helps in the healing of wounds and plays a part in forming collagen.

Where you find it: Found in red berries, kiwi, red and green bell peppers, tomatoes, broccoli, spinach, and orange and grapefruit juice.

Vitamin D

Why you need it: Vitamin D strengthens bones by aiding in the body's absorption of calcium.

Where you find it: Uniquely, this vitamin is manufactured when your skin is exposed to sunlight. It also is found in egg yolks, fish oils, and fortified foods such as milk.

Vitamin E

Why you need it: An antioxidant, Vitamin E helps protect cells from damage and keeps red blood cells healthy.

Where you find it: Found in many foods, such as vegetable oils, nuts, avocados, wheat germ, whole grains, and green leafy vegetables.

Vitamin K

Why you need it: Regulating normal blood clotting, Vitamin K is part of the synthesis process of several proteins that are necessary for coagulation and anticoagulation. Also, it prevents the hardening of arteries, so can reduce the occurrence of heart disease and failure.

Where you find it: Found in green leafy vegetables, in particular the dark ones such as spinach and kale, as well as in cabbage, cauliflower, broccoli, and sprouts, and fruits such as avocado and kiwi. Parsley is full of Vitamin K.

Top 5 Minerals

Unlike vitamins and other nutrients, minerals are different in that they are inorganic compounds. Typically, a mineral is usually nothing more than a molecule, or a couple of molecules, of an element. Minerals help maintain normal function of the nervous system, cellular reactions, structural and skeletal systems, and water balance in the body.

Many minerals are found within the human body, but at least 16 "essential" minerals are known. Here are my Top 5.

5. Potassium

Why you need it: Potassium is an electrolyte that works alongside another mineral, sodium, to regulate the body's water levels. A poor potassium/sodium balance ultimately can lead to dehydration and weakness.

Where you find it: Potassium is commonly found in all balanced diets (for example, orange juice, potatoes, bananas, avocados, tomatoes, broccoli, apricots).

4. Iron

Why you need it: Iron is a constituent of hemoglobin, which is responsible for transporting oxygen around your body. Thus, with a healthy amount of iron in the body, you can get more oxygen to your muscles, and you will recover much, much faster.

Where you find it: Red meat, fish, poultry, lentils, beans, tofu, chickpeas, black-eyed peas, fortified bread, and breakfast cereals. Iron in meat is absorbed more easily than iron in vegetables.

3. Sodium

Why you need it: The human requirement for sodium in the diet is about 500 mg per day. Yet, many people consume far more sodium than is needed, so this may be a case of balancing your intake of sodium to get just the right amount. Together with potassium, this electrolyte plays an important role in the body.

Where you find it: Table salt.

2. Zinc

Why you need it: Zinc is necessary for sustaining all life. And it's critical for all phases of growth; without it, you are susceptible to numerous chronic diseases.

Where you find it: In pill form, but also naturally occurring in oysters, beans, nuts, almonds, whole grains, pumpkin seeds, and sunflower seeds.

1. Calcium

Why you need it: Great for teeth and bone building. Calcium is also needed for healthy muscles, heart, and digestive system.

Where you find it: Dairy products, calcium-fortified foods, canned fish with bones (salmon, sardines), and green leafy vegetables.

Balanced Diet

Find a balance with vitamins and minerals—make sure your intake is just right, so that you get enough but not too much of one alone. Some turn to nutritional supplements, such as a multivitamin, to guarantee the consumption of a sufficient quantity of selected nutrients. However, when you are mixing and matching supplements, there is a chance that you might overdose or underdose on certain vitamins and minerals, which is a recipe for disaster.

Too much of one mineral, for instance, could cause a functional imbalance of another, or even negative side effects. As an example, if you consume too much zinc, you can inadvertently lower your HDL levels (the "good" cholesterol).

At the end of the day, the secret to getting a well-balanced proportion of nutrients is eating a healthy diet. Strive to follow the "Five-a-Day" rule of five portions of fruit and vegetables. Whole grain breads and cereals, low-fat poultry and meat, non-fried fish, and low-fat milk, cheese, and yogurt are key factors in a balanced diet. It sounds simple, because it is!

Protein Power

Illness and injury take a nutritional toll on the body. People who have had surgery need extra protein, calories, and other nutrients that support this repair and recovery.

Those who are well nourished are likely to recover from illness, injury, and surgery better and more quickly than those who are poorly nourished. Medical research has shown, time and again, that people who are not well nourished take longer to recover, are more likely to have complications, and are more likely to be rehospitalized.

Protein is especially important for healing. The body uses the amino acids in protein to build and repair body cells and tissues. Those who are undernourished may not have the nutritional resources, especially the protein, that they need for the body's "extra" work of healing.

Four Tips for a Protein-Packed Day

Extra protein can be especially beneficial if you're embarking on a major healing process, such as during postsurgery recovery. These suggestions will help you get more protein and extra calories in about the same amount of food you usually eat:

1. Add nonfat dry milk or powdered protein supplements to regular whole milk. You also can add them to sauces and gravies or use them for breading meat, fish, or poultry. Cook cereals with milk instead of water. Use milk, half-and-half, and evaporated milk when making instant cocoa, canned soups, mashed potatoes, and puddings. Add extra ice cream to milk shakes. One cup of whole or nonfat milk contains about 8 g of protein.

2. Add small pieces of meat, fish, or poultry to soups and to vegetable, noodle, and rice casseroles. A 3-oz portion of meat, fish, or poultry contains approximately 21 g of protein.

3. Add grated cheese to cream sauces, casseroles, or vegetables. Melt sliced cheese over hot apple pie. Combine cottage cheese and cream cheese with fruit. Use cream cheese and margarine on hot bread or rolls. A 1-oz slice of American cheese contains about 5 g of protein. One-half cup of cottage cheese has approximately 12 g of protein.

4. Blend finely chopped hard-boiled eggs into sauces, gravies, chopped meats, or salad dressings, or sprinkle over salads. One very large egg contains about 6 g of protein.

Ultimately, changing to a healthier lifestyle is key to getting better after surgery, and onward for the rest of your life, leading to increased wellness and longevity, as well as peak physical fitness.

Eating the right things and exercising regularly isn't a big secret. But the real secret to success is finding your passions—the foods that taste great and deliver vitamins, proteins, and minerals, and the lifestyle exercises that you enjoy, like playing tennis, golf, or squash, or going swimming and jogging with a friend. Only then will you give your body what it needs, while putting a smile on your face.

Index